Genome Medicine

Genome Medicine

Edited by Stuart Gates

hayle
medical

New York

Hayle Medical,
750 Third Avenue, 9th Floor,
New York, NY 10017, USA

Visit us on the World Wide Web at:
www.haylemedical.com

ISBN: 978-1-63241-654-4

Cataloging-in-Publication Data

Genome medicine / edited by Stuart Gates.
    p. cm.
Includes bibliographical references and index.
ISBN 978-1-63241-654-4
1. Medical genetics. 2. Genomics. 3. Genomes. 4. Human genome. I. Gates, Stuart.
RB155 .G46 2019
616.042--dc23

Table of Contents

Preface

Over the recent decade, advancements and applications have progressed exponentially. This has led to the increased interest in this field and projects are being conducted to enhance knowledge. The main objective of this book is to present some of the critical challenges and provide insights into possible solutions. This book will answer the varied questions that arise in the field and also provide an increased scope for furthering studies.

The field of genome medicine involves the application of the understanding of genetics to medical care. Besides, its immediate relevance in the diagnosis and management of genetic disorders, it also contributes to revealing etiologies for the incidence of neurological, pulmonary, psychiatric, cardiovascular and endocrine conditions. Various diagnostic chromosome studies, molecular studies and basic metabolic studies are used to form a diagnosis of genetic diseases. Biochemical studies that screen for imbalances of metabolites can be done through quantitative amino acid analysis, acylcarnitine combination profile, urine organic acid analysis, etc. A number of different methods such as fluorescence in situ hybridization (FISH), array comparative genomic hybridization and chromosome analysis, are used for determining the cause of birth defects and developmental delay, autism, etc. Advanced molecular techniques of DNA sequencing and DNA methylation analysis provide insights into the underlying condition. This book is compiled in such a manner, that it will provide in-depth knowledge about the theory and practice of genome medicine. It presents researches and studies performed by experts across the globe. It will prove to be immensely beneficial to students and researchers in this field.

I hope that this book, with its visionary approach, will be a valuable addition and will promote interest among readers. Each of the authors has provided their extraordinary competence in their specific fields by providing different perspectives as they come from diverse nations and regions. I thank them for their contributions.

Editor

Local adaptation in European populations affected the genetics of psychiatric disorders and behavioral traits

Renato Polimanti[1*], Manfred H. Kayser[2] and Joel Gelernter[1,3]

Abstract

Background: Recent studies have used genome-wide data to investigate evolutionary mechanisms related to behavioral phenotypes, identifying widespread signals of positive selection. Here, we conducted a genome-wide investigation to study whether the molecular mechanisms involved in these traits were affected by local adaptation.

Methods: We performed a polygenic risk score analysis in a sample of 2455 individuals from 23 European populations with respect to variables related to geo-climate diversity, pathogen diversity, and language phonological complexity. The analysis was adjusted for the genetic diversity of European populations to ensure that the differences detected would reflect differences in environmental exposures.

Results: The top finding was related to the association between winter minimum temperature and schizophrenia. Additional significant geo-climate results were also observed with respect to bipolar disorder (sunny daylight), depressive symptoms (precipitation rate), major depressive disorder (precipitation rate), and subjective well-being (relative humidity). Beyond geo-climate variables, we also observed findings related to pathogen diversity and language phonological complexity: openness to experience was associated with protozoan diversity; conscientiousness and extraversion were associated with language consonants.

Conclusions: We report that common variation associated with psychiatric disorders and behavioral traits was affected by processes related to local adaptation in European populations.

Keywords: Evolution, Natural selection, Genetic diversity, GWAS, Polygenicity, Psychiatry

Background

Recent studies have used genome-wide data to investigate evolutionary mechanisms related to behavioral phenotypes, identifying widespread signals of positive selection (i.e., variants with beneficial effects on individual fitness increase in population frequency) in the predisposition to psychiatric disorder and behavioral traits [1–3]. Brain-related phenotypes have undergone polygenic adaptation (adaptation that occurs by simultaneous selection on variants at many loci) during different phases of human evolutionary history [4] including to the present day [5]. This is consistent with several other investigations that found evidence of polygenic adaptation for predisposition to

a wide range of complex traits [6–9]. These genome-wide signals of positive selection are the signatures of adaptation processes that occurred in response to environmental pressures. Single-variant analyses identified loci affected by local adaption (i.e., adaptation in response to selective pressure related to the local environment) to diet, pathogens, and geo-climate variables [10, 11]. Polygenic mechanisms have also been observed in response to local environments. The observed difference in height between northern and southern Europeans appears to be related to a highly polygenic mechanism [12]. Polygenic risk scores (PRSs) for height, skin pigmentation, body mass index, type 2 diabetes, Crohn's disease, and ulcerative colitis were tested with respect to geo-climate variables in worldwide populations, with the discovery of putative signals of local adaptation [9]. However, a recent analysis demonstrated that PRSs derived from genome-wide association studies (GWASs) on populations

---
* Correspondence: renato.polimanti@yale.edu
[1]Department of Psychiatry, Yale School of Medicine and VA CT Healthcare Center, 950 Campbell Avenue, West Haven, CT 06516, USA
Full list of author information is available at the end of the article

of European descent generate biased results when applied to non-European samples [13]. PRS analysis should thus be limited to training and target datasets with the same ancestry backgrounds; we were therefore able to investigate local adaption only in European populations. To investigate whether molecular mechanisms at the basis of psychiatric/behavioral traits (Table 1) were affected by local-adaptation processes that occurred during the colonization of Europe [14], we conducted a PRS analysis based on GWASs of psychiatric disorders and behavioral traits (Table 1) from the Psychiatric Genomics Consortium [15–17], the Genetics of Personality Consortium [18–20], and the Social Science Genetic Association Consortium [21] in a sample of 2455 individuals from 23 European populations. Then, we conducted a Gene Ontology (GO) enrichment analysis based on PRS results to provide information regarding the specific molecular mechanisms involved in the polygenic signatures of local adaptation observed.

Methods
Study population
The cohort used in the present study was previously investigated to analyze the genetic structure of European populations [22]. The sample included individuals from 23 different sampling sites located in one of 20 different European countries (Additional file 1: Table S1). The GeneChip Human Mapping 500K Array Set (Affymetrix) was used to genotype 500,568 single nucleotide polymorphisms (SNPs) according to the instructions provided by the manufacturer as reported previously [22]. The analysis of identity-by-state values permitted us to exclude the possibility of the presence of related individuals (i.e., individuals who were genetically more similar than expected to another member of the same subpopulation) and outliers (i.e., individuals who were far less genetically similar than expected to the rest of the subpopulation). We used this genotype information for imputation to

maximize a consistent SNP panel between this cohort and the GWAS summary statistics used for the PRS analysis. Pre-imputation quality control criteria were minor allele frequency $\geq 1\%$, missingness per marker $\leq 5\%$, missingness per individual $\leq 5\%$, and Hardy-Weinberg equilibrium $p > 10^{-4}$. We used SHAPEIT [23] for pre-phasing, IMPUTE2 [24] for imputation, and the 1000 Genomes Project reference panel [25]. We retained imputed SNPs with high imputation quality (genotype call probability ≥ 0.8), minor allele frequency $\geq 1\%$, missingness per marker $\leq 5\%$, and missingness per individual $\leq 5\%$. After applying the post-imputation quality control criteria, we retained information regarding 3,416,230 variants in a final sample of 2455 individuals. Principal component analysis of the final sample was conducted using PLINK 1.9 [26] after linkage disequilibrium (LD) pruning ($R^2 < 0.2$) of the genotyped data. Principal components derived from genetic information were included in the regression model to adjust the analysis for population genetic background, which reflects the demographic history of European populations [27]. In line with previous PRS analyses [28–32], the initial analysis was conducted including the top 10 principal components. To verify whether residual population stratification affected our analysis, the top 20 principal components were included as covariates to confirm the reliability of the significant findings.

Local-adaptation variables
We extracted information regarding local adaptation by considering the location of the 23 sampling sites used to recruit the cohort investigated. Specifically, we considered three different types of variables: geo-climate (geographical coordinates, temperature, daylight, precipitation rate, and humidity), pathogen diversity (bacteria, protozoa, and virus), and language phonological complexity (consonants, segments, and vowels) (Table 2). Geo-climate information was extracted from ClimaTemps (available at http://

Table 1 GWASs of psychiatric disorders and behavioral traits used to generate polygenic risk scores

Consortium	Trait	Abbreviation	Sample size	Publication year	Link
Psychiatric Genomics Consortium	Autism spectrum disorder	ASD	5305 cases	2015	https://www.med.unc.edu/pgc/results-and-downloads
	Bipolar disorder	BD	7481 cases	2011	
	Major depressive disorder	MDD	9240 cases	2013	
	Schizophrenia	SCZ	36,989 cases	2014	
Genetics of Personality Consortium	Neuroticism	gpcNEURO	63,661	2015	http://www.tweelingenregister.org/GPC/
	Extraversion	EXTRA	63,030	2016	
	Openness to experience	OPEN	17,375	2012	
	Agreeableness	AGREE	17,375	2012	
	Conscientiousness	CONS	17,375	2012	
Social Science Genetic Association Consortium	Subjective well-being	SWB	298,420	2016	https://www.thessgac.org/data
	Depressive symptoms	DS	161,460	2016	
	Neuroticism	ssgacNEURO	170,911	2016	

Table 2 Variables related to local adaptation tested

Category	Variable	Abbreviation	Source	Link
Geo-climate	Latitude	LAT	ClimaTemps	http://www.climatemps.com/
	Longitude	LON		
	Altitude	ALT		
	Summer temperature (Max-Min)	SumMaxTemp SumMinTemp		
	Winter temperature (Max-Min)	WinMaxTemp WinMinTemp		
	Precipitation rate (Max-Min)	MaxPrecipRate MinPrecipRate		
	Relative humidity (Max-Min)	MaxRelHumidity MinRelHumidity		
	Sunny daylight (Max-Min)	MaxSunnyDaylight MinSunnyDaylight		
Pathogen diversity	Virus	VirusDiversity	GIDEON	https://www.gideononline.com/
	Bacteria	BacteriaDiversity		
	Protozoa	ProtozoaDiversity		
Language phonological complexity	Segments	Segments	PHOIBLE	http://phoible.org/
	Vowels	Vowels		
	Consonants	Consonants		

www.climatemps.com/), which contains more than 12.5 million climate comparison reports providing information for more than 4000 locations worldwide. Data regarding pathogen diversity were extracted from the GIDEON (Global Infectious Diseases and Epidemiology Online Network) database (available at https://www.gideononline.com/). This includes information regarding 350 infectious diseases and 1700 microbial taxa in 231 countries. Information about the phonological complexity of European languages was extracted from PHOIBLE Online (available at http://phoible.org/), which is a repository of cross-linguistic phonological inventory data including 2155 inventories that contain 2160 segment types found in 1672 distinct languages [33]. Correlations among local-adaptation variables were estimated using Spearman's correlation test.

Polygenic risk score analysis

We conducted a PRS analysis using PRSice software [34] (available at http://prsice.info/). For polygenic profile scoring, we used summary statistics generated from multiple large-scale GWASs of psychiatric disorders and behavioral traits (Table 1) conducted by the Psychiatric Genomics Consortium [15–17], the Genetics of Personality Consortium [18–20], and the Social Science Genetic Association Consortium [21]. None of the GWASs used in the present study showed evidence of inflation due to population stratification or other possible confounders. Since none of the samples included in our target dataset was used in the GWAS considered to generate the PRS, no systematic overlap is expected between training and target datasets.

We considered multiple association p-value thresholds ($PT = 5 \times 10^{-8}$, 10^{-7}, 10^{-6}, 10^{-5}, 10^{-4}, 0.001, 0.01, 0.05, 0.1, 0.3, 0.5, 1) for SNP inclusion and calculated multiple PRSs for each trait investigated. The PRSs were calculated after using p-value-informed clumping with an LD cutoff of $R^2 = 0.3$ within a 500-kb window, and excluding the major histocompatibility complex region of the genome because of its complex LD structure. The PRSs that were generated were fitted in regression models with adjustments for the top 10 ancestry principal components. Before being entered into the analysis, local-adaptation variables were normalized using appropriate Box-Cox power transformations to avoid biases due to the distribution of the phenotypes tested. We applied a false discovery rate (FDR) correction ($q < 0.05$) to correct for the multiple testing for the psychiatric/behavioral PRS × local-adaptation variables tested [35]. To verify that no systematic bias inflated our analyses, we also conducted a permutation analysis. Specifically, considering the significant datasets, we performed 10,000 permutations of the PRSs with respect to their associated variables and verified whether the observed differences were significantly different from the null distribution of the permuted results. To estimate the genetic correlation among psychiatric disorders and behavioral traits, we considered the information provided by LD Hub v1.3.1 [36] (available at http://ldsc.broadinstitute.org/ldhub/) and used the LD score regression method [37] for the missing pair-wise comparisons. Heritability statistics of the GWAS considered are reported in Additional file 2: Table S2.

Gene Ontology enrichment analysis

To provide information regarding the molecular mechanisms involved in the signatures of local adaptation in psychiatric and behavioral traits, a GO enrichment analysis was conducted based on the PRS results; the variants included in the significant PRS and with nominally significant concordant direction with PRS direction were considered in the enrichment analysis. A description of the GO analysis based on PRS results was reported in previous studies [28–30]. Variants were then entered in the enrichment analysis performed using eSNPO [38]. This method permits one to conduct enrichment analysis based on information related to expression quantitative trait loci (eQTLs) rather than physical positions of SNPs and genes, integrating the eQTL data and GO, constructing associations between SNPs and GO terms, and then performing functional enrichment analysis. An FDR correction was applied to the enrichment results for multiple testing ($q < 0.05$). To validate the results further, we conducted a permutation analysis based on the variants obtained from the major depressive disorder (MDD)-altitude result (the one that gave the highest number of significant GO enrichments). Based on this SNP set, we generated 100 SNP sets using SNPsnap (available at https://data.broadinstitute.org/mpg/snpsnap/match_snps.html) [39] and the following matching criteria: minor allele frequency ± 5%, gene density ± 50%, distance to nearest gene ± 50%, LD independence ($R^2 = 0.3$) ± 50%. The SNP sets generated were entered in the eSNPO analysis and the distribution of their results compared with those obtained from the SNP sets from the PRS analyses.

Natural and Orthogonal InterAction (NOIA) model

The NOIA model [40] was applied to validate the results related to single-locus and oligogenic signals identified by our PRS analysis. NOIA is able to estimate the interaction between genes (or epistasis), which is a key process in determining the effect of genomic variants in complex diseases and the adaptation and evolution of natural populations [41]. We performed NOIA analysis testing the genotypes of the variants included in the significant PRSs with respect to local-adaptation variables identified. The NOIA analysis was conducted using the R package *noia* (available at https://cran.r-project.org/web/packages/noia/index.html).

Data sources

Data supporting the findings of this study are available within this article and its additional files. GWAS summary association data used to calculate PRSs in this study were obtained from the Psychiatric Genomics Consortium (available at https://www.med.unc.edu/pgc/results-and-downloads/), the Genetics of Personality Consortium (available at http://www.tweelingenregister.org/GPC/), and the Social Science Genetic Association Consortium (available at https://www.thessgac.org/data).

Results

As expected, the set of variables related to the local environment were strongly intercorrelated (Fig. 1; Additional file 3: Table S3). Similarly, psychiatric disorders and behavioral traits showed strong genetic correlations (Fig. 2; Additional file 4: Table S4). We considered multiple GWAS significance thresholds to test PRSs [34], investigating both oligogenic and polygenic mechanisms (i.e., local-adaptation processes affecting few and many loci, respectively). To adjust our analysis for population genetic background, which reflects the demographic history of European populations [27], we included the top 10 principal components reflecting population ancestry variation as covariates in the regression models. This approach was considered on the basis of the experience of many GWAS and PRS analyses conducted on samples containing populations of different European descents. The use of 10 principal components is generally considered a standard approach to adjust within ancestry population stratification. However, to demonstrate that our findings are not due to the genetic relationships among European populations, we recalculated the significant PRS results (Table 3) considering 20 principal components in the regression models, and then tested for differences with respect to the original model: we did not observe significant differences between the two models (Additional file 5: Table S5).

Considering the results that survived FDR multiple testing correction ($q < 0.05$; Additional file 6: Table S6), we observed 13 variables related to local adaptation: 11 geo-climate variables, one related to pathogen diversity, and one related to language phonological complexity. Table 3 reports the top associations that survived FDR multiple testing correction for each of these 13 local-adaptation variables. Figure 3 reports full visualization of the results for all comparisons (psychiatric/behavioral PRS × local-adaptation variables). We confirmed the reliability of the significant results empirically by generating a null distribution from 10,000 permutations of the original datasets and comparing the permuted results with the observed ones (Additional file 7: Figure S1). Since polygenic signatures of local adaptation have previously been reported in height genetics of European populations [12], we used this trait as a positive control for our approach. With this analysis, we replicated the presence of adaptation signals in the genetics of this trait ($p < 0.05$; Additional file 8: Table S7).

The strongest result was observed between the schizophrenia (SCZ) PRS and winter minimum temperature

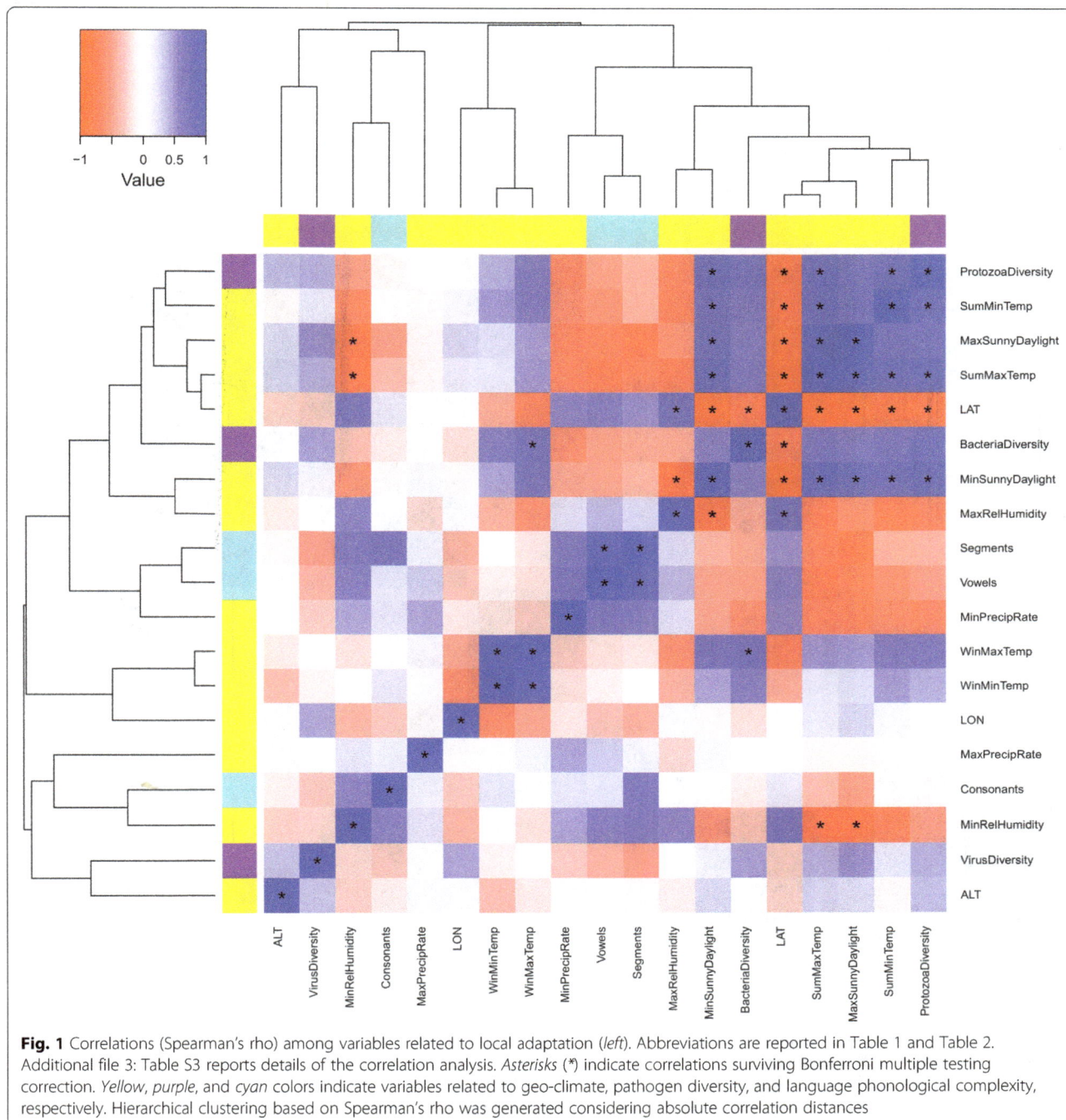

Fig. 1 Correlations (Spearman's rho) among variables related to local adaptation (*left*). Abbreviations are reported in Table 1 and Table 2. Additional file 3: Table S3 reports details of the correlation analysis. *Asterisks* (*) indicate correlations surviving Bonferroni multiple testing correction. *Yellow, purple,* and *cyan* colors indicate variables related to geo-climate, pathogen diversity, and language phonological complexity, respectively. Hierarchical clustering based on Spearman's rho was generated considering absolute correlation distances

(WinMinTemp): higher WinMinTemp correlates with increased SCZ genetic risk (SNP N = 104,106, Nagelkerke's R^2 = 0.40%, Z = 3.84, p = 1.28 × 10^{-4}, q = 0.029). Higher WinMinTemp was also associated with increased MDD PRS (SNP N = 8160, Nagelkerke's R^2 = 0.30%, Z = 3.34, p = 8.46 × 10^{-4}, q = 0.029) and increased extraversion PRS (SNP N = 7, Nagelkerke's R^2 = 0.26%, Z = 3.14, p = 1.75 × 10^{-3}, q = 0.037). While the MDD result is concordant with the SCZ-MDD genetic correlation, the

extraversion finding seems to be independent of the SCZ and MDD results. The SCZ PRS was also associated with winter maximum temperature (WinMaxTemp) and longitude; the three environmental variables are highly correlated, and the results are driven by the same mechanism related to winter temperature. Covarying these three local-adaptation variables, WinMaxTemp appears to be the driving signal among the correlated results (p < 0.05; Additional file 9: Table S8).

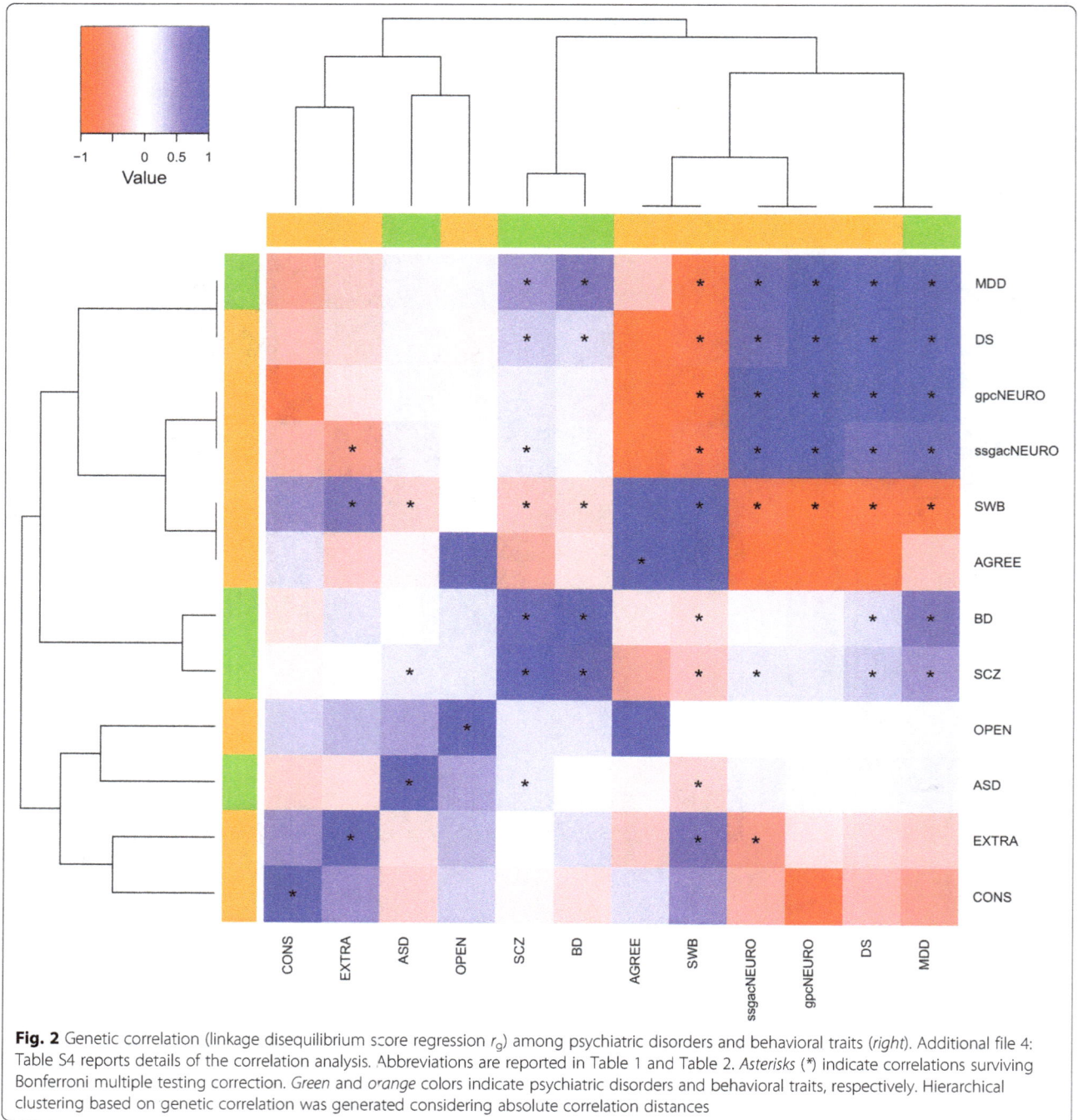

Fig. 2 Genetic correlation (linkage disequilibrium score regression r_g) among psychiatric disorders and behavioral traits (*right*). Additional file 4: Table S4 reports details of the correlation analysis. Abbreviations are reported in Table 1 and Table 2. *Asterisks* (*) indicate correlations surviving Bonferroni multiple testing correction. *Green* and *orange* colors indicate psychiatric disorders and behavioral traits, respectively. Hierarchical clustering based on genetic correlation was generated considering absolute correlation distances

To understand better the molecular processes involved in this association, we conducted a GO enrichment analysis based on the PRS result. We observed 16 GOs that survived FDR multiple testing correction ($q < 0.05$; Additional file 10: Table S9). Among the other significant PRS associations, we observed significant GO enrichments ($N = 54$; Additional file 11: Table S10) in the negative association between altitude and MDD PRS (SNP $N = 97,481$, Nagelkerke's $R^2 = 0.31\%$, $Z = -3.13$, p = 1.79×10^{-3}, $q = 0.037$) only. Five GO enrichments are significant in both SCZ and MDD analyses (GO:0008285~negative regulation of cell proliferation, GO:0017147~Wnt-protein binding, GO:2000041~negative regulation of planar cell polarity pathway involved in axis elongation, GO:0071481~cellular response to X-ray, and GO:0090244~Wnt signaling pathway involved in somitogenesis); two of these are related to the Wnt signaling pathway. To confirm empirically that these

Table 3 Top significant associations of psychiatric and behavioral polygenic risk scores (PRSs) with the 13 local-adaptation variables identified. Abbreviations are reported in Table 1 and Table 2

Local-adaptation variable	PRS	PT	SNP N	R^2	Z score	p value	q value
MaxSunnyDaylight	BD	0.01	2833	0.09%	−2.93	3.42×10^{-3}	0.043
Consonants	CONS	0.5	60,620	0.28%	−2.97	2.98×10^{-3}	0.043
Latitude	DS	10^{-7}	1	0.09%	3.47	5.38×10^{-4}	0.029
SumMaxTemp				0.12%	−3.40	6.91×10^{-4}	0.029
MinPrecipRate		0.05	12,832	0.27%	−3.29	1.03×10^{-3}	0.029
MaxPrecipRate	MDD	0.3	39,390	0.31%	−3.21	1.33×10^{-3}	0.034
Altitude		1	97,481	0.31%	−3.13	1.79×10^{-3}	0.037
ProtozoaDiversity	OPEN	10^{-6}	2	0.18%	3.56	3.82×10^{-4}	0.029
SumMinTemp		5×10^{-8}	1	0.18%	2.7	3.02×10^{-3}	0.043
WinMinTemp	SCZ	0.5	104,106	0.40%	3.84	1.28×10^{-4}	0.029
Longitude				0.13%	−3.29	1.01×10^{-3}	0.029
WinMaxTemp				0.12%	2.96	3.09×10^{-3}	0.043
MinRelHumidity	SWB	10^{-6}	4	0.21%	−2.95	3.22×10^{-3}	0.043

enrichment results are not false positives, we conducted a permutation analysis: we generated 100 random sets of LD-independent variants derived from the SNPs included in the MDD analysis (which was the one that gave the highest number of GO enrichments), considering minor allele frequency, gene density, distance to nearest gene, and LD independence as matching criteria. There was no permuted set with more than two significant GO enrichments (i.e., the empirical probability to observe a random set with more than two significant GO enrichments is $p <$ 0.01; Additional file 12: Figure S2); the overall probability to observe a significant GO enrichment from a permuted set is $p = 6.69*10^{-5}$ (Additional file 13: Figure S3); and none of the four GOs shared by SCZ and MDD results resulted in significance in the permuted sets ($q > 0.18$).

Among the psychiatric disorders investigated, MDD and depressive symptoms (DS) showed a very strong genetic correlation ($r_g = 1$, $p = 1.77 \times 10^{-36}$). In accordance with this genetic overlap, we observed a convergence in the local-adaptation findings that survived multiple testing correction. The MDD and DS PRS showed concordant negative associations with precipitation rate (PR): maximum PR (SNP $N = 39,390$, Nagelkerke's $R^2 = 0.31\%$, $Z = -3.21$, $p = 1.33 \times 10^{-3}$, $q = 0.034$) and minimum PR (SNP $N = 12,832$, Nagelkerke's $R^2 = 0.27\%$, $Z = -3.29$, $p = 1.03 \times 10^{-3}$, $q = 0.029$), respectively. The same DS PRS also nominally replicated the negative association with maximum PR (SNP $N = 12,832$, Nagelkerke's $R^2 = 0.16\%$, $Z = -2.28$, $p = 0.022$).

An additional polygenic signature of local adaptation was observed between bipolar disorder (BD) and maximum sunny daylight, where increased daylight is associated with reduced BD genetic risk (SNP $N = 2833$, Nagelkerke's $R^2 = 0.09\%$, $Z = -2.93$, $p = 3.42 \times 10^{-3}$, $q = 0.043$).

The results discussed above are related to highly polygenic local-adaptation mechanisms (i.e., thousands of variants involved). However, we also observed some instances of local adaptation involving few loci. Among them, the strongest signal was the positive association between protozoa diversity and openness-to-experience (OPEN) score including the top two associated variants (rs1477268 and rs10932966; SNP $N = 2$, Nagelkerke's $R^2 = 0.18\%$, $Z = 3.56$, $p = 3.82 \times 10^{-4}$, $q = 0.029$). An OPEN score including only rs1477268 showed a positive association with summer minimum temperature (SNP $N = 1$, Nagelkerke's $R^2 = 0.18\%$, $Z = 2.7$, $p = 3.02 \times 10^{-3}$, $q = 0.043$). Another single-locus result was observed between rs6992714, which is associated with DS risk, and latitude (SNP $N = 1$, Nagelkerke's $R^2 = 0.09\%$, $Z = 3.47$, $p = 5.38 \times 10^{-4}$, $q = 0.029$) and summer maximum temperature (SNP $N = 1$, Nagelkerke's $R^2 = 0.12\%$, $Z = -3.40$, $p = 6.91 \times 10^{-4}$, $q = 0.029$). According to GTEx data [42], rs6992714 is associated with *GGH* (*gamma-glutamyl hydrolase*) gene expression (beta = −0.13, $p = 3.3 \times 10^{-5}$; Additional file 14: Figure S4). NOIA analysis confirmed the presence of additive effects in the models based on the single-locus and oligogenic PRS with respect to the local-adaptation variables identified as significant ($p < 0.05$; Additional file 15: Table S11).

Finally, we observed a genetic association with respect to language phonological complexity: the number of consonants in European languages is positively associated with genome-wide PRS of conscientiousness (SNP $N = 60,620$, Nagelkerke's $R^2 = 0.28\%$, $Z = -2.97$, $p = 2.98 \times 10^{-3}$, $q = 0.043$) and extraversion (SNP $N = 3261$, Nagelkerke's $R^2 = 0.26\%$, $Z = 2.87$, $p = 4.13 \times 10^{-3}$, $q = 0.049$).

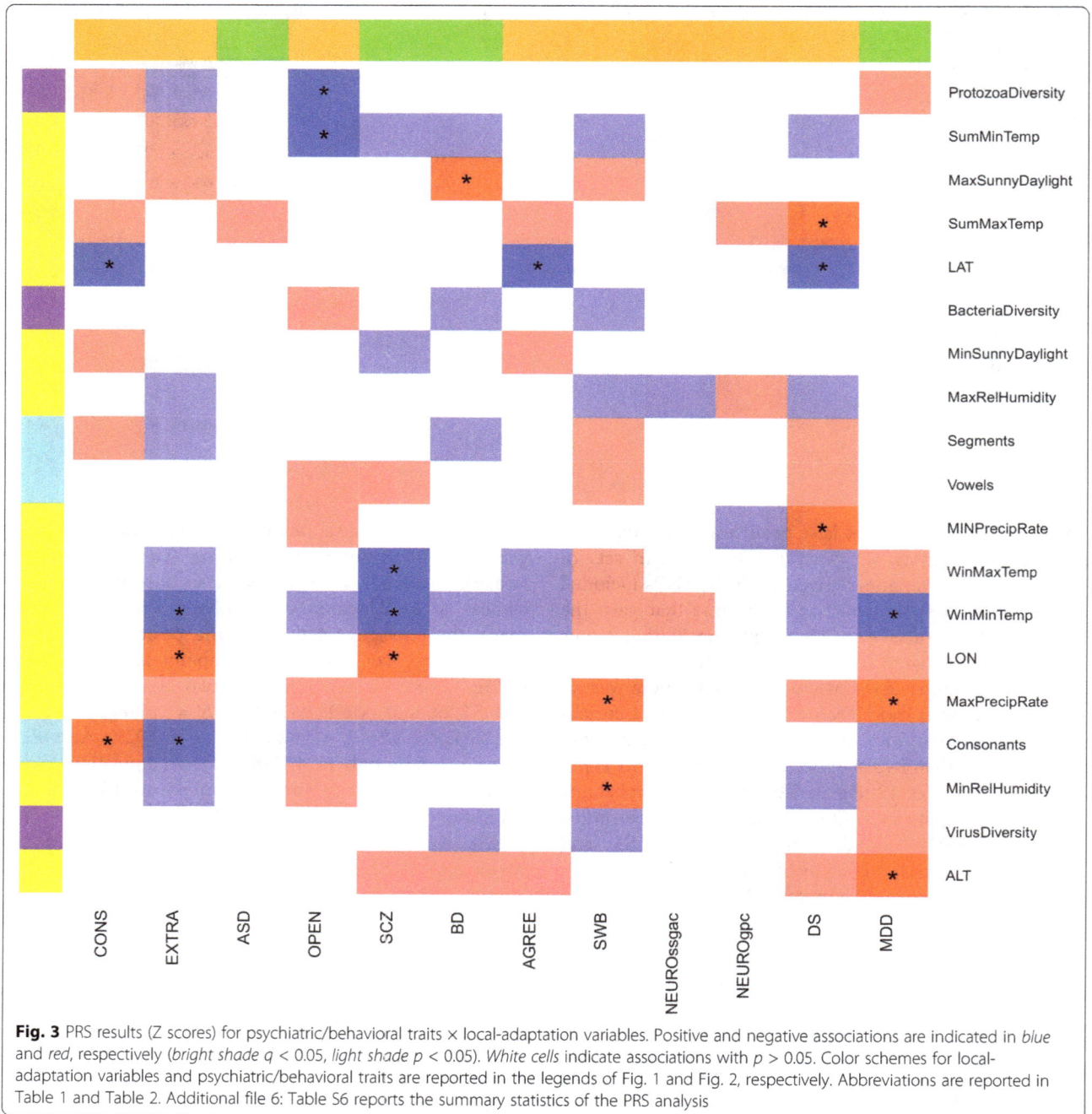

Fig. 3 PRS results (Z scores) for psychiatric/behavioral traits × local-adaptation variables. Positive and negative associations are indicated in *blue* and *red*, respectively (*bright shade q* < 0.05, *light shade p* < 0.05). *White cells* indicate associations with *p* > 0.05. Color schemes for local-adaptation variables and psychiatric/behavioral traits are reported in the legends of Fig. 1 and Fig. 2, respectively. Abbreviations are reported in Table 1 and Table 2. Additional file 6: Table S6 reports the summary statistics of the PRS analysis

Discussion

There are many datasets available with information regarding positive selection signatures in reference European populations [43, 44]. We previously used these available data, observing a significant enrichment for positive selection in the genetics of psychiatric disorders [1]. Comparable results have been observed by independent groups using different approaches [2, 3]. Our current analysis provides novel data with respect to local-adaptation differences among European populations. Indeed,

considering positive selection signals in a reference European population, the signatures of positive selection are those shared by European populations and those specific for that particular population. With local-adaptation analysis, we are investigating the differences in selective pressures among a set of distinct European populations. Thus, the signals detected in the reference population may not overlap with those related to the local-adaptation mechanisms. To be able to use tests for positive selection (e.g., haplotype-based methods), we would need a larger sample in each of the populations considered.

Our PRS analysis identified 20 associations that survived FDR multiple testing correction (Additional file 5: Table S5). The specific characteristics of the sample investigated may generate false positive results due to several factors (e.g., different sample sizes at the different populations and non-random spatial sampling). However, our permutation analysis of the significant PRS results (i.e., we permuted the genetic scores with respect to the environmental variables) indicated that there is little possibility of bias due to the composition of the sample investigated.

Our findings appear to indicate that psychiatric and behavioral traits are not necessarily the outcomes selected by evolutionary pressures; some of the molecular pathways involved in their predisposition were affected by local adaptation. We observed some convergence between our local-adaptation findings and known epidemiological evidence. However, our findings should be related to evolutionary forces that acted on a population level, while epidemiological evidence should be due to mechanisms that acted on an individual level. We hypothesize that evolutionary forces shaped the genetic diversity of European populations, while individual-level changes should be due to post-genetic changes (e.g., epigenetic modifications) or the interaction of social-psychological risk factors on loci affected by local adaptation.

The strongest result observed between the SCZ PRS and WinMinTemp is in line with previous epidemiological studies. Season of birth is a widely recognized SCZ risk factor, where there is significantly increased risk associated with winter birth [45]. Our current finding may justify a molecular hypothesis: loci associated with increased SCZ risk may have undergone local adaptation related to winter conditions. The same environmental pressure may be responsible for the winter-birth risk through epigenetic mechanisms in line with the convergence between regional DNA methylation changes and signals of local adaptation reported for other loci [46]. Our GO enrichment analysis highlighted Wnt signaling as one of the molecular processes affected by this local-adaptation mechanism. This biological pathway is well studied in relation to both psychiatric disorders and human evolution; synaptic Wnt signaling is implicated as a possible contributor to several major psychiatric disorders due its involvement in neural differentiation processes [47]. Signatures of positive selection were reported in relation to the Wnt signaling pathway in multiple species [48]. Our present findings indicate that risk loci for psychiatric disorders involved in this molecular pathway could have been under local adaptation in European populations.

Another result in line with a known epidemiological association is the negative association between maximum

sunny daylight period and BD (bipolar disorder) PRS. Seasonality of BD symptoms is common and, in particular, light exposure during early life may have important consequences for those who are susceptible to bipolar disorder [49]. More generally, lack of daylight is implicated in mood change in seasonal affective disorder [50]. Our finding indicates that daylight may have acted as a local selective pressure with respect to molecular pathways involved in BD pathogenesis.

As mentioned above, we also observed some instances of local adaptation involving oligogenic and single-locus signals. Although top results from GWASs of psychiatric and behavioral traits do not explain a large percentage of the variance, loci surviving stringent significance cut-offs usually show larger effect sizes, suggesting that they may be involved in key mechanisms involved in the pathogenesis of the traits investigated. Among the oligogenic signals, the strongest finding is the association of OPEN PRS, including the top two associated variants (rs1477268 and rs10932966), with protozoa diversity and summer minimum temperature. These two results appear concordant with the strong positive correlation between summer minimum temperature and protozoa diversity (Spearman's rho = 0.75, $p = 4.51 \times 10^{-5}$), which is consistent with the relationship between temperature and pathogen diversity [51]. rs1477268 is located near *RAS1*, which was implicated by previous studies as being involved in pathogen response [52]. From GTEx data [42], rs10932966 is significantly associated with *RP11-16P6.1* gene expression in multiple human tissues (Additional file 16: Table S12), but no information regarding its function is available. We hypothesize that these loci have been under local selective adaption in response to pathogen-related selective pressure. This is in line with the consistent literature regarding the role of selective pressures induced by pathogen diversity in shaping human genome diversity [6].

Another single-locus result was observed between rs6992714, which is associated with DS risk, with latitude and summer maximum temperature. This genetic variant is associated with *GGH* gene expression, which was previously implicated as involved in the pathogenesis of tropical sprue, a malabsorption syndrome commonly found in tropical regions [53]. According to our data, *GGH* may have been under local adaptation in relation to selective pressures induced by summer temperatures. The associations discussed appear to be related to the effect of selective pressures induced by geo-climate and pathogen-related variables on the human genome.

The relationship between genetic and language diversities has been investigated from several perspectives [54], and genetic associations with language phonological complexity require careful consideration. Our data indicate that there is at least a partial relationship between genetic variation and language diversity that is not driven by their shared association with human demographic history (which should be reflected by the genetic diversity accounted for by the adjustment for principal components derived from genetic data). This supports two possible converse scenarios: (1) genetic variation may have contributed to shape European language diversity; (2) European language diversity may have been a local selective pressure that shaped the genetics of behavioral traits. Although it is not possible to establish causality or a mechanism based on our current data, phonological working memory appears to be associated with extraversion and conscientiousness [55], in agreement with the relationship highlighted by our results.

Conclusions

We report the first evidence regarding the role of local adaptation in shaping the genetic architecture of psychiatric disorders and behavioral traits. We hypothesize that most of our findings are due to the effects of local selective pressure on molecular pathways involved in the predisposition to these complex traits. Due to the presence of pervasive pleiotropy among them, some of the "evolutionary selected" pathways (e.g., the Wnt signaling pathway identified in the present study) are shared by multiple traits. Although our analysis was adjusted for human demographic history through principal components, we cannot exclude that genes involved in behavioral traits may have had a role in population migrations. Further analyses will be needed to explore this hypothesis. The main limitation of our current investigation is the impossibility of investigating local-adaptation mechanisms in non-European populations due to the general lack of large GWASs in individuals of African, Middle Eastern, Central Asian, East Asian, Native American, and Oceanic descents. Additionally, larger target cohorts with more individuals per population and more populations may permit one to detect further signals of local adaptation in the genetics of psychiatric and behavioral traits.

Additional files

Additional file 1: Table S1. Details of the European samples investigated.

Additional file 2: Table S2. Heritability statistics (LD score regression) of the GWASs considered.

Additional file 3: Table S3. Correlations (Spearman's rho, upper triangular; p value, lower triangular) among variables related to local adaptation. p values surviving Bonferroni multiple testing correction are reported in red. Abbreviations are reported in Table 1 and Table 2.

Additional file 4: Table S4. Genetic correlation (r_g, upper triangular; p value, lower triangular) among psychiatric disorders and behavioral traits.

p values surviving Bonferroni multiple testing correction are reported in red. Abbreviations are reported in Table 1 and Table 2.

Additional file 5: Table S5. Comparisons of regression models including 10 principal components (10PC) vs. 20 principal components (20PC). The 10PC model is the model tested in the main analysis and included as covariates 10 principal components derived from genetic information. The 20PC model was run on the top significant findings and included as covariates 20 principal components derived from genetic information. P10vs20 is the p value calculated testing the difference between these two models. Abbreviations are reported in Table 1 and Table 2.

Additional file 6: Table S6. Best associations for each of the PRS × local-adaptation variables tested. Abbreviations are reported in Table 1 and Table 2.

Additional file 7: Figure S1. Null distribution generated from 10,000 random permutations of the significant PRS datasets. Blue lines represent the observed results. Abbreviations are reported in Table 1 and Table 2.

Additional file 8: Table S7. Association between height PRS and local-adaptation variables. Abbreviations are reported in Table 2.

Additional file 9: Table S8. Covariate analysis of SCZ PRS with respect to winter minimum temperature (WMinTemp), winter maximum temperature (WMaxTemp), and longitude (LON). We report top PRS cutoff and cutoff obtained from the main analysis.

Additional file 10: Table S9. Gene Ontology (GO) enrichment in the SCZ-WinMinTemp (Abbreviations are reported in Table 1 and Table 2) result that survived FDR multiple testing correction (q < 0.05).

Additional file 11: Table S10. Gene Ontology (GO) enrichment in the MDD-altitude result that survived FDR multiple testing correction (q < 0.05). Abbreviations are reported in Table 1 and Table 2.

Additional file 12: Figure S2. Distribution of the results of GO enrichment analysis from 100 random sets. Orange line represents q < 0.05.

Additional file 13: Figure S3. Overall distribution of q values generated from the GO enrichment analysis of 100 random sets. The red line represents q < 0.05.

Additional file 14: Figure S4. Significant association of rs6992714 with GGH gene expression.

Additional file 15: Table S11. Addictive effects in variants included in single-locus and oligogenic PRS from NOIA analysis.

Additional file 16: Table S12. Significant associations of rs10932966 with RP11-16P6.1 gene expression in multiple tissues.

Abbreviations

BD: Bipolar disorder; DS: Depressive symptoms; eQTL: Expression quantitative trait locus; FDR: False discovery rate; GGH: Gamma-glutamyl hydrolase; GIDEON: Global Infectious Diseases and Epidemiology Online Network; GO: Gene Ontology; GWAS: Genome-wide association study; LD: Linkage disequilibrium; MDD: Major depressive disorder; NOIA: Natural and Orthogonal InterAction; OPEN: Openness to experience; PRS: Polygenic risk score; SCZ: Schizophrenia; WinMaxTemp: Winter maximum temperature; WinMinTem: Winter minimum temperature

Acknowledgements
All volunteers included in the cohort of individuals of European descent are gratefully acknowledged for sample donation. We thank Oscar Lao for his useful comments on the manuscript. The authors are also grateful to the research groups of the Psychiatric Genomics Consortium, the Genetics of Personality Consortium, and the Social Science Genetic Association Consortium for their publicly available GWAS summary statistics.

Funding
This study was supported by National Institutes of Health grants R01 DA12690, R01 AA017535, P50 AA012870, U01 MH109532, and R21 AA024404, the Veterans Affairs Connecticut Mental Illness Research Education Clinical Centers of Excellence, a National Alliance for Research on Schizophrenia and

Depression Young Investigator (NARSAD) Award from the Brain & Behavior Research Foundation, and an Explorer Grant from the Simons Foundation Autism Research Initiative (SFARI).

Authors' contributions

RP and JG were involved in the study design. MHK was involved in cohort ascertainment and recruitment. RP carried out the statistical analysis. RP wrote the first draft of the manuscript, and all authors contributed to the final version of the manuscript. All authors read and approved the final manuscript.

Competing interests

The authors declare that they have no competing interests.

Author details

[1]Department of Psychiatry, Yale School of Medicine and VA CT Healthcare Center, 950 Campbell Avenue, West Haven, CT 06516, USA. [2]Department of Genetic Identification, Erasmus University Medical Center, Rotterdam, Rotterdam, the Netherlands. [3]Departments of Genetics and Neuroscience, Yale School of Medicine, New Haven, CT, USA.

References

1. Polimanti R, Gelernter J. Widespread signatures of positive selection in common risk alleles associated to autism spectrum disorder. PLoS Genet. 2017;13:e1006618.
2. Xu K, Schadt EE, Pollard KS, Roussos P, Dudley JT. Genomic and network patterns of schizophrenia genetic variation in human evolutionary accelerated regions. Mol Biol Evol. 2015;32:1148–60.
3. Srinivasan S, Bettella F, Mattingsdal M, Wang Y, Witoelar A, Schork AJ, Thompson WK, Zuber V, Schizophrenia Working Group of the Psychiatric Genomics Consortium TIHGC, Winsvold BS, et al. Genetic markers of human evolution are enriched in schizophrenia. Biol Psychiatry. 2016;80:284–92.
4. Beiter ER, Khramtsova EA, van der Merwe C, Chimusa ER, Simonti C, Stein J, Thompson P, Fisher S, Stein DJ, Capra JA, et al. Polygenic selection underlies evolution of human brain structure and behavioral traits. bioRxiv. 2017. https://doi.org/10.1101/164707.
5. Mullins N, Ingason A, Porter H, Euesden J, Gillett A, Olafsson S, Gudbjartsson DF, Lewis CM, Sigurdsson E, Saemundsen E, et al. Reproductive fitness and genetic risk of psychiatric disorders in the general population. Nat Commun. 2017;8:15833.
6. Daub JT, Hofer T, Cutivet E, Dupanloup I, Quintana-Murci L, Robinson-Rechavi M, Excoffier L. Evidence for polygenic adaptation to pathogens in the human genome. Mol Biol Evol. 2013;30:1544–58.
7. Hansen ME, Hunt SC, Stone RC, Horvath K, Herbig U, Ranciaro A, Hirbo J, Beggs W, Reiner AP, Wilson JG, et al. Shorter telomere length in Europeans than in Africans due to polygenetic adaptation. Hum Mol Genet. 2016;25: 2324–30.
8. Polimanti R, Yang BZ, Zhao H, Gelernter J. Evidence of polygenic adaptation in the systems genetics of anthropometric traits. PLoS One. 2016;11: e0160654.
9. Berg JJ, Coop G. A population genetic signal of polygenic adaptation. PLoS Genet. 2014;10:e1004412.
10. Hancock AM, Witonsky DB, Gordon AS, Eshel G, Pritchard JK, Coop G, Di Rienzo A. Adaptations to climate in candidate genes for common metabolic disorders. PLoS Genet. 2008;4:e32.
11. Polimanti R, Piacentini S, Iorio A, De Angelis F, Kozlov A, Novelletto A, Fuciarelli M. Haplotype differences for copy number variants in the 22q11. 23 region among human populations: a pigmentation-based model for selective pressure. Eur J Hum Genet. 2015;23:116–23.
12. Turchin MC, Chiang CW, Palmer CD, Sankararaman S, Reich D, Genetic Investigation of ATC, Hirschhorn JN. Evidence of widespread selection on standing variation in Europe at height-associated SNPs. Nat Genet. 2012;44: 1015–9.

13. Martin AR, Gignoux CR, Walters RK, Wojcik GL, Neale BM, Gravel S, Daly MJ, Bustamante CD, Kenny EE. Human demographic history impacts genetic risk prediction across diverse populations. Am J Hum Genet. 2017;100:635–49.
14. Key FM, Fu Q, Romagne F, Lachmann M, Andres AM. Human adaptation and population differentiation in the light of ancient genomes. Nat Commun. 2016;7:10775.
15. Psychiatric GWAS Consortium Bipolar Disorder Working Group. Large-scale genome-wide association analysis of bipolar disorder identifies a new susceptibility locus near ODZ4. Nat Genet. 2011;43:977–83.
16. Major Depressive Disorder Working Group of the Psychiatric GWAS Consortium, Ripke S, Wray NR, Lewis CM, Hamilton SP, Weissman MM, Breen G, Byrne EM, Blackwood DH, Boomsma DI, et al. A mega-analysis of genome-wide association studies for major depressive disorder. Mol Psychiatry. 2013;18:497–511.
17. Schizophrenia Working Group of the Psychiatric Genomics Consortium. Biological insights from 108 schizophrenia-associated genetic loci. Nature. 2014;511:421–7.
18. de Moor MH, Costa PT, Terracciano A, Krueger RF, de Geus EJ, Toshiko T, Penninx BW, Esko T, Madden PA, Derringer J, et al. Meta-analysis of genome-wide association studies for personality. Mol Psychiatry. 2012;17: 337–49.
19. van den Berg SM, de Moor MH, Verweij KJ, Krueger RF, Luciano M, Arias Vasquez A, Matteson LK, Derringer J, Esko T, Amin N, et al. Meta-analysis of genome-wide association studies for extraversion: findings from the Genetics of Personality Consortium. Behav Genet. 2016;46:170–82.
20. Genetics of Personality Consortium, de Moor MH, van den Berg SM, Verweij KJ, Krueger RF, Luciano M, Arias Vasquez A, Matteson LK, Derringer J, Esko T, et al. Meta-analysis of genome-wide association studies for neuroticism, and the polygenic association with major depressive disorder. JAMA Psychiatry. 2015;72:642–50.
21. Okbay A, Baselmans BM, De Neve JE, Turley P, Nivard MG, Fontana MA, Meddens SF, Linner RK, Rietveld CA, Derringer J, et al. Genetic variants associated with subjective well-being, depressive symptoms, and neuroticism identified through genome-wide analyses. Nat Genet. 2016;48:624–33.
22. Lao O, Lu TT, Nothnagel M, Junge O, Freitag-Wolf S, Caliebe A, Balascakova M, Bertranpetit J, Bindoff LA, Comas D, et al. Correlation between genetic and geographic structure in Europe. Curr Biol. 2008;18:1241–8.
23. Delaneau O, Marchini J, Zagury JF. A linear complexity phasing method for thousands of genomes. Nat Methods. 2011;9:179–81.
24. Howie B, Marchini J, Stephens M. Genotype imputation with thousands of genomes. G3 (Bethesda). 2011;1:457–70.
25. 1000 Genomes Project Consortium, Auton A, Brooks LD, Durbin RM, Garrison EP, Kang HM, Korbel JO, Marchini JL, McCarthy S, McVean GA, Abecasis GR. A global reference for human genetic variation. Nature. 2015; 526:68–74.
26. Chang CC, Chow CC, Tellier LC, Vattikuti S, Purcell SM, Lee JJ. Second-generation PLINK: rising to the challenge of larger and richer datasets. Gigascience. 2015;4:7.
27. Galinsky KJ, Bhatia G, Loh PR, Georgiev S, Mukherjee S, Patterson NJ, Price AL. Fast principal-component analysis reveals convergent evolution of ADH1B in Europe and East Asia. Am J Hum Genet. 2016;98:456–72.
28. Polimanti R, Amstadter AB, Stein MB, Almli LM, Baker DG, Bierut LJ, Bradley B, Farrer LA, Johnson EO, King A, et al. A putative causal relationship between genetically determined female body shape and posttraumatic stress disorder. Genome Med. 2017;9:99.
29. Polimanti R, Chen CY, Ursano RJ, Heeringa SG, Jain S, Kessler RC, Nock MK, Smoller JW, Sun X, Gelernter J, Stein MB. Cross-phenotype polygenic risk score analysis of persistent post-concussive symptoms in U.S. Army soldiers with deployment-acquired traumatic brain injury. J Neurotrauma. 2017;34:781–9.
30. Polimanti R, Kaufman J, Zhao H, Kranzler HR, Ursano RJ, Kessler RC, Stein MB, Gelernter J. Trauma exposure interacts with the genetic risk of bipolar disorder in alcohol misuse of US soldiers. Acta Psychiatr Scand. 2018;137: 148–56.
31. Zhou H, Polimanti R, Yang BZ, Wang Q, Han S, Sherva R, Nunez YZ, Zhao H, Farrer LA, Kranzler HR, Gelernter J. Genetic risk variants associated with comorbid alcohol dependence and major depression. JAMA Psychiatry. 2017;74:1234–41.
32. Wang Q, Polimanti R, Kranzler HR, Farrer LA, Zhao H, Gelernter J. Genetic factor common to schizophrenia and HIV infection is associated with risky sexual behavior: antagonistic vs. synergistic pleiotropic SNPs enriched for distinctly different biological functions. Hum Genet. 2017;136:75–83.

33. Moran S, McCloy D, Wright R. PHOIBLE Online. Leipzig: Max Planck Institute for Evolutionary Anthropology; 2014.

34. Euesden J, Lewis CM, O'Reilly PF. PRSice: polygenic risk score software. Bioinformatics. 2015;31:1466–8.

35. Benjamini Y, Hochberg Y. Controlling the false discovery rate: a practical and powerful approach to multiple testing. J R Stat Soc Ser B Methodol. 1995;57:289–300.

36. Zheng J, Erzurumluoglu AM, Elsworth BL, Kemp JP, Howe L, Haycock PC, Hemani G, Tansey K, Laurin C, Early G, et al. LD Hub: a centralized database and web interface to perform LD score regression that maximizes the potential of summary level GWAS data for SNP heritability and genetic correlation analysis. Bioinformatics. 2017;33:272–9.

37. Bulik-Sullivan B, Finucane HK, Anttila V, Gusev A, Day FR, Loh PR, ReproGen C, Psychiatric Genomics C, Genetic Consortium for Anorexia Nervosa of the Wellcome Trust Case Control C, Duncan L, et al. An atlas of genetic correlations across human diseases and traits. Nat Genet. 2015;47:1236–41.

38. Li J, Wang L, Jiang T, Wang J, Li X, Liu X, Wang C, Teng Z, Zhang R, Lv H, Guo M. eSNPO: An eQTL-based SNP ontology and SNP functional enrichment analysis platform. Sci Rep. 2016;6:30595.

39. Pers TH, Timshel P, Hirschhorn JN. SNPsnap: a Web-based tool for identification and annotation of matched SNPs. Bioinformatics. 2015;31:418–20.

40. Alvarez-Castro JM, Carlborg O. A unified model for functional and statistical epistasis and its application in quantitative trait loci analysis. Genetics. 2007; 176:1151–67.

41. Harris RA, Alcott CE, Sullivan EL, Takahashi D, McCurdy CE, Comstock S, Baquero K, Blundell P, Frias AE, Kahr M, et al. Genomic variants associated with resistance to high fat diet induced obesity in a primate model. Sci Rep. 2016;6:36123.

42. GTEx Consortium. The Genotype-Tissue Expression (GTEx) project. Nat Genet. 2013;45:580–5.

43. Pybus M, Luisi P, Dall'Olio GM, Uzkudun M, Laayouni H, Bertranpetit J, Engelken J. Hierarchical boosting: a machine-learning framework to detect and classify hard selective sweeps in human populations. Bioinformatics. 2015;31:3946–52.

44. Field Y, Boyle EA, Telis N, Gao Z, Gaulton KJ, Golan D, Yengo L, Rocheleau G, Froguel P, McCarthy MI, Pritchard JK. Detection of human adaptation during the past 2000 years. Science. 2016;354:760–4.

45. Mortensen PB, Pedersen CB, Westergaard T, Wohlfahrt J, Ewald H, Mors O, Andersen PK, Melbye M. Effects of family history and place and season of birth on the risk of schizophrenia. N Engl J Med. 1999;340:603–8.

46. Racimo F, Gokhman D, Fumagalli M, Ko A, Hansen T, Moltke I, Albrechtsen A, Carmel L, Huerta-Sanchez E, Nielsen R. Archaic adaptive introgression in TBX15/WARS2. Mol Biol Evol. 2017;34:509–24.

47. Okerlund ND, Cheyette BN. Synaptic Wnt signaling—a contributor to major psychiatric disorders? J Neurodev Disord. 2011;3:162–74.

48. Holstein TW. The evolution of the Wnt pathway. Cold Spring Harb Perspect Biol. 2012;4:a007922.

49. Bauer M, Glenn T, Alda M, Andreassen OA, Angelopoulos E, Ardau R, Baethge C, Bauer R, Baune BT, Bellivier F, et al. Influence of light exposure during early life on the age of onset of bipolar disorder. J Psychiatr Res. 2015;64:1–8.

50. Dauphinais DR, Rosenthal JZ, Terman M, DiFebo HM, Tuggle C, Rosenthal NE. Controlled trial of safety and efficacy of bright light therapy vs. negative air ions in patients with bipolar depression. Psychiatry Res. 2012;196:57–61.

51. Cohen JM, Civitello DJ, Brace AJ, Feichtinger EM, Ortega CN, Richardson JC, Sauer EL, Liu X, Rohr JR. Spatial scale modulates the strength of ecological processes driving disease distributions. Proc Natl Acad Sci U S A. 2016;113:E3359–64.

52. Xie JL, Grahl N, Sless T, Leach MD, Kim SH, Hogan DA, Robbins N, Cowen LE. Signaling through Lrg1, Rho1 and Pkc1 governs Candida albicans morphogenesis in response to diverse cues. PLoS Genet. 2016;12:e1006405.

53. Tomkins A. Tropical malabsorption: recent concepts in pathogenesis and nutritional significance. Clin Sci (Lond). 1981;60:131–7.

54. Creanza N, Ruhlen M, Pemberton TJ, Rosenberg NA, Feldman MW, Ramachandran S. A comparison of worldwide phonemic and genetic variation in human populations. Proc Natl Acad Sci U S A. 2015;112:1265–72.

55. Moyer A. Exceptional outcomes in L2 phonology: the critical factors of learner engagement and self-regulation. Appl Linguist. 2014;35:418–40.

2

Exploring the pre-immune landscape of antigen-specific T cells

Mikhail V. Pogorelyy[1], Alla D. Fedorova[1], James E. McLaren[2], Kristin Ladell[2], Dmitri V. Bagaev[1], Alexey V. Eliseev[1,3], Artem I. Mikelov[1,4], Anna E. Koneva[1], Ivan V. Zvyagin[1,3], David A. Price[2,6], Dmitry M. Chudakov[1,3,4,5] and Mikhail Shugay[1,3,4*] (iD)

Abstract

Background: Adaptive immune responses to newly encountered pathogens depend on the mobilization of antigen-specific clonotypes from a vastly diverse pool of naive T cells. Using recent advances in immune repertoire sequencing technologies, models of the immune receptor rearrangement process, and a database of annotated T cell receptor (TCR) sequences with known specificities, we explored the baseline frequencies of T cells specific for defined human leukocyte antigen (HLA) class I-restricted epitopes in healthy individuals.

Methods: We used a database of TCR sequences with known antigen specificities and a probabilistic TCR rearrangement model to estimate the baseline frequencies of TCRs specific to distinct antigens epitopespecificT-cells. We verified our estimates using a publicly available collection of TCR repertoires from healthy individuals. We also interrogated a database of immunogenic and non-immunogenic peptides is used to link baseline T-cell frequencies with epitope immunogenicity.

Results: Our findings revealed a high degree of variability in the prevalence of T cells specific for different antigens that could be explained by the physicochemical properties of the corresponding HLA class I-bound peptides. The occurrence of certain rearrangements was influenced by ancestry and HLA class I restriction, and umbilical cord blood samples contained higher frequencies of common pathogen-specific TCRs. We also identified a quantitative link between specific T cell frequencies and the immunogenicity of cognate epitopes presented by defined HLA class I molecules.

Conclusions: Our results suggest that the population frequencies of specific T cells are strikingly non-uniform across epitopes that are known to elicit immune responses. This inference leads to a new definition of epitope immunogenicity based on specific TCR frequencies, which can be estimated with a high degree of accuracy in silico, thereby providing a novel framework to integrate computational and experimental genomics with basic and translational research efforts in the field of T cell immunology.

Keywords: Antigen, Immune repertoire, Immunogenicity, T cell receptor

Background

The availability of huge volumes of repertoire sequencing (RepSeq) [1] data and a growing curated list of T cell receptor (TCR) sequences with known antigen specificities [2] have enabled quantitative exploration of the adaptive immune system. Previous large-scale studies of immune repertoire structure in health and disease have been limited in the main to analyses of basic parameters, such as repertoire diversity and somatic rearrangement patterns incorporating variable (V), diversity (D), and joining (J) segments of the TCR [3–6]. However, it is now possible to extract potentially more useful information from these rich datasets by stratifying for antigen specificity, as exemplified recently in the settings of cytomegalovirus (CMV) infection [7] and ankylosing spondylitis [8].

Theoretical [9] and experimental [10] studies have indicated that the ability of the T cell repertoire to recognize any novel antigen is essentially determined by the frequency of antigen-specific clonotypes prior to immune challenge. The

* Correspondence: mikhail.shugay@gmail.com
[1]Department of Genomics of Adaptive Immunity, IBCH RAS, Moscow, Russia
[3]Department of Molecular Technologies, Pirogov Russian National Research Medical University, Moscow, Russia
Full list of author information is available at the end of the article

emergence of sensitive major histocompatibility complex (MHC) multimer staining protocols has further permitted the accurate measurement of specific T cell populations in the naive pool [11]. Using this approach, it has been shown that the absolute numbers of specific T cells in the pre-immune repertoire vary greatly across different epitopes, yet remain largely conserved across individuals [12, 13]. Moreover, the frequency of antigen-specific T cells in the naive pool determines both the magnitude and the kinetics of the cognate immune response [10].

Recent estimates suggest that naïve T cell clone can be as small as ~ 5 cells, which constitutes a negligible fraction of ~ 3×10^{11} T cells in the human body [14]. This leads to the observation that naive T cells specific for certain antigens are often present at very low frequencies, in some cases around one cell per million sampled T cells [10], which makes them hard to detect reliably, even using modern high-throughput RepSeq techniques. Accurate quantification via flow cytometry is a similarly challenging task [15]. However, recently developed computational methods based on probabilistic models of the VDJ re-arrangement process have allowed surprisingly precise estimates of generation frequency for individual nucleotide [16] and amino acid [17] sequences, which in turn dictate the antigen specificity of a TCR repertoire. These approaches can be used in conjunction with RepSeq data and TCR specificity annotation to characterize the pre-immune landscape of antigen-specific T cells.

We hypothesized that a growing knowledge base of antigen-specific TCR sequences, together with recent advances in RepSeq techniques and theoretical models of the TCR repertoire formation might allow in silico enumeration of T cells specific for different epitopes. An analytical framework that integrates these various datasets could provide quantitative answers to several intriguing questions regarding the organization of the adaptive immune system. For example, one could ask if major differences exist among epitope-specific T cell frequencies and how any such differences relate to the biochemical and structural properties of the targeted epitopes. One could also ask if specific T cell frequencies vary depending on the origin of T cells (for example, between cells derived from peripheral and umbilical cord blood) and individual ancestry. In addition, one could define the concept of immunogenicity in terms of the ability of the adaptive immune system to field specific T cells as a function of individual and population-level biases in repertoire structure determined by stochasticity and variability in the VDJ rearrangement process.

In this study, we report the first comprehensive analysis of baseline frequencies and population incidence rates for TCRs with known specificities that target human leukocyte antigen (HLA) class I-restricted epitopes derived from eight different pathogens. We developed a computational model that accurately predicts the baseline frequency of individual antigen-specific TCR amino acid variants curated in a publicly available database (VDJdb). This model was verified using 859 unfiltered RepSeq datasets from healthy donors [3, 7]. Accordingly, our computational framework provided a solid basis to quantify the population frequencies of antigen-specific TCRs, explore the phenomenon of shared ("public") clonotypes [18–20], and perform in silico analyses of various factors that shape the pre-immune repertoire. Using this approach, we further assessed the impact of ancestry and HLA class I type on antigen-specific T cell frequencies and characterized the specificity landscape in umbilical cord blood samples, which allowed unique insights into a convergent and highly stable "core" repertoire of naive T cells [3]. Finally, we mined a large dataset of epitopes with known immunogenicity scores [21] to derive a probabilistic measure of antigenic potential. This novel variable was used to refine our understanding of epitope specificity and develop a hierarchical view of adaptive immune responses.

Methods
Datasets and pre-processing
We used two publicly available human TCRβ RepSeq datasets: (i) data from Emerson et al. [7] (available at [https://clients.adaptivebiotech.com/immuneaccess]) and (ii) data from Britanova et al. [3] (available at [https://zenodo.org/record/826447]). TCR reads from Emerson et al. were re-mapped using MiXCR software v2.1.5 with default settings (no clonotype assembly was performed, only read mapping using the MiXCR Align routine) [22] to provide V, D, and J segment assignments consistent with Britanova et al. and IMGT nomenclature [23]. The resulting clonotype tables were then processed using VDJtools software v1.1.6 with default settings [6]. Samples were corrected for sequencing errors (VDJtools Correct routine), split into coding and non-coding clonotypes (VDJtools FilterNonFunctional routine), and VJ segment use was computed to model TCR rearrangements (VDJtools CalcSegmentUsage routine). Clonotypes were pooled by CDR3 amino acid sequence using the VDJtools PoolSamples routine to determine population frequency and the total number of TCR nucleotide sequence variants. Identical variants were counted if they were observed in different individuals. The number of nucleotide variants was used as a measure of baseline TCR frequency. Although expanded memory T cells occupy a major fraction of the repertoire, they account for only a minor fraction of unique variants [3]. Analyses based on counting unique rearrangements are therefore relatively unbiased by clone size.

T cell repertoire annotation

Human TCRβ sequences known to bind certain HLA class I-restricted epitopes were obtained from the VDJdb database [2]. CDR3 amino acid sequence matching that allowed at most one amino acid substitution and no indels was used to assign antigen specificities to RepSeq data. Of note, exact matching that required CDR3 sequence and V/J gene identity resulted in far fewer hits, rendering this approach unfeasible for currently available TCR datasets. Application of this procedure to the VDJdb data increased matches with concordant antigen by an additional ~ 20%, while allowing more substitutions linearly increased the number of discordant matches, which became greater than the concordant match frequency at three substitutions [2]. This procedure is stricter than those proposed in other analyses [24, 25]. The method used by Dash et al. allowed both substitutions and indels, while the method used by Glanville et al. operated with k-mers, allowing several substitutions.

It is important to note that our method does not require V or J segment matches, yet in most cases, it also does not allow mismatches in germline-encoded regions of the CDR3. The latter can determine the J segment accurately and narrow the list of possible V segment variants. The implicit matching of V and J segments resulting from our annotation method is reflected in the strong correlation observed between annotated TCR sequencing data and

the TCR rearrangement model (described below) that uses both V and J segment information (see Fig. 1b).

Estimating rearrangement probabilities for TCR amino acid variants

The probabilistic model for TCR sequence generation was described previously [26]. Briefly, the probability of recombination scenario is represented as the product of probabilities of distinct events in the VDJ recombination process:

$$P^{\beta}_{\text{rearr}}(r) = P(V)P(D,J)P(\text{del}V|V)P(\text{ins}VD)$$
$$\times P(\text{del}Dl, \text{del}Dr|D)P(\text{ins}DJ)P(\text{del}J|J). \quad (1)$$

$$P_{gen}(n) = \sum_{r \in r_n} P^{\beta}_{\text{rearr}}(r) \quad (2)$$

$$P_{gen}(a) = \sum_{n \in n_a} P_{gen}(n) \quad (3)$$

where P(V) and P(D,J) are the probabilities of V and D,J pair choices, P(delV|V) is the probability of a certain number of 3′ nucleotide deletions from the V segment at the VD junction, P(delJ|J) is the probability of a certain number of 5′ nucleotide deletions from the J segment at the DJ junction, P(delDl,delDr) accounts for 3′ and 5′ D segment deletions, and P(insVD) and P(insDJ) are the probabilities of certain insertion sequences at the

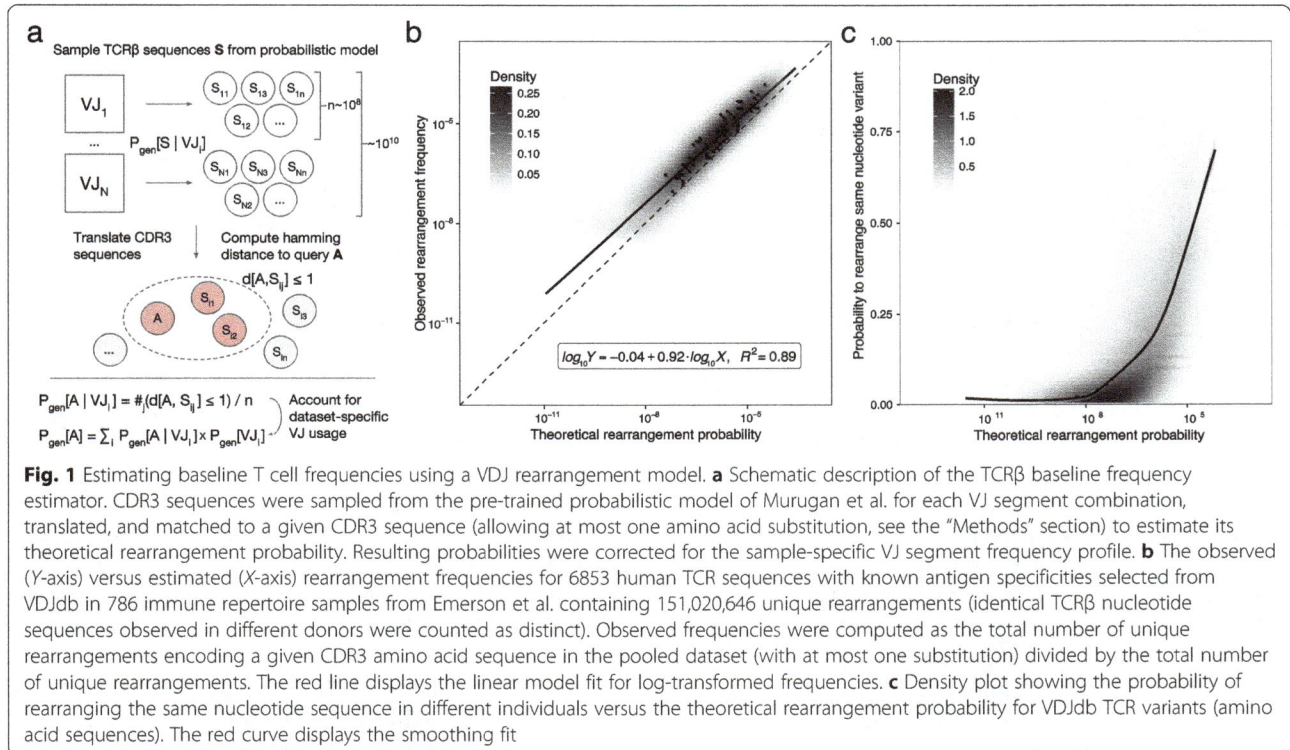

Fig. 1 Estimating baseline T cell frequencies using a VDJ rearrangement model. **a** Schematic description of the TCRβ baseline frequency estimator. CDR3 sequences were sampled from the pre-trained probabilistic model of Murugan et al. for each VJ segment combination, translated, and matched to a given CDR3 sequence (allowing at most one amino acid substitution, see the "Methods" section) to estimate its theoretical rearrangement probability. Resulting probabilities were corrected for the sample-specific VJ segment frequency profile. **b** The observed (Y-axis) versus estimated (X-axis) rearrangement frequencies for 6853 human TCR sequences with known antigen specificities selected from VDJdb in 786 immune repertoire samples from Emerson et al. containing 151,020,646 unique rearrangements (identical TCRβ nucleotide sequences observed in different donors were counted as distinct). Observed frequencies were computed as the total number of unique rearrangements encoding a given CDR3 amino acid sequence in the pooled dataset (with at most one substitution) divided by the total number of unique rearrangements. The red line displays the linear model fit for log-transformed frequencies. **c** Density plot showing the probability of rearranging the same nucleotide sequence in different individuals versus the theoretical rearrangement probability for VDJdb TCR variants (amino acid sequences). The red curve displays the smoothing fit

VD and DJ junctions, respectively. Probability tables used in this study were identical to those provided in [26], with the exception of P(V) and P(D,J), which were obtained by computing the V/J frequencies of non-functional clonotypes in the Emerson et al. and Britanova et al. datasets. The latter were calculated to account for potential V/J biases arising from methodological differences in the procedure used to generate TCR amplicon libraries (Emerson et al. used multiplexed polymerase chain reactions, and Britanova et al. used 5′ rapid amplification of cDNA ends).

To calculate the generative probability for a given nucleotide sequence, we summed the probabilities of all possible scenarios that can generate that nucleotide sequence (see Eq. 2). Amino acid sequence generation probability was then computed as the sum of probabilities of all possible underlying nucleotide sequences (see Eq. 3). Exact calculation of the probability of generating a particular amino acid sequence is computationally expensive, mostly due to the presence of a short D segment, so we used the previously described Monte Carlo approach [17]. Briefly, we generated a large set of possible rearrangements from the model, translated the resulting nucleotide sequences, and counted the number of matches to the CDR3 amino acid sequence of interest, allowing a fixed number of mismatches.

It has been shown previously that the profiles of randomly added and deleted nucleotides are very stable across repertoires sequenced using different technologies, in contrast to identification of the V and J segments [16], which are subject to amplification bias during library preparation. This leads to differences in the P(V) and P(D,J) distributions, which can be accounted for by computing P(CDR3aa) in two steps: (i) compute P(CDR3aa|V,J) by simulating recombination scenarios for a fixed VJ combination (J unambiguously determines possible D); and (ii) calculate P(CDR3aa) as a sum of P(CDR3aa|V,J) times P(V,J), where P(V,J) is estimated from non-functional sequences in the dataset of interest. In this study, we simulated 10^8 recombination scenarios for each VJ combination, generating more than 10^{10}-sequences in total. We then scaled the estimated frequencies by VJ usage in the corresponding RepSeq dataset. Of note, the final probabilities can fall below 10^{-10}, because some VJ combinations have a frequency of less than 10^{-2}.

Analysis of amino acid features
The physicochemical properties of CDR3 loops and peptide epitopes were estimated using sums of ten Kidera factors (see [27] for more details and corresponding values) across all residues. Kidera factors were originally derived as principal components of various physicochemical properties of individual amino acids and encode features such as volume and hydropathy (as

determined by the origin of the largest term in a factor). In our analysis, we computed the Pearson correlation between raw factor values and the variable of interest (e.g., rearrangement probability) and used an ANOVA test for the values of a given Kidera factor partitioned into four quantiles. The partitioning was done based on the whole spectrum of Kidera factor sums observed for all VDJdb epitopes with the first (Q1) and last (Q4) quantiles corresponding to the highest and lowest factor values, respectively.

Statistical analysis
All statistical testing was performed in R using standard packages for T test, ANOVA, Mann–Whitney U test, and Kolmogorov–Smirnov test. R markdown templates for all analysis steps are available at [https://github.com/antigenomics/public-epitope].

Results
Modelling baseline frequencies of specific TCR amino acid sequences
It has been shown previously that the chance of a certain TCR nucleotide sequence being produced by the VDJ rearrangement process can be efficiently recaptured with a probabilistic model that considers V, D, and J gene choices, the number of bases trimmed from the rearranged germline sequences, and the number and composition of random insertions [26]. This model can be applied reliably to a given TCR repertoire using an expectation maximization algorithm, and the results are extremely stable across individuals [16, 26]. However, estimating the probability of TCR variants and their amino acid translations requires traversing a large tree of possible rearrangement scenarios, which can be computationally inefficient. We therefore chose to compute approximate probabilities using the Monte Carlo method, which operates in a two-step manner: (i) it counts the expected number of matches to a given CDR3 amino acid sequence within a given V(D)J combination by sampling rearrangements using corresponding V/D/J trimming and random insert probabilities [26] and (ii) it scales match frequencies to account for a specific V(D)J combination frequency profile in a given dataset and computes the final probability value by summarizing frequencies across different V(D)J combinations (see the "Methods" section and Fig. 1a). This method was used to estimate the probability of observing a certain TCR beta chain (TCRβ) CDR3 amino acid sequence with a maximum discrepancy of one amino acid substitution, which in turn was used as a proxy to estimate specific T cell frequency throughout this study.

Baseline frequencies of TCR variants estimated using this method were in good agreement with those observed in a dataset of 786 repertoires (Fig. 1b). The intercept of the model was close to zero (− 0.04 ± 0.03) after correcting for the percentage of non-coding sequences (either out-of-frame or containing a stop codon) generated by the probabilistic model (24.3 ± 0.1%). A slope of 0.920 ± 0.005 could be attributed to sampling effects, because the frequencies observed in the real dataset exhibited a lower bound of 10^{-7} to 10^{-8}, which was much higher than the corresponding range in the theoretical model.

The case where multiple TCR nucleotide sequences encode the same TCR amino acid sequence (also known as convergent recombination) has previously been linked to the phenomenon of "public" TCRs, which are shared across multiple individuals [18]. As can be seen from Fig. 1c, this process was also observed for TCR variants with high rearrangement frequencies, in some instances exceeding previous estimates. Moreover, for the most

frequent TCR amino acid variants, as many as three in four separate rearrangement events generated the same TCR nucleotide sequence.

Rearrangement probabilities and population frequencies vary greatly across T cells specific for different antigens

Next, we applied this model to explore frequency differences across distinct antigen-specific T cell populations. As can be seen from Fig. 2a, the median frequencies of TCR variants associated with different epitopes varied significantly, and the difference between the highest and lowest associated frequencies was almost two orders of magnitude. Nonetheless, the intra-epitope frequency variance reached six orders of magnitude, suggesting that each epitope featured both public and rare antigen-specific TCRs. These differences were also present when TCR variants were grouped by epitope origin (Fig. 2b). Interestingly,

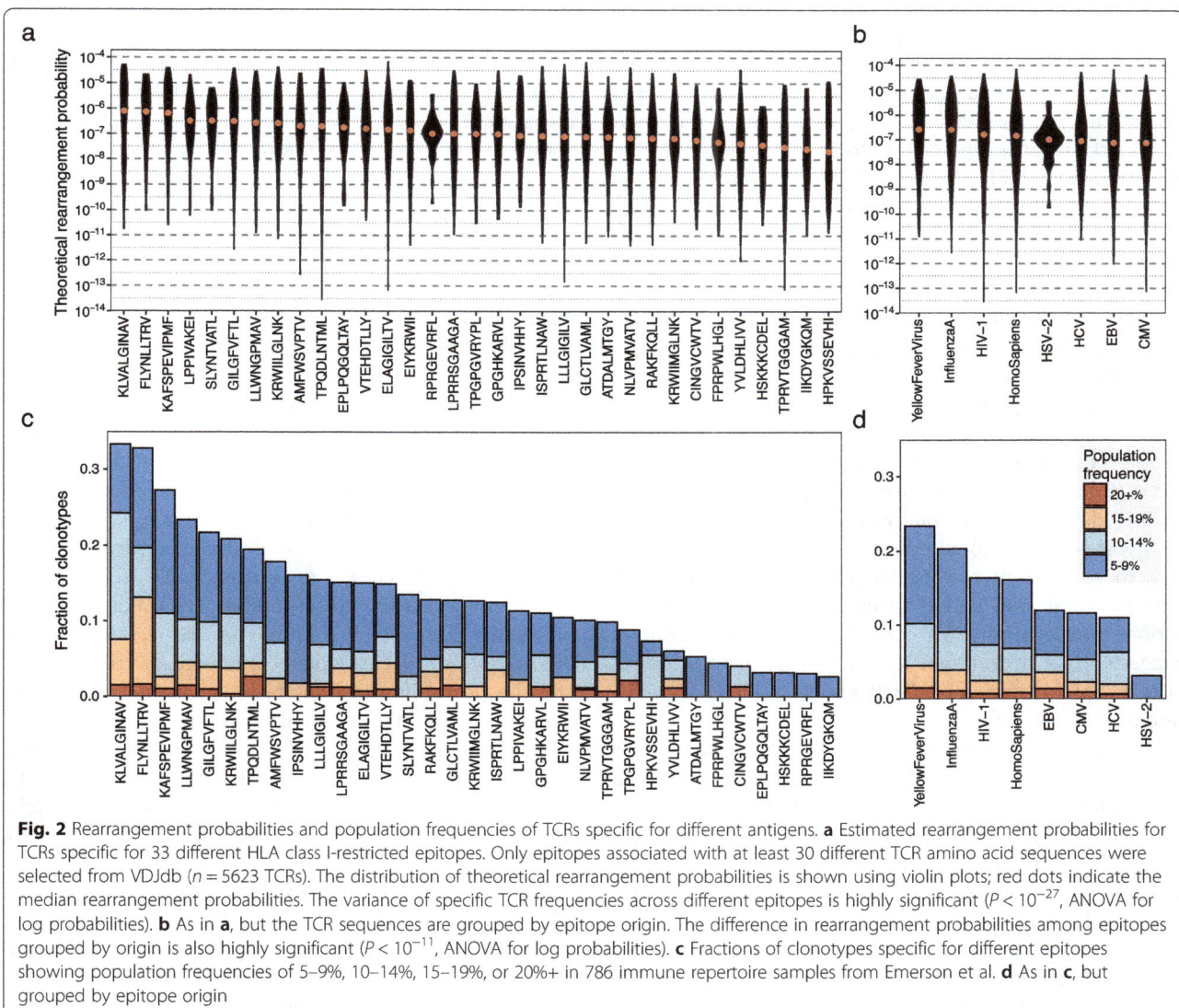

Fig. 2 Rearrangement probabilities and population frequencies of TCRs specific for different antigens. **a** Estimated rearrangement probabilities for TCRs specific for 33 different HLA class I-restricted epitopes. Only epitopes associated with at least 30 different TCR amino acid sequences were selected from VDJdb ($n = 5623$ TCRs). The distribution of theoretical rearrangement probabilities is shown using violin plots; red dots indicate the median rearrangement probabilities. The variance of specific TCR frequencies across different epitopes is highly significant ($P < 10^{-27}$, ANOVA for log probabilities). **b** As in **a**, but the TCR sequences are grouped by epitope origin. The difference in rearrangement probabilities among epitopes grouped by origin is also highly significant ($P < 10^{-11}$, ANOVA for log probabilities). **c** Fractions of clonotypes specific for different epitopes showing population frequencies of 5–9%, 10–14%, 15–19%, or 20%+ in 786 immune repertoire samples from Emerson et al. **d** As in **c**, but grouped by epitope origin

TCR variants specific for CMV or Epstein–Barr virus (EBV) were the least frequent, ruling out the hypothesis that the VDJ rearrangement machinery is biased towards targeting common pathogens [28].

Of note, these results translated into population frequencies of specific TCR variants. The fraction of individuals with a specific TCR variant shown in Fig. 2c, d closely mirrored the theoretical frequencies shown in Fig. 2a, b, and the Spearman rank correlation coefficient between median rearrangement probability and the fraction of epitope-specific TCRs found in at least 5% samples was $\rho = 0.71$ $(P = 4 \times 10^{-6})$. This finding suggests that differences in baseline frequencies resulting from intrinsic features of the VDJ recombination machinery may have a profound effect on immunity at the population level.

Epitope sequence features can predict the population frequency of specific T cells

To explore the source of large differences in the baseline frequencies of specific TCRs across epitopes, we analyzed the underlying amino acid sequence features of epitopes present in VDJdb, focusing on epitope lengths and their physicochemical properties modelled by sums of ten Kidera factors [27]. We performed correlation analysis and ANOVA. For the latter, values of each Kidera factor were categorized into four quantiles. Epitope length, net partial specific volume, and net surrounding hydrophobicity were significantly associated with specific TCR frequency $(P < 0.01$ after Benjamini–Hochberg correction for both correlation and ANOVA; Fig. 3a). Of note, the latter two Kidera factors were independent of epitope length $(P > 0.2$ for net partial specific volume, and $P > 0.49$ for net surrounding hydrophobicity, one-way ANOVA). Moreover, significant associations were observed between these Kidera factors and baseline frequencies of specific TCRs (adjusted $P < 0.01$, one-way ANOVA) when the analysis was restricted to an epitope length of 9 amino acids (the most frequent epitope length in VDJdb). Although epitope length and partial specific volume were not described previously in this context, multiple studies have suggested that hydrophobicity is an important feature related to epitope immunogenicity and TCR–peptide–MHC interactions [21, 29].

The correlation between epitope length and baseline frequencies of specific TCRs is especially interesting in the context of a recent study, which demonstrated that TCR specificity is restricted by epitope length [30]. This observation can be explained by structural constraints on the corresponding TCR–peptide–MHC interactions. Specifically, we observed that longer epitopes were recognized by TCRs with shorter CDR3 loops and vice versa (Fig. 3b) and that shorter CDR3 sequences were easier to assemble during VDJ rearrangement (Fig. 3c).

Structural constraints then follow from the fact that longer CDR3 loops and epitopes are more bulged (as can be seen from the structural data analysis shown in Fig. 3d, e), such that a certain balance of CDR3 versus epitope lengths is required to allow tight docking of specific TCRs onto cognate peptide–MHC complexes. Tight docking in the context of longer epitopes may also limit the amino acid positions available for cognate TCR interactions. Following the logic shown in Fig. 3f, we can further hypothesize that longer epitopes are generally recognized by more public and less specific repertoires of TCRs.

Exploring HLA-mediated effects on specific T cell frequencies

Thymic selection allows the passage of T cells that recognize peptides bound by donor HLA molecules (positive selection), yet do not interact strongly with self-peptides (negative selection) [31]. The complex interplay between positive and negative selection is therefore shaped by the ability of a TCR to bind certain HLA molecules and the pool of self-peptides presented by the donor-specific array of HLA molecules. Defining an HLA-specific TCR sequence as a TCR sequence known to recognize at least one epitope in a given HLA context according to VDJdb, we computed the extent of positive selection as the degree of association between donor HLAs and specific HLA-restricted TCRs (Fig. 4a). We detected a significant $(P = 0.004)$ association between donor HLAs and the frequencies of TCRs that recognize specific epitopes in a matched HLA context, yet the effect size of this association was very small (1.02-fold increase on average). This observation suggests that HLA restriction plays a minimal role in thymic selection of the functional TCR repertoire, as described previously at the protein level [32]. As a consequence, T cells are free to recognize both HLA-matched and HLA-mismatched epitopes, which is highly pertinent in the setting of allogeneic stem cell transplantation.

To confirm this finding, we used a hypergeometric test to compare the frequencies of specific TCRs in samples with and without the corresponding HLA allele, as listed in VDJdb (Fig. 4b). We found no association between the probability of enrichment in any given HLA context and the probability of TCR rearrangement (Fig. 4b, left panel), suggesting minimal bias as a function of under-sampling certain TCRs. However, we also found that the vast majority of significantly enriched TCRs were present in samples carrying an HLA allele matching the restriction element reported in VDJdb (Fig. 4b, left panel). Of note, TCR enrichment was most prominent for epitopes derived from EBV and influenza virus (Fig. 4b, right panel).

The effect of HLA restriction on T cell selection should not be confused with HLA-restricted clonal expansions, which can be quantified by comparing sequence read

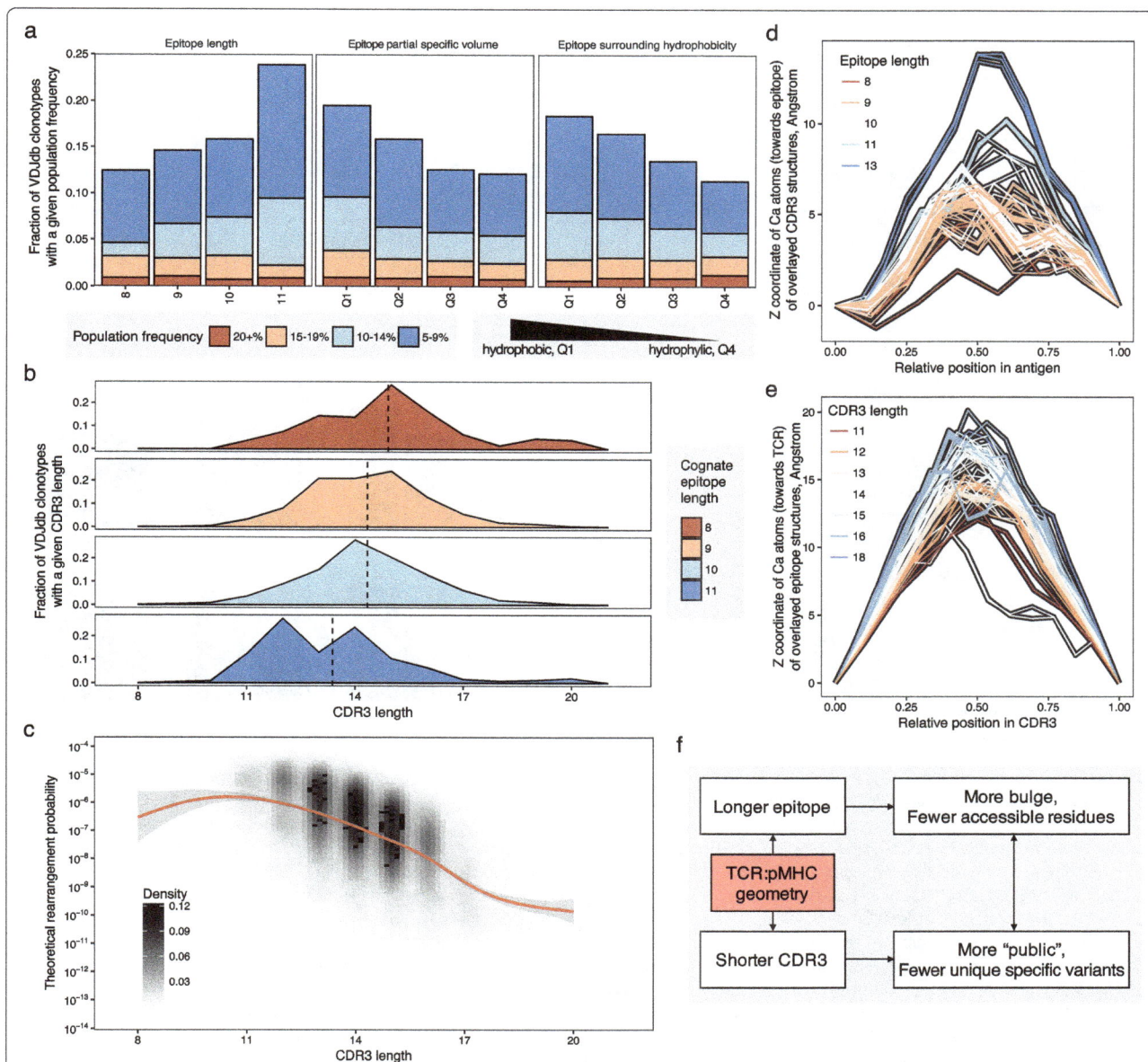

Fig. 3 Epitope features that affect the rearrangement probabilities of specific TCRs. **a** Population frequencies of TCRs specific for epitopes of different length, net partial specific volume (sixth Kidera factor), and net surrounding hydrophobicity (tenth Kidera factor). Fractions of public clonotypes (found in 5%+ of samples) are shown with population frequencies as in Fig. 2b. The association and correlation between these features and the theoretical rearrangement probabilities is highly significant: $P_{ANOVA} = 10^{-8}$, $P_{corr} = 4 \times 10^{-6}$ for length; $P_{ANOVA} = 8 \times 10^{-9}$, $P_{corr} = 10^{-6}$ for partial specific volume; $P_{ANOVA} = 4 \times 10^{-10}$, $P_{corr} = 4 \times 10^{-8}$ for surrounding hydrophobicity (P values were corrected for multiple testing using the Benjamini–Hochberg method). Only epitope lengths of 8 to 11 amino acids were considered in the first subplot, as other lengths were represented by fewer than 30 TCRs. Partial specific volume and surrounding hydrophobicity were categorized into four quantiles (Q1 to Q4, from smallest to largest standardized value) according to their levels among VDJdb epitopes. See main text for details of feature selection. **b** CDR3 length distributions for epitope lengths of 8 to 11 amino acids. **c** Density plot of rearrangement probabilities for VDJdb TCRs with different CDR3 lengths. **d**, **e** Projection of epitope and CDR3 structures on a plane passing through the line connecting their C- and N-terminal residues and the center of mass of all Cα atoms. Longer epitope and CDR3 sequences result in more bulged structures. Data were obtained from a manually curated list of 125 PDB structures [https://github.com/antigenomics/tcr-pmhc-study]. **f** Schematic representation of the association between CDR3 and epitope lengths and the potential consequences for TCR cross-reactivity and specificity

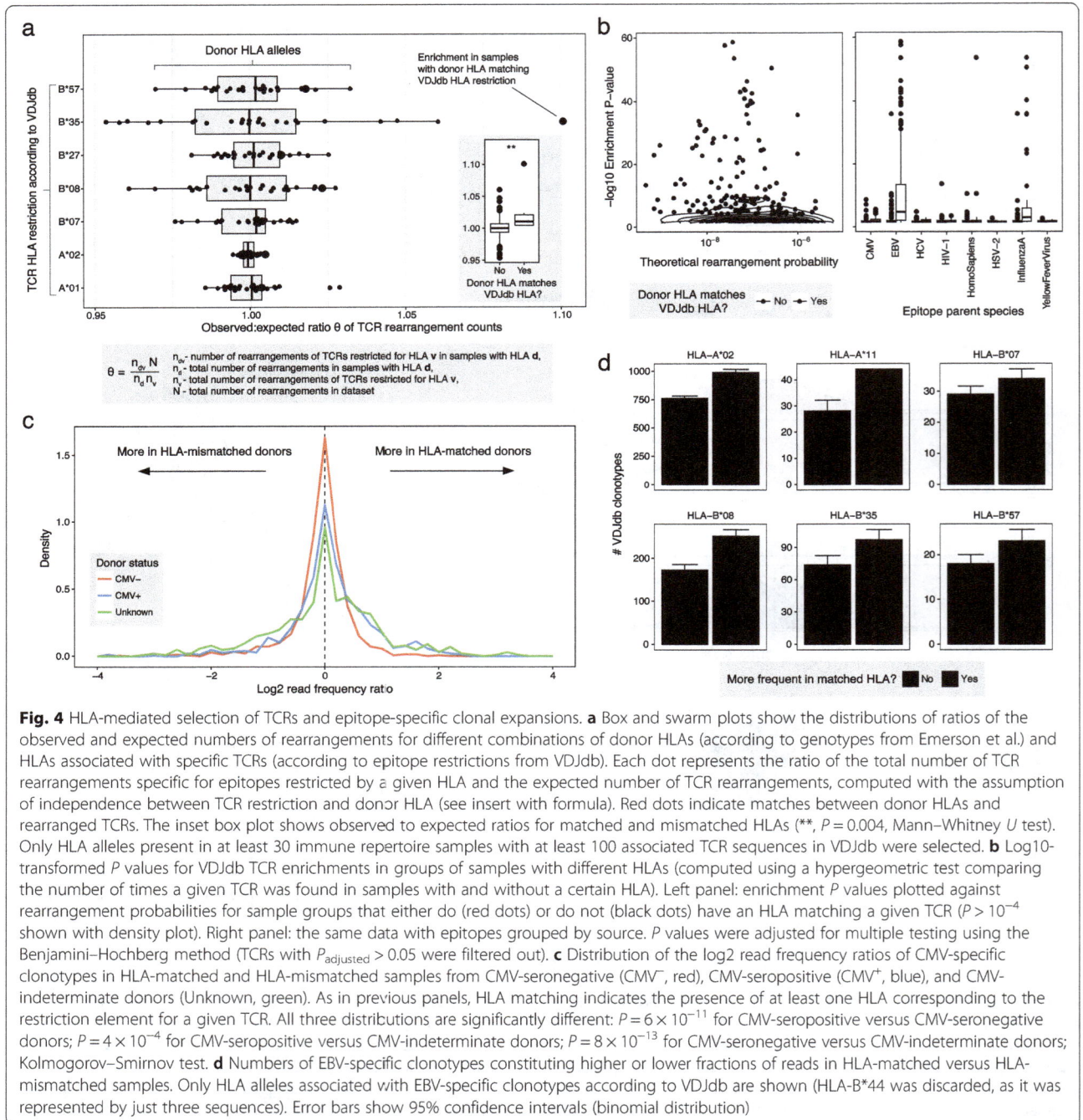

Fig. 4 HLA-mediated selection of TCRs and epitope-specific clonal expansions. **a** Box and swarm plots show the distributions of ratios of the observed and expected numbers of rearrangements for different combinations of donor HLAs (according to genotypes from Emerson et al.) and HLAs associated with specific TCRs (according to epitope restrictions from VDJdb). Each dot represents the ratio of the total number of TCR rearrangements specific for epitopes restricted by a given HLA and the expected number of TCR rearrangements, computed with the assumption of independence between TCR restriction and donor HLA (see insert with formula). Red dots indicate matches between donor HLAs and rearranged TCRs. The inset box plot shows observed to expected ratios for matched and mismatched HLAs (**, $P = 0.004$, Mann–Whitney U test). Only HLA alleles present in at least 30 immune repertoire samples with at least 100 associated TCR sequences in VDJdb were selected. **b** Log10-transformed P values for VDJdb TCR enrichments in groups of samples with different HLAs (computed using a hypergeometric test comparing the number of times a given TCR was found in samples with and without a certain HLA). Left panel: enrichment P values plotted against rearrangement probabilities for sample groups that either do (red dots) or do not (black dots) have an HLA matching a given TCR ($P > 10^{-4}$ shown with density plot). Right panel: the same data with epitopes grouped by source. P values were adjusted for multiple testing using the Benjamini–Hochberg method (TCRs with $P_{adjusted} > 0.05$ were filtered out). **c** Distribution of the log2 read frequency ratios of CMV-specific clonotypes in HLA-matched and HLA-mismatched samples from CMV-seronegative (CMV$^-$, red), CMV-seropositive (CMV$^+$, blue), and CMV-indeterminate donors (Unknown, green). As in previous panels, HLA matching indicates the presence of at least one HLA corresponding to the restriction element for a given TCR. All three distributions are significantly different: $P = 6 \times 10^{-11}$ for CMV-seropositive versus CMV-seronegative donors; $P = 4 \times 10^{-4}$ for CMV-seropositive versus CMV-indeterminate donors; $P = 8 \times 10^{-13}$ for CMV-seronegative versus CMV-indeterminate donors; Kolmogorov–Smirnov test. **d** Numbers of EBV-specific clonotypes constituting higher or lower fractions of reads in HLA-matched versus HLA-mismatched samples. Only HLA alleles associated with EBV-specific clonotypes according to VDJdb are shown (HLA-B*44 was discarded, as it was represented by just three sequences). Error bars show 95% confidence intervals (binomial distribution)

frequencies (Fig. 4c, d). This phenomenon was clearly demonstrated in CMV-seropositive versus CMV-seronegative donors (Fig. 4c). As the vast majority (almost 90%) of individuals are infected with EBV by adulthood [33], one can also expect to observe HLA-restricted expansions of EBV-specific clonotypes (Fig. 4d). In line with this expectation, EBV-derived epitope-specific clonal expansions were highly discriminatory for certain HLA alleles (Additional file 1: Figure S1), explaining the accuracy of an HLA classification

technique that relies on the detection of certain "predictor" TCR sequences [7].

Umbilical cord blood is enriched for known antigen-specific TCR variants

Umbilical cord blood (UCB) contains predominantly naive but fully functional T cells that shape the TCR repertoire early in life [3, 34]. Previous studies have shown that antigen-specific TCR repertoires in UCB samples are distinct from those in peripheral blood mononuclear cell (PBMC) samples [15], featuring lower numbers of N-bases and higher numbers of public TCRs [3]. Moreover, T cells of fetal origin persist in an individual for long periods of time, with a half-life of approximately 42 years [35]. These substantial differences in repertoire structure between T cells derived from UCB and PBMC samples prompted a suggestion that these populations may also differ with respect to the recognition of certain epitopes, potentially affecting immune competence. We have therefore used our framework to quantify the epitope specificity profile of T cells in UCB versus PBMC samples.

Comparison of the fraction of unique TCR rearrangements matched with VDJdb records in samples from Britanova et al. showed that UCB samples contained ~ 1.3 times more specific TCR matches than PBMC samples ($P = 0.0015$, two-tailed T test, Additional file 1: Figure S2). This difference could not be attributed to the CD4/CD8 ratio bias in UCB samples, because the same effect was observed for HLA class II-restricted epitopes ($P = 0.0008$, two-tailed T test; Additional file 1: Figure S2). The probable explanation here is that UCB clonotypes are more likely to be observed in antigen-specific responses as a function of simpler rearrangements and prolonged persistence. Moreover, there were notable differences between the specificity profiles observed in UCB versus PBMC samples. In particular, the relative abundance of specific TCR rearrangements was significantly different for 7 of 33 epitopes (Additional file 1: Figure S3 and Table S1).

Evidence of ancestry-associated differences in baseline frequencies of specific T cells

Ancestry is a major determinant of population-specific differences in susceptibility to immune-related diseases and various pathogens [36, 37]. In line with these observations, previous studies have documented ancestry-related differences in T cell immunity [38, 39]. However, to the best of our knowledge, there have been no previous attempts to link these findings to the composition of the T cell repertoire. We took advantage of the racially diverse cohort used in the Emerson et al. study to explore this possibility. For 9 of 33 epitopes, there was a significant variance in TCR frequencies across individuals of Caucasian, African, and Asian descent (Additional file 1: Figure S4 and Table S2). These results suggest that substantial differences may exist among populations with respect to T cell antigen specificity.

Linking specific T cell frequencies and epitope immunogenicity

A recently published study [21] provided a large set of immunogenic and non-immunogenic epitopes, allowing us to test for an association between epitope-specific TCR frequency and immunogenicity. Epitope immunogenicity is not defined in VDJdb. However, it is still possible to score immunogenicity on a continuous scale, either by comparing the distance between each epitope and those categorized as immunogenic or non-immunogenic in the Chowell et al. dataset with respect to discriminatory features in amino acid sequence space or by training an immunogenic epitope classifier and using it to compute "immunogenicity" scores.

Immunogenic and non-immunogenic epitopes were efficiently separated in Kidera factor feature space by transforming every epitope sequence into a vector of sums for each of the ten Kidera factors that encode the physicochemical properties of amino acids (Fig. 5a). As can be seen from Fig. 5b, c, theoretical epitope-specific T cell frequencies estimated using our models correlated positively with VDJdb epitope similarity to those defined as immunogenic by Chowell et al. and with the probabilities of VDJdb epitopes being classified as immunogenic, which in turn correlated positively with the median rearrangement probabilities determined for the corresponding epitope-specific TCRs (Fig. 5d). Conversely, when using the link between epitope features and TCR frequencies introduced previously (Fig. 3) and predicting TCR frequencies using a simple linear model (log TCR frequency fit using values of ten Kidera factor sums) for the Chowell et al. data, we found that significantly higher TCR frequencies were predicted for immunogenic epitopes (Fig. 5e). It is also important to note that higher TCR frequencies were associated with epitopes located closer to the "core" set of immunogenic epitope sequences (i.e., inside a denser region of immunogenic epitope feature space) (Additional file 1: Figure S5). Thus, a degree of variance can be expected in the T cell "view" of epitopes defined as immunogenic on the basis of physicochemical determinants.

Concerning the effect of missing TCRα chain information on the overall analysis

One caveat of our study is that it does not account for the paired TCRα chain. This limitation stems from the fact that most of the sequence data available in the public domain were generated via bulk analyses and largely restricted to the TCRβ chain, which nonetheless allow an empirical assessment of clonotypically distributed TCRs. It is clear from previous studies that TCRα chain bias dictates immune recognition of several epitopes, such as HLA-A*02-ELA [15, 40]. We therefore expect that additional data from single-cell sequencing approaches and dedicated methods for paired-chain TCR sequencing will lead to substantial improvements in our ability to estimate baseline antigen-specific TCR frequencies [41, 42]. To assess the validity of our approach in this light, we conducted similar analyses using Pair-SEQ data [42]. As can be seen from Fig. 6a, b, there was a significant correlation between epitope-specific TCRα

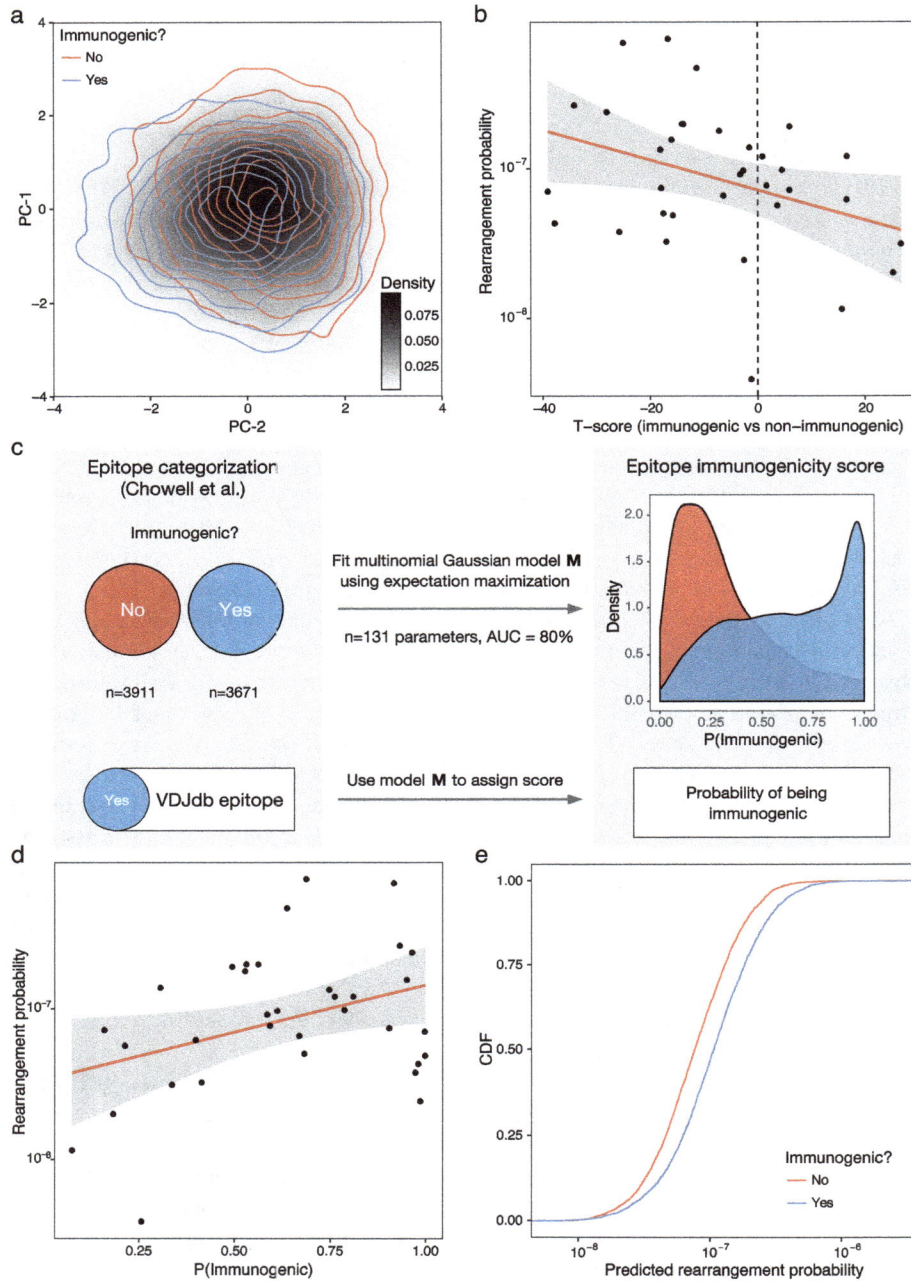

Fig. 5 (See legend on next page.)

(See figure on previous page.)
Fig. 5 Specific T cell frequencies at baseline correlate with epitope immunogenicity profiles. **a** Principal component analysis of epitope space for immunogenic and non-immunogenic epitopes from Chowell et al. Dimensionality reduction was performed on 10-dimensional vectors of Kidera factor sums for each epitope, and the first two principal components were used to plot each epitope into a 2D plane using the Euclidean distance between Kidera factor vectors. The density map shows the overall epitope repertoire space. Red and blue contour maps show densities for immunogenic and non-immunogenic epitopes, respectively. **b** Correlation of median theoretical rearrangement probabilities of TCRs specific for certain epitopes and T-scores for the Euclidean distance of each VDJdb epitope to the immunogenic and non-immunogenic epitopes computed in Kidera factor space ($R = 0.35$, $P = 0.039$). T-scores were computed by comparing distances from a given epitope to immunogenic versus non-immunogenic epitopes. Only epitopes with more than 30 associated TCRs were selected from VDJdb. **c** A schematic representation of the algorithm used to transform categorical representation of immunogenicity (yes/no for data from Chowell et al., and yes/unknown for VDJdb epitopes) into a continuous set of probability values using an immunogenicity classifier to enable a correlation analysis between immunogenicity and TCR repertoire structure. **d** Correlation of median theoretical rearrangement probabilities of TCRs specific for certain epitopes and the probability of a given epitope being immunogenic as estimated using an expectation maximization classifier ($R = 0.37$, $P = 0.031$). **e** Cumulative distribution function plot for median rearrangement probabilities predicted for immunogenic and non-immunogenic epitopes using a simple linear model based on Kidera factor sums. The difference in predicted values for all data from Chowell et al. is highly significant ($P < 2 \times 10^{-16}$, Kolmogorov–Smirnov test)

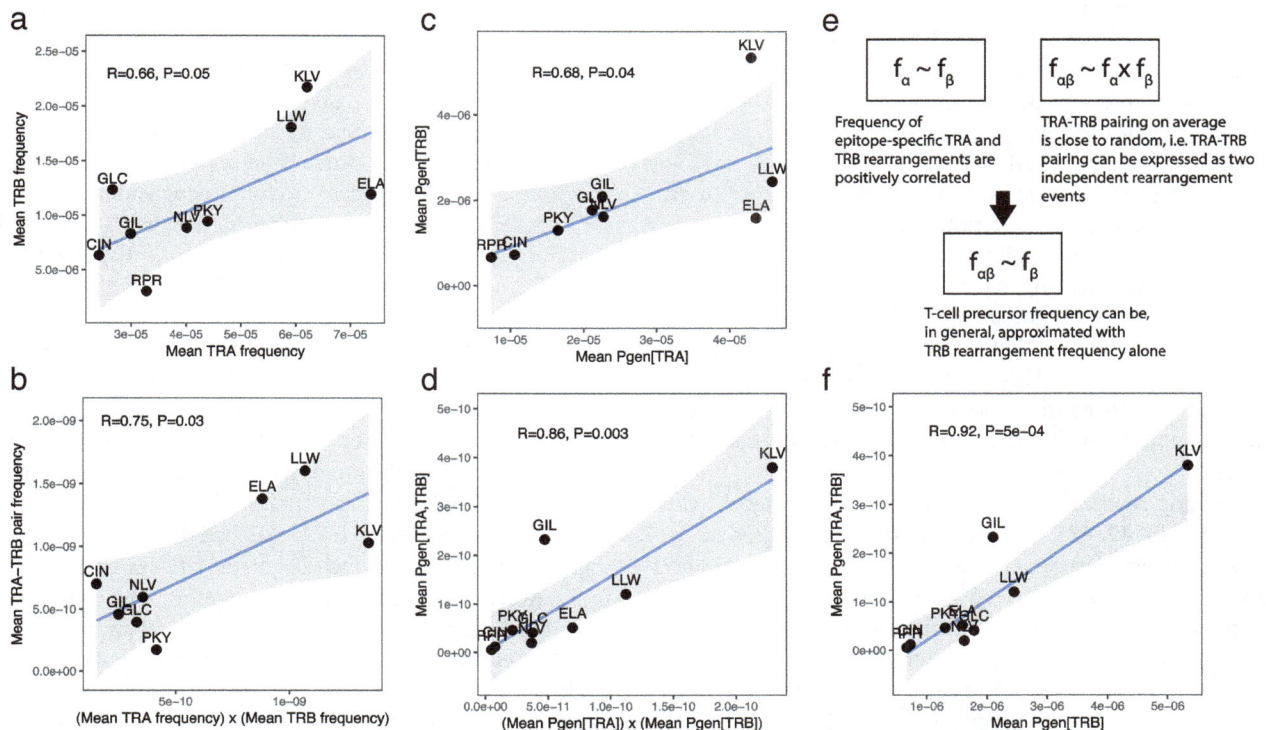

Fig. 6 Epitope-specific TCRα-TCRβ heterodimer frequencies can be estimated using TCRβ clonotype frequencies. **a, b** Matching paired TCRα-TCRβ sequencing data (PairSEQ assay, Howie et al.) against VDJdb. **a** Scatter plot of TCRα and TCRβ chain rearrangement frequencies matching a given epitope. **b** Product of marginal frequencies of TCRα and TCRβ chain rearrangements (i.e., TCR heterodimer frequencies assuming independent pairing) plotted against the frequencies of paired-chain records matching the same epitopes. Mean frequencies were computed as follows: (number of matching rearrangements)/(number of records in VDJdb for a given epitope)/(total number of rearrangements in the PairSEQ dataset). **c** As in **a**, but using TCRα and TCRβ frequencies estimated using the TCR rearrangement model. **d** As in **b**, but using TCRα and TCRβ frequencies estimated using the TCR rearrangement model. **e** Conditions required to estimate baseline T cell frequencies using TCRβ rearrangement frequencies alone. **f** Scatter plot of the mean theoretical rearrangement probabilities for TCRβ chain and paired TCRα-TCRβ chain rearrangements matching a given epitope. Epitopes lacking paired TCRα-TCRβ sequences, as well as epitopes represented by less than 30 TCRα or TCRβ sequences according to VDJdb, were excluded from the analysis. This figure uses 3-letter epitope abbreviations (see Additional file 1: Table S3 for full epitope names)

and TCRβ chain rearrangement frequencies, and paired TCRα-TCRβ chain rearrangement frequencies approximated the corresponding independent TCRα and TCRβ chain rearrangement frequencies. These results were reproduced using the TCR rearrangement model (Fig. 6c, d), suggesting that the estimates reported in this paper can be extrapolated to TCRα chain and paired TCRα-TCRβ chain data (Fig. 6e, f).

Discussion

Numerous studies have shown that antigen presentation by MHC molecules is a critical determinant of immunogenicity [24, 25, 43]. More recently, advances in the field of immune repertoire informatics [4, 5, 44–46] have allowed us to look at this problem from another angle, taking the perspective of the host immune system represented by an array of specific TCRs. In this study, we used TCR repertoire sequencing data to investigate how antigen-specific T cells discriminate among epitopes presented by HLA class I molecules.

The baseline frequencies of antigen-specific T cells were found to vary substantially from epitope to epitope in tight linkage with the presence of public TCRs. Across individual epitopes, these frequencies varied by several orders of magnitude, in line with previous estimates based on the use of MHC multimers [12, 15, 34]. For each epitope, we observed both extremely common and extremely rare TCRs. Of note, we did not find greater numbers of public TCRs specific for epitopes derived from common pathogens, such as CMV and EBV, although we did find that amalgamated clonotype frequencies varied considerably among pathogens, grouping epitopes by source. However, this latter finding should be treated with caution, because VDJdb still lists a relatively small fraction of known epitopes for each host species.

Immune repertoire diversity can be computed in various ways [5, 47, 48]. Although used with a degree of success in several RepSeq studies, the number of unique T cell clones (either observed in a sample or estimated to be present in the entire repertoire) is in no way the same as the number of antigen specificities encoded in the overall repertoire. This limitation can be solved by moving to the concept of "functional" diversity [2, 14], which accounts for the similarity of TCR sequences and their antigen binding profiles. Moreover, while the TCRβ repertoire of an individual can feature more than $\sim 10^9$ unique clones [14], the probability of a specific T cell encountering an antigen-presenting cell bearing a cognate epitope is proportional to the fraction of specific cells rather than the number of specific TCR variants. Thus, although we sampled just a minor fraction of each individual T cell pool ($\sim 10^6$ from up to $\sim 10^{12}$ individual T cells) and could not accurately estimate the total diversity of

the T cell repertoire, this did not limit our ability to estimate baseline frequencies and functional diversity. It is also important to note that VDJdb lists only a sample of specific clonotypes for each epitope, but again, this likely did not introduce significant bias into our median baseline frequency estimates, because there was no correlation between these frequency estimates and the number of epitope-specific TCRs (Additional file 1: Figure S6). In addition, potential confounders lurked in the origins of the RepSeq data, which were generated using bulk PBMCs. The resulting sequences therefore emanated from both naive and antigen-experienced T cells. As a consequence of clonal expansion, the latter almost invariably contribute the majority of sequence reads, but these sequences generally represent just a small fraction of the total number of unique rearrangements [3]. Accordingly, our approach most probably yielded results' characteristics of the naïve T cell compartment, because we focused on counting unique TCRs.

Studying the incidence of T cells specific for different epitopes across the repertoires of individuals with different HLA genotypes can provide insights into the behavior of the cellular immune system during transplantation. The enrichment observed for TCRs known to engage certain HLA class I molecules in HLA-matched samples highlights the effect of positive selection in thymus. However, the effect size of this phenomenon was dwarfed by the magnitude of HLA-restricted clonal expansions observed for specific epitopes derived from CMV or EBV. We can therefore speculate that positive selection in the thymus is more focused on general features of TCR–peptide–MHC interactions rather than the specific features of individual HLA molecules. As shown previously [3, 20], the naive T cell repertoire was highly similar across individuals with respect to the relative abundance of public TCR variants, including those inherited from the fetal period [35]. We also detected T cells known to recognize certain HLA class I molecules at just slightly lower frequencies in HLA-mismatched versus HLA-matched donors. Collectively, these findings suggest a high degree of HLA cross-reactivity, in line with an overall requirement to cover the universe of potential antigens within a limited individual framework of germline-encoded antigen-presenting molecules [49, 50].

Three other features of our analysis are particularly noteworthy. First, we identified differences in the TCR specificity profiles of repertoires isolated from UCB versus PBMC samples. Substantial fractions of T cells specific for all surveyed epitopes were nonetheless present in UCB samples, highlighting the remarkable pre-immune reservoir of virus-specific T cells [51]. This result demonstrates the capability of our analytical framework to identify different T cell populations and reveals potential differences in immune coverage among T cells derived from UCB and PBMCs. Second, we found differences in the baseline frequencies of specific T cells across individuals with different ancestries, potentially indicating genetic variance in the VDJ rearrangement machinery and/or thymic selection in the context of different HLA molecules. Although further studies are required to characterize this phenomenon in more detail, such differences may have important consequences for population-level immunity and rational vaccine design. Of note, we did not find any significant gender-related differences using data from the Britanova et al. and Emerson et al. studies. Finally, we refuted a long-standing concern that analyses reliant on TCRβ sequence data alone are inherently uninformative or biased, at least for the purposes of our study. Indeed, both TCRα and TCRβ chain frequencies specific for a given epitope were concordant, allowing the use of TCRβ sequences in isolation to derive meaningful conclusions regarding the antigen-specific landscape of heterodimeric TCRs.

Conclusions
In summary, our data indicate that the pre-immune landscape of antigen-specific T cells is a major determinant of epitope immunogenicity. As the numbers of annotated epitopes and cognate TCR sequences deposited in the VDJdb database continue to grow, we expect that our ability to characterize novel antigens in terms of immunogenicity will increase rapidly. In addition, we note that our work provides proof-of-concept for a new type of analysis that combines high-throughput T cell repertoire sequencing and in silico testing of TCR sequences across a wide range of antigen specificities to inform our basic and translational understanding of adaptive immune reactivity.

Abbreviations
CDR3: Complementarity-determining region 3 of the T cell receptor; CMV: Cytomegalovirus; EBV: Epstein–Barr virus; HCV: Hepatitis C virus; HIV: Human immunodeficiency virus; HLA: Human leukocyte antigen; MHC: Major histocompatibility complex; PBMC: Peripheral blood mononuclear cell; RepSeq: Immune repertoire sequencing technology; TCR: T cell receptor; TCRα and TCRβ: Alpha and beta chains of the T cell receptor; UCB: Umbilical cord blood; VDJ: Variable, diversity, and joining segments of the T cell receptor

Acknowledgements
The authors would like to thank Nili Tickotsky, Nir Friedman, Can Kesmir, Thierry Mora, and Andrew Sewell for helpful discussions. D.A.P. is a Wellcome Trust Senior Investigator.

Funding
The study received funding from the Russian Science Foundation grant 17-15-01495.

Authors' contributions
MVP, IVZ, DMC, and MS developed the concept. MVP implemented the TCR rearrangement model. MVP, ADF, JEM, KL, DVB, AVE, AIM, AEK, DAP, and MS acquired, pre-processed, and analyzed the data. MVP, IVZ, DAP, DMC, and MS prepared the manuscript. DMC and MS supervised the study. All authors read and approved the final manuscript.

Competing interests
The authors declare that they have no competing interests.

Author details
[1]Department of Genomics of Adaptive Immunity, IBCH RAS, Moscow, Russia. [2]Division of Infection and Immunity, Cardiff University School of Medicine, Cardiff, UK. [3]Department of Molecular Technologies, Pirogov Russian National Research Medical University, Moscow, Russia. [4]Center for Data-Intensive Biomedicine and Biotechnology, Skoltech, Moscow, Russia. [5]Central European Institute of Technology, CEITEC, Brno, Czech Republic. [6]Systems Immunity Research Institute, Cardiff University School of Medicine, Cardiff, UK.

References
1. Benichou J, Ben-Hamo R, Louzoun Y, Efroni S. Rep-Seq: uncovering the immunological repertoire through next-generation sequencing. Immunology. 2012;135:183–91.
2. Shugay M, Bagaev DV, Zvyagin IV, Vroomans RM, Crawford JC, Dolton G, Komech EA, Sycheva AL, Koneva AE, Egorov ES, et al. VDJdb: a curated database of T-cell receptor sequences with known antigen specificity. Nucleic Acids Res. 2017;46:D419–27.
3. Britanova OV, Shugay M, Merzlyak EM, Staroverov DB, Putintseva EV, Turchaninova MA, Mamedov IZ, Pogorelyy MV, Bolotin DA, Izraelson M, et al. Dynamics of individual T cell repertoires: from cord blood to centenarians. J Immunol. 2016;196:5005–13.
4. Greiff V, Miho E, Menzel U, Reddy ST. Bioinformatic and statistical analysis of adaptive immune repertoires. Trends Immunol. 2015;36:738–49.
5. Heather JM, Ismail M, Oakes T, Chain B. High-throughput sequencing of the T-cell receptor repertoire: pitfalls and opportunities. Brief Bioinform. 2018; 19(4):554-65.
6. Shugay M, Bagaev DV, Turchaninova MA, Bolotin DA, Britanova OV, Putintseva EV, Pogorelyy MV, Nazarov VI, Zvyagin IV, et al. VDJtools: unifying post-analysis of T cell receptor repertoires. PLoS Comput Biol. 2015;11: e1004503.
7. Emerson RO, DeWitt WS, Vignali M, Gravley J, Hu JK, Osborne EJ, Desmarais C, Klinger M, Carlson CS, et al. Immunosequencing identifies signatures of cytomegalovirus exposure history and HLA-mediated effects on the T cell repertoire. Nat Genet. 2017;49:659–65.
8. Faham M, Carlton V, Moorhead M, Zheng J, Klinger M, Pepin F, Asbury T, Vignali M, Emerson RO, Robins HS, et al. Discovery of T cell receptor beta motifs specific to HLA-B27-positive ankylosing spondylitis by deep repertoire sequence analysis. Arthritis Rheumatol. 2017;69:774–84.
9. Mayer A, Balasubramanian V, Mora T, Walczak AM. How a well-adapted immune system is organized. Proc Natl Acad Sci U S A. 2015;112:5950–5.
10. Jenkins MK, Moon JJ. The role of naive T cell precursor frequency and recruitment in dictating immune response magnitude. J Immunol. 2012; 188:4135–40.
11. Blattman JN, Antia R, Sourdive DJ, Wang X, Kaech SM, Murali-Krishna K, Altman JD, Ahmed R. Estimating the precursor frequency of naive antigen-specific CD8 T cells. J Exp Med. 2002;195:657–64.
12. Alanio C, Lemaitre F, Law HK, Hasan M, Albert ML. Enumeration of human antigen-specific naive CD8+ T cells reveals conserved precursor frequencies. Blood. 2010;115:3718–25.
13. Obar JJ, Khanna KM, Lefrancois L. Endogenous naive CD8+ T cell precursor frequency regulates primary and memory responses to infection. Immunity. 2008;28:859–69.
14. Mora T, Walczak A. Quantifying lymphocyte receptor diversity. ArXiv e-prints. 2016;1604:00487.
15. Neller MA, Ladell K, McLaren JE, Matthews KK, Gostick E, Pentier JM, Dolton G, Schauenburg AJ, Koning D, Fontaine Costa AI, et al. Naive CD8+ T-cell precursors display structured TCR repertoires and composite antigen-driven selection dynamics. Immunol Cell Biol. 2015;93:625–33.
16. Marcou Q, Mora T, Walczak AM. High-throughput immune repertoire analysis with IGoR. Nat Commun. 2018;9:561.
17. Pogorelyy MV, Minervina AA, Chudakov DM, Mamedov IZ, Lebedev YB, Mora T, Walczak AM. Method for identification of condition-associated public antigen receptor sequences. Elife. 2018;7:e33050.
18. Venturi V, Price DA, Douek DC, Davenport MP. The molecular basis for public T-cell responses? Nat Rev Immunol. 2008;8:231–8.

19. Bagaev DV, Zvyagin IV, Putintseva EV, Izraelson M, Britanova OV, Chudakov DM, Shugay M. VDJviz: a versatile browser for immuncgenomics data. BMC Genomics. 2016;17:453.
20. Shugay M, Bolotin DA, Putintseva EV, Pogorelyy MV, Mamedov IZ, Chudakov DM. Huge overlap of individual TCR beta repertoires. Front Immunol. 2013;4:466.
21. Chowell D, Krishna S, Becker PD, Cocita C, Shu J, Tan X, Greenberg PD, Klavinskis LS, Blattman JN, Anderson KS. TCR contact residue hydrophobicity is a hallmark of immunogenic CD8+ T cell epitopes. Proc Natl Acad Sci U S A. 2015;112(14):E1754–62.
22. Bolotin DA, Poslavsky S, Mitrophanov I, Shugay M, Mamedov IZ, Putintseva EV, Chudakov DM. MiXCR: software for comprehensive adaptive immunity profiling. Nat Methods. 2015;12:380–1.
23. Lefranc MP, Giudicelli V, Ginestoux C, Jabado-Michaloud J, Folch G, Bellahcene F, Wu Y, Gemrot E, Brochet X, Lane J, et al. IMGT, the international ImMunoGeneTics information system. Nucleic Acids Res. 2009;37:D1006–12.
24. Fleri W, Paul S, Dhanda SK, Mahajan S, Xu X, Peters B, Sette A. The immune epitope database and analysis resource in epitope discovery and synthetic vaccine design. Front Immunol. 2017;8:278.
25. Hackl H, Charoentong P, Finotello F, Trajanoski Z. Computational genomics tools for dissecting tumour-immune cell interactions. Nat Rev Genet. 2016;17:441–58.
26. Murugan A, Mora T, Walczak AM, Callan CG Jr. Statistical inference of the generation probability of T-cell receptors from sequence repertoires. Proc Natl Acad Sci U S A. 2012;109:16161–6.
27. Kidera A, Konishi Y, Oka M, Ooi T, Scheraga HA. Statistcal analysis of the physical properties of the 20 naturally occurring amino acids. J Protein Chem. 1985;4:23–55.
28. Attaf M, Huseby E, Sewell AK. Alphabeta T cell receptors as predictors of health and disease. Cell Mol Immunol. 2015;12:391–9.
29. Calis JJ, Maybeno M, Greenbaum JA, Weiskopf D, De Silva AD, Sette A, Kesmir C, Peters B. Properties of MHC class I presented peptides that enhance immunogenicity. PLoS Comput Biol. 2013;9:e1003266.
30. Ekeruche-Makinde J, Miles JJ, van den Berg HA, Skowera A, Cole DK, Dolton G, Schauenburg AJ, Tan MP, Pentier JM, Llewellyn-Lacey S, et al. Peptide length determines the outcome of TCR/peptide-MHCI engagement. Blood. 2013;121:1112–23.
31. Yates AJ. Theories and quantification of thymic selection. Front Immunol. 2014;5:13.
32. Melenhorst JJ, Lay MD, Price DA, Adams SD, Zeilah J, Sosa E, Hensel NF, Follmann D, Douek DC, Davenport MP, et al. Contribution of TCR-beta locus and HLA to the shape of the mature human Vbeta repertoire. J Immunol. 2008;180:6484–9.
33. Balfour HH Jr, Sifakis F, Sliman JA, Knight JA, Schmeling DO, Thomas W. Age-specific prevalence of Epstein-Barr virus infection among individuals aged 6-19 years in the United States and factors affecting its acquisition. J Infect Dis. 2013;208:1286–93.
34. Garderet L, Dulphy N, Douay C, Chalumeau N, Schaeffer V, Zilber MT, Lim A, Even J, Mooney N, Gelin C, et al. The umbilical cord blood alphabeta T-cell repertoire: characteristics of a polyclonal and naive but completely formed repertoire. Blood. 1998;91:340–6.
35. Pogorelyy MV, Elhanati Y, Marcou Q, Sycheva AL, Komech EA, Nazarov VI, Britanova OV, Chudakov DM, Mamedov IZ, Lebedev YB, et al. Persisting fetal clonotypes influence the structure and overlap of adult human T cell receptor repertoires. PLoS Comput Biol. 2017;13:e1005572.
36. Nedelec Y, Sanz J, Baharian G, Szpiech ZA, Pacis A, Dumaine A, Grenier JC, Freiman A, Sams AJ, Hebert S, et al. Genetic ancestry and natural selection drive population differences in immune responses to pathogens. Cell. 2016; 167:657–69. e621
37. Quach H, Rotival M, Pothlichet J, Loh YE, Dannemann M, Zidane N, Laval G, Patin E, Harmant C, Lopez M, et al. Genetic adaptation and Neandertal admixture shaped the immune system of human populations. Cell. 2016; 167:643–56. e617
38. Haralambieva IH, Ovsyannikova IG, Kennedy RB, Larrabee BR, Shane Pankratz V, Poland GA. Race and sex-based differences in cytokine immune responses to smallpox vaccine in healthy individuals. Hum Immunol. 2013;74:1263–6.
39. Tan AT, Loggi E, Boni C, Chia A, Gehring AJ, Sastry KS, Goh V, Fisicaro P, Andreone P, Brander C, et al. Host ethnicity and virus genotype shape the hepatitis B virus-specific T-cell repertoire. J Virol. 2008;82:10986–97.
40. Cole DK, Yuan F, Rizkallah PJ, Miles JJ, Gostick E, Price DA, Gao GF, Jakobsen BK, Sewell AK. Germ line-governed recognition of a cancer epitope by an immunodominant human T-cell receptor. J Biol Chem. 2009;284:27281–9.
41. Eltahla AA, Rizzetto S, Pirozyan MR, Betz-Stablein BD, Venturi V, Kedzierska K, Lloyd AR, Bull RA, Luciani F. Linking the T cell receptor to the single cell transcriptome in antigen-specific human T cells. Immunol Cell Biol. 2016;94:604–11.
42. Howie B, Sherwood AM, Berkebile AD, Berka J, Emerson RO, Williamson DW, Kirsch I, Vignali M, Rieder MJ, Carlson CS, et al. High-throughput pairing of T cell receptor alpha and beta sequences. Sci Transl Med. 2015;7:301ra131.
43. Stronen E, Toebes M, Kelderman S, van Buuren MM, Yang W, van Rooij N, Donia M, Boschen ML, Lund-Johansen F, Olweus J, et al. Targeting of cancer neoantigens with donor-derived T cell repertoires. Science. 2016;352:1337–41.
44. Dash P, Fiore-Gartland AJ, Hertz T, Wang GC, Sharma S, Souquette A, Crawford JC, Clemens EB, Nguyen THO, Kedzierska K, et al. Quantifiable predictive features define epitope-specific T cell receptor repertoires. Nature. 2017;547:89–93.
45. Glanville J, Huang H, Nau A, Hatton O, Wagar LE, Rubelt F, Ji X, Han A, Krams SM, Pettus C, et al. Identifying specificity groups in the T cell receptor repertoire. Nature. 2017;547:94–8.
46. Rossjohn J, Gras S, Miles JJ, Turner SJ, Godfrey DI, McCluskey J. T cell antigen receptor recognition of antigen-presenting molecules. Annu Rev Immunol. 2015;33:169–200.
47. Six A, Mariotti-Ferrandiz ME, Chaara W, Magadan S, Pham HP, Lefranc MP, Mora T, Thomas-Vaslin V, Walczak AM, Boudinot P. The past, present, and future of immune repertoire biology - the rise of next-generation repertoire analysis. Front Immunol. 2013;4:413.
48. Laydon DJ, Melamed A, Sim A, Gillet NA, Sim K, Darko S, Kroll JS, Douek DC, Price DA, Bangham CR, et al. Quantification of HTLV-1 clonality and TCR diversity. PLoS Comput Biol. 2014;10:e1003646.
49. Degauque N, Brouard S, Soulillou JP. Cross-reactivity of TCR repertoire: current concepts, challenges, and implication for allotransplantation. Front Immunol. 2016;7:89.
50. Sewell AK. Why must T cells be cross-reactive? Nat Rev Immunol. 2012;12:669–77.
51. Dave H, Luo M, Blaney JW, Patel S, Barese C, Cruz CR, Shpall EJ, Bollard CM, Hanley PJ. Toward a rapid production of multivirus-specific T cells targeting BKV, adenovirus, CMV, and EBV from umbilical cord blood. Mol Ther Methods Clin Dev. 2017;5:13–21.

3

Disease-specific regulation of gene expression in a comparative analysis of juvenile idiopathic arthritis and inflammatory bowel disease

Angela Mo[1], Urko M. Marigorta[1], Dalia Arafat[1], Lai Hin Kimi Chan[2], Lori Ponder[2], Se Ryeong Jang[2], Jarod Prince[2], Subra Kugathasan[2], Sampath Prahalad[2] and Greg Gibson[1*]

Abstract

Background: The genetic and immunological factors that contribute to differences in susceptibility and progression between sub-types of inflammatory and autoimmune diseases continue to be elucidated. Inflammatory bowel disease and juvenile idiopathic arthritis are both clinically heterogeneous and known to be due in part to abnormal regulation of gene activity in diverse immune cell types. Comparative genomic analysis of these conditions is expected to reveal differences in underlying genetic mechanisms of disease.

Methods: We performed RNA-Seq on whole blood samples from 202 patients with oligoarticular, polyarticular, or systemic juvenile idiopathic arthritis, or with Crohn's disease or ulcerative colitis, as well as healthy controls, to characterize differences in gene expression. Gene ontology analysis combined with Blood Transcript Module and Blood Informative Transcript analysis was used to infer immunological differences. Comparative expression quantitative trait locus (eQTL) analysis was used to quantify disease-specific regulation of transcript abundance.

Results: A pattern of differentially expressed genes and pathways reveals a gradient of disease spanning from healthy controls to oligoarticular, polyarticular, and systemic juvenile idiopathic arthritis (JIA); Crohn's disease; and ulcerative colitis. Transcriptional risk scores also provide good discrimination of controls, JIA, and IBD. Most eQTL are found to have similar effects across disease sub-types, but we also identify disease-specific eQTL at loci associated with disease by GWAS.

Conclusion: JIA and IBD are characterized by divergent peripheral blood transcriptomes, the genetic regulation of which displays limited disease specificity, implying that disease-specific genetic influences are largely independent of, or downstream of, eQTL effects.

Keywords: Juvenile idiopathic arthritis, Inflammatory bowel disease, eQTL, Gene expression

Background

While genomic analyses have clearly established a high degree of shared genetic susceptibility across autoimmune and inflammatory disorders, the reasons for disease-specific effects of particular loci are yet to be understood [1]. Likely explanations range from the technical, such as variable statistical power across studies, to the biological, including restriction of effects to relevant cell types for each condition, and interactions between genotypes and either the environment or genetic background. Since the majority of genome-wide association study (GWAS) associations are likely regulatory, attention has focused on mapping genetic effects on gene expression and/or epigenetic marks, namely discovery of expression quantitative trait locus (eQTL) and their methylation counterparts, mQTL [2]. With a few exceptions, most studies attempting to relate GWAS to

* Correspondence: greg.gibson@biology.gatech.edu
[1]Center for Integrative Genomics and School of Biological Sciences, Georgia Institute of Technology, Engineered Biosystems Building, EBB 2115, 950 Atlantic Drive, Atlanta, GA 30332, USA
Full list of author information is available at the end of the article

functional genomics have utilized large public eQTL and epigenetic datasets of peripheral blood-derived profiles of healthy volunteers. These implicitly assume equivalence of eQTL across health and disease, despite recent findings that eQTL can be modified by ex vivo treatments which mimic perturbations corresponding to disease states [3, 4]. In order to evaluate the ratio of common to disease-specific effects in inflammatory autoimmune disease, here we describe side-by-side comparative eQTL analysis of juvenile idiopathic arthritis (JIA) and inflammatory bowel disease (IBD), also comparing the transcriptomes among major sub-types within both JIA and IBD.

IBD has been extensively studied using a variety of genomic approaches, but despite several early publications, JIA has been less well characterized [5–8]. JIA is the most common rheumatic disease of childhood, with an estimated prevalence of approximately 1.2 individuals per 1000 in the USA [9]. It comprises multiple clinically and genetically distinct forms of arthritis with onset prior to age 16. Although all forms of JIA are characterized by persistent swelling of the joints, the disease is further classified into sub-types based on clinical presentation [10]. Oligoarticular JIA affects four or fewer joints and is the most common and typically the mildest form of JIA [10, 11]. Polyarticular JIA involves five or more joints and is intermediate in severity. Both oligoarticular and polyarticular JIA disproportionately affect females. Systemic JIA (sJIA) is distinct from other JIA sub-types, displaying unique symptoms and no bias towards females [10, 12]. Diagnosis is based on presentation of arthritis accompanied by spiking fever, rash, and lymphadenopathy. Approximately 10% of sJIA patients are also diagnosed with life-threatening macrophage activation syndrome, and about 50% experience a persistent course of disease and are unable to achieve remission [12, 13].

The categorization of sub-types based primarily on clinical criteria reflects uncertainty about the biological factors that contribute to the heterogeneity of the disease. The immune system is thought to play a critical role in the pathogenesis of JIA. Levels of immune-related cells like lymphocytes, monocytes, and neutrophils are differentially elevated between sub-types [14], as is also seen in other autoimmune and autoinflammatory diseases such as rheumatoid arthritis (RA) and inflammatory bowel disease [15]. Evidence of T cell activation has been described in oligoarticular and polyarticular patients, suggesting the importance of adaptive immunity in these sub-types [11, 16], but there is considerable heterogeneity in immune profiles that masks differences between levels of severity [17, 18], with age-of-onset also an important factor influencing gene expression [19]. In contrast, sJIA is thought to be more characterized by activation of innate immunity and upregulated monocytes, macrophages, and neutrophils [12, 20].

Extensive genome-wide association studies have been performed across autoimmune classes and are conveniently summarized on the ImmunoBase website, which as of February 2018 lists 23 validated loci for JIA, 81 for RA, 102 for ulcerative colitis (UC), and 122 for Crohn's disease (CD) [21]. Previous studies have demonstrated familial aggregation of JIA, supporting the idea that genetics plays a role in susceptibility [22] as well as sub-type development. Studies of genetic variants within the major histocompatibility complex region have uncovered associations between various human leukocyte antigen (HLA) polymorphisms and sub-types of JIA [23, 24]. HLA-independent loci such as PTPN22 and STAT4 have also been repeatedly found in genome-wide association studies to be associated with oligoarticular and RF-negative polyarticular JIA at genome-wide significance levels [25–28], while polymorphisms in interleukins 1 and 10 were early on identified as occurring at higher frequencies in sJIA patients [29, 30]. The most recent international GWAS of 982 children with sJIA concluded that the systemic form of JIA engages more inflammatory than autoimmune-related genes [31], consistent with clinical observations of the course of disease.

Diverse autoimmune conditions certainly are attributable in part to intrinsic aspects of the focal tissue and in part to gene activity in the immune system, some of which should be detectable in peripheral blood samples. It is thus surprising that side-by-side comparisons of immune gene expression across disease sub-types have not been reported. Transcriptomic studies of disease are for practical reasons orders of magnitude smaller than GWAS, typically involving fewer than 200 patients, but these are nevertheless sufficient to identify eQTL given the relatively large effect of regulatory polymorphisms on local gene expression. Numerous blood- and tissue-specific susceptibility loci and eQTL have previously been discovered [32–34]. It is likely that sJIA in particular shares associated risk polymorphisms with IBD given the auto-inflammatory component of both diseases. For instance, a mutation in LACC1 that was initially associated with Crohn's disease was later found also to be associated with sJIA [35, 36]. Thus, IBD is an attractive candidate for comparison with JIA to elucidate the mechanisms behind each of the sub-types. Here we contrast healthy controls; patients with oligoarticular, polyarticular, or systemic JIA; and patients with two forms of IBD, CD, or UC. As well as evaluating overall transcriptome differences among sub-types, we evaluate the disease specificity of whole blood eQTL effects in order to infer what fraction of risk can be attributed to differences in genetic regulation of gene expression.

Methods

Cohorts

In total, there were 190 patients and 12 controls. Protocols including signed consent of all participants and/or assent of parents in the case of minors were approved by the IRBs of Emory University and Georgia Institute of Technology. All patient cohorts were comprised of individuals of European ($n = 141$) or African ($n = 49$) ancestry from the USA. The cohorts are further divided into IBD and JIA subgroups. Within the IBD subgroup, 60 individuals were CD patients while 15 were UC patients. The average age of disease onset for CD and UC patients was approximately 14 years, with ages of onset ranging from less than 1 to 26 years. The JIA subgroup was comprised of 43 oligoarticular, 46 polyarticular, and 26 systemic JIA patients. The average age of disease onset for JIA patients was 8 years, with onset ages ranging from 0.7 to 17 years.

RNA-Seq processing and differential gene expression analysis

RNA was isolated from whole blood, and RNA-Seq was used to determine profiles of gene expression. The paired-end 100 bp reads were mapped to human genome hg19 using TopHat2 [37] with default parameters, with 90.4% success rate. The aligned reads were converted into number of reads per gene using SAMtools and HTSeq with the default union mode [38, 39]. The raw counts were then processed by trimmed mean of M-values normalization via the edgeR R package into normalized counts [40]. To further normalize and remove batch effects from gene expression data, surrogate variable analysis (SVA) combined with supervised normalization was used [41]. First, FPKM was calculated and all genes with greater than 10 individuals with greater than six read counts and FPKM > 0.1 were extracted. Expression of the sex-specific genes RPS4Y1, EIF1AY, DDX3Y, KDM5D, and XIST was used to verify the gender of each individual. The SVA R package [41] was used to identify 15 latent confounding factors, and these were statistically removed without compromising known disease variables using the supervised normalization procedure in the SNM R package [42]. Pairwise comparisons between control, CD, UC, oligoarticular JIA, polyarticular JIA, and systemic JIA were performed to quantify the extent of differential expression. Using edgeR's generalized linear model likelihood ratio test function, the log fold change and Benjamini-Hochberg adjusted p value were obtained for all genes within each contrast [40].

Gene ontology analysis was performed using the GOseq R package, which incorporates RNA-Seq read length biases into its testing [43]. Genes with an edgeR-calculated FDR of < 0.01 were considered to be differentially expressed and input into the GOseq software. Genes were distinguished by positive and negative log fold change to classify upregulation in specific sub-types. Only pathways within the biological processes and molecular function gene ontology branches were called.

Analysis of established immune-related gene sets was performed using BIT (Blood Informative Transcript) and BTM (Blood Transcript Module) gene expression [44, 45]. The BITs are highly co-regulated genes which define seven axes of blood immune activity that are highly conserved across whole blood gene expression datasets. Standard PCA analysis including multiple PC captures most of the variance also described by the BIT, but it does so in a study-specific manner in which the actual PC have little biological meaning. By contrast, the BIT axes, as originally characterized by Preininger et al. [44], capture components of variation that are consistently observed across all peripheral blood gene expression studies, for the most part independent of platform. We simply take PC1 for the representative genes for each axis and note that this typically explains upwards of 70% of variance of those transcripts, so it is highly representative of overall gene expression in the axis. Whereas in previous work [44] we labelled nine axes BIT axis 1 through 9, subsequent analyses and comparison with BTMs has led to affirmation of the immunological functions captured by six of the axes, which we here rename reflecting these functions as axis T (T cell-related, formerly 1), axis B (B cell-related, formerly 3), axis N (neutrophil-related, formerly 5), axis R (reticulocyte-related, formerly 2), axis I (interferon-responsive, formerly 7), and axis G (general cellular biosynthesis, formerly 4). axis 6 remains of uncertain function, while axes 8 and 9 are dropped since they are derivative and less consistent. Finally, a newly identified axis C captures numerous cell cycle-related aspects of gene activity. Each of these axes clusters with a subset of the 247 BTMs identified by Li et al. in their machine-learning meta-analysis of 30,000 peripheral blood gene expression samples from over 500 studies [45], and these relationships were visualized by hierarchical cluster analysis performed using Ward's method in SAS/JMP Genomics [46].

SNP data processing and eQTL analysis

The Affymetrix Axiom BioBank and Illumina Immunochip arrays were used to perform genotyping, at Akesogen Inc. (Norcross, GA). Quality control was performed using PLINK, with parameters set to remove non-biallelic variants, SNPs not in Hardy-Weinberg equilibrium at $P < 10^{-3}$, minor allele frequency < 1%, and rate of missing data across individuals > 5% [47].

The Affymetrix Axiom BioBank array, which has a coverage of 800 k SNPs, was utilized to genotype the 115 JIA samples and 27 IBD samples. The Immunochip, which includes a high density of genotypes at loci containing markers known to be associated with various autoimmune and inflammatory diseases, including CD and UC, was used to genotype the remaining IBD samples. Following QC, imputation was performed using the SHAPEIT and IMPUTE2 software in order to merge the datasets [48, 49]. However, due to the nature of the Immunochip, imputation failed to generate reliable results for sites outside of the densely genotyped regions. Consequently, the eQTL analysis was initially performed independently on the JIA and IBD datasets, and then, overlapping loci significant in either study were pooled for the interaction testing. For JIA, following QC, we analyzed 109 individuals with 5,522,769 variants. For IBD, the available Affymetrix samples were merged with the remaining 27 IBD samples from the Immunochip dataset by selecting overlapping SNPs, which following QC resulted in 54 individuals with 58,788 variants in the vicinity of the 186 immune-related loci, plus the HLA complex, included on the Immunochip. In summary, 27 IBD samples were genotyped on the Affymetrix array, while 27 were typed on the Immunochip, and the remaining 21 IBD samples had expression but not genotype data.

Using the genes from the SVA and SNM adjusted expression data and the separate compiled variants from JIA and IBD, a list of genes and SNPs within 250 kb upstream and downstream of the stop and start coordinates of the gene was generated. eQTL mapping was performed using the linear mixed modelling method in GEMMA [50], which generated a final file of 16,913,152 SNP-gene pairs for JIA samples and 338,005 SNP-gene pairs for IBD samples. Since there are on average close to five candidate genes per SNP, between the two diseases, 263,575 SNP-gene pairs were shared that were analyzed jointly. A common p value threshold of $p < 0.0001$ corresponding to an empirical FDR $< 5\%$ was chosen, yielding 814 SNP-gene univariate associations. Conditional analysis was underpowered to detect secondary signals consistently, so we simply retained the peak eSNP associations defining 142 eGenes. Since low minor allele frequencies can drive spurious eQTL signatures if the minor homozygotes have outlier gene expression, we checked for an overall relationship between MAF and eQTL significance. None was observed, implying that rare variants are not driving the results in general, but we also examined each of the loci with significant interaction effects manually, identifying a small number of false positives. A notable example is IL10, which had an anomalously high disease-by-interaction ($p \sim 10^{-7}$) driven by a large effect size in IBD (beta = 2.7) that turns out to be due to a single outlier, removal of which abrogates any eQTL effect at the locus (also consistent with the blood eQTL browser report [51]).

The eQTL×disease interaction effect which evaluates whether the genotype contribution is the same in JIA and IBD was modeled by combining the imputed rsID genotypes for the lead SNP in either disease into a joint linear model with gene expression as a function of genotype, disease, and genotype-by-disease interaction, assuming the residuals are normally distributed with a mean of zero. A caveat to this analysis is that the lead SNP (i.e., the one with the smallest p value) is not necessarily the causal variant, and secondary SNPs in one or other condition may skew the single-site evaluations. Post hoc analyses revealed that secondary eQTLs are evident at three loci reported (*PAM*, *SLC22A5*, and *GBAP1*).

Adjustments for medication and disease duration

Because the JIA patients in our study were not recruited from a single cohort, therapeutic interventions and duration of disease vary between individuals. Environmental factors include exposure to medications and impact gene expression profiles [52]. In addition, it has previously been shown that gene expression networks are altered over the first 6 months of therapy for JIA patients [53]. To characterize the effects of these covariates, our JIA patients were classified by three non-exclusive categories of medication: known treatment with DMARDs, biologics, and steroids at the time of sample collection, as well as three categories of disease duration prior to sampling: less than 180 days, 180–360 days, and greater than 360 days. Nearly all IBD patients were sampled at diagnosis, so this stratification was only necessary for JIA patients. Medication and time variables were then modeled and removed using SNM, resulting in an adjusted gene expression dataset [42]. The previously described BIT axis analysis was performed again using this adjusted dataset and compared with results from the unadjusted dataset (Additional file 1: Figure S1A). Additional file 1: Figure S1B shows the correlation between unadjusted gene expression and category of disease duration. In addition, the JIA eQTL study was rerun using the adjusted expression dataset. The correlation of betas from the unadjusted and adjusted analyses is depicted in Additional file 1: Figure S2.

Furthermore, we were able to replicate the major trends in gene expression observed in our dataset in a published Affymetrix microarray study of samples from the various subsets of JIA [54]. They studied PBMC gene expression for 29 controls, 30 oligoarticular, 49 polyarticular, and 18 systemic JIA patients all obtained prior to initiation of therapy [54]. As shown in Additional file 1: Figure S3, axes R, B, N, I, and C give very similar results whereas the T cell signature which is mildly reduced in more severe JIA in our data does not differentiate their sample types. Additionally, axis G reverses the sign of effect, as it does upon adjustment for medication usage, reinforcing the conclusion that general cellular metabolic processes are affected by medication. By contrast, Hu et al. [55] report effects of anti-TNF biologic therapy specifically on certain neutrophil-related pathways, a result not recapitulated in our data, likely due to differences in experimental design.

Colocalization and transcriptional risk score (TRS) analysis

Colocalization analysis was performed using JIA and IBD eQTL data and prior IBD, rheumatoid arthritis, and JIA GWAS study data. The coloc R package uses a Bayesian model to determine posterior probabilities for five hypotheses on whether a shared causal variant is present for two traits [56]. The analysis considered all SNPs associated with IBD ($n = 232$), RA ($n = 101$), or JIA ($n = 28$) as discovered by GWAS, where $n = 198, 57, 21$ and $n = 198, 83, 20$ were present in SNP-gene eQTL datasets for IBD and JIA, respectively. Cross-comparisons between both of the eQTL datasets and each of the GWAS studies' reported loci was performed, following which select SNP-gene pairs with high probabilities of hypothesis 3 (same locus but different eQTL and GWAS peaks) and 4 (same causal variant driving the signal at the eQTL and GWAS peaks) were plotted using LocusZoom [57] to visualize the region surrounding the variants.

Two independent transcriptional risk scores (TRS) were generated using GWAS results for IBD [58] and RA [59] as a proxy for JIA (since the JIA pool of variants is currently too small). As previously described, TRS sums the z-scores of gene expression polarized by the direction of effect of the eQTL relative to the GWAS risk allele [60]. Thus, if the risk genotype is associated with decreased expression, we invert the z-score in the summation such that positive TRS represents elevated risk. We only used genotypes that are validated as both eQTL and GWAS by H4 in the coloc analysis, taking the eQTL list from the blood eQTL browser since it has much higher power than the small disease samples. Thirty-nine and 23 genes were included in the IBD and RA TRS, respectively, as listed in Additional file 2: Table S1. ANOVA was performed between groups to establish whether the TRS can be used to predict disease from blood gene expression.

Results

Heterogeneity of gene expression within and among disease sub-types

In order to contrast the nature of differential gene expression between three sub-types of JIA and two sub-types of IBD as well as relative to healthy controls, we conducted whole blood gene expression profiling on a combined sample of 202 children with disease onset between the ages of 0.7 and 17. The sample included 43 cases of oligoarticular JIA, 46 of polyarticular JIA, 26 of systemic JIA, 60 of Crohn's disease, and 15 of ulcerative colitis. RNA-Seq analysis was performed with a median of 19.6 million paired-end 100 bp reads per sample. After normalization and quality control as described in the "Methods" section, a total of 11,614 genes remained for analysis.

Previous microarray-based gene expression profiling of JIA has established significant mean differences among disease sub-types, as well as heterogeneity within sub-types [6–9]. A heat map of two-way hierarchical clustering of all genes in all individuals reveals six major clusters of individuals (rows in Fig. 1a) who share co-regulation of at least nine sets of genes (columns). For example, the top cluster labeled in dark blue consists of individuals with generally high innate immunity gene expression and low lymphocyte gene expression, whereas the bottom two clusters labeled in pale blue and green have the opposite profile, though with differences in T cell-related expression. Individuals in each of the six health and disease categories are dispersed throughout the matrix but with highly significant tendencies for enrichment of specific expression clusters in each sub-type, as shown in Fig. 1b. Eighty percent of the healthy controls are in the pale green cluster, which accounts for just one quarter of the oligo-JIA sub-type and less than 15% of each of the others. The two IBD sub-types are more likely to be in the dark blue cluster, as are sJIA cases, consistent with these being more inflammatory conditions, but in each case, the majority of individuals from each disease sub-type are dispersed throughout the other clusters. JIA in general has high membership in the red cluster, while there is an apparent gradient with oligo-JIA more control-like and sJIA more IBD-like. As with other autoimmune diseases, although there are certainly disease-related trends, the overall blood gene expression pattern is dominated by heterogeneity without ambiguous separation by disease type. Figure 1c shows that 9.5% of the gene expression captured by the first five principal components is among disease categories and another 7.3% among the sub-types within JIA and IBD, with a small component also attributable to age-of-onset less than 6.

Functional characterization of the gradient of differential expression

Contrasts of significant differential expression performed between healthy controls and sub-types of JIA as well as combined IBD and sub-types of JIA confirm the gradient of differential expression between disease groups of different severities. Additional file 2: Table S2 lists the significantly differentially expressed genes at the 5% Benjamini-Hochberg false discovery rate, for each comparison of two disease groups from the six under

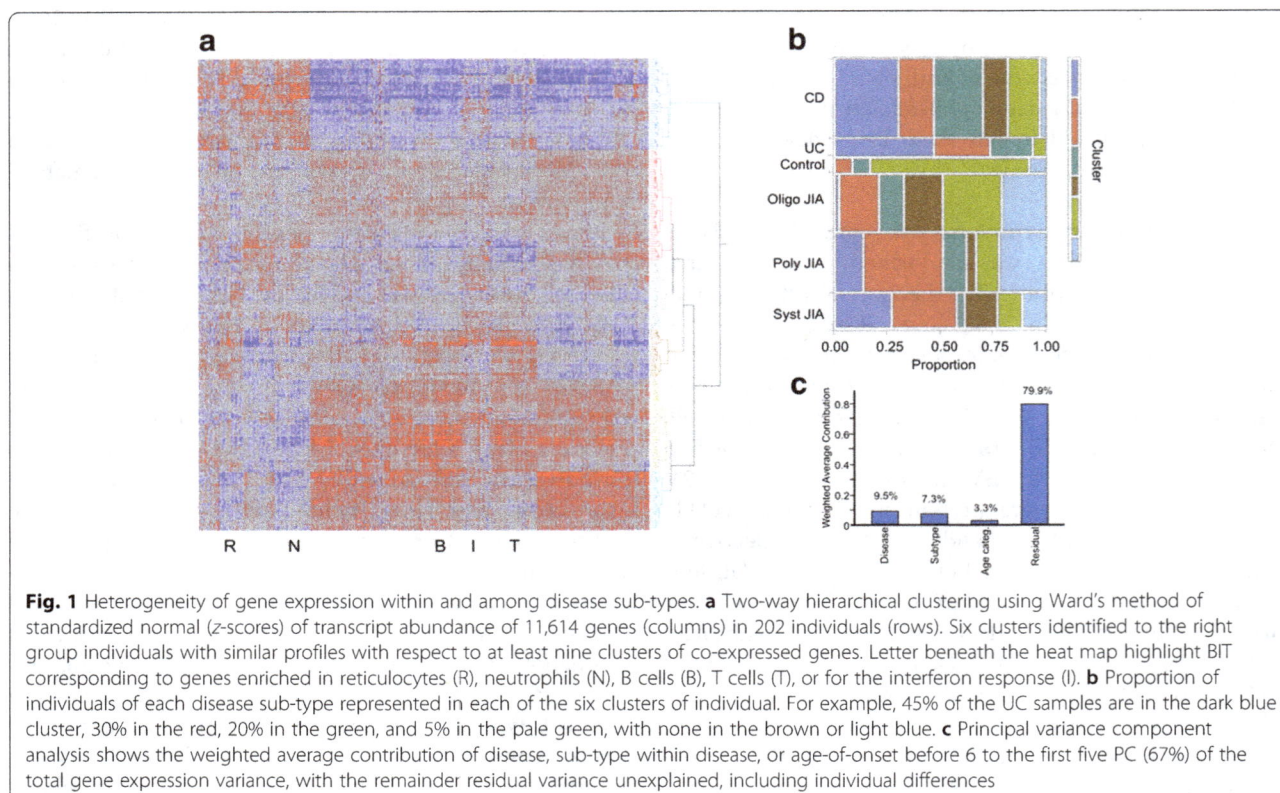

Fig. 1 Heterogeneity of gene expression within and among disease sub-types. **a** Two-way hierarchical clustering using Ward's method of standardized normal (z-scores) of transcript abundance of 11,614 genes (columns) in 202 individuals (rows). Six clusters identified to the right group individuals with similar profiles with respect to at least nine clusters of co-expressed genes. Letter beneath the heat map highlight BIT corresponding to genes enriched in reticulocytes (R), neutrophils (N), B cells (B), T cells (T), or for the interferon response (I). **b** Proportion of individuals of each disease sub-type represented in each of the six clusters of individual. For example, 45% of the UC samples are in the dark blue cluster, 30% in the red, 20% in the green, and 5% in the pale green, with none in the brown or light blue. **c** Principal variance component analysis shows the weighted average contribution of disease, sub-type within disease, or age-of-onset before 6 to the first five PC (67%) of the total gene expression variance, with the remainder residual variance unexplained, including individual differences

consideration. In the comparison between healthy controls and oligoarticular JIA, 82 genes were significantly upregulated in healthy controls, and 7 were upregulated in oligoarticular JIA. These numbers are lower than the 136 and 36 differentially expressed genes found in the contrasts between healthy controls and polyarticular JIA, and the 216 and 547 upregulated genes found between healthy controls and sJIA. A similar graded pattern of differentiation was found in comparisons of IBD and JIA. The fewest differentially expressed genes were found in the contrast between IBD and sJIA, with 73 upregulated genes in IBD and 170 upregulated genes in systemic JIA. Between IBD and polyarticular JIA, 934 upregulated IBD genes and 767 upregulated polyarticular genes were discovered, while the biggest differentiation was observed between IBD and oligoarticular JIA, where 2038 upregulated IBD genes and 1751 upregulated oligoarticular genes were discovered. These patterns of differential expression also confirm that of the three JIA sub-types, systemic JIA is the most similar to IBD.

The biological meaning of these differentially expressed genes was investigated through gene ontology and modular analysis. Contrasts between healthy controls and JIA subtypes implied a variety of classes of differential pathway regulation. Overall, all subtypes of JIA showed downregulation of transmembrane signaling and

G-protein-coupled receptor activity. However, oligoarticular JIA showed primarily upregulation of protein and phospholipid metabolic processes while polyarticular JIA showed upregulation in secretion, exocytosis, and granulocyte activation, as well as neutrophil activation. Systemic JIA showed an even more strongly significant upregulation of immune pathways, notably general immune response and myeloid activation. In contrast, for the comparisons between IBD and JIA subtypes, all JIA subtypes showed upregulation of nucleic acid processes compared with IBD. Both oligoarticular and polyarticular JIA showed strongly significant downregulation of myeloid, neutrophil, and leukocyte activity compared with IBD, whereas sJIA showed downregulation of general metabolic processes albeit at a much lower significance level.

Clustering by BTMs and BITs further reveals enriched immune pathways

Decades of blood gene expression analysis have highlighted the existence of modules of co-expressed genes that reflect a combination of joint regulation within cell types and variable abundance of the major leukocyte classes [61]. Seven highly conserved axes of blood variation [44] are composed of genes broadly capturing immune activity related to T and B cells, reticulocytes and neutrophils, interferon response, general biosynthesis, and the cell cycle. Figure 2 shows clear trend expression along these axes correlating with disease sub-type, each panel indicating the level of activation in each immune component in, from left to right, healthy control, oligoarticular JIA, polyarticular JIA, systemic JIA, Crohn's disease, and ulcerative colitis. Axis T, representing T cell expression, and axis B, representing B cell expression, show a trend of decreasing PC1 values correlating with severity of disease, suggesting downregulation of adaptive immunity in systemic JIA, CD, and UC. In contrast, axis R, representing reticulocytes, and axis N, representing neutrophils, show trends of increasing PC1 values with disease severity that indicates upregulation of the innate immune system in systemic JIA, CD, and UC. Axis I represents interferon-responsive gene expression and has a more parabolic trend, being elevated in polyarticular and systemic JIA and Crohn's disease, but not ulcerative colitis, reflecting the interferon response's dual roles in both adaptive and innate immunity. Axes G and C represent general and cell cycle expression, and show trends of higher PC1 values in inflammatory bowel disease and systemic JIA. Despite sample sizes of around 30 patients in each group, ANOVA indicates that the differences are significant in each case.

These disease-specific trends are confirmed by hierarchical clustering of 247 Blood Transcript Modules (BTMs) [45] in Fig. 3, tabulated in Additional file 2: Table S3, further supporting the gradient of disrupted gene expression based on disease severity. Healthy controls and oligoarticular JIA show largely similar expression, except for apparent elevation of NK cell gene expression in controls. IBD most resembles sJIA, although with some key differences. Myeloid gene expression tends to be elevated in IBD and lymphoid gene expression suppressed, with JIA intermediate. In addition, ulcerative colitis appears to have a specific deficit in NK cell-biased gene expression, sJIA has a unique signature including inositol metabolism, and JIA in general shows reduced mitochondrial gene activity.

Transcriptional risk scores differentiate healthy controls, JIA, and IBD

We recently proposed the notion of a transcriptional risk score (TRS), which is analogous to a cumulative burden of genotypic risk, but evaluates cumulative burden of risk due to elevated or suppressed gene expression relevant to disease [60, 62]. By just focusing on genes with shared eQTL and GWAS associations, the analysis is restricted to genes most likely to have a causal role in pathology, whether because the risk allele directly promotes disease or fails to provide sufficient protection. A TRS based on eQTL detected in blood but with gene expression measured in ileum was highly predictive of Crohn's disease progression, whereas a corresponding genetic risk score was not. Figure 4 shows similarly that the 39-gene IBD TRS measured in peripheral blood provides significant discrimination of cases and controls (difference in standard deviation units of TRS; Δs.d. = 1.10, $p = 0.0003$); notably, sJIA is elevated to the same degree as both CD and UC. By contrast, oligoarticular JIA and polyarticular JIA have intermediate TRS that are nevertheless significantly greater than healthy controls (Δs.d. = 1.04, $p = 0.0031$). For comparison, a TRS based on genes that are likely to be causal in driving the signal at 23 genome-wide significant associations for RA does not discriminate between healthy controls and IBD as a group (Δs.d. = 0.11, $p = 0.63$) but does trend toward discrimination of JIA as a category (Δs.d. = 0.42, $p = 0.09$). This RA TRS is mostly enhanced in sJIA (Δs.d. = 0.86, $p = 0.008$ relative to healthy controls), suggesting that it is capturing the effects of inflammatory gene contributions to this most severe form of JIA.

Evaluation of disease specificity of eQTL

We next addressed the degree of sharing of the local genetic control of gene expression in the two classes of disease (namely JIA and IBD) by performing comparative eQTL analysis. Whole genome genotypes were ascertained on the Immunochip (CD and UC samples) or the Affymetrix Axiom Biobank array (see the "Methods" section). As far as possible, SNPs were imputed onto the 1000 Genomes reference, allowing cross-comparison of the disease subsets, noting that this was not possible for loci not included on the Immunochip. Since genotypes were generated on different platforms, the eQTL assessment was first performed independently for the two broad disease classes, after which significant effects were evaluated jointly. Here we only consider genes located within the vicinity of the Immunochip loci.

For JIA, 107 independent eSNPs were identified within 500 kb of a transcript at an FDR of 5% (approximate $p < 10^{-4}$), and for IBD, which had a smaller sample size, 52 independent eSNPs were identified. These are listed in Additional file 2: Table S4. Twelve of the loci overlap between the two diseases, but failure to detect an eQTL in one condition does not necessarily imply absence of the effect, since the small sample size results in relatively low power. Overall, the correlation in effect sizes is high, ~ 0.7 ($p = 5 \times 10^{-20}$ in JIA; $p = 2 \times 10^{-8}$ in IBD), which is remarkable given the small sample sizes, and strongly implies that most eQTL effects in whole blood are consistent across the diseases. Nevertheless, the plots in Fig. 5 depicting the estimated eQTL effect sizes in IBD relative to JIA provide some support for disease-biased effects in so far as the eQTL discovered in JIA (red points, panel a) tend to have

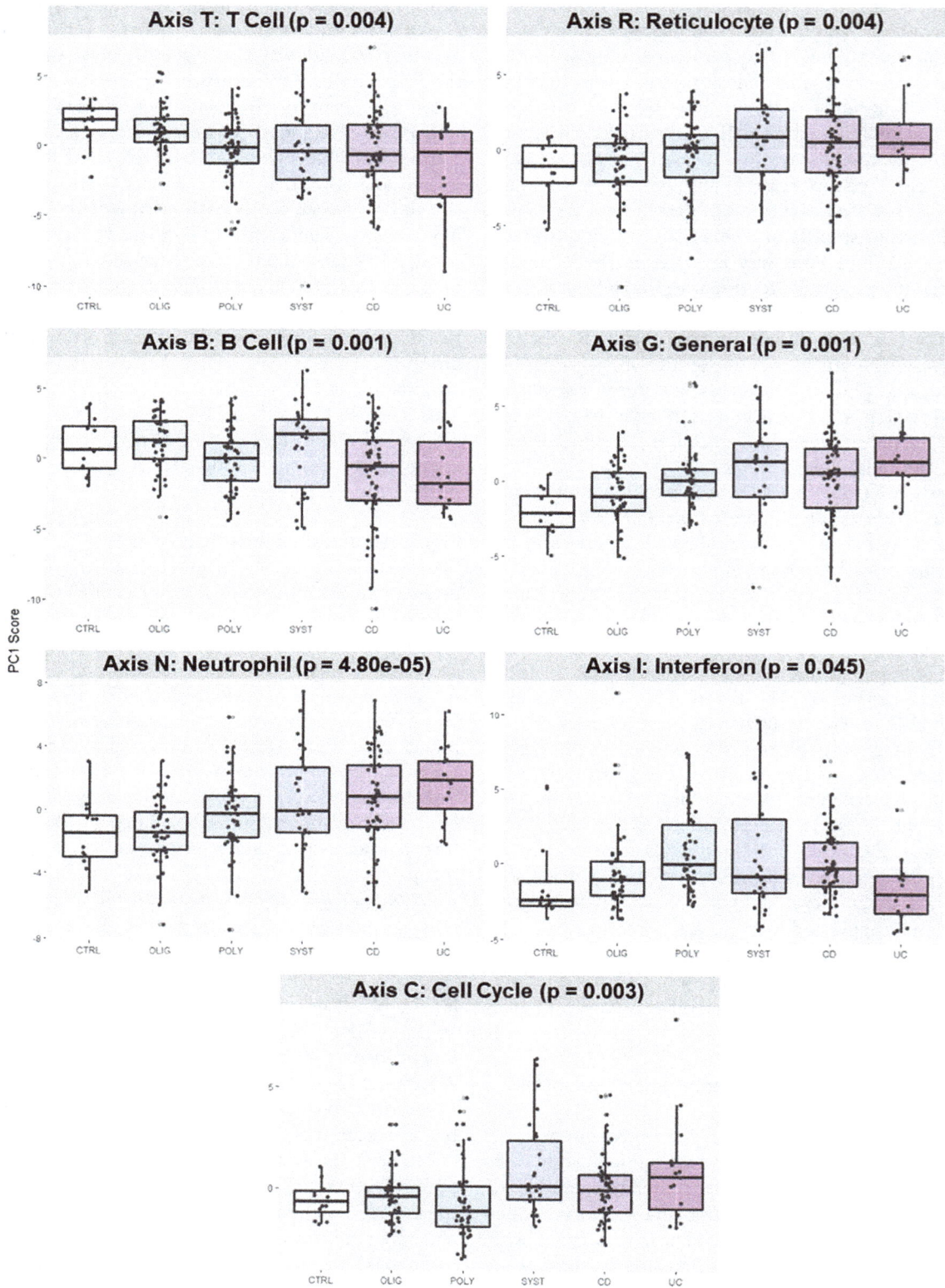

Fig. 2 (See legend on next page.)

(See figure on previous page.)
Fig. 2 Axes of variation across disease sub-types. Axes of variation defined by the first PC of the Blood Informative Transcripts (BIT) highlight variation in types of immune activity across disease sub-types. Each individual data point represents PC1 score for 10 BIT for the indicated axis, with box and whisker plots showing the median and interquartile range as well as 95% confidence intervals for the sub-types. Indicated p values are from one-way ANOVA contrasting the six sub-types of sample

larger effects on JIA (beta values) than those observed in IBD and hence lie between the diagonal and the x-axis. Conversely, the eQTL discovered in IBD (blue points, panel b) tend to have larger effects on IBD than those observed in JIA and hence lie between the diagonal and the y-axis. This result is biased by winner's curse, the tendency to over-estimate effect sizes upon discovery, so we also evaluated all associations jointly in order to also identify interaction effects. At an FDR of 10%, 34 of the 147 independent eQTL, highlighted in panel , show nominally significant interaction effects ($p < 0.02$), implying different effect sizes in the two broad classes of disease. Example box plots of genotypic effects on transcript abundance across the two disease classes are provided in Additional file 1: Figure S4. These genotype-by-disease interaction effects remain significant after accounting for ancestry (see Additional file 1: Figure S5).

As expected, many of the detected eQTLs affect expression of genes in the vicinity of established GWAS hits for autoimmune disease. Table 1 lists 25 lead eSNPs that regulate expression in cis of 22 target genes that are listed on ImmunoBase as potential causal genes for IBD or arthritis (JIA or RA). Half of these associations are with IBD only, but this bias may simply reflect increased power of the IBD GWAS to date. Several of the SNPs show evidence of disease-specific or disease-biased

effects. Naively, we might expect the eQTL to be seen only in the disease(s) for which the association with disease is seen, as this would be consistent with allele-specific expression driving pathology. Three cases (*ARPC2*, *CPTP* for IBD, and the secondary eQTL in *PAM* for JIA) fit the expected pattern, but three others have the counter-intuitive relationship where the eQTL is observed in one disease but the established GWAS association is with the opposite disease (*PRDX6* and *ADAM1A* for RA, the secondary eQTL in *GBAP1* for CD). Three more cases (*SLC22A5*, *CD226*, and *RNASET2*) have possibly disease-biased eQTL effects where the eQTL is absent from or much less in one disease, although the interaction effect is only significant in one of these cases. Despite the small sample, there is not an intuitive pattern to the relationship between disease-biased regulation of gene expression and association with disease.

One reason for divergent effect sizes may be that different causal variants in variable degrees of linkage disequilibrium could be responsible for the differential expression in the two disease sub-types. To investigate this, we performed colocalization analysis using coloc [56] to visualize the locus-wide SNP effects across all loci reported in IBD, RA, and JIA GWAS and present in our SNP-gene datasets for IBD or JIA and compared these with the distribution of GWAS summary statistics.

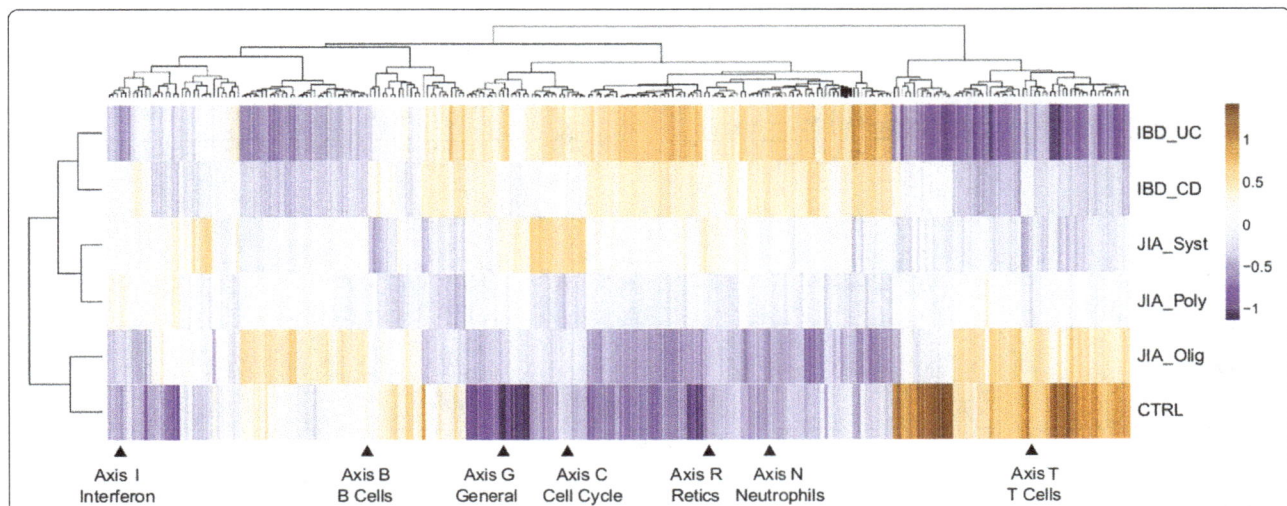

Fig. 3 Blood Transcript Modules. Hierarchical clustering of blood transcription modules across disease sub-types. The heat map shows the mean PC1 scores for 247 BTM identified in [45], as well seven BIT axes. Note how the BTM form ~ 10 clusters, seven of which co-cluster with one orthogonally determined axis. See Additional file 2: Table S3 for a complete listing of BTM scores in each disease sub-type

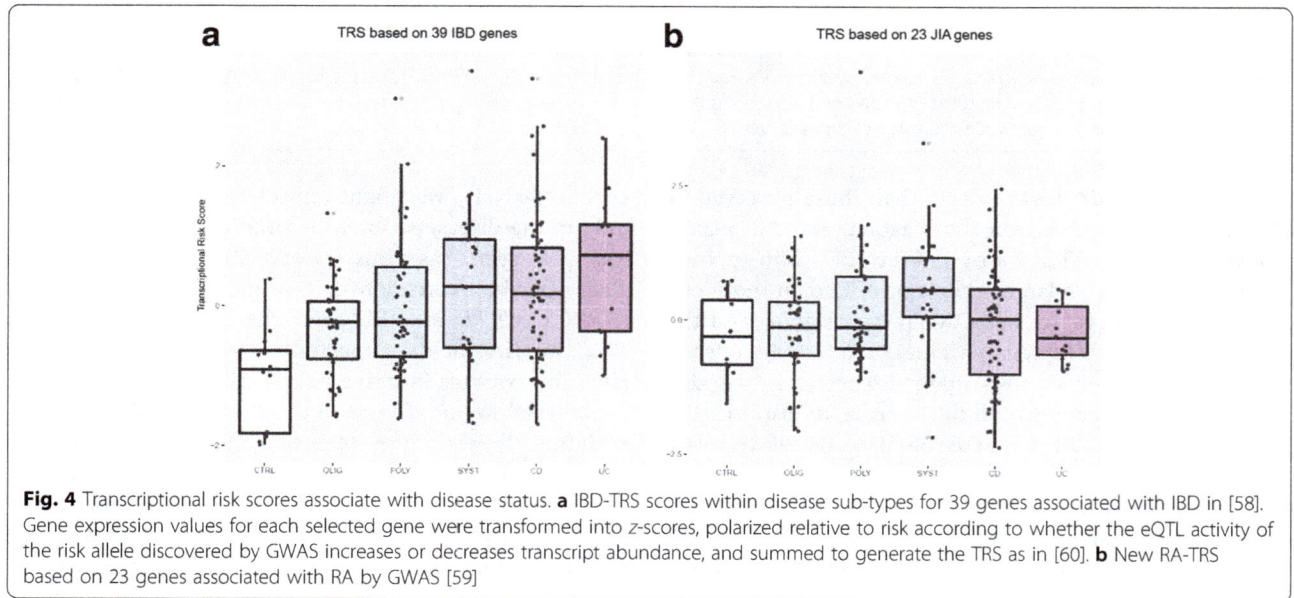

Fig. 4 Transcriptional risk scores associate with disease status. **a** IBD-TRS scores within disease sub-types for 39 genes associated with IBD in [58]. Gene expression values for each selected gene were transformed into z-scores, polarized relative to risk according to whether the eQTL activity of the risk allele discovered by GWAS increases or decreases transcript abundance, and summed to generate the TRS as in [60]. **b** New RA-TRS based on 23 genes associated with RA by GWAS [59]

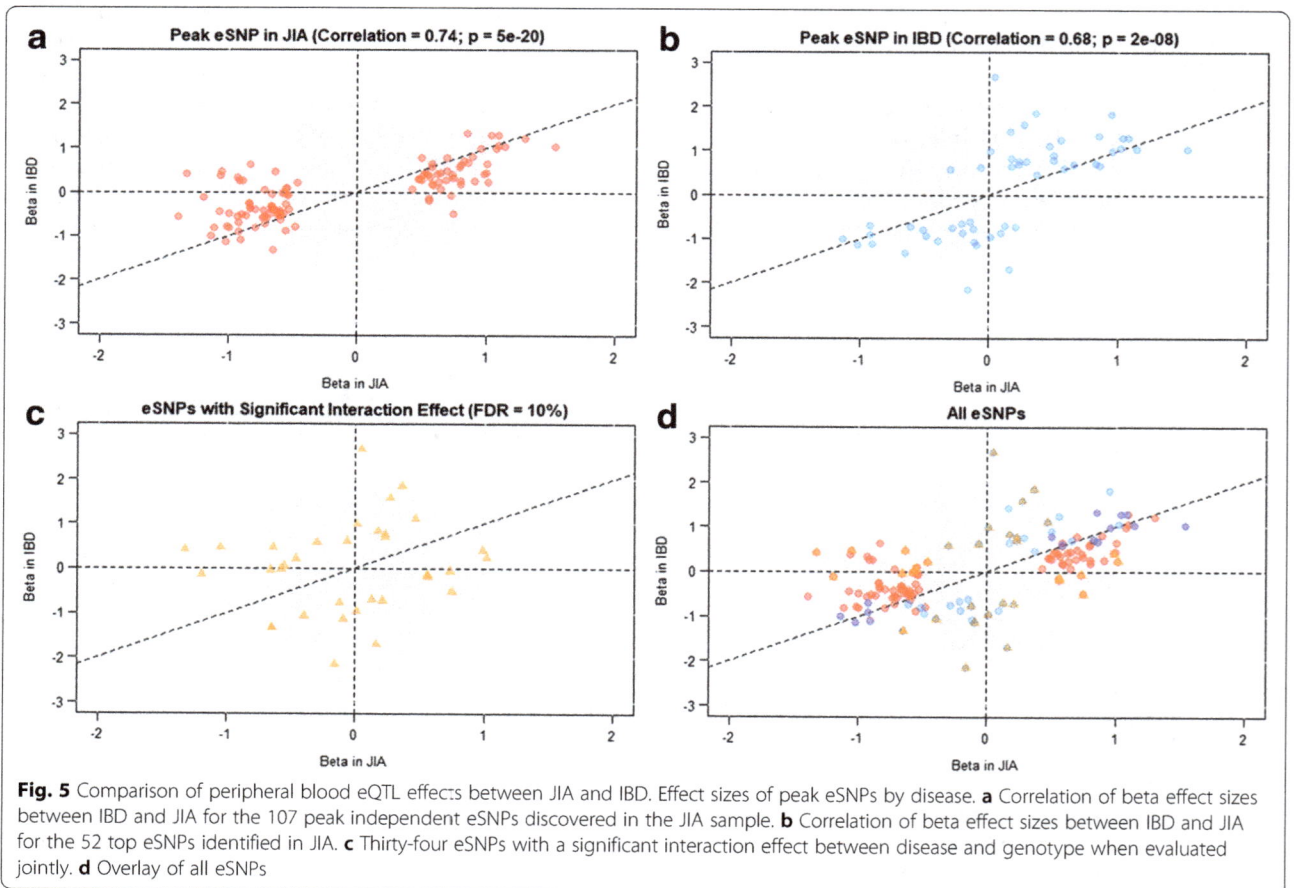

Fig. 5 Comparison of peripheral blood eQTL effects between JIA and IBD. Effect sizes of peak eSNPs by disease. **a** Correlation of beta effect sizes between IBD and JIA for the 107 peak independent eSNPs discovered in the JIA sample. **b** Correlation of beta effect sizes between IBD and JIA for the 52 top eSNPs identified in JIA. **c** Thirty-four eSNPs with a significant interaction effect between disease and genotype when evaluated jointly. **d** Overlay of all eSNPs

Table 1 GWAS eQTL

Gene	rsID	IBD β	IBD p val	JIA β	JIA p val	IBD-GWAS	ATH-GWAS	Interact p
ARPC2	rs13429408	0.82	6.60E−05	0.18	0.22	CD, UC	–	0.01
CPTP	rs11809901	− 1.08	9.80E−05	− 0.12	0.69	CD, UC	–	0.04
PAM	rs2431321	1.04	3.80E−09	1.15	2.10E−23	–	RA	0.48
PAM	rs32677	0.21	0.3	0.94	5.30E−15	–	RA	9.60E−05
C5	rs1468673	0.39	0.02	0.74	3.10E−07	–	RA	0.34
PRDX6	rs4279882	1.84	3.80E−05	0.36	0.05	–	RA	0.001
ADAM1A	rs11066027	1.22	2.40E−05	0.61	5.30E−03	–	JIA, RA	0.09
RNASET2	rs385863	− 0.68	1.30E−04	− 1.05	1.40E−14	CD, UC	RA	0.3
GSDMB	rs11078926	− 0.51	5.90E−03	− 0.56	9.90E−07	CD, UC	RA	0.87
SLC22A5	rs11739135	0.09	0.6	− 0.8	9.80E−10	CD, UC	JIA	4.00E−05
SLC22A5	rs11950562	− 0.53	8.00E−04	− 0.86	6.10E−14	CD, UC	JIA	0.07
ORMDL3	rs1565923	1.11	8.80E−07	0.47	6.20E−04	CD, UC	RA	0.01
ICAM4	rs3093029	1.22	4.80E−04	1.3	2.90E−08	CD, UC	JIA	0.69
RMI2	rs11644184	− 0.58	7.60E−04	− 0.7	3.00E−07	CD, UC	JIA	0.54
PLTP	rs7275164	− 0.56	2.10E−04	− 0.71	7.00E−07	CD, UC	RA	0.58
CD226	rs12969613	0.63	2.20E−07	0.18	0.15	CD, UC	RA	0.11
NOD2	rs1981760	1.28	2.70E−08	1.05	2.30E−16	CD	–	0.23
GBAP1	rs914615	0.6	3.20E−04	0.8	7.80E−10	CD	–	0.62
GBAP1	rs3814319	0.16	0.33	0.7	1.20E−06	CD	–	0.05
KSR1	rs2945378	− 0.48	6.20E−03	− 0.6	4.40E−07	CD	–	0.52
SULT1A1	rs7191548	− 0.49	6.50E−03	− 0.61	5.30E−07	CD, UC	–	0.93
PNKD	rs13430006	0.34	0.14	0.57	6.80E−07	CD, UC	–	0.41
NLRP2	rs12975582	0.56	0.01	0.8	1.20E−06	CD, UC	–	0.43
SLC11A1	rs78846874	− 0.35	0.36	− 0.83	3.90E−06	CD, UC	–	0.22
LGALS9	rs1984547	− 0.88	2.40E−05	− 0.55	4.10E−05	CD, UC	–	0.16

Coloc assigns a posterior probability that the same SNP is responsible for both an eQTL effect and the disease association (H4) or that different SNPs are responsible for the two effects (H3). Since the power of this mode of analysis is limited when sample sizes are small, we identified cases from either disease with relatively strong H3 or H4 posterior probabilities and plotted representative examples in Fig. 6. The full results are summarized in Additional file 2: Table S5.

Figure 6a shows results for association of rs12946510 with IBD from GWAS (bottom panel) and the eQTL profiles for the JIA (top panel) and IBD (middle panel) gene expression. Although coloc calls both cases as H4, the correspondence of SNP profiles in high LD with the lead SNP is more notable in JIA. The light blue SNPs suggest a second, independent, eQTL which does not produce a GWAS signal. Hence, the gene expression difference may be mediated by two different SNPs, possibly with different effect sizes in the two diseases, only one of which appears to contribute strongly to disease risk. Figure 6b shows a clear H3 case in JIA where the eQTL

effect on expression of *PAM* appears to be mediated by a cluster of variants to the left of the lead GWAS cluster. Figure 6c shows a classical H4 where the fine mapping supports a single causal locus for both the gene expression and disease, although the precise identity of the causal variant is impossible to ascertain from the statistical data alone owing to the extensive block of variants in high LD.

Discussion
Disease-specific associations with autoimmune disease
There are multiple technical reasons why GWAS may fail to detect associations that are shared across multiple autoimmune diseases. These include differences in sample size and clinical heterogeneity, and with respect to eQTL analysis, differences in expression profiling platform, statistical methodology, and effects of pharmacological interventions could all obscure associations. However, it is also clear that the genetic correlation across diseases is significantly less than one, establishing the expectation that some effects must be disease-specific [63]. The most

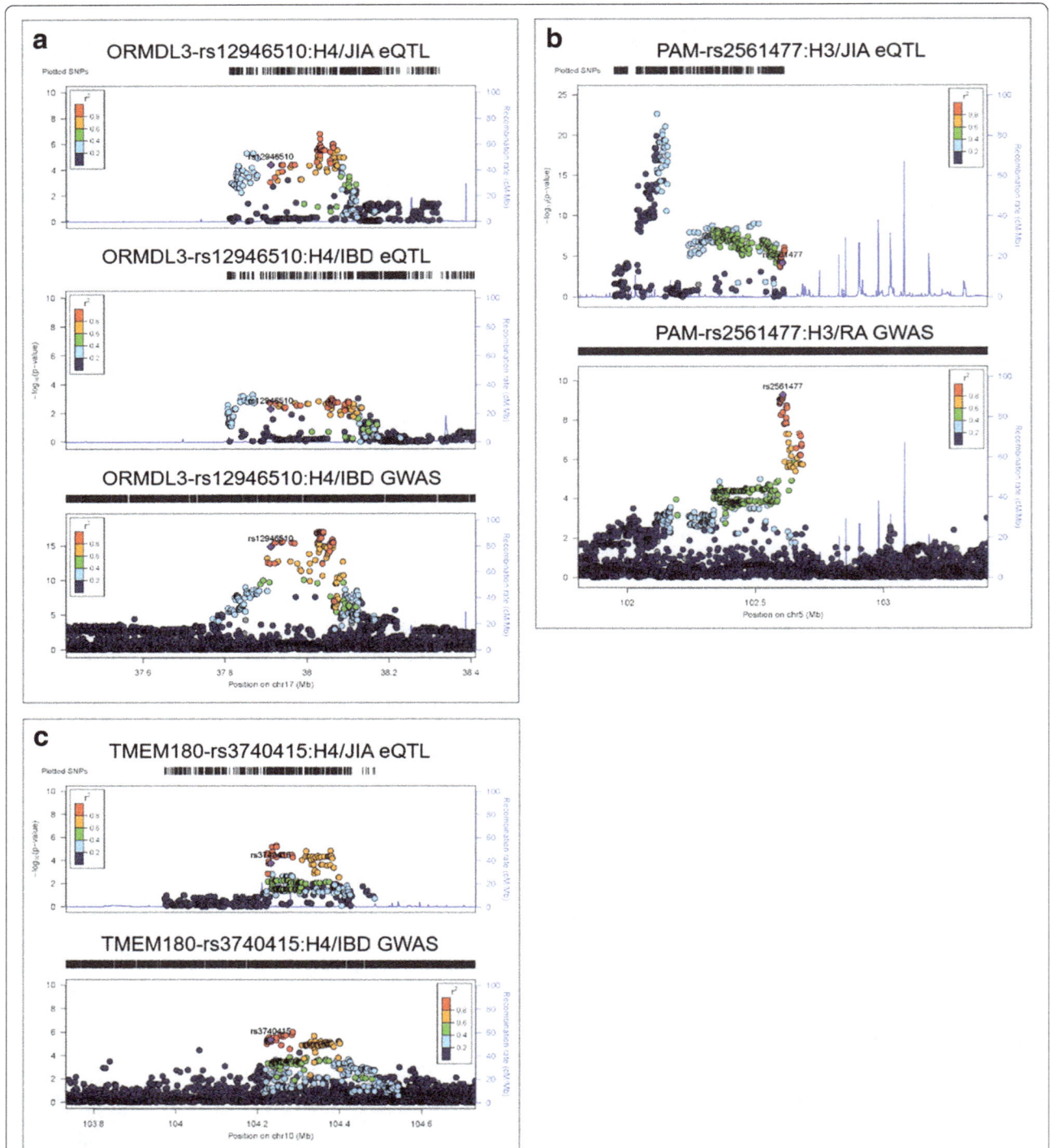

Fig. 6 Colocalization of eQTL and GWAS signatures. LocusZoom plots show the univariate SNP-wise association statistics for each genotyped SNP either with the abundance of the indicated trasncript (eQTL effects) or from the GWAS for IBD or RA. Color coding indicates the r^2 measure of linkage disequilibrium of each SNP with the relevant peak GWAS SNP. **a** rs12946510 is most likely a shared causal variant for *ORMDL3* gene expression in both IBD and JIA, as well as in the IBD GWAS. However, a likely secondary signal in the light blue region is not associated with IBD. **b** rs2561477 is the peak causal variant in RA but clearly does not colocalize with the peak eQTL for JIA. **c** rs3740415 is most likely a shared causal variant for expression of *TMEM180* and in the IBD GWAS despite an extensive LD block at the locus (though it does not meet the strict GWAS threshold)

appropriate framework for detecting such effects is evaluation of the significance of genotype-by-disease interaction terms, which motivated the current study.

The core result of the comparative eQTL component of this study is that the majority of genetic influences on transcript abundance measured in whole blood are consistent across IBD and JIA. A major caveat to this conclusion is that immune cell sub-type specific effects will often go undetected in both whole blood and PBMC studies [14, 18]. It is though important to note that while neutrophils, lymphocytes, macrophages, and monocytes certainly do have unique and disease-relevant eQTL, comparative studies also confirm that over three quarters of eQTL are shared by the majority of immune cells [64, 65].

Just as importantly, equivalence of genetic influences on gene expression does not necessarily mean equivalence of genetic influences on disease susceptibility. Among the shared eQTL, some numbers are still likely to be specific to CD, UC, JIA, or other conditions by virtue of other influences. These may include disease-specific contributions of the critical cell type, environmental differences (for example, microbial infection of the gut may elevate or suppress expression of the gene to a degree that renders the eQTL meaningful or irrelevant), or interactions with the genetic background (for example, elevated expression of a gene may only matter in the context of other genetic risk factors). Although there is little evidence that two-locus genotype-by-genotype interactions contribute meaningfully to heritability [66], renewed interest in influences of overall genetic risk on the impact of specific genotypes makes sense given the context of gene expression heterogeneity [67].

Our analyses do provide evidence that as many as 20% of eQTL effects in peripheral blood may at least show disease-specific biases. Such differences in effect sizes are likely to trace to differences in the expression of transcription factors and epigenetic modifications between diseases and/or to differences in the relative abundance of contributing cell types. Methods exist for deconvoluting effects of cell-type abundance [68], but they are low resolution and in our opinion unreliable when applied to sample sizes of the order of 100; next-generation studies incorporating single-cell RNA-Seq will be much more informative.

The relationship between disease-specific eQTL and GWAS association at the same locus is less straightforward than might be expected under the assumption that the effect of a polymorphism on disease is mediated through its effect on transcription of the associated gene. It is not immediately clear why an eQTL may only be detected in one disease while the GWAS association is in another disease, yet multiple instances are found in our data. This observation adds to a growing body of data questioning whether detected eQTL effects explain causal associations. Two fine mapping studies of IBD published in 2017 [69, 70] both found less than 30% identity between mapped eQTL and GWAS causal intervals, one suggesting that there is more significant overlap with methylation QTL and both arguing that the relevant effects may be specific to particular cell types or activation conditions, including immune activity at the sight of the pathology. Additionally, we described a meaningful number of "incoherent" associations, where mean differential expression between cases and controls is in the opposite direction to that predicted by the effect of the risk allele on gene expression [60]. Such results highlight the need for a combination of fine structure mapping of causal variants and detailed mechanistic studies of immune cell-type contributions if we are to fully understand how segregating polymorphisms contribute to disease susceptibility and progression.

Disease- and sub-type-specific gene expression

Numerous other studies have described gene expression profiles in a variety of inflammatory autoimmune diseases, but we are aware of just a single side-by-side comparison of two or more diseases on the same platform [65]. Straightforward cluster analysis shows that both IBD and JIA subjects tend to differ from healthy controls, but they have overall transcriptome profiles that may belong to a half dozen types. Blood Transcript Module and BIT axis analyses, both based on comprehensive analysis of existing whole blood gene expression datasets, confirm that these types broadly reflect differences in gene activity in the major immune sub-types, partly reflecting cell abundance, but also innate states of activity of biosynthetic, cell cycle, and cytokine signaling. Immunoprofiling by flow cytometry has established that individuals have baseline profiles, or omic personalities [71], to which they return after immunological perturbation but which are also influenced by such environmental factors as child-rearing [72]. Sub-type-specific blood gene expression should be seen in light of this immunological elasticity, as the heterogeneity among subjects may be more meaningful for disease risk than individual eQTL effects.

Juvenile idiopathic arthritis is the most prevalent childhood rheumatic disease, encompassing multiple physically, immunologically, and genetically different sub-types of disease. Although diagnosis and classification is based upon largely clinical criteria, the genetic complexity of JIA has been well documented [27, 28]. While the oligoarticular and polyarticular sub-types demonstrate activation of adaptive immunity, systemic JIA appears to be mediated more heavily through innate immunity, and profiles of immune cell activity between sub-types differ [73–75]. These findings at the gene expression level are consistent with emerging GWAS results suggesting that systemic JIA is etiologically a quite different disease. It is particularly noteworthy that both of the transcriptional risk scores we document show that systemic JIA is divergent from the articular forms, being close to the IBD profiles for the IBD-TRS, and uniquely elevated for the RA-TRS.

In this study, we performed cross-sub-type and disease comparisons of gene expression and eQTLs to characterize the similarities and differences between the forms of JIA. Differential gene expression analysis revealed a gradient of order among the JIA sub-types and IBD, from healthy controls, to oligoarticular, polyarticular, and systemic JIA, to Crohn's disease and ulcerative colitis. Numbers of differentially expressed genes, gene ontology pathway types, and significance levels agree with this pattern of ordering. Consistent with previous research, oligoarticular and polyarticular JIA exhibits a trend of activated T cell gene expression relative to systemic JIA [17–20, 23]. As a group, JIA also demonstrates increased expression of B cell-related genes. There is also an ordered increase in neutrophil gene expression from oligoarticular to systemic JIA, which concurs with systemic JIA being closely tied with innate immunity. In addition, the elevation of oligoarticular and polyarticular JIA over controls points to involvement of neutrophils in these sub-types as well, which has been previously suggested [5]. Taken as a whole, these findings suggest that JIA sub-types are mediated through a complex relationship between adaptive and innate immunity, and neither disease can be fully characterized by simply one or the other.

Limitations
This study has three major limitations. Firstly, since the subjects were not a part of any single-cohort study, they were treated with different medications or had samples taken at later time points after diagnosis. The sample size, though larger than many published studies, is still too small to partition the effects of plausible technical covariates or of environmental mediators of gene expression such as those described by Favé et al. and Idaghdour et al. [52, 76]. The results of the covariate-adjustment analyses presented in Additional file 1: Figures S1 and S2 suggest that the effects on our dataset are minimal compared with the consistent effect of disease subtype, but therapeutic effects should still be considered in interpretations of our findings. Secondly, whole blood samples were utilized to measure gene expression. Because whole blood is composed of multiple cell types, there will inherently be some mixture and dilution of gene signatures. Although it is well established that whole blood expression profiles are capable of illuminating aspects of autoimmune pathology, immune cell sub-type analyses will have higher resolution [18]. Single-cell RNA-Seq has great potential both to trace general features of peripheral blood gene expression to specific cell types and to foster accurate eQTL analysis

at the sub-type level. Thirdly, we describe just a cross-sectional snap shot of the transcriptome of each subject, whereas longitudinal profiling has the promise of correlating personalized transcriptional shifts to clinical response [77].

Conclusions
Gene expression and genotyping data can help to categorize sub-types of JIA and IBD beyond just clinical features. The gradient of gene expression from healthy controls to oligoarticular, polyarticular, and systemic JIA to IBD reflects a complex interplay between adaptive and innate immunity responsible for differentiation between JIA sub-types. Individuals have sub-type-specific probabilities of having one of a small number of global gene expression profiles. Since the majority of eQTL appear to have similar effect sizes across disease sub-types, disease-specific eQTL effects only explain a small fraction of disease-specific genetic influences on disease. Considerably more fine mapping and functional analysis will be required before personalized therapeutic interventions for patients with distinct forms of JIA or IBD become commonplace.

Abbreviations
BIT: Blood Informative Transcript; BTM: Blood Transcription Module; CD: Crohn's disease; eQTL: Expression quantitative trait locus; GWAS: Genome-wide association study; HLA: Human leukocyte antigen; IBD: Inflammatory bowel disease; JIA: Juvenile idiopathic arthritis; mQTL: Methylation quantitative trait locus; RA: Rheumatoid arthritis; TRS: Transcriptional risk score; UC: Ulcerative colitis

Acknowledgements
We thank the study participants for their willingness to engage in this research.

Funding
This research was funded by US NIH grants 1-P01-GM099568 (Project 3) to GG and 2-R01-DK087694 to SK and GG. AM is supported by T32-GM105490. SP is supported by Marcus Foundation Inc. Atlanta, GA.

Authors' contributions
The study was conceived and designed by GG and SP. LKC, LP, and JP coordinated sample acquisition and patient enrollment under the supervision of SP (JIA) and SK (IBD). DA processed the RNA samples for sequencing. AM and UMM performed the statistical and bioinformatics analyses under the supervision of GG. AM, UMM, and GG wrote the manuscript which was further revised by SP and SK. All authors read and approved the final manuscript.

Competing interests
The authors declare that they have no competing interests.

Author details
[1]Center for Integrative Genomics and School of Biological Sciences, Georgia Institute of Technology, Engineered Biosystems Building, EBB 2115, 950 Atlantic Drive, Atlanta, GA 30332, USA. [2]Department of Pediatrics, Emory University School of Medicine and Children's Healthcare of Atlanta, 1760 Haygood Dr NE, Atlanta, GA 30322, USA.

References

1. Gutierrez-Arcelus M, Rich SS, Raychaudhuri S. Autoimmune diseases—connecting risk alleles with molecular traits of the immune system. Nat Rev Genet. 2016;17:160–74.
2. McGovern DP, Kugathasan S, Cho JH. Genetics of inflammatory bowel diseases. Gastroenterology. 2015;149:1163–1176.e2.
3. Nédélec Y, Sanz J, Baharian G, Szpiech ZA, Pacis A, Dumaine A, et al. Genetic ancestry and natural selection drive population differences in immune responses to pathogens. Cell. 2016;167:657–69. e21
4. Ye CJ, Feng T, Kwon HK, Raj T, Wilson MT, Asinovski N, et al. Intersection of population variation and autoimmunity genetics in human T cell activation. Science. 2014;345:1254665.
5. Jarvis JN, Petty HR, Tang Y, Frank MB, Tessier PA, Dozmorov I, et al. Evidence for chronic, peripheral activation of neutrophils in polyarticular juvenile rheumatoid arthritis. Arthritis Res Ther. 2006;8(5):R154.
6. Ogilvie EM, Khan A, Hubank M, Kellam P, Woo P. Specific gene expression profiles in systemic juvenile idiopathic arthritis. Arthritis Rheumatol. 2007;56: 1954–65.
7. Barnes MG, Grom AA, Thompson SD, Griffin TA, Pavlidis P, Itert L, et al. Subtype-specific peripheral blood gene expression profiles in recent-onset juvenile idiopathic arthritis. Arthritis Rheumatol. 2009;60:2102–12.
8. Jiang K, Sawle AD, Frank MB, Chen Y, Wallace CA, Jarvis JN. Whole blood gene expression profiling predicts therapeutic response at six months in patients with polyarticular juvenile idiopathic arthritis. Arthritis Rheumatol. 2014;66:1363–71.
9. Prahalad S, Zeft AS, Pimentel R, Clifford B, McNally B, Mineau GP, et al. Quantification of the familial contribution to juvenile idiopathic arthritis. Arthritis Rheumatol. 2010;62(8):2525–9.
10. Ravelli A, Martini A. Juvenile idiopathic arthritis. Lancet. 2007;369:767–78.
11. Macaubas C, Nguyen K, Milojevic D, Park JL, Mellins ED. Oligoarticular and polarticular JIA: epidemiology and pathogenesis. Nat Rev Rheumatol. 2009;5: 616–26.
12. Mellins ED, Macaubas C, Grom AA. Pathogenesis of systemic juvenile idiopathic arthritis: some answers, more questions. Nat Rev Rheumatol. 2011;7:416–26.
13. Singh-Grewal D, Schneider R, Bayer N, Feldman BM. Predictors of disease course and remission in systemic juvenile idiopathic arthritis: significance of early clinical and laboratory features. Arthritis Rheumatol. 2006;54:1595–601.
14. Cui A, Quon G, Rosenberg AM, Yeung RSM, Morris Q, BBOP Study Consortium. Gene expression deconvolution for uncovering molecular signatures in response to therapy in juvenile idiopathic arthritis. PLoS One 2016;11:e0156055.
15. Jarvis JN, Frank MB. Functional genomics and rheumatoid arthritis: where have we been and where should we go? Genome Med. 2010;2:44.
16. Wouters CH, Ceuppens JL, Stevens EA. Different circulating lymphocyte profiles in patients with different sub-types of juvenile idiopathic arthritis. Clin Exp Rheumatol. 2002;20:239–48.
17. Griffin TA, Barnes MG, Ilowite NT, Olson JC, Sherry DD, Gottlieb BS, et al. Gene expression signatures in polyarticular juvenile idiopathic arthritis demonstrate disease heterogeneity and offer a molecular classification of disease subsets. Arthritis Rheum. 2009;60:2113–23.
18. Wong L, Jiang K, Chen Y, Hennon T, Holmes L, Wallace CA, Jarvis JN. Limits of peripheral blood mononuclear cells for gene expression-based biomarkers in juvenile idiopathic arthritis. Sci Rep. 2016;6:29477.
19. Barnes MG, Grom AA, Thompson SD, Griffin TA, Luyrink LK, Colbert RA, Glass DN. Biologic similarities based on age at onset in oligoarticular and polyarticular sub-types of juvenile idiopathic arthritis. Arthritis Rheumatol. 2010;62:3249–58.
20. Macaubas C, Nguyen K, Deshpande C, Phillips C, Peck A, Lee T, et al. Distribution of circulating cells in systemic juvenile idiopathic arthritis across disease activity states. Clin Immunol. 2010;134:206–16.
21. ImmunoBase. Juvenile Diabetes Research Foundation/Wellcome Trust Diabetes and Inflammation Laboratory 2018. https://www.immunobase.org. Accessed 5 Feb 2018.
22. Prahalad S, O-Brien E, Fraser AM, Kerber RA, Mineau GP, Pratt D, et al. Familial aggregation of juvenile idiopathic arthritis. Arthritis Rheumatol. 2004;50:4022–7.
23. Hinks A, Bowes J, Cobb J, Ainsworth HC, Marion MC, Comeau ME, et al. Fine-mapping the MHC locus in juvenile idiopathic arthritis (JIA) reveals genetic heterogeneity corresponding to distinct adult inflammatory arthritic diseases. Ann Rheum Dis. 2017;76:765–72.
24. Hersh AO, Prahalad S. Immunogenetics of juvenile idiopathic arthritis: a comprehensive review. J Autoimmun. 2015;64:113–24.
25. Thompson SD, Sudman M, Ramos PS, Marion MC, Ryan M, Tsoras M, et al. The susceptibility loci juvenile idiopathic arthritis shares with other autoimmune diseases extend to PTPN2, COG6, and ANGPT1. Arthritis Rheumatol. 2010;62:3265–76.
26. Thompson SD, Marion MC, Sudman M, Ryan M, Tsoras M, Howard TD, et al. Genome-wide association analysis of juvenile idiopathic arthritis identifies a new susceptibility locus at chromosomal region 3q13. Arthritis Rheumatol. 2012;64:2781–91.
27. Hinks A, Cobb J, Marion MC, Prahalad S, Sudman M, Bowes J, et al. Dense genotyping of immune-related disease regions identifies 14 new susceptibility loci for juvenile idiopathic arthritis. Nat Genet. 2013;45:664–9.
28. McIntosh LA, Marion MC, Sudman M, Comeau ME, Becker ML, Bohnsack JF, et al. Genome-wide association meta-analysis reveals novel juvenile idiopathic arthritis susceptibility loci. Arthritis Rheumatol. 2017;69:2222–32.
29. Stock CJ, Ogilvie EM, Samuel JM, Fife M, Lewis CM, Woo P. Comprehensive association study of genetic variants in the IL-1 gene family in systemic juvenile idiopathic arthritis. Genes Immun. 2008;9:349–57.
30. Fife MS, Gutierrez A, Ogilvie EM, Stock CJ, Samuel JM, Thomson W, et al. Novel IL10 gene family associations with systemic juvenile idiopathic arthritis. Arthritis Res Ther. 2006;8:R148.
31. Ombrello MJ, Arthur VL, Remmers EF, Hinks A, Tachmazidou I, Grom AA, et al. Genetic architecture distinguishes systemic juvenile idiopathic arthritis from other forms of juvenile idiopathic arthritis: clinical and therapeutic implications. Ann Rheum Dis. 2017;76:906–13.
32. Di Narzo AF, Peters LA, Argmann C, Stojmirovic A, Perrigoue J, Li K, et al. Blood and intestine eQTLs from an anti-TNF-resistant Crohn's disease cohort inform IBD genetic association loci. Clin Transl Gastroenterol. 2016;7:e177.
33. Singh T, Levine AP, Smith PJ, Smith AM, Segal AW, Barrett JC. Characterization of expression quantitative trait loci in the human colon. Inflamm Bowel Dis. 2015;21:251–6.
34. Kabakchiev B, Silverberg MS. Expression quantitative trait loci analysis identifies associations between genotype and gene expression in human intestine. Gastroenterology. 2013;144:1488–96. e1–3
35. Wakil SM, Monies DM, Abouelhoda M, Al-Tassan N, Al-Dusery H, Naim EA, et al. Association of a mutation in LACC1 with a monogenic form of systemic juvenile idiopathic arthritis. Arthritis Rheumatol. 2015;67:288–95.
36. Assadi G, Saleh R, Hadizadeh F, Vesterlund L, Bonfiglio F, Halfvarson J, et al. LACC1 polymorphisms in inflammatory bowel disease and juvenile idiopathic arthritis. Genes Immun. 2016;17:261–4.
37. Kim D, Pertea G, Trapnell C, Pimentel H, Kelley R, Salzberg SL. TopHat2: accurate alignment of transcriptomes in the presence of insertions, deletions and gene fusions. Genome Biol. 2013;14:R36.
38. Li H, Handsaker B, Wysoker A, Fennell T, Ruan J, Homer N, et al. 1000 Genome Project Data Processing Subgroup. The sequence alignment/map format and SAMtools. Bioinformatics 2009;25:2078–2079.
39. Anders S, Pyl PT, Huber W. HTSeq—a Python framework to work with high-throughput sequencing data. Bioinformatics. 2015;31:166–9.
40. Robinson MD, McCarthy DJ, Smyth GK. edgeR: a Bioconductor package for differential expression analysis of digital gene expression data. Bioinformatics. 2010;26:139–40.
41. Leek J, Johnson WE, Jaffe A, Parker H, Storey JD. The SVA package for removing batch effects and other unwanted variation in high-throughput experiments. Bioinformatics. 2012;28:882–3.
42. Mecham BH, Nelson PS, Storey JD. Supervised normalization of microarrays. Bioinformatics. 2010;26:1308–15.
43. Young MD, Wakefield MJ, Smyth GK, Oshlack A. Gene ontology analysis for RNA-seq: accounting for selection bias. Genome Biol. 2010;11:R14.
44. Preininger M, Arafat D, Kim J, Nath AP, Idaghdour Y, Brigham KL, et al. Blood-informative transcripts define nine common axes of peripheral blood gene expression. PLoS Genet. 2013;9:e1003362.
45. Li S, Rouphael N, Duraisingham S, Romero-Steiner S, Presnell S, Davis C, et al. Molecular signatures of antibody responses derived from a systems biological study of 5 human vaccines. Nat Immunol. 2014;15:195–204.

46. JMP® Genomics, Version 8.0. SAS Institute Inc., Cary, NC, 1989–2015.

47. Purcell S, Neale B, Todd-Brown K, Thomas L, Ferreira MAR, Bender D, et al. PLINK: a tool set for whole-genome association and population-based linkage analyses. Am J Hum Genet. 2007;81:559–75.

48. Delaneau O, Coulonges C, Zagury JF. Shape-IT: new rapid and accurate algorithm for haplotype inference. BMC Bioinformatics. 2008;9:540.

49. Howie BN, Donnelly P, Marchini J. A flexible and accurate genotype imputation method for the next generation of genome-wide association studies. PLoS Genet. 2009;5:e1000529.

50. Zhou X, Stephens M. Genome-wide efficient mixed-model analysis for association studies. Nat Genet. 2012;44:821–4.

51. Westra HJ, Peters MJ, Esko T, Yaghootkar H, Schurmann C, Kettunen J, et al. Systematic identification of trans eQTLs as putative drivers of known disease associations. Nat Genet. 2014;45:1238–43.

52. Favé MJ, Lamaze FC, Soave D, Hodgkinson A, Gauvin H, Bruat V, et al. Gene-by-environment interactions in urban populations modulate risk phenotypes. Nat Commun. 2018;9(1):827.

53. Du N, Jiang K, Sawle AD, Frank MB, Wallace CA, Zhang A, et al. Dynamic tracking of functional gene modules in treated juvenile idiopathic arthritis. Genome Med. 2015;7:109.

54. Hinze CH, Fall N, Thornton S, Mo JQ, Aronow BJ, Layh-Schmitt G, et al. Immature cell populations and an erythropoiesis gene-expression signature in systemic juvenile idiopathic arthritis: implications for pathogenesis. Arthritis Res Ther. 2010;12(3):R123.

55. Hu Z, Jiang K, Frank MB, Chen Y, Jarvis JN. Modeling transcriptional rewiring in neutrophils through the course of treated juvenile idiopathic arthritis. Sci Rep. 2018;8:7805.

56. Giambartolomei C, Vukcevic D, Schadt EE, Franke L, Hingorani AD, Wallace C, et al. Bayesian test for colocalisation between pairs of genetic association studies using summary statistics. PLoS Genet. 2014; 10:e1004383.

57. Pruim RJ, Welch RP, Sanna S, Teslovich TM, Chines PS, Gliedt TP, et al. LocusZoom: regional visualization of genome-wide association scan results. Bioinformatics. 2010;26:2336–7.

58. Liu JZ, van Sommeren S, Huang H, Ng SC, Alberts R, Takahashi A, et al. Association analyses identify 38 susceptibility loci for inflammatory bowel disease and highlight shared genetic risk across populations. Nat Genet. 2015;47:979–86.

59. Okada Y, Wu D, Trynka G, Raj T, Terao C, Ikari K, et al. Genetics of rheumatoid arthritis contributes to biology and drug discovery. Nature. 2014;506:376–81.

60. Marigorta UM, Denson LA, Hyams JS, Mondal K, Prince J, Walters TD, et al. Transcriptional risk scores link GWAS to eQTLs and predict complications in Crohn's disease. Nat Genet. 2017;49:1517–21.

61. Chaussabel D, Quinn C, Shen J, Patel P, Glaser C, Baldwin N, et al. A modular analysis framework for blood genomics studies: application to systemic lupus erythematosus. Immunity. 2008;29:150–64.

62. Gibson G, Powell JE, Marigorta UM. Expression quantitative trait locus analysis for translational medicine. Genome Med. 2015;7:60.

63. Ellinghaus D, Jostins L, Spain SL, Cortes A, Bethune J, Han B, et al. Analysis of five chronic inflammatory diseases identifies 27 new associations and highlights disease-specific patterns at shared loci. Nat Genet. 2016;48:510–8.

64. Fairfax BP, Makino S, Radhakrishnan J, Plant K, Leslie S, Dilthey A, et al. Genetics of gene expression in primary immune cells identifies cell type-specific master regulators and roles of HLA alleles. Nat Genet. 2012;44:502–10.

65. Peters JE, Lyons PA, Lee JC, Richard AC, Fortune MD, Newcombe PJ, et al. Insight into genotype-phenotype associations through eQTL mapping in multiple cell types in health and immune-mediated disease. PLoS Genet. 2016;12:e1005908.

66. Hemani G, Shakhbazov K, Westra HJ, Esko T, Henders AK, McRae AF, et al. Detection and replication of epistasis influencing transcription in humans. Nature. 2012;508:249–53.

67. Mäki-Tanila A, Hill WG. Influence of gene interaction on complex trait variation with multilocus models. Genetics. 2014;198:355–67.

68. Newman AM, Liu CL, Green MR, Gentles AJ, Feng W, Xu Y, et al. Robust enumeration of cell subsets from tissue expression profiles. Nat Methods. 2015;12:453–7.

69. Huang H, Fang M, Jostins L, Umićević Mirkov M, Boucher G, et al. Fine-mapping inflammatory bowel disease loci to single-variant resolution. Nature. 2017;547:173–8.

70. Chun S, Casparino A, Patsopoulos NA, Croteau-Chonka DC, Raby BA, De Jager PL, et al. Limited statistical evidence for shared genetic effects of eQTLs and autoimmune-disease-associated loci in three major immune-cell types. Nat Genet. 2017;49:600–5.

71. Tabassum R, Sivadas A, Agrawal V, Tian H, Arafat D, Gibson G. Omic personality: implications of stable transcript and methylation profiles for personalized medicine. Genome Med. 2015;7:88.

72. Carr EJ, Dooley J, Garcia-Perez JE, Lagou V, Lee JC, Wouters C, et al. The cellular composition of the human immune system is shaped by age and cohabitation. Nat Immunol. 2016;17:461–8.

73. Lin YT, Wang CT, Gershwin ME, Chiang BL. The pathogenesis of oligoarticular/polyarticular vs systemic juvenile idiopathic arthritis. Autoimmun Rev. 2011;10:482–9.

74. McGonagle D, Aziz A, Dickie LJ, McDermott MF. An integrated classification of pediatric inflammatory diseases, based on the concepts of autoinflammation and the immunological disease continuum. Pediatr Res. 2009;65(5, pt 2):38R–45R.

75. Jiang K, Wong L, Sawle AD, Frank MB, Chen Y, Wallace CA, et al. Whole blood expression profiling from the TREAT trial: insights for the pathogenesis of polyarticular juvenile idiopathic arthritis. Arthritis Res Ther. 2016;18:157.

76. Idaghdour Y, Storey JD, Jadallah SJ, Gibson G. A genome-wide gene expression signature of environmental geography in leukocytes of Moroccan Amazighs. PLoS Genet. 2008;4:e1000052.

77. Banchereau R, Hong S, Cantarel B, Baldwin N, Baisch J, Edens M, et al. Personalized immunomonitoring uncovers molecular networks that stratify lupus patients. Cell. 2016;165:1548–50.

4

Functional and genomic analyses reveal therapeutic potential of targeting β-catenin/CBP activity in head and neck cancer

Vinay K. Kartha[1,2,†], Khalid A. Alamoud[3,†], Khikmet Sadykov[3], Bach-Cuc Nguyen[3], Fabrice Laroche[4], Hui Feng[4], Jina Lee[5], Sara I. Pai[5], Xaralabos Varelas[6], Ann Marie Egloff[7], Jennifer E. Snyder-Cappione[8,9], Anna C. Belkina[8], Manish V. Bais[3], Stefano Monti[1,2] and Maria A. Kukuruzinska[3*]

Abstract

Background: Head and neck squamous cell carcinoma (HNSCC) is an aggressive malignancy characterized by tumor heterogeneity, locoregional metastases, and resistance to existing treatments. Although a number of genomic and molecular alterations associated with HNSCC have been identified, they have had limited impact on the clinical management of this disease. To date, few targeted therapies are available for HNSCC, and only a small fraction of patients have benefited from these treatments. A frequent feature of HNSCC is the inappropriate activation of β-catenin that has been implicated in cell survival and in the maintenance and expansion of stem cell-like populations, thought to be the underlying cause of tumor recurrence and resistance to treatment. However, the therapeutic value of targeting β-catenin activity in HNSCC has not been explored.

Methods: We utilized a combination of computational and experimental profiling approaches to examine the effects of blocking the interaction between β-catenin and cAMP-responsive element binding (CREB)-binding protein (CBP) using the small molecule inhibitor ICG-001. We generated and annotated in vitro treatment gene expression signatures of HNSCC cells, derived from human oral squamous cell carcinomas (OSCCs), using microarrays. We validated the anti-tumorigenic activity of ICG-001 in vivo using SCC-derived tumor xenografts in murine models, as well as embryonic zebrafish-based screens of sorted stem cell-like subpopulations. Additionally, ICG-001-inhibition signatures were overlaid with RNA-sequencing data from The Cancer Genome Atlas (TCGA) for human OSCCs to evaluate its association with tumor progression and prognosis.

Results: ICG-001 inhibited HNSCC cell proliferation and tumor growth in cellular and murine models, respectively, while promoting intercellular adhesion and loss of invasive phenotypes. Furthermore, ICG-001 preferentially targeted the ability of subpopulations of stem-like cells to establish metastatic tumors in zebrafish. Significantly, interrogation of the ICG-001 inhibition-associated gene expression signature in the TCGA OSCC human cohort indicated that the targeted β-catenin/CBP transcriptional activity tracked with tumor status, advanced tumor grade, and poor overall patient survival.

Conclusions: Collectively, our results identify β-catenin/CBP interaction as a novel target for anti-HNSCC therapy and provide evidence that derivatives of ICG-001 with enhanced inhibitory activity may serve as an effective strategy to interfere with aggressive features of HNSCC.

Keywords: HNSCC, β-Catenin/CBP transcriptional activity, Aggressive tumor cells, ICG-001, TCGA

* Correspondence: mkukuruz@bu.edu
†Vinay K. Kartha and Khalid A. Alamoud contributed equally to this work.
³Department of Molecular and Cell Biology, Goldman School of Dental Medicine, Boston University School of Medicine, 72 East Concord Street, E4, Boston, MA 02118, USA
Full list of author information is available at the end of the article

Background

The Wnt/β-catenin signaling pathway plays pivotal roles in development, tissue injury and regeneration, hematopoiesis, and maintenance of somatic stem cell niches in multiple tissue types [1–3]. Under normal conditions of development and homeostasis, the transcriptional activity of β-catenin is subject to negative regulatory controls [4, 5]. In contrast, persistent activation of β-catenin signaling due to somatic inactivating mutations in the upstream regulatory components of the Wnt pathway, or as a result of activating mutations in the β-catenin gene, *CTNNB1*, can contribute to the development of many cancers [1, 6–9].

In head and neck cancer, which presents primarily as head and neck squamous cell carcinoma (HNSCC), mutations in *CTNNB1* are relatively infrequent. Instead, β-catenin activity is induced by the more common mutations in negative regulators of Wnt/β-catenin signaling, specifically in *NOTCH1*, *FAT1*, and *AJUBA* [9, 10], where the inappropriate stabilization of β-catenin has been correlated with de-differentiation and poor prognosis [11]. A large fraction of HNSCC arises in the oral cavity as oral squamous cell carcinoma (OSCC), an aggressive malignancy associated with high morbidity and mortality [12–14]. Although the mechanisms underlying OSCC pathobiology and resistance to therapeutic interventions remain less-understood, mounting evidence suggests that Wnt/β-catenin signaling contributes to advanced OSCC disease and resistance to current therapies [6, 7, 10, 15]. In addition to activating genes with tumor promoting activities, Wnt/β-catenin signaling has been shown to advance aggressive cancer phenotypes through the maintenance of cancer stem cells (CSCs). These CSCs are highly resistant to conventional therapies and are linked to cancer cell expansion, locoregional spread with lymph node metastasis, and tumor recurrence following treatment [16–19]. Recently, CSCs with increased β-catenin transcriptional activity were identified in HNSCC [20], suggesting that targeting β-catenin has the potential to inhibit and eliminate treatment-resistant CSCs, thereby intercepting this malignancy.

The important roles played by Wnt/β-catenin signaling in cancer prompted the development of targeted agents directed at different components of the Wnt/β-catenin pathway. During the past decade, numerous Wnt/β-catenin inhibitors have been tested in preclinical models of different cancers, with some moving on to clinical trials [1, 4, 21]. In particular, several protein and small molecule inhibitors have displayed modest efficacy in vivo [22–24], with those blocking β-catenin activity that impacts its transcriptional targets demonstrating more promise. However, to date, no inhibitors of β-catenin have entered clinical trials for head and neck cancer patients.

In a search for an antagonist of Wnt/β-catenin signaling in OSCC, we have focused on a small molecule inhibitor that preferentially blocks the interaction between β-catenin and cAMP-response element-binding (CREB)-binding protein (CBP) in the nucleus [25]. First identified for its anti-tumorigenic effects in pre-clinical models of colorectal cancer [25], ICG-001 has been shown to have a beneficial role in interfering with multiple cancers and fibrosis [26–30] and to specifically target subpopulations of aggressive HNSCC CSCs [20, 31]. Nonetheless, the activity of ICG-001 has not been investigated in the context of changes in global genomic and cellular programs and their significance to the prognosis and treatment of human HNSCC patients.

To identify an effective strategy to target OSCC cells and to interfere with overall tumor growth and metastasis, we have focused on targeting β-catenin/CBP transcriptional activity using a combination of in vitro and in vivo models coupled with the interrogation of a large high-throughput human OSCC dataset derived from The Cancer Genome Atlas (TCGA). We align molecular and functional approaches with computational interrogation of large data sets for human head and neck cancer cell lines and tumor specimens to comprehensively characterize phenotypic and transcriptional consequences of ICG-001-mediated targeting β-catenin/CBP activity in HNSCC. Our studies provide evidence that inhibition of β-catenin/CBP activity in a panel of OSCC and pharyngeal cell lines by ICG-001 interfered with cell proliferation concomitant with an acquisition of an epithelial-like phenotype. In response to ICG-001, patient OSCC cell line-derived tumor xenografts in nude mice displayed reduced growth and loss of invasive characteristics while acquiring prominent junctional E-cadherin and β-catenin. Further, ICG-001 effectively and preferentially inhibited rapid tumor metastases of aggressive subpopulations of OSCC cells in zebrafish embryos. Importantly, we demonstrate the association between ICG-001 treatment signatures and clinical outcomes in primary human OSCCs. Collectively, our studies align β-catenin/CBP transcriptional activity with OSCC aggressive traits and suggest that targeting β-catenin-CBP interaction represents a potential novel treatment for this malignancy.

Methods

Cell lines and EC$_{50}$ measurements

Cell lines were obtained from the following sources: human CAL27, SCC9, and SCC25 cells were purchased from ATCC, and human HSC-3 cells were obtained from XenoTech, Japan. All cell lines were authenticated by short tandem repeat DNA profiling every 6 months either by ATCC or Genetica, with last validation in October, 2016. Cells were grown at 37 °C under 5% CO_2 to 70% confluence in DMEM (Invitrogen) supplemented with 10% fetal bovine serum, penicillin, and streptomycin, as described [32]. Determination of the half-maximal effective concentration (EC$_{50}$) in response to ICG-001 treatment at different concentrations of the drug was carried out using IncuCyte live-cell imaging per manufacturer's instructions (Essen BioScience). Briefly, OSCC cells were grown in T75 flasks, collected by trypsin digestion and washed in 5–10 ml DMEM media containing 10% FCS. Cells were seeded in Essen Bioscience 96-well Image Lock plate (Bioscience 96-well ImageLock Microplate no. 4379) at a density of 2000–3000 cells/well and allowed to attach for 12–24 h. Next, cells were treated with different concentrations of ICG-001 (Selleckchem):0.1, 0.3, 1, 3, 10, 20, and 30 μM and examined at 6-h time intervals. After 72 h, data were transferred to the Excel format and analyzed using the GraphPad Prism program.

Nude mice and orthotopic xenograft experiments

HSC-3 cells were lentivirally transduced with DsRed and suspended in serum-free Dulbecco's Modified Eagle Medium (DMEM). For orthotopic tongue xenografts, 0.5×10^6 cells in 40 μl of DMEM were injected into each tongue of 2-month-old nude mice (Taconic Farms, Hudson, NY) that were anesthetized with isoflurane. Anesthesia was administered in an induction chamber with 2.5% isoflurane in 100% oxygen at a flow rate of 1 L/min and then maintained with a 1.5% mixture at 0.5 L/min. Two days following injection, mice ($n = 16$) were equally divided into two groups: vehicle (DMSO control) and ICG-001-treated. For tumor inhibition studies, ICG-001 was diluted in 0.1% DMSO and administered via oral gavage at a concentration of 80 mg/kg into treatment-group mice via the tongue daily. Digital caliper measurements were performed at 2–3 day intervals to monitor the volumes of all tumors. Mice were imaged for DsRed protein expression on day 17 using an IVIS 200 system (Xenogen, Alameda, CA, USA). The fluorescence signals were optimized for the DsRed protein at excitation 570 and emission 620. Fluorescence region of interest (ROI) data were calibrated and normalized fluorescence efficiency $(p/s/cm^2/sr)/(\mu W/cm^2)$ determined as per the instructions (Perkin Elmer, USA). The data are reported as normalized fluorescence intensity (FU) from a defined region of interest for oral tongue tumors or systemic metastases compared to control vehicle-injected mice. Mice were sacrificed at day 20, and tumors were harvested and processed for further analyses.

Immunocompetent SCC mouse model

HPV-16 E6 and E7-expressing TC-1 tumor cells were used which were generated as previously described [33]. In brief, the HPV-16 E6, E7, and *ras* oncogene were used to transform primary C57BL/6 mice lung epithelial cells to generate the TC-1 tumor cell line. TC-1 has been reliably used as a preclinical model to study HPV16 E7-specific CD8$^+$ T cell responses for the evaluation of

novel immunotherapeutic agents to support phase I clinical trials in human subjects [34]. The cells were maintained in RPMI medium supplemented with 2 mM glutamine, 1 mM sodium pyruvate, 100 U/ml penicillin, 100 lg/ml streptomycin, and 10% fetal bovine serum. C57BL/6 mice were inoculated subcutaneously in the right flank with 1×10^5 TC-1 cells per mouse. When the tumor volume reached 50 mm^3 (7 days post-inoculation), mice were treated daily with either 50 μl of ICG-001 (0.04 mg/μl; 80 mg/kg BW) or a mixture of 10% DMSO + 90% vegetable oil (vehicle control group) administered orally using a 16-gauge oral feeding tube daily for 7 days. Mice were sacrificed, and tumors were dissected and processed as described below.

Mouse tumor sample processing

Tumors were harvested at sacrifice at day 20, weighed and either snap-frozen, and processed for histology, immunohistochemistry, immunoblot, and flow cytometry analyses. Tumors were paraffin-embedded and 5 μm sections were placed on Fisherbrand Superfrost Plus Microscope Slides (Fisher Scientific), deparaffinized, treated with Retrievit-6 Target Retrieval Solution (BioGenex), and processed for immunofluorescence and histological analyses (see below). Frozen tumor tissues were used for immunoblot analyses. In addition, portions of mouse tumors were minced and digested with 0.1% collagenase I (Worthington) at 37 °C for 1 h. Cells were passed through 70 μm mesh and washed twice, and the resulting single-cell suspension was used for flow cytometric analysis and sorting.

Immunofluorescence analysis

Morphologies of OSCC cell lines comprising CAL27, HSC-3, SCC9, and SCC25 cells treated with ICG-001 or DMSO vehicle control were examined using a Nikon Eclipse TE300 microscope. For indirect immunofluorescence analyses, cells were grown to 70% confluence on Nunc Lab-Tek II Chamber Slide (Thermo Fisher Scientific), fixed in 3.7% paraformaldehyde, permeabilized with 0.1% Triton X-100, blocked with 10% goat serum, and incubated with primary antibodies to β-catenin (Abcam, rabbit polyclonal AB followed by secondary antibody, goat anti-rabbit conjugated with Alexa Fluor 488 (Jackson ImmunoResearch). Cells were counterstained for nuclei with 4′6-diamidino-2-phenylindole, dihydrochloride (DAPI) (Molecular Probes), mounted in ProLong Gold Antifade, (Molecular Probes), and images were analyzed with a Zeiss LSM 710-Live Duo Scan confocal microscope. The observed changes in cellular phenotypes in response to the ICG-001 treatment were quantified using two independent criteria: cell size (area occupied by cell, $n = 15$) and junctional organization of β-catenin at the membrane (width of membrane localization, $n = 10$). All images were quantified using the ImageJ software. Mouse tumor tissue sections were blocked with 10% goat serum, mouse IgG blocking reagent (Vector) and incubated with antibodies against β-catenin, E-cadherin (Abcam, rabbit), and vimentin (Sigma, mouse) followed by secondary antibodies, goat anti-rabbit and goat anti-mouse conjugated with Alexa Fluor 488. Negative controls lacked primary antibodies. The slides were mounted in ProLong Gold Antifade, and optical sections (0.5 μm intervals) were analyzed by confocal microscopy using a Zeiss LSM710-Live Due Scan confocal microscope. To compare fluorescence intensities between samples, settings were fixed to the most highly stained sample with all other images acquired at those settings. Images were processed with ZEN 2 and ImageJ imaging software.

Immunoblot analysis

Total tissue lysate (TTL) from harvested mouse orthotopic tongue tumors was prepared by grinding tumors to a fine powder in liquid nitrogen and extracting total tissue proteins with Triton/β-octylglucoside buffer. Protein concentrations for TTL were determined using BCA assay (Pierce). For immunoblot analyses, TTL (20–30 μg of total protein) were fractionated on 7.5% SDS-PAGE, transferred onto polyvinylidene difluoride membranes, blocked with 5% nonfat dry milk, and incubated with primary antibodies to either E-cadherin or β-catenin (Abcam, rabbit) and GAPDH (Novus Biologicals). Protein-specific detection was carried out with horseradish peroxidase-labeled secondary antibodies conjugated to horseradish peroxidase (Bio-Rad) and Enhanced Chemiluminescence Plus (Amersham Biosciences). Signal intensities were normalized to GAPDH (Novus Biologicals).

Histology

Mouse tumor tissues were fixed overnight in 4% paraformaldehyde in PBS and dehydrated. Samples were embedded in paraffin and sectioned (5 μm thickness) and stained with hematoxylin and eosin (H&E) at the Boston University Medical Campus Pathology Core Facility. Digital images of stained slides were acquired with a TE 300 microscope (Nikon). Quantification of the effects of ICG-001 on tumor spread in harvested tongue tumors was carried out by measuring tumor area (region occupied by cancer cells) relative to the total section on the slide.

Zebrafish transplantation and ICG-001 treatment

Zebrafish husbandry was performed as described [35]. *Casper x Fli-GFP* fish breeders were crossed, and embryos overexpressing GFP in their vasculature were obtained. For micro-injections of zebrafish embryos, OSCC cells were either stained with a CellTracker™ dye (Molecular Probes) or lentivirally transduced with red fluorescent protein (RFP), trypsinized, and resuspended at a concentration of 50×10^6 cells/ml in DMEM containing 10% FBS. One day post-fertilization (dpf) embryos were enzymatically dechorionated using Pronase (Roche Diagnostics) and allowed to recover overnight at 28 °C, in the dark and in sterilized egg water. The two-dpf zebrafish larvae were anesthetized with Tricaine and immobilized before injections. The borosilicate glass capillaries (World Precision Instruments) 1.0 mm O.D. × 0,78 mm (I.D. Harvard Apparatus) used for micro-injection were pulled using 500 V (pull = 100, velocity = 250) in a capillary machine (Sutter Instrument). The OSCC cell transplantations were performed by injection of ~ 1 nL directly into the perivitelline space [36] of the embryo using a needle holder and a micro-injection station (World Precision Instruments). The transplanted zebrafish embryos were treated with ICG-001 or vehicle and incubated in the dark at 34.6 °C. Zebrafish embryos were individually mounted in a low melting 1.5% agarose gel (Fisher BioReagents) for a side view and imaged using an Olympus MVX10 fluorescence stereomacroscope or a Leica SP5 laser scanning confocal microscope at Boston University cellular imaging core. For comparison of metastases in CAL27 and HSC-3 cell-injected fish, metastases were measured by scoring numbers of CellTracker™-labeled fish outside the injection site. To quantify the extent of metastases in zebrafish injected with RFP-labeled HSC-3 cells, individual fish were scored for numbers of cells.

Flow cytometry and fluorescence-activated cell sorting (FACS)

For characterization of cells from immunocompetent SCC mouse model by multicolor flow cytometry staining, cells were first incubated with Zombie Aqua Live-dead dye (Biolegend) in PBS for 20 min, washed, pre-blocked with mouse antiCD16/32 FcBlock (Biolegend), and stained with the cocktail of conjugated fluorescent anti-mouse antibodies: CD29 eFluor 450, CD166 PE and CD133 PerCP-e710 (eBioscience), CD44 BV786, EpCAM FITC, E-Cadherin PE-Cy7, CD24 Alexa Fluor 647, and CD45 APC-750 (BioLegend) for 30 min. Cells were washed and immediately run on the BD FACSARIA II flow cytometry sorter for sorting and analysis. At least 200,000 events were recorded per sample. Data were analyzed in FACSDiva v6.2.0 (BD) and FlowJo v10.2 (FlowJo).

For zebrafish studies, cells were prepared for flow cytometry as a single-cell suspension and stained with Zombie Aqua Live-Dead dye (Biolegend) in DPBS for 20 min in the dark according to manufacturer's protocol, then washed and pelleted by centrifugation. The cell pellet was resuspended in DPBS/BSA/EDTA buffer containing Brilliant Buffer (BD Biosciences) and fluorochrome-conjugated antibodies to human CD29 (Alexa Fluor 700, Biolegend), human CD24 (BUV395, BD Biosciences), human EpCAM (BV650, BD Biosciences), and human CD44 (BV421,

Biolegend), incubated for 30 min in the dark, then washed and pelleted twice. The resulting cell pellet was resuspended in DPBS/BSA/EDTA buffer and immediately analyzed on a BD FACSAria II SORP sorter located in the Flow Cytometry Core Facility at Boston University Medical Center (BUMC) using the BD FACSDiva 6.2 software. For analysis, at least 100,000 events per sample were recorded and data were subsequently analyzed with FlowJo 10.2 software (FlowJo, Inc). For quality controls, purity of the sorts was confirmed to be > 95%.

Microarray gene expression analysis

Three separate wells (triplicate) from 6-well plates were seeded by HSC-3 and CAL27 cells (around 5×10^4/well). After 12–24 h (i.e., approximately 50% confluency), the cells were treated with either 0.1% DMSO or 10 μM ICG-001. After 48–64 h, the cells were trypsinized and harvested for RNA purification using miRNeasy Micro Kit (QIAGEN no. 217084). Gene expression profiling was performed in triplicates per treatment group ($n = 3$) using Affymetrix Human Gene 2.0ST arrays. Raw expression values were normalized together using the Robust Multiarray Average (RMA) with the affy R package. A BrainArray Chip Definition File (CDF) was used to map the probes on the array to unique Entrez Gene identifiers (http://brainarray.mbni.med.umich.edu/Brainarray/Database/CustomCDF). Differential gene expression analysis with respect to ICG-001 treatment was performed for each cell line using the Limma R package v3.14.4 [37]. Filtered false discovery rate (FDR) q values were recomputed based on the Benjamini-Hochberg method [38] after removing genes that were not expressed above the array-wise median value of at least one array. Only genes with absolute linear fold-change ≥ 1.5 and filtered FDR $q \leq 0.01$ were considered and used for further analysis as the ICG-001 treatment signature.

CCLE and TCGA data processing and analysis

Microarray gene expression data from the Cancer Cell Line Encyclopedia (CCLE) was processed as previously described [39]. Only data for cell lines annotated as originating in the upper aerodigestive tract (UAT; $n = 32$) was used. RNA-sequencing (RNASeq) expression and matched clinical data pertaining to The Cancer Genome Atlas (TCGA) OSCC samples ($n = 352$) was obtained and processed as previously described [40]. For gene set projection analyses, TCGA OSCC RNASeq and CCLE UAT microarray data were separately projected onto the "core" set of genes downregulated by ICG-001 in both HSC-3 and CAL27 cells ($n = 104$) using ASSIGN [41], yielding sample stratification based on a score representing the coordinated expression of ICG-001-downregulated genes (referred to as the ICG-001-*inhibition* score). For TCGA OSCCs, only samples with known tumor grade information were retained

when comparing scores with respect to tumor grade. Survival analysis was performed using the survival package in R (https://cran.r-project.org/). Patient survival information pertaining to the February 4th 2015 Firehose release was used to compute overall survival for TCGA OSCC patients. Patients were divided into two groups (ICG-001-high and -low) based on the median ICG-001 inhibition scores. AE and metastatic tumor samples were filtered out for this analysis (i.e., only the primary tumor-associated inhibition scores were used to bin samples into ICG-001 high, and low groups).

Statistical analyses

Statistics for all pairwise comparisons of quantitative measurements, including relative abundances from TTL obtained using immunoblot assays, tumor volume, relative tumor area within harvested tumor sections, and relative radiant efficiency measurements in orthotopic mice, as well as metastases quantification in injected zebrafish, were obtained using an unpaired two-tailed t test between comparison groups (ICG-001 versus DMSO vehicle, unsorted versus sorted cells etc.). Mouse tumor volume measurements were compared between groups per time point. All bar plots are represented as means ± S.D. ICG-001 ASSIGN scores for OSCC versus AE TCGA samples were compared using an unpaired two-tailed t test. Analysis of scores with respect to tumor grade was done using a pairwise one-sided t test between adjacent grade groups (g2 versus g1, g3 versus g2, and g4 versus g3), with their corresponding p values combined as previously described [42]. A log-rank test was used to compare survival rates between the ICG-001-high and ICG-001-low patient groups.

Results

Inhibition of β-catenin/CBP-activity interferes with OSCC cell growth and promotes membrane localization of β-catenin

The small molecule inhibitor, ICG-001, has been shown to inhibit the interaction between β-catenin and CBP in the nucleus and to affect transcription of a subset of β-catenin target genes [25, 43]. We first verified the inhibitory effect of ICG-001 on transcriptional activity of β-catenin using the TOPflash-driven Renilla luciferase reporter assay (Additional file 1: Figure S1). Given that intrinsic activity of β-catenin has been associated with treatment-resistant features of carcinomas, we examined whether ICG-001 would impact phenotypes of OSCC cells. Thus, we examined β-catenin localization in response to ICG-001 in a panel of cell lines including CAL27, HSC-3, SCC9, and SCC25 cells using immunofluorescence staining and high-resolution confocal microscopy. Remarkably, while vehicle-treated cells displayed a broad distribution of β-catenin at the membrane, ICG-001 promoted a more focused localization of β-catenin in all four cell lines evaluated (Fig. 1a). This was accompanied by a more compact epithelial cell phenotype, as indicated by reduced average cell size (Fig. 1b). Additionally, examination of junctional β-catenin by immunofluorescence imaging in Fig. 1a revealed tighter organization as indicated by its diminished thickness at the membrane, a feature that accompanies more mature E-cadherin junctions (Fig. 1c). To better visualize the effects of ICG-001 on β-catenin localization and OSCC cell morphology, we imaged CAL27 cells at a higher power and found that in vehicle-treated cells, β-catenin was localized at widespread membrane projections that formed loose cell-cell contacts. These cells displayed a mesenchymal morphology with prominent stress fibers and little co-localization between β-catenin and F-actin at the membrane (Additional file 1: Figure S2a, DMSO). In contrast, in ICG-001-treated cells, β-catenin

was enriched at membrane domains with reduced projections, where it co-localized with F-actin (Additional file 1: Figure S2a, ICG-001). The differences in cell size and β-catenin junctional organization in response to ICG-001 treatment in CAL27 and HSC-3 cells did not involve major changes in E-cadherin and β-catenin transcript or protein levels (Additional file 1: Figure S2b), suggesting altered distribution of these components rather than expression. Instead, we found that the CBP abundance was substantially reduced following the ICG-001 treatment (Additional file 1: Figure S2b), a result supported by the fractionation of β-catenin and CBP from HSC-3 cells into cytoplasmic and nuclear fractions (Additional file 1: Figure S3). Interestingly, with this approach, we detected majority of β-catenin in the cytosolic compartment with only a small fraction in the nucleus. Collectively, these results strongly suggest that

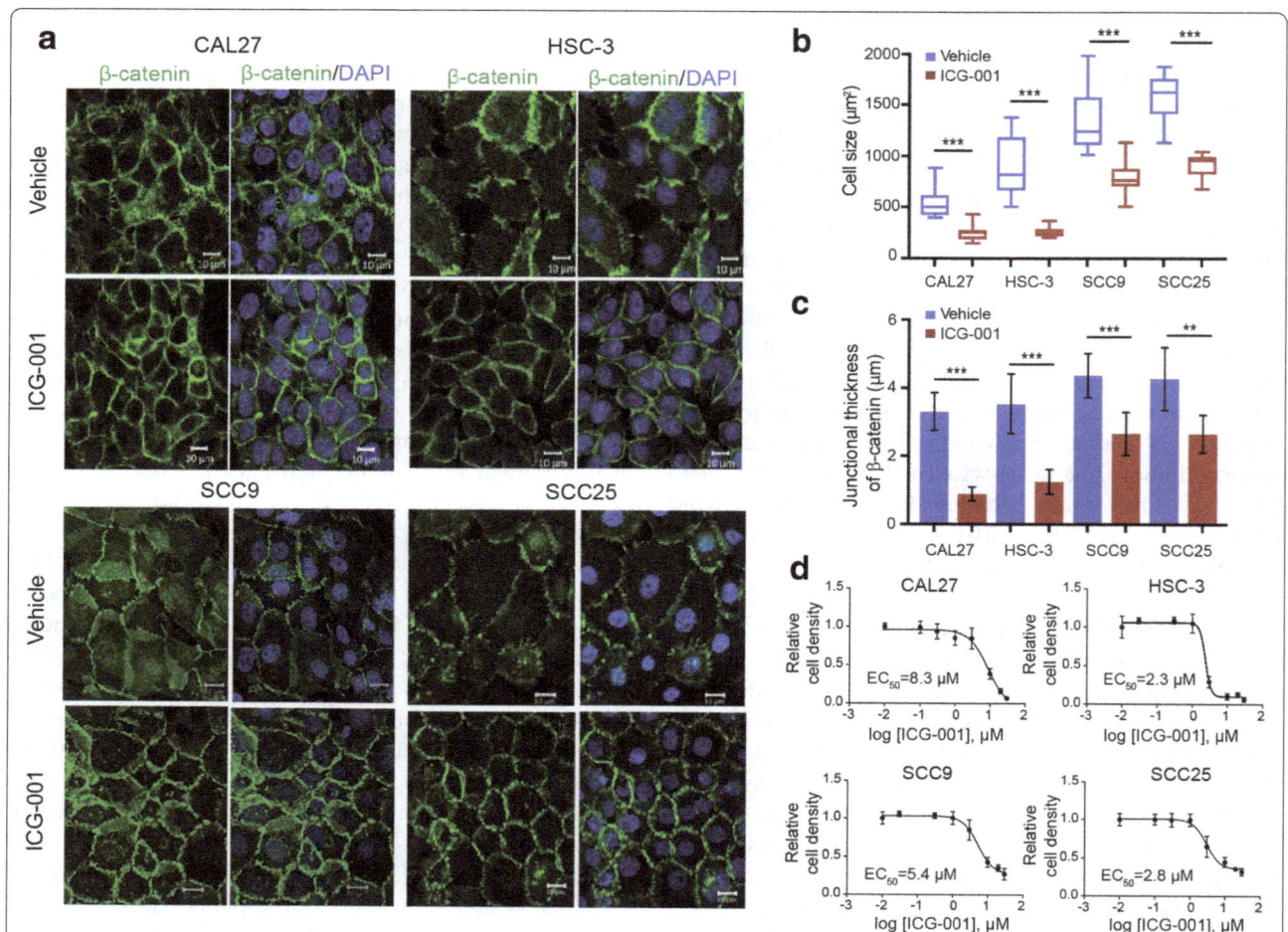

Fig. 1 ICG-001 inhibits growth of OSCC cell lines and promotes an epithelial phenotype. a Immunofluorescence imaging of β-catenin localization in OSCC cell lines in response to ICG-001 treatment showing more focused membrane localization of β-catenin, increased intercellular adhesion with a more pronounced epithelial phenotype. Size bars, 10 μm. b ICG-001 treatment promotes cell compaction as measured by the average cell size ($n = 15$) captured in 1a. c Increased junctional organization of β-catenin in immunofluorescence images shown in 1a was determined based on the thickness of β-catenin at the membrane ($n = 10$). d Determination of half maximal effective concentration (EC_{50}) for ICG-001 effects in OSCC cell lines. Shown are graded dose response curves for ICG-001 in CAL27, HSC-3, SCC9, and SCC25 cell lines for 72 h of treatment. Immunofluorescence images were quantified using ImageJ and compared using PRISM GraphPad. **$P < 0.001$; ***$P < 0.0001$ unpaired t test

treatment of OSCC cells with ICG-001 promoted junctional localization of β-catenin and enhanced their epithelial-like morphology.

We next determined the in vitro sensitivity of the four OSCC cell lines to ICG-001 using incuCyte live imaging. Dose-dependent inhibition of cell growth was observed for all cell lines examined following 72 h of treatment with ICG-001, with EC_{50} values of 2.3, 2.8, 5.4, and 8.3 μM for HSC-3, SCC25, SCC9, and CAL27 cells, respectively (Fig. 1d). Notably, the most aggressive metastatic cell line exhibited the greatest sensitivity to ICG-001, especially when compared to the non-metastatic CAL27 cells (Fig. 1d).

ICG-001 impacts expression of genes involved in Wnt signaling, cell proliferation, survival, and intercellular adhesion

For the subsequent studies, we selected CAL27 and HSC-3 cells to represent non-metastatic and metastatic OSCC phenotypes, respectively. To determine the effects of disrupting β-catenin/CBP-mediated activity with ICG-001 in OSCC cell lines, we performed gene expression profiling of RNA isolated from CAL27 and HSC-3 cells treated with either vehicle (DMSO) control or ICG-001 using microarrays. Differential gene expression testing between ICG-001 treatment and control groups yielded cell type-specific ICG-001 treatment signatures (Fig. 2a and Additional file 2). Consistent with EC_{50} values in vitro, which demonstrated greater ICG-001 treatment sensitivity of HSC-3 cells as compared to CAL27, HSC-3 cells showed a greater transcriptional response to treatment (1390 upregulated and 1238 downregulated genes) than CAL27 cells (246 upregulated and 256 downregulated genes) (Fig. 2b). Importantly, genes known to be targets of Wnt/β-catenin signaling (*DKK1*, *WNT5B*, *CCND2*, *CDK1*, *LEF1*, and *SKP2*) and to play a role in cell survival and proliferation (*BIRC5*, *CCNE1*, *CCNE2*, *CCNB1*, *CCNB2*, *CDKN3*, and *CDCA7*) were significantly downregulated, while genes with key roles in intercellular adhesion and epithelial differenetiation (*CLDN1*, *CLDN4*, *CLDN9*, *CLDN16*, *CDH4*, and *ICAM1*) were upregulated, with greater effect in HSC-3 cells than in CAL27 cells (Fig. 2c and Fig. 3a). Of significance, cell markers that were previously identified to be associated with a more stem cell-like state in HNSCC (*DNAJC6*, *NR5A2*, *HELLS*, *KRT5*, and *KRT14*), and characterized by elevated β-catenin activity [20, 44], were also found to be significantly downregulated by ICG-001 in HSC-3 cells (Fig. 2c and Fig. 3a). Treatment effects of ICG-001 on selected genes within these functional groups in CAL27 and HSC-3 cells were confirmed using quantitative real-time PCR (Fig. 3b). This includes the significant upregulation of cell-cell adhesion genes in HSC-3 cells, *CDH4* and *CLDN1*, further supporting the observed phenotypic effects of ICG-001 (Fig. 1a–c) and convergence between Wnt/

β-catenin signaling and intercellular adhesion [45]. Immunoblot analyses of protein products of genes impacted by ICG-001 in CAL27 and HSC-3 revealed reduction in the steady-state levels of survivin, the *BIRC5* gene protein product, and products of genes associated with stem cell-like-phenotypes, *HELLS* and *KRT14* (Additional file 1: Figures S4 and S5). Also, expression of a differentiation marker, claudin 1, was increased substantially in HSC-3 cells, while it was not altered in non-malignant CAL27 cells consistent with no significant changes detected in *CLDN1* transcript levels in CAL27 cells (Additional file 1: Figures S4 and S5).

To examine if the inhibition of β-catenin/CBP activity by ICG-001 has a broader relevance, we aligned the activity of genes repressed by ICG-001 in CAL27 and HSC-3 cells relative to additional cancer cell lines. Specifically, we interrogated gene expression data pertaining to a "core signature" comprising genes significantly downregulated by ICG-001 in both HSC-3 and CAL27 cells ($n = 104$ genes; Fig. 2b) in a panel of UAT cell lines from the CCLE (see "Methods"). Using the ASSIGN algorithm [41], we projected gene expression data for these cells in the space of the core gene signature, scoring each sample based on the coordinated expression of the gene set (referred to as the "ICG-001 inhibition score"; Additional file 1: Figure S6). Of the panel of OSCC cell lines assessed for sensitivity to ICG-001 treatment (Fig. 1d), HSC-3 cells displayed the highest ICG-001 inhibition score, followed by SCC25 cells, similar the trend observed based on EC_{50} values. Further, as per EC_{50} values, CAL27 and SCC9 cells were ranked lower (Fig. 1d; Additional file 1: Figure S6). In addition, we observed that hypopharygeal SCC FaDu cells clustered next to HSC-3 cells (rank = 1/32), suggesting that, although these cells are derived from a different anatomic site, they may also exhibit sensitivity to ICG-001 treatment. While FaDu cells did show sensitivity to treatment ($EC_{50} = 3.5$ μM; Additional file 1: Figure S7), it was lower compared to the EC_{50} values for HSC-3 and SCC25 cells, most likely reflecting differences arising from cell-specific and anatomical site-specific treatment effects. Importantly, treatment with ICG-001 of FaDu cells led to downregulation of CBP steady-state levels, consistent with CAL27 and HSC-3 cells (Additional file 1: Figure S7). In addition, levels of survivin were reduced in response to ICG-001 in FaDu cells. However, we did not detect changes in proteins encoded by *HELLS* and *CLDN1*, while the protein product of *KRT14* was not detectable.

To assess whether transcriptional effects of ICG-001 treatment correlated with that induced by β-catenin knockdown in OSCC in vitro, we first generated a gene list ranked by differential expression of β-catenin siRNA knockdown (KD) versus control in HSC-3 cells (Additional file 3). We then

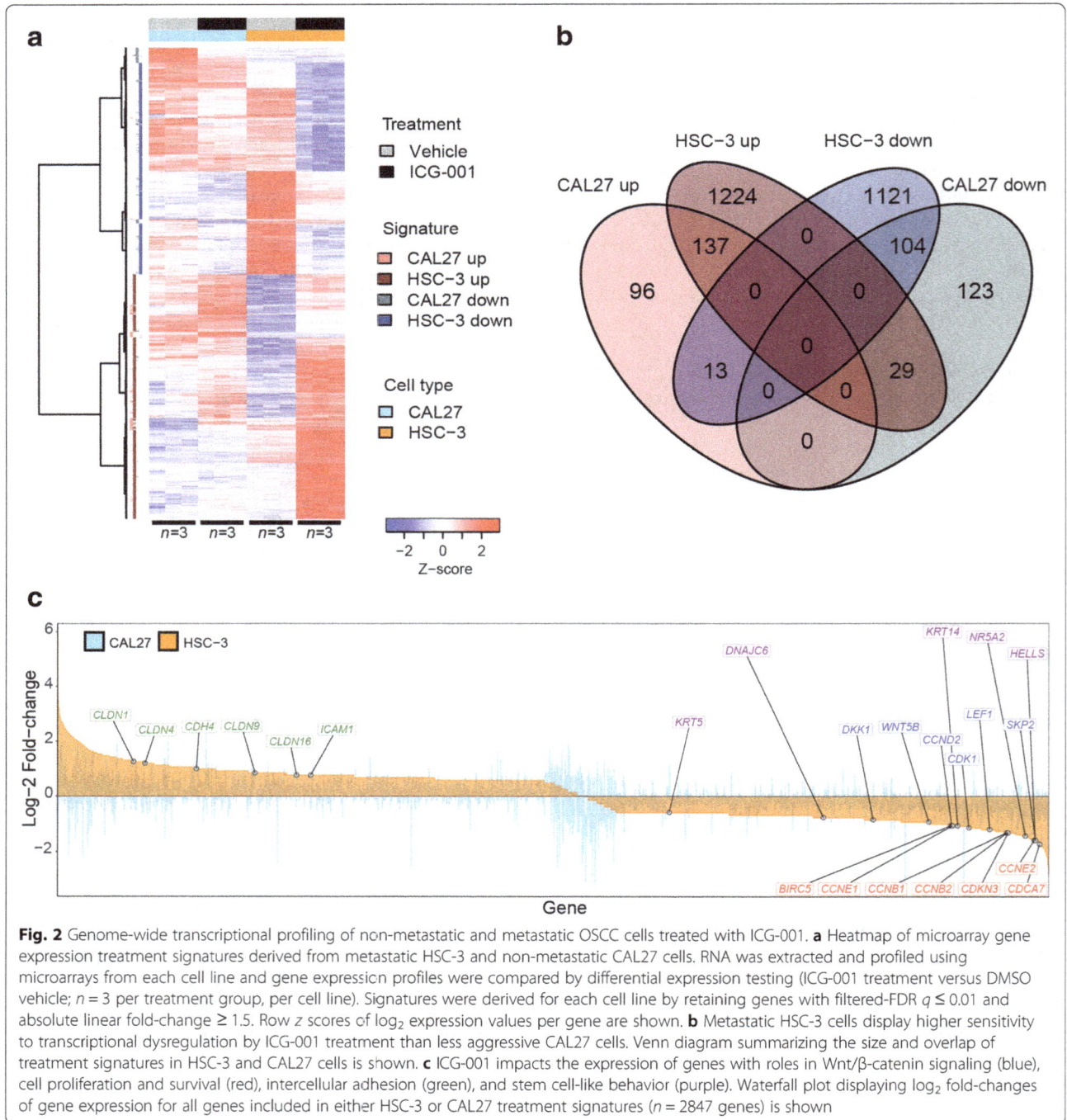

Fig. 2 Genome-wide transcriptional profiling of non-metastatic and metastatic OSCC cells treated with ICG-001. **a** Heatmap of microarray gene expression treatment signatures derived from metastatic HSC-3 and non-metastatic CAL27 cells. RNA was extracted and profiled using microarrays from each cell line and gene expression profiles were compared by differential expression testing (ICG-001 treatment versus DMSO vehicle; $n = 3$ per treatment group, per cell line). Signatures were derived for each cell line by retaining genes with filtered-FDR $q \leq 0.01$ and absolute linear fold-change ≥ 1.5. Row z scores of $\log_2$ expression values per gene are shown. **b** Metastatic HSC-3 cells display higher sensitivity to transcriptional dysregulation by ICG-001 treatment than less aggressive CAL27 cells. Venn diagram summarizing the size and overlap of treatment signatures in HSC-3 and CAL27 cells is shown. **c** ICG-001 impacts the expression of genes with roles in Wnt/β-catenin signaling (blue), cell proliferation and survival (red), intercellular adhesion (green), and stem cell-like behavior (purple). Waterfall plot displaying $\log_2$ fold-changes of gene expression for all genes included in either HSC-3 or CAL27 treatment signatures ($n = 2847$ genes) is shown

queried the derived ICG-001 treatment signatures against this reference list using Gene Set Enrichment Analysis (GSEA; see Additional file 1 for methods). We observed a significant skewedness of ICG-001 down and upregulated genes towards negative and positive fold-change of gene expression associated with β-catenin KD, respectively (FDR q < 0.001; Additional file 1: Figure S8a), suggesting that the ICG-001 treatment targeted specific β-catenin-mediated transcriptional activity in aggressive OSCC cells.

ICG-001 inhibits OSCC tumor growth and aggressive phenotypes in vivo

Our previous studies have shown that while CAL27 cells form orthotopic tongue tumors in nude mice, these tumors do not metastasize to distant sites. In contrast, HSC-3 cell-driven tumors undergo significant metastases in nude mice [46]. To determine whether ICG-001 treatment impacted growth and metastasis of HSC-3 xenografts, we treated mice ($n = 16$) with either ICG-001

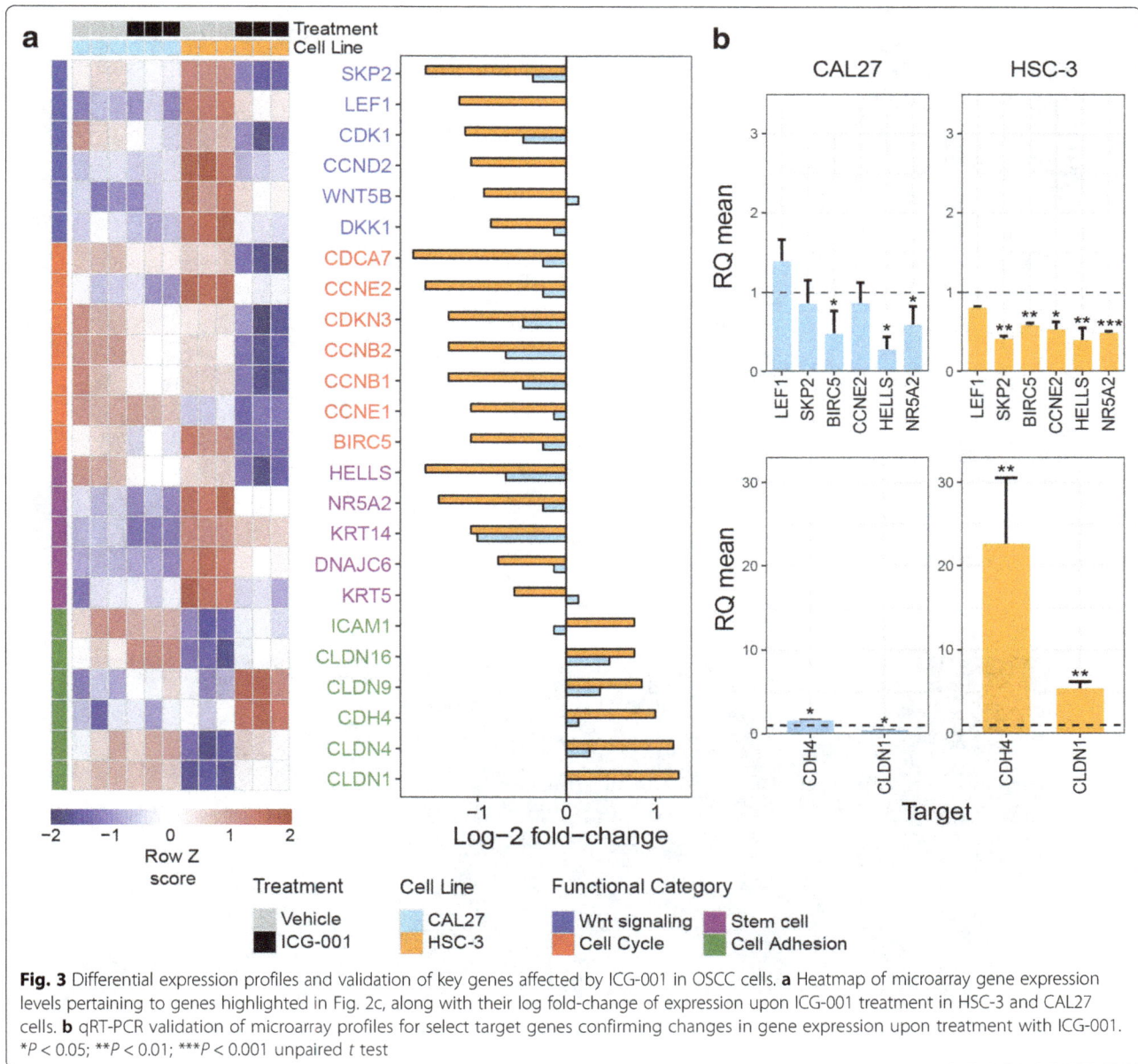

Fig. 3 Differential expression profiles and validation of key genes affected by ICG-001 in OSCC cells. **a** Heatmap of microarray gene expression levels pertaining to genes highlighted in Fig. 2c, along with their log fold-change of expression upon ICG-001 treatment in HSC-3 and CAL27 cells. **b** qRT-PCR validation of microarray profiles for select target genes confirming changes in gene expression upon treatment with ICG-001. *$P < 0.05$; **$P < 0.01$; ***$P < 0.001$ unpaired t test

($n = 8$) or DMSO vehicle ($n = 8$) by oral gavage beginning on day 3 following cell implantation into the tongues of nude mice, with treatment repeated every day. For these studies, cells were transduced with red fluorescent protein (DsRed) to track tumor growth and metastasis prior to orthotopic inoculation. Primary tumor growth was monitored every 2–3 days using caliper measurements. In addition, in vivo imaging system (IVIS) was used to follow localization of DsRed-expressing cells. Comparison of relative radiance efficiencies at day 17 post-inoculation revealed significantly reduced primary tumor growth ($P = 4.65e–3$, two-tailed t test) and whole body metastases ($P = 0.013$, two-tailed t test) associated radiance intensities in the

treated versus control groups (Fig. 4a). Further, starting at 13 days post-inoculation, we observed a significant reduction in tumor volume ($P < 0.005$, two-tailed t test) following treatment with ICG-001, relative to vehicle treated-control mice (Fig. 4b). Histological hematoxylin and eosin (H&E) analysis of vehicle-treated tumors revealed streaks of invasive cells growing out from primary tumors into the tongue stroma, while ICG-001-treated tumors displayed a capsular phenotype (Fig. 4c). Quantification of the tumor cross-sectional area taken up by squamous carcinoma cells was significantly reduced relative to the control condition ($P = 0.005$, two-tailed t test; Fig. 4c). Interestingly, examination of E-cadherin protein levels by immunoblot revealed that ICG-001-treated

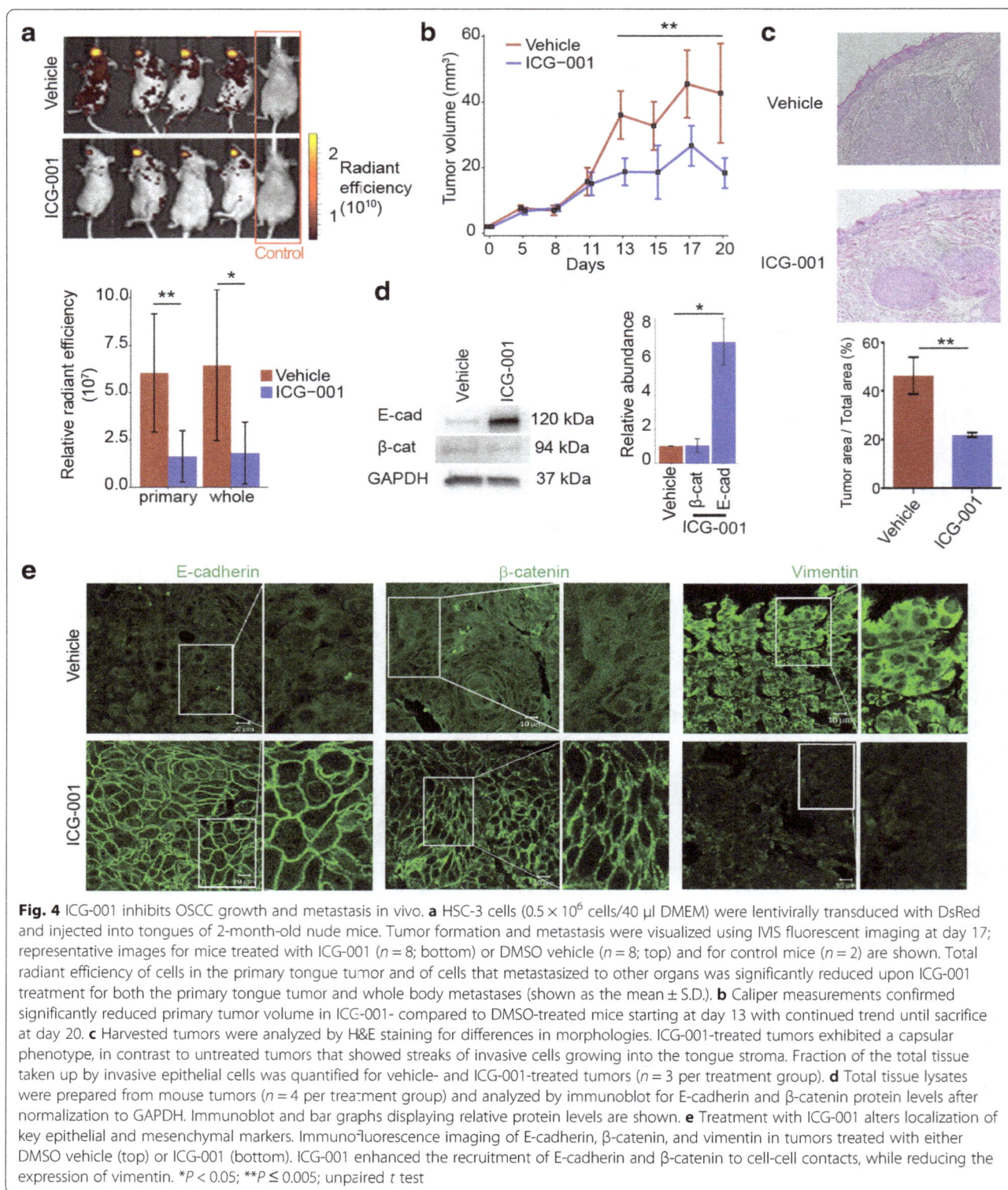

Fig. 4 ICG-001 inhibits OSCC growth and metastasis in vivo. **a** HSC-3 cells (0.5×10^6 cells/40 μl DMEM) were lentivirally transduced with DsRed and injected into tongues of 2-month-old nude mice. Tumor formation and metastasis were visualized using IMS fluorescent imaging at day 17; representative images for mice treated with ICG-001 ($n = 8$; bottom) or DMSO vehicle ($n = 8$; top) and for control mice ($n = 2$) are shown. Total radiant efficiency of cells in the primary tongue tumor and of cells that metastasized to other organs was significantly reduced upon ICG-001 treatment for both the primary tongue tumor and whole body metastases (shown as the mean ± S.D.). **b** Caliper measurements confirmed significantly reduced primary tumor volume in ICG-001- compared to DMSO-treated mice starting at day 13 with continued trend until sacrifice at day 20. **c** Harvested tumors were analyzed by H&E staining for differences in morphologies. ICG-001-treated tumors exhibited a capsular phenotype, in contrast to untreated tumors that showed streaks of invasive cells growing into the tongue stroma. Fraction of the total tissue taken up by invasive epithelial cells was quantified for vehicle- and ICG-001-treated tumors ($n = 3$ per treatment group). **d** Total tissue lysates were prepared from mouse tumors ($n = 4$ per treatment group) and analyzed by immunoblot for E-cadherin and β-catenin protein levels after normalization to GAPDH. Immunoblot and bar graphs displaying relative protein levels are shown. **e** Treatment with ICG-001 alters localization of key epithelial and mesenchymal markers. Immunofluorescence imaging of E-cadherin, β-catenin, and vimentin in tumors treated with either DMSO vehicle (top) or ICG-001 (bottom). ICG-001 enhanced the recruitment of E-cadherin and β-catenin to cell-cell contacts, while reducing the expression of vimentin. *$P < 0.05$; **$P \leq 0.005$; unpaired t test

tumors exhibited increased E-cadherin abundance compared to vehicle control-treated tumors ($P = 0.016$, two-tailed t test), while levels of β-catenin were not significantly altered ($P = 0.67$, two-tailed t test; Fig. 4d). Immunofluorescence

analyses of these tumors showed that the ICG-001-treated tumors phenocopied ICG-001-treated OSCC cell lines in vitro and displayed robust E-cadherin and β-catenin junctional localization with an almost complete loss of a mesenchymal protein vimentin, further indicating that ICG-001 promoted an epithelial phenotype (Fig. 4e).

Given that our in vivo model was based on an immuno-compromised mouse, it was possible that the observed tumor-inhibitory effects of ICG-001 were enhanced by the absence of the immune system. We therefore further tested whether ICG-001 inhibited aggressive phenotypes and promoted membrane localization of β-catenin in an immunocompetent mouse model of squamous cell carcinoma (SCC) [47]. Specifically, we assessed the effects of

ICG-001 treatment on lung squamous cell carcinoma TC-1-derived tumor xenografts from syngeneic C57BL/6 mice. Strikingly, we found that treatment with ICG-001 completely abrogated aggressive mesenchymal-like pheno-types of dissociated tumor cells coincident with the acqui-sition of a cuboidal epithelial-like morphology (Fig. 5a). We next searched for subpopulations of cells with imma-ture cell surface markers from TC-1-derived tumors by flow cytometry using a panel of primitive epithelial cell surface markers that included CD44, CD29, CD24,

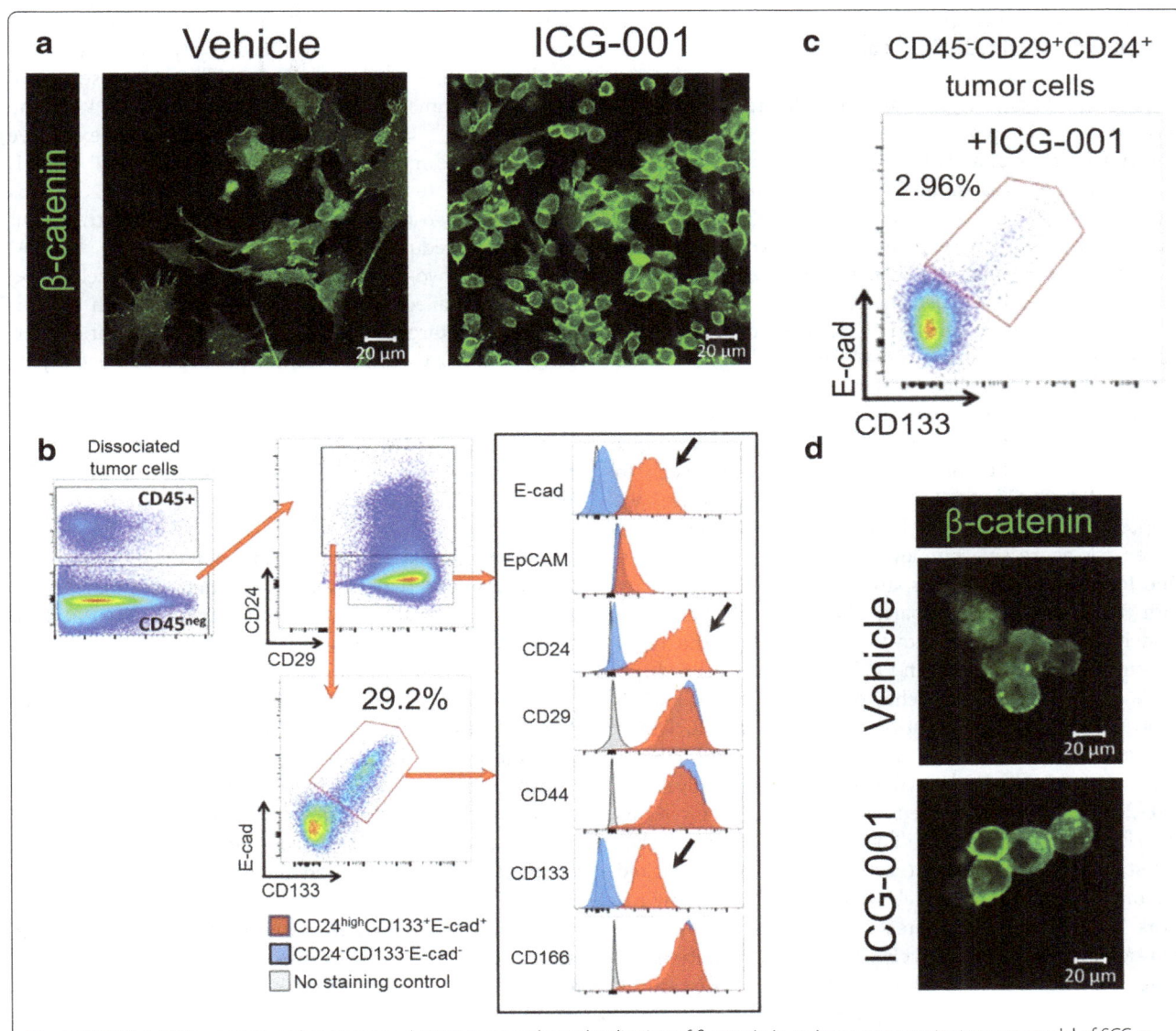

Fig. 5 ICG-001 inhibits aggressive phenotypes and promotes membrane localization of β-catenin in an immunocompetent mouse model of SCC. **a** Immunofluorescence imaging of β-catenin in HPV-16 E6 and E7-expressing TC-1 tumor cells. ICG-001 induces a cuboidal phenotype in cells dissociated from TC-1 tumors and promotes expression of junctional β-catenin. Representative images are shown for ICG-001 treatment versus DMSO (vehicle) control conditions. **b** Flow cytometry phenotyping of TC-1 tumor cells. Live, single cells were further gated based on expression of CD45, CD24, CD29, CD133, and E-cadherin (E-cad) as shown (red arrows), and expression profiles of stem cell-like CD24^{high}CD133$^+$E-cad$^+$ (red histograms, black arrows) were compared to CD24$^-$CD133$^-$E-cad$^-$ (blue histograms). **c** Stem cell-like CD24^{high}CD133$^+$E-cad$^+$ population in ICG-001-treated group is greatly diminished. Gating was performed as shown in panel **b**. **d** Localization of β-catenin in FACS-sorted CD24^{high}CD133$^+$E-cad$^+$ cells. Treatment of CD24^{high}CD133$^+$E-cad$^+$ cells with ICG-001 resulted in increased membrane distribution of β-catenin compared to vehicle-treated cells

CD166, and CD133. Phenotyping these tumor cells identi-fied a subpopulation of CD29$^+$ and E-cadherin-expressing (CD29$^+$E-cad$^+$) cells enriched for cell surface antigenic markers of primitive cell phenotypes, namely CD24 and CD133 (CD24^{high}CD133$^+$E-cad$^+$; Fig. 5b). Treatment with ICG-001 dramatically reduced the abundance of this stem-like cell population (Fig. 5c). Further, immuno-fluorescence staining for β-catenin of FACS-isolated CD29$^+$CD24^{high}CD133$^+$E-cad$^+$ cells from those tumors confirmed that ICG-001 treatment promoted membrane localization of β-catenin (Fig. 5d). Thus, ICG-001 inhib-ited aggressive phenotypes of TC-1 cells in a manner simi-lar to its effects on OSCC cells and tumors.

ICG-001 selectively targets a stem cell-like tumor subpopulation in vivo

The transcriptional activity of β-catenin has been shown to promote the expansion of subpopulations of cells with immature stem-cell-like phenotypes [20, 43]. These cells exhibit the ability to self-renew are capable of seeding tumors at low numbers in mouse xenografts and driving tumor progression to metastasis. In particular, a subset of β-catenin-positive cells from HNSCC, expressing the tumor stem cell marker CD44, were also shown to co-express CD24 and CD29 and to promote non-adherent tumor sphere growth and seed tumors at low numbers in mice [20]. Thus, to assess if ICG-001 inhibited the ability of CD44$^+$CD24^{high}CD29$^+$ cells to drive rapid OSCC tumor growth and metastases, we adapted an embryonic zebrafish xenograft model to screen for aggressive human stem cell-like OSCC cells. Due to its small size, transparency, and close homology with its human counterpart, the zebrafish xenograft model possesses unique advantages enabling the rapid screens of aggressive human OSCC stem-like cells [48].

We first examined the behavior of CAL27 and HSC-3 cells in 2-day post-fertilization (2-dpf) zebrafish, which lack an adaptive immune system. CAL27 and HSC-3 cells were labeled with a fluorescent tracker dye and 100–200 cells were injected into zebrafish embryos as described (see "Methods"). The behavior of cell tracker dye-stained OSCC cells in zebrafish closely mimicked our orthotopic mouse models in their ability to grow tu-mors without and with metastatic properties ($P < 00001$; two-tailed t test), respectively (Fig. 6a–c). Additionally, treatment with ICG-001 significantly reduced metastasis in zebrafish tumors induced by HSC-3 cells ($P < 0.0001$, two-tailed t test; Fig. 6b–c), as it did in murine models.

Since it has been shown that a specific subpopulation of aggressive tumor cells is associated with stem cell-like properties [20], we assessed CD24, CD29, and CD44 ex-pression in HSC-3 cells by flow cytometry. HSC-3 cells, transduced with lentiviral red fluorescent protein (RFP), displayed high levels of CD44 and CD29 expression but

varying levels of CD24 expression. To determine the role of β-catenin on aggressive behavior of OSCC cell subpopula-tions, we used fluorescence-activated cell sorting (FACS) to isolate CD44$^+$CD24^{low}CD29$^+$ and CD44$^+$CD24^{high}CD29$^+$ cells from RFP-expressing HSC-3 cells (Fig. 6d). After sort-ing, CD44$^+$CD24^{low}CD29$^+$, CD44$^+$CD24^{high}CD29$^+$, and un-sorted HSC-3 cells were cultured for 12 h and then treated with either vehicle control (DMSO) or 10 μM ICG-001 for 24 h. Remarkably, untreated CD44$^+$CD24^{high}CD29$^+$ cells showed rapid growth and metastasis within the first 2 h following injection. This was in sharp contrast to CD44$^+$CD24^{low}CD29$^+$ cells ($P = 0.002$, two-tailed t test) and unsorted cells ($P = 0.002$, two-tailed t test), which produced smaller tumors with no detectable metastases until 24 h post-transplantation (Fig. 6e). After 24 h, the CD44$^+$CD24^{high}CD29$^+$ cells exhibited more extensive metastases compared to both the unsorted ($P = 0.001$, two-tailed t test) and CD44$^+$CD24^{low}CD29$^+$ groups ($P = 0.0001$, two-tailed t test). Notably, ICG-001 treatment significantly reduced metastasis of CD44$^+$CD24^{high}CD29$^+$ ($P < 0.0001$, two-tailed t test) and unsorted cells ($P < 0.0001$, two-tailed t test; Fig. 6e), consistent with its pro-posed role in targeting β-catenin activity in immature can-cer cells [20, 24]. Thus, inhibition of β-catenin activity by treatment with ICG-001 virtually eliminated metastasis of CD44$^+$CD24^{high}CD29$^+$ cells in zebrafish embryos, con-firming that β-catenin/CBP-mediated transcriptional ac-tivity was critical for the maintenance of aggressive human OSCC CSCs in vivo.

ICG-001 treatment signature is associated with tumor progression and patient survival in primary human OSCC

To align the activity of genes repressed by ICG-001 with clinically aggressive OSCC, we assessed the derived ICG-001-inhibited gene signature in primary human OSCC samples by querying RNA-sequencing (RNASeq) data from the cancer genome atlas (TCGA). Specifically, we projected the TCGA OSCC data ($n = 352$ samples) in the space of the core ICG-001 inhibition signature de-scribed earlier, thus capturing shared inhibitory activity over broader OSCC phenotypes (see "Methods"). TCGA samples were scored based on the coordinated expres-sion of the signature genes, with a high (low) score cor-responding to coordinated up(down) regulation of the signature genes, which in turn, reflected the level of po-tential ICG-001 inhibition (i.e., the ICG-001 inhibition score) per sample (Fig. 7a). The expectation was that samples with high inhibition score (i.e., with coordinated upregulation of the signature genes) would be more re-sponsive to ICG-001 treatment. Thus, we tested whether ICG-001 inhibition scores were predictive of patient out-come, as measured by the overall survival (OS) estimates for OSCC patients ($n = 318$). Comparison of the survival curves corresponding to patients with high (> median)

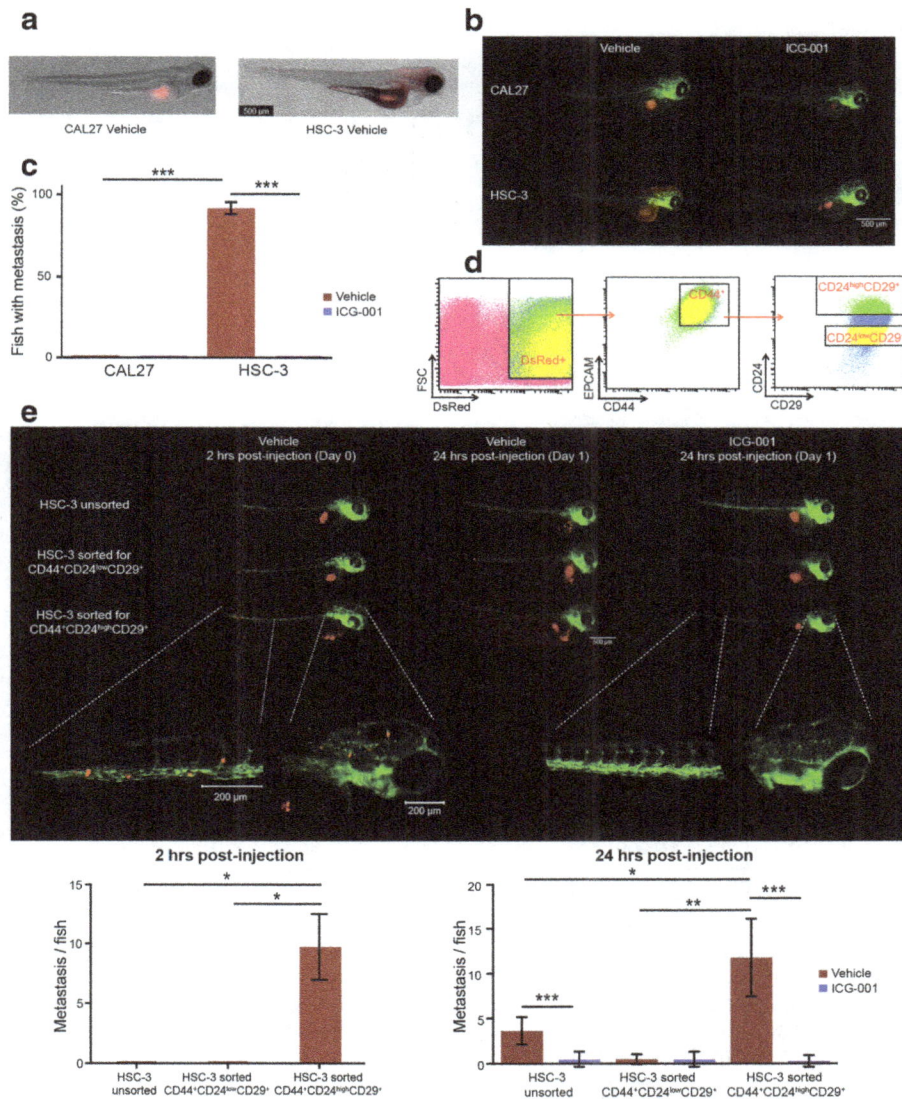

Fig. 6 Zebrafish embryos facilitate rapid detection of an aggressive stem-like subpopulation of OSCC cells and of the effects of ICG-001 inhibition. **a** HSC-3 and CAL27 cells were transduced with a CellTracker™, and 100–200 cells in ~ 1 nL were injected directly into the periviteline space of the embryo. After 24 h, CAL27 cells formed tumors that did not metastasize, whereas HSC-3 cells produced larger tumors that metastasized to the tail and to the craniofacial region. **b** Immunofluorescence imaging of CellTracker™-labeled CAL27 and HSC-3 cells revealed that treatment with ICG-001 inhibited CAL27 cell-driven tumor growth, as well as growth and metastasis of HSC-3-derived tumors. **c** Percent of injected fish exhibiting metastasis was quantified and displayed as the mean (± S.D.) per cell type and per treatment group. Majority of vehicle-treated HSC-3-driven tumors ($n = 86$) metastasized relative to vehicle-treated CAL27-driven tumors ($n = 68$). ICG-001 treatment prior to injection resulted in a significant reduction in percent fish displaying HSC-3-driven metastasis ($n = 104$). **d** Identification of subpopulations of RFP-transduced HSC-3 cells with primitive antigenic cell markers CD44$^+$CD24^{high}CD29$^+$ by flow cytometry. **e** Subpopulations of CD44$^+$CD24^{high}CD29$^+$ and CD44$^+$CD24^{low}CD29$^+$ cells were isolated by FACS, grown in culture for 12 h followed by treatment with either DMSO (vehicle) control or ICG-001 for 24 h. Unsorted HSC-3 cells were used as control. Immunofluorescence imaging of tumor xenografts derived from unsorted RFP HSC-3 cells ($n = 3$), RFP CD44$^+$CD24^{low}CD29$^+$ cells ($n = 3$), or CD44$^+$CD24^{high}CD29$^+$ cells ($n = 3$) revealed that only CD44$^+$CD24^{high}CD29$^+$ cells formed tumors that metastasized rapidly within 2 h to the tail and craniofacial regions (left panel). After 24 h, metastases were detected from tumors derived from CD44$^+$CD24^{high}CD29$^+$ ($n = 5$) as well as unsorted cells ($n = 6$), and to a much lesser extent, from CD44$^+$CD24^{low}CD29$^+$ cells ($n = 6$; middle panel). We note that a substantial population of zebrafish injected with CD44$^+$CD24^{high}CD29$^+$ cells died within the 24 h (middle panel). Treatment of CD44$^+$CD24^{high}CD29$^+$ cells ($n = 11$) as well as unsorted cells ($n = 6$) with ICG-001 inhibited tumor growth and significantly abrogated metastases (right panel). In each case, metastasis was quantified as number of metastasis per fish (see "Methods"), and displayed as the mean (± S.D.). *$P < 0.01$; **$P < 0.001$; ***$P < 0.0001$; unpaired t test

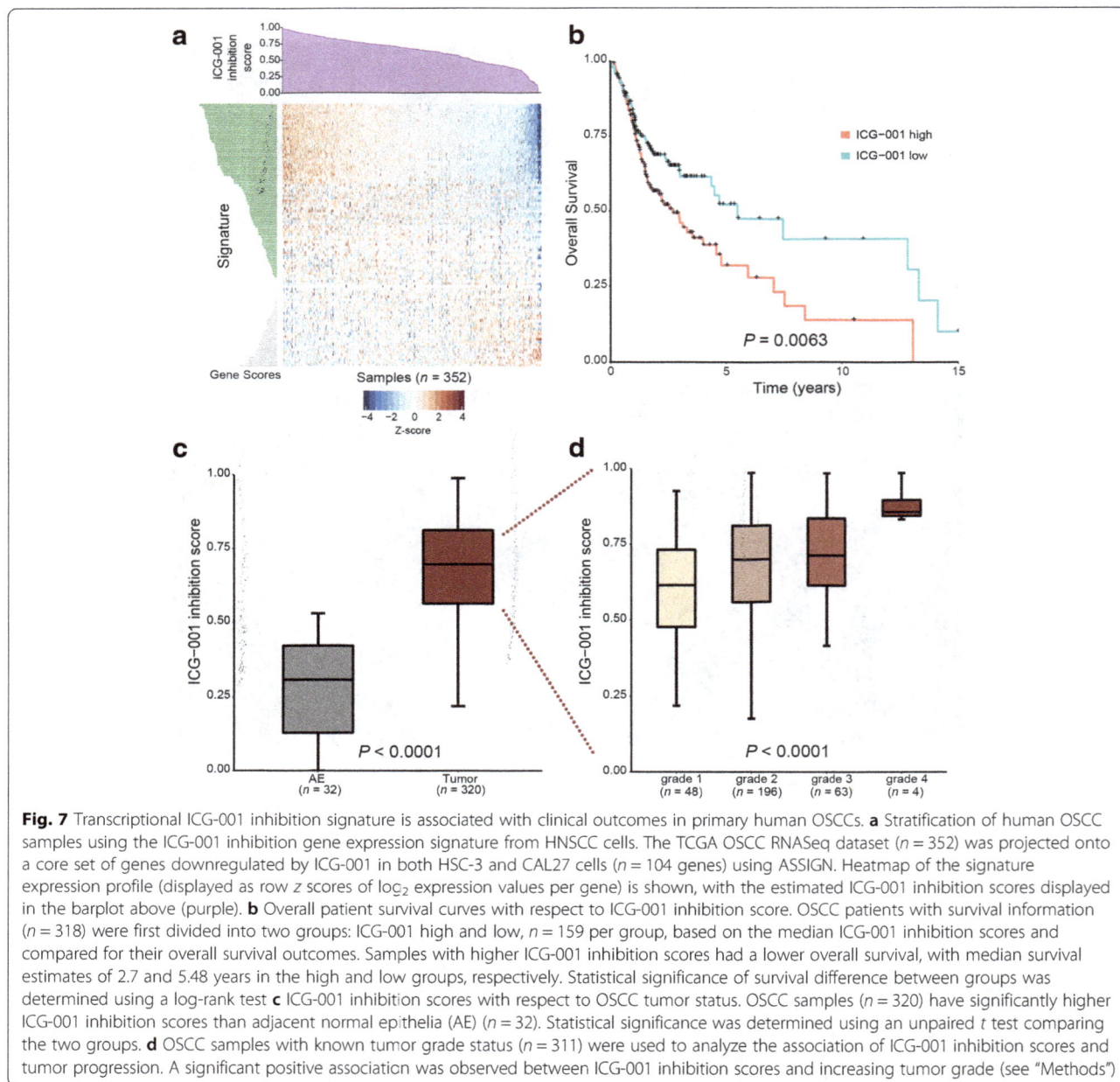

Fig. 7 Transcriptional ICG-001 inhibition signature is associated with clinical outcomes in primary human OSCCs. **a** Stratification of human OSCC samples using the ICG-001 inhibition gene expression signature from HNSCC cells. The TCGA OSCC RNASeq dataset ($n = 352$) was projected onto a core set of genes downregulated by ICG-001 in both HSC-3 and CAL27 cells ($n = 104$ genes) using ASSIGN. Heatmap of the signature expression profile (displayed as row z scores of $\log_2$ expression values per gene) is shown, with the estimated ICG-001 inhibition scores displayed in the barplot above (purple). **b** Overall patient survival curves with respect to ICG-001 inhibition score. OSCC patients with survival information ($n = 318$) were first divided into two groups: ICG-001 high and low, $n = 159$ per group, based on the median ICG-001 inhibition scores and compared for their overall survival outcomes. Samples with higher ICG-001 inhibition scores had a lower overall survival, with median survival estimates of 2.7 and 5.48 years in the high and low groups, respectively. Statistical significance of survival difference between groups was determined using a log-rank test **c** ICG-001 inhibition scores with respect to OSCC tumor status. OSCC samples ($n = 320$) have significantly higher ICG-001 inhibition scores than adjacent normal epithelia (AE) ($n = 32$). Statistical significance was determined using an unpaired t test comparing the two groups. **d** OSCC samples with known tumor grade status ($n = 311$) were used to analyze the association of ICG-001 inhibition scores and tumor progression. A significant positive association was observed between ICG-001 inhibition scores and increasing tumor grade (see "Methods")

or low (≤ median) ICG-001 inhibition scores showed a significantly lower OS in the former group (Fig. 7b; $P = 0.0063$, log-rank test), with median survival estimates of 2.7 and 5.48 years in the high and low groups, respectively. This confirmed that the ICG-001 inhibition signature was predictive of patient prognosis in OSCC and suggested that patients with high inhibition scores were likely to be responsive to the treatment targeting β-catenin/CBP activity. Furthermore, comparison of the ICG-001 inhibition scores in OSCCs ($n = 320$) versus normal adjacent epithelial (AE) samples ($n = 32$) yielded significantly higher scores in OSCCs than in AE's (Fig. 7c;

$P < 0.0001$, two-tailed t test), thus showing that ICG-001 inhibition was associated with tumor status. We then assessed samples with known tumor grade information ($n = 311$) to determine the association between ICG-001 inhibition scores and tumor progression. Remarkably, ICG-001 inhibition scores were found to significantly increase with advanced tumor grade (Fig. 7d; combined $P < 0.0001$), suggesting a correlation with tumor progression. Taken together, these results show that higher inhibition scores in primary tissues are associated with tumor status and positively associated with tumor progression and suggest that more aggressive/advanced tumors would be more responsive/susceptible to inhibition by ICG-001.

Discussion

Identifying oncogenic activities that drive HNSCC and represent bona fide therapeutic targets is paramount to finding effective treatments for patients with this malignancy. The challenge to identifying new biomarkers and targets for therapeutic interventions is exacerbated by the intra-tumoral heterogeneity of HNSCC and diversity of anatomical sites and subsites, many with different underlying biology. Emerging computational methodologies coupled with genomic analyses have provided powerful tools for the identification of molecular circuitries, new druggable targets, and biomarkers relevant to disease progression and treatment response. We have reported previously that integrating in vitro treatment signatures with high-throughput data from consortia such as the TCGA network facilitated decoding their significance in OSCC when coupled with functional analyses [40, 49]. Here, we applied computational approaches to interrogate gene expression signatures in response to the disruption of β-catenin-CBP interaction with a small molecule antagonist, ICG-001, in OSCC cell lines and to align them with patho-clinical features of human OSCC tumors. We further validate anti-tumor effects of ICG-001 in vivo using tumor xenografts in zebrafish and mouse models and show that this antagonist of β-catenin/CBP activity specifically targets subpopulations of cells expressing stem-like cell surface markers. Our studies highlight the significance of β-catenin/CBP signaling in the pathobiology of OSCC and suggest that inhibition of β-catenin-CBP activity with ICG-001 promotes epithelial differentiation program. By investigating TCGA OSCCs, we demonstrate that gene expression changes resulting from ICG-001 inhibition are associated with higher tumor grade and lower overall survival, suggesting that transcriptional signature associated with the disruption of β-catenin-CBP interaction has prognostic value. Our work provides new evidence for the feasibility of using inhibitors of β-catenin/CBP activity for the treatment of head and neck cancer patients.

One important outcome of this study is the identification of a shared transcriptional program associated with the inhibition of β-catenin/CBP with ICG-001 in OSCC. Using microarray data from CCLE, we show that the core ICG-001 inhibition signature derived from OSCC cells can be used to predict sensitivity of additional cell lines to ICG-001 based on coordinated expression of these core genes. To this end, we show that pharyngeal SCC FaDu cells are indeed sensitive to ICG-001, although not all gene products we show to be repressed by this antagonist in OSCC HSC-3 cells are altered in FaDu cells, suggesting cell- and tumor site-specific

differences. Nonetheless, similar to OSCC CAL27 and HSC-3 cells, the ICG-001 treatment led to downregulation of the CBP steady-state levels in FaDu cells. The acetyltransferase activity of CBP promotes an open chromatin structure by acetylation of histone and non-histone proteins [50], and when complexed with β-catenin, it induces the expression of stem-like, proliferation and survival genes [20]. Thus, inhibition of β-catenin/CBP signaling by ICG-001 would be expected to counteract epigenetic changes aligned with immature states and promote a chromatin structure associated with cellular differentiation. Accordingly, our genomic and biochemical analyses show that in OSCC cell lines, ICG-001 suppresses stem cell-like and survival markers and enhances the expression of epithelial differentiation genes. Besides CLDN1, CLDN4, CDH4, and ICAM1, ICG-001 induced the expression of additional genes associated with epithelial differentiation, including SLP1, KLK7, KLK10, and KRT7 in HSC-3 cells [51]. In mouse models of tongue OSCC, ICG-001 inhibited invasive tumor growth and promoted a capsular phenotype along with cellular characteristics consistent with enhanced intercellular adhesion that accompanies cellular differentiation. Further, ICG-001 abrogated the ability of subpopulations of human OSCC cells with stem cell-like properties to induce rapid tumor formation and metastases in zebrafish. Notably, the ICG-001 treatment-associated inhibition signature stratified primary OSCCs based on tumor grade and overall survival. We thus hypothesize that the ICG-001 inhibition signature represents a transcriptional program of patients more likely to respond to the inhibitor. Although current diagnoses and treatment decisions for patients with HNSCC rely on tumor stage rather than grade, recent single-cell RNA–sequencing-based characterization of human HNSCCs revealed a new partial epithelial-to-mesenchymal transition program associated with loco-regional invasion and metastases, as well as higher tumor grade but not tumor size [51]. Further, epithelial differentiation was negatively associated with metastases. Therefore, our observation that ICG-001 inhibition signatures track with tumor grade may prove important to future therapies.

Another novel finding from this study is that disruption of the β-catenin-CBP interaction with ICG-001 in OSCC cell lines destabilizes CBP without greatly affecting E-cadherin or β-catenin transcript or protein levels. Previous analyses mapped the binding of ICG-001 to the 111N-terminal amino acids of CBP, required for the interaction with the C-terminal domain of β-catenin to induce TCF/LEF-mediated expression of target genes [25]. Given that CBP is involved in the co-activation of different transcription factors, these mapping studies revealed a selectivity of ICG-001 for a fraction of genes impacted by the interaction of CBP with β-catenin. The dramatic inhibition of CBP levels by ICG-001 in OSCC and pharyngeal SCC cell lines suggests that these cells depend on β-catenin-CBP signaling for proliferation and survival. CBP has been suggested to be rate limiting in its transcriptional activities [25], although how the steady-state levels of CBP align with aggressive HNSCC cell phenotypes is unclear. While further investigation is needed to determine the exact mechanism underlying downregulation of nuclear CBP protein levels by ICG-001, our studies suggest that the binding of its N-terminal region to β-catenin provides protection from degradation.

In addition to directly inhibiting β-catenin/CBP signaling, our studies show that ICG-001 affects activities of other pathways that converge on the Wnt/β-catenin pathway. We have previously demonstrated that the transcriptional activities of two Hippo pathway effectors, YAP and its paralog TAZ, track with OSCC development and progression to advanced state [49]. GSEA of the YAP/TAZ-associated signature revealed a significant positive correlation between ICG-001 treatment and YAP/TAZ knockdown in HSC-3 cells (Additional file 1: Figure S8b; FDR $q < 0.001$), suggesting potential convergence between YAP/TAZ and CBP and/or β-catenin in OSCC [52]. Moreover, in our prior studies, we showed that Wnt/β-catenin signaling contributed to the induction of the Wnt/Planar Cell Polarity (Wnt/PCP) pathway in oral cancer [32]. Thus, it is likely that ICG-001 also interferes with the Wnt/PCP pathway along with its associated oncogenic features.

The effects of ICG-001 inhibition in OSCC resemble those initially described in colorectal cancer (CRC) with some exceptions. Similar to OSCC, ICG-001 inhibited β-catenin/TCF signaling and reduced CRC cell growth in vitro and in nude mouse xenografts in vivo. Furthermore, in CRC cell lines, ICG-001 inhibited the expression of the *BIRC5* gene product, survivin, coincident with upregulation of caspase 3 activity [25]. While *BIRC5* transcript and survivin protein levels were inhibited by ICG-001 in OSCC cell lines, we did not detect apoptosis or increased caspase 3 levels, indicating that in OSCC, ICG-001 was cytostatic. Also, analogous to OSCC, ICG-001 did not impact β-catenin levels in CRC cell lines but, unlike OSCC, ICG-001 did not inhibit CBP levels, indicating tumor tissue-specific differences in response to this inhibitor.

Current FDA-approved targeted therapies for HNSCC are limited to cetuximab, a monoclonal antibody directed at the epidermal growth factor receptor (EGFR), and pembrolizumab and nivolumab, anti-programmed cell death-1 (PD-1) targeted immunotherapies [53]. These therapies have modest clinical response rates, and there are few biomarkers available to predict response. Our genomic and functional analyses provide evidence that β-catenin/CBP activity plays a pivotal role in the pathobiology of OSCC and is associated with poor clinical outcomes. Given that no inhibitors of β-catenin activity have entered clinical trials for the treatment of head and neck cancer, our studies may facilitate the development of therapies targeting β-catenin/CBP activity in human patients.

Conclusions

Although HNSCC is a devastating disease that continues to mount a major global health problem [13, 14], current clinical management of this malignancy remains limited by factors such as treatment-associated morbidity, resistance to conventional therapy, and disease persistence/recurrence [54]. Decoding the underlying molecular mechanisms involved in HNSCC development and progression to aggressive disease is critical to the discovery of new druggable targets and effective treatment paradigms. Using cellular and animal models, as well as human data, we highlight the contribution of the β-catenin/CBP signaling axis to HNSCC and provide evidence that targeting this signaling activity may be a useful strategy to intercept this malignancy.

Additional files

Additional file 1: Document describing Supplemental Materials and Methods, also including **Table S1.** and **Figures S1-S8.**

Additional file 2: Tabular spreadsheet file containing both table of differential gene expression results comparing ICG-001 treatment ($n = 3$) versus DMSO (vehicle) control ($n = 3$) in HSC-3 and CAL27 OSCC cell lines, as well as the ICG-001 treatment gene expression signatures derived thereof (see manuscript "Methods").

Additional file 3: Tabular ranked gene list file (viewable in Excel) pertaining to differential gene expression testing comparing siRNA-mediated knockdown of β-catenin versus scrambled siRNA control in HSC-3 cells used for GSEA. Fields indicate gene symbol and t test statistic of differential expression, respectively, used as input to the pre-ranked GSEA tool.

Abbreviations
ASSIGN: Adaptive Signature Selection and Integration; CBP: cAMP response element-binding (CREB)-binding protein; CCLE: Cancer Cell Line Encyclopedia; CSCs: Cancer stem cells; FDR: False discovery rate; GSEA: Gene Set Enrichment Analysis; HNSCC: Head and neck squamous cell carcinoma; OS: Overall survival; OSCC: Oral squamous cell carcinoma; RNASeq: RNA-sequencing; SCC: Squamous cell carcinoma; TCGA: The Cancer Genome Atlas; UAT: Upper aerodigestive tract

Acknowledgements
We acknowledge dbGap for granting access to the TCGA data (phs000178.v9.p8) and the BUMC Flow Cytometry and CTSI Core facilities for providing services related to cell sorting and microarray gene expression profiling, respectively.

Funding
This study was supported by the National Institutes of Health grants R01DE015304 (MAK), F31DE025536 (VKK), R01DE025340 (SIP), R01HL124392 (XV), and R03DE025274 (MVB). Additional funding was provided by the Evans Center for Interdisciplinary Biomedical Research Affinity Research Collaborative no. 9950000118 (MAK). We further acknowledge funding from the Clinical and Translational Science Institute (supported by Clinical and Translational Research Award CTSA grant UL1-TR001430) for microarray experiments and in vitro assays (AME). Funding sources

played no role in the design of the study and collection, analysis, and interpretation of data and in the writing of the manuscript.

Authors' contributions
MAK, SM, and VKK conceived and designed the study. VKK, SM, KAA, ACB, JESC, MVB, AME, FL, HF, and SIP developed the methodology of the study. VKK, KAA, KS, BCN, AME, MVB, ACB, FL, JL, and SIP acquired the data (cellular, mice, zebrafish, flow cytometry) of the study. VKK, KAA, MVB, FL, AME, SM, and MAK analyzed and interpreted the data (statistical and computational analyses) of the study. VKK, KAA, SM, XV, AME, ACB, JESC, HF, MAK, and SIP contributed to the writing, review, and revision of the study. KS, BCN, SM, and MAK helped in the administrative, technical, and material support of the study. VKK, KAA, SM, and MAK supervised the study. All authors read and approved the final manuscript.

Competing interests
The authors declare that they have no competing interests.

Author details
[1]Bioinformatics Program, Boston University, Boston, MA, USA. [2]Division of Computational Biomedicine, Boston University School of Medicine, Boston, MA, USA. [3]Department of Molecular and Cell Biology, Goldman School of Dental Medicine, Boston University School of Medicine, 72 East Concord Street, E4, Boston, MA 02118, USA. [4]Department of Pharmacology & Experimental Therapeutics, Boston University School of Medicine, Boston, MA, USA. [5]Department of Surgery, Massachusetts General Hospital, Harvard Medical School, Boston, MA, USA. [6]Department of Biochemistry, Boston University School of Medicine, Boston, MA, USA. [7]Department of Surgery, Brigham and Women's Hospital, Boston, MA, USA. [8]Flow Cytometry Core Facility, Boston University School of Medicine, Boston, MA, USA. [9]Department of Microbiology, Boston University School of Medicine, Boston, MA, USA.

References
1. Nusse R, Clevers H. Wnt/β-catenin signaling, disease, and emerging therapeutic modalities. Cell. 2017;169:985–99. Elsevier Inc. Available from: http://dx.doi.org/10.1016/j.cell.2017.05.016
2. Lien WH, Fuchs E. Wnt some lose some: transcriptional governance of stem cells by Wnt/β-catenin signaling. Genes Dev. 2014;28:1517–32.
3. Wend P, Holland JD, Ziebold U, Birchmeier W. Wnt signaling in stem and cancer cells. Semin Cell Dev Biol. 2010;21:855–63.
4. Zhan T, Rindtorff N, Boutros M. Wnt signaling in cancer. Oncogene; 2016; 4(5). Nature Publishing Group. Available from: http://cshperspectives.cshlp.org/content/4/5/a008052.long%5Cnhttp://www.nature.com/doifinder/10.1038/onc.2016.304
5. Brembeck FH, Rosário M, Birchmeier W. Balancing cell adhesion and Wnt signaling, the key role of beta-catenin. Curr. Opin. Genet. Dev. 2006;16:51–9. Available from: http://www.ncbi.nlm.nih.gov/pubmed/16377174
6. Castilho RM, Gutkind JS. The Wnt/β-catenin signaling circuitry in head and neck cancer; 2014. p. 199–214.
7. Zhou, G. Wnt/β-catenin signaling and oral cancer metastasis. In Oral Cancer Metastasis. Springer New York. 2010;pp. 231–64. https://doi.org/10.1007/978-1-4419-0775-2_11.
8. Morin PJ, Sparks AB, Korinek V, Barker N, Clevers H, Vogelstein B, et al. Activation of β-catenin-Tcf signaling in colon cancer by mutations in β-catenin or APC. Science. 1997;275: 1784–90.
9. Haraguchi K, Ohsugi M, Abe Y, Semba K, Akiyama T, Yamamoto T. Ajuba negatively regulates the Wnt signaling pathway by promoting GSK-3beta-mediated phosphorylation of beta-catenin. Oncogene. 2008; 27:274–84.
10. TCGA Network. Comprehensive genomic characterization of head and neck squamous cell carcinomas. Nature. 2015;517:576–82. Available from: http://www.nature.com/doifinder/10.1038/nature14129
11. Padhi S, Saha A, Kar M, Ghosh C, Adhya A, Baisakh M, et al. Clinico-pathological correlation of β-catenin and telomere dysfunction in head and neck squamous cell carcinoma patients. J Cancer. 2015;6:192–202. Available from: http://www.jcancer.org/v06p0192.htm
12. Rothenberg SM, Ellisen LW. The molecular pathogenesis of head and neck squamous cell carcinoma. J Clin Invest. 2012;122:1951–7. Available from: http://www.pubmedcentral.nih.gov/articlerender.fcgi?artid=3589176&tool=pmcentrez&rendertype=abstract
13. Siegel R, Miller K, Jemal A. Cancer statistics , 2015. CA Cancer J Clin. 2015;65: 29. Available from: http://onlinelibrary.wiley.com/doi/10.3322/caac.21254/pdf
14. Rosebush MS, Rao SK, Samant S, Gu W, Handorf CR, Pfeffer LM, et al. Oral cancer: enduring characteristics and emerging trends. J Tenn Dent Assoc. 2011;91:24–7. quiz 28-29
15. Lee SH, Koo BS, Kim JM, Huang S, Rho YS, Bae WJ, et al. Wnt/β-catenin signalling maintains self-renewal and tumourigenicity of head and neck squamous cell carcinoma stem-like cells by activating Oct4. J Pathol. 2014; 234:99–107.
16. Visvader JE, Lindeman GJ. Cancer stem cells: current status and evolving complexities. Cell Stem Cell. 2012;10(6):717–28. https://doi.org/10.1016/j.stem.2012.05.007
17. Shiozawa Y, Nie B, Pienta KJ, Morgan TM, Taichman RS. Cancer stem cells and their role in metastasis. Pharmacol Ther. 2013;138:285–93. Available from: http://www.sciencedirect.com/science/article/pii/S0163725813000260
18. Holland JD, Klaus A, Garratt AN, Birchmeier W. Wnt signaling in stem and cancer cells. Curr Opin Cell Biol. 2013;25:254–64.
19. Song J, Chang I, Chen Z, Kang M, Wang CY. Characterization of side populations in HNSCC: highly invasive, chemoresistant and abnormal Wnt signaling. PLoS One. 2010;5. https://doi.org/10.1371/journal.pone.0011456
20. Wend P, Fang L, Zhu Q, Schipper JH, Loddenkemper C, Kosel F, et al. Wnt/β-catenin signalling induces MLL to create epigenetic changes in salivary gland tumours. EMBO J. 2013;32:1977–89. Available from: http://www.pubmedcentral.nih.gov/articlerender.fcgi?artid=3715856&tool=pmcentrez&rendertype=abstract
21. Krishnamurthy N, Kurzrock R. Targeting the Wnt/beta-catenin pathway in cancer: update on effectors and inhibitors. Cancer Treat. Rev. 2018;62:50–60. Elsevier Ltd. Available from: https://doi.org/10.1016/j.ctrv.2017.11.002
22. Anastas JN, Moon RT. WNT signalling pathways as therapeutic targets in cancer. Nat. Rev. Cancer. 2013;13:11–26. Available from: http://www.ncbi.nlm.nih.gov/pubmed/23258168
23. Voronkov A, Krauss S. Wnt/beta-catenin signaling and small molecule inhibitors. Curr Pharm Des. 2013;19:634–64.
24. Kahn M. Can we safely target the WNT pathway? Nat. Rev. Drug Discov. 2014;13:513–32. Nature Publishing Group. Available from: http://dx.doi.org/10.1038/nrd4233
25. Emami KH, Nguyen C, Ma H, Kim DH, Jeong KW, Eguchi M, et al. A small molecule inhibitor of β-catenin/CREB-binding protein transcription. Proc Natl Acad Sci. 2004;101:12682–87.
26. Arensman MD, Telesca D, Lay AR, Kershaw KM, Wu N, Donahue TR, et al. The CREB-binding protein inhibitor ICG-001 suppresses pancreatic cancer growth. Mol. Cancer Ther. 2014;13:2303–14. Available from: http://www.ncbi.nlm.nih.gov/pubmed/25082960
27. Stiles BLG. Inhibiting the expansion of hepatic cancer stem cells by targeting beta-catenin/CBP interaction with ICG-001 in liver Pten deficient mice. Cancer Res. 2011;Conference.
28. Sasaki T, Hwang H, Nguyen C, Kloner RA, Kahn M. The small molecule Wnt signaling modulator ICG-001 improves contractile function in chronically infarcted rat myocardium. PLoS One. 2013;8. http://journals.plos.org/plosone/article?id=10.1371/journal.pone.00750h0.
29. Grigson ER, Ozerova M, Pisklakova V, Liu H, Sullivan DM, Nefedova Y. Canonical Wnt pathway inhibitor ICG-001 induces cytotoxicity of multiple myeloma cells in Wnt-independent manner. PLoS One. 2015;10. http://journahs.plos.org/plosone/article?id=10.1371/journal.pone.0117693.
30. Lafyatis R, Mantero JC, Gordon J, Kishore N, Carns M, Dittrich H, et al. Inhibition of β-catenin signaling in the skin rescues cutaneous adipogenesis in systemic sclerosis: a randomized, double-blind, placebo-controlled trial of C-82. J Invest Dermatol. 2017;137:2473–83.
31. Chan KC, Chan LS, Ip JCY, Lo C, Yip TTC, Ngan RKC, et al. Therapeutic targeting of CBP/β-catenin signaling reduces cancer stem-like population and synergistically suppresses growth of EBV-positive nasopharyngeal carcinoma cells with cisplatin. Sci Rep. 2015;5. https://www.nature.com/articles/srep09979.

32. Liu G, Sengupta PK, Jamal B, Yang HY, Bouchie MP, Lindner V, et al. N-glycosylation induces the CTHRC1 protein and drives oral cancer cell migration. J Biol Chem. 2013;288:20217–27.

33. Lin KY, Guarnieri FG, Staveley-O'Carroll KF, Levitsky HI, August JT, Pardoll DM, et al. Treatment of established tumors with a novel vaccine that enhances major histocompatibility class II presentation of tumor antigen. Cancer Res. 1996;56:21–6.

34. Kim TW, Hung C-F, Kim JW, Juang J, Chen P-J, He L, et al. Vaccination with a DNA vaccine encoding herpes simplex virus type 1 VP22 linked to antigen generates long-term antigen-specific CD8-positive memory T cells and protective immunity. Hum Gene Ther. 2004;15:167–77.

35. Westerfield M. The zebrafish book. A guide for the laboratory use of zebrafish (*Danio rerio*). 5th ed. Eugene: Univ. Oregon Press; 2007.

36. Nicoli S, Presta M. The zebrafish/tumor xenograft angiogenesis assay. Nat. Protoc. 2007;2:2918–23. Available from: http://www.ncbi.nlm.nih.gov/pubmed/18007628

37. Ritchie ME, Phipson B, Wu D, Hu Y, Law CW, Shi W, et al. limma powers differential expression analyses for RNA-sequencing and microarray studies. Nucleic Acids Res. 2015;43:e47.

38. Benjamini Y, Hochberg Y. Controlling the false discovery rate: a practical and powerful approach to multiple testing. J. R. Stat. Soc. B. 1995;57:289–300. Available from: http://www.stat.purdue.edu/~doerge/BIOINFORM.D/FALL06/Benjamini and Y FDR.pdf%5Cnhttp://engr.case.edu/ray_soumya/mlrg/controlling_fdr_benjamini95.pdf

39. Barretina J, Caponigro G, Stransky N, Venkatesan K, Margolin AA, Kim S, et al. The Cancer Cell Line Encyclopedia enables predictive modelling of anticancer drug sensitivity. Nature. 2012;483:603–7.

40. Kartha VK, Stawski L, Han R, Haines P, Gallagher G, Noonan V, et al. PDGFRβ is a novel marker of stromal activation in oral squamous cell carcinomas. PLoS One. 2016;11:e0154645. Available from: http://journals.plos.org/plosone/article?id=10.1371/journal.pone.0154645

41. Shen Y, Rahman M, Piccolo SR, Gusenleitner D, El-Chaar NN, Cheng L, et al. ASSIGN: context-specific genomic profiling of multiple heterogeneous biological pathways. Bioinformatics. 2015;1–9. Available from: http://bioinformatics.oxfordjournals.org/cgi/doi/10.1093/bioinformatics/btv031

42. Dai H, Leeder JS, Cui Y. A modified generalized fisher method for combining probabilities from dependent tests. Front Genet. 2014;5:1–10.

43. Ma H, Nguyen C, Lee K, Kahn M. Differential roles for the coactivators CBP and p300 on TCF/b-catenin-mediated survivin gene expression. Oncogene. 2005;24:3619–31.

44. Alam H, Sehgal L, Kundu ST, Dalal SN, Vaidya MM. Novel function of keratins 5 and 14 in proliferation and differentiation of stratified epithelial cells. Mol. Biol. Cell. 2011;22:4068–78. Available from: http://www.molbiolcell.org/cgi/doi/10.1091/mbc.E10-08-0703

45. Brembeck FH, Rosário M, Birchmeier W. Balancing cell adhesion and Wnt signaling, the key role of β-catenin. Curr Opin Genet Dev. 2006;16:51–9.

46. Bais MV, Kukuruzinska M, Trackman PC. Orthotopic non-metastatic and metastatic oral cancer mouse models. Oral Oncol. 2015;51:476–82.

47. Peng S, Wang JW, Karanam B, Wang C, Huh WK, Alvarez RD, et al. Sequential cisplatin therapy and vaccination with HPV16 E6E7L2 fusion protein in saponin adjuvant GPI-0100 for the treatment of a model HPV16+ cancer. PLoS One. 2015;10:1–25.

48. Ignatius MS, Chen E, Elpek NM, Fuller AZ, Tenente IM, Clagg R, et al. In vivo imaging of tumor-propagating cells, regional tumor heterogeneity, and dynamic cell movements in embryonal rhabdomyosarcoma. Cancer Cell. 2012;21:680–93.

49. Hiemer SE, Zhang L, Kartha VK, Packer TS, Almershed M, Noonan V, et al. A YAP/TAZ-regulated molecular signature is associated with oral squamous cell carcinoma. Mol. Cancer Res. 2015;13:957–68. [cited 2015 Jul 1]. Available from: http://mcr.aacrjournals.org/content/13/6/957.long

50. Ogryzko VV, Schiltz RL, Russanova V, Howard BH, Nakatani Y. The transcriptional coactivators p300 and CBP are histone acetyltransferases. Cell. 1996;87:953–9.

51. Puram SV, Tirosh I, Parikh AS, Patel AP, Yizhak K, Gillespie S, et al. Single-cell transcriptomic analysis of primary and metastatic tumor ecosystems in head and neck cancer. Cell. 2017;171:1611–24. e24. Elsevier Inc. Available from: https://doi.org/10.1016/j.cell.2017.10.044

52. Rosenbluh J, Nijhawan D, Cox AG, Li X, Neal JT, Schafer EJ, et al. β-Catenin-driven cancers require a YAP1 transcriptional complex for survival and tumorigenesis. Cell. 2012;151:1457–73. Elsevier Inc. Available from: http://dx.doi.org/10.1016/j.cell.2012.11.026

53. Moreira J, Tobias A, O'Brien MP, Agulnik M. Targeted therapy in head and neck cancer: an update on current clinical developments in epidermal growth factor receptor-targeted therapy and immunotherapies. Drugs. 2017;77:843–57.

54. Aminuddin A, Ng PY. Promising druggable target in head and neck squamous cell carcinoma: Wnt signaling. Front. Pharmacol. 2016;7:244. Available from: http://www.ncbi.nlm.nih.gov/pubmed/27570510%0Ahttp://www.pubmedcentral.nih.gov/articlerender.fcgi?artid=PMC4982242

5

Increased DNA methylation variability in rheumatoid arthritis-discordant monozygotic twins

Amy P. Webster[1,2]* , Darren Plant[3], Simone Ecker[2], Flore Zufferey[4], Jordana T. Bell[4], Andrew Feber[2,5], Dirk S. Paul[6], Stephan Beck[2], Anne Barton[1,3], Frances M. K. Williams[4†] and Jane Worthington[1,3*†]

Abstract

Background: Rheumatoid arthritis is a common autoimmune disorder influenced by both genetic and environmental factors. Epigenome-wide association studies can identify environmentally mediated epigenetic changes such as altered DNA methylation, which may also be influenced by genetic factors. To investigate possible contributions of DNA methylation to the aetiology of rheumatoid arthritis with minimum confounding genetic heterogeneity, we investigated genome-wide DNA methylation in disease-discordant monozygotic twin pairs.

Methods: Genome-wide DNA methylation was assessed in 79 monozygotic twin pairs discordant for rheumatoid arthritis using the HumanMethylation450 BeadChip array (Illumina). Discordant twins were tested for both differential DNA methylation and methylation variability between rheumatoid arthritis and healthy twins. The methylation variability signature was then compared with methylation variants from studies of other autoimmune diseases and with an independent healthy population.

Results: We have identified a differentially variable DNA methylation signature that suggests multiple stress response pathways may be involved in the aetiology of the disease. This methylation variability signature also highlighted potential epigenetic disruption of multiple RUNX3 transcription factor binding sites as being associated with disease development. Comparison with previously performed epigenome-wide association studies of rheumatoid arthritis and type 1 diabetes identified shared pathways for autoimmune disorders, suggesting that epigenetics plays a role in autoimmunity and offering the possibility of identifying new targets for intervention.

Conclusions: Through genome-wide analysis of DNA methylation in disease-discordant monozygotic twins, we have identified a differentially variable DNA methylation signature, in the absence of differential methylation in rheumatoid arthritis. This finding supports the importance of epigenetic variability as an emerging component in autoimmune disorders.

Keywords: Autoimmune disease, Rheumatoid arthritis, Epigenetics, DNA methylation, Twins

Background

Low disease concordance rates between monozygotic (MZ) twins (~ 15%) have revealed that environmental exposures are important in rheumatoid arthritis (RA) [1]. Many putative environmental risk factors have been investigated, including exposure to cigarette smoke, hormone influences, infection, vitamin D intake and dietary factors [2, 3], but few have been robustly confirmed.

Epigenetics is the study of heritable modifications of DNA which can alter gene expression without changing the DNA sequence and which can be influenced by environmental factors, such as smoking [4]. The most widely studied epigenetic phenomenon is DNA methylation, which may act as a composite measure of numerous environmental exposures, making it an intriguing candidate for investigation of diseases that involve both genetic and environmental factors, such as RA.

* Correspondence: a.webster@ucl.ac.uk; jane.worthington@manchester.ac.uk
†Frances M. K. Williams and Jane Worthington contributed equally to this work.
[1]Arthritis Research UK Centre for Genetics and Genomics, Centre for Musculoskeletal Research, The University of Manchester, Manchester, UK
Full list of author information is available at the end of the article

Current evidence suggests that DNA methylation changes are associated with RA [5–10] but whether this is due to intrinsic genetic differences, which can also influence DNA methylation, is not yet known. Disease-discordant MZ twin pairs offer an ideal study design as they are matched for many factors, including genetic variation and as such they offer a crucial advantage in epigenetic studies [11]. Differences in methylation between MZ twins may capture the effects of environmentally driven mechanisms, independent of genetically driven changes. Two small epigenome-wide association studies (EWAS) of DNA methylation in MZ twins discordant for RA have reported conflicting results. The first ($n = 5$ pairs) identifying no significant changes associated with RA using the GoldenGate assay [12], while the second ($n = 7$ pairs) identified no significant differentially methylated positions (DMPs), but one significantly differentially methylated region (DMR) using the CHARM platform [13]. Due to the small sample sizes of both studies, they were underpowered to detect subtle methylation differences [14] and have limited scope to characterise the epigenomic landscape of RA-discordant twins.

To our knowledge, all studies of DNA methylation in relation to RA have focussed on the identification of DMPs or DMRs, which describe differential DNA methylation levels at a particular CpG site or closely spaced group of CpG sites, respectively. In DMPs and DMRs, one group has a consistently higher level of DNA methylation than the comparison group (e.g. when comparing RA patients with healthy controls). Differentially variable positions (DVPs) are another type of epigenetic variation, the importance of which has recently been elucidated in type 1 diabetes (T1D) and cervical and breast cancer [15–18]. DVPs are CpG sites that do not necessarily have a large difference in mean DNA methylation and therefore may not be classed as DMPs;

however, they have a difference in the range of DNA methylation values between comparison groups.

We have examined genome-wide DNA methylation in both a DMP and DVP context using the Infinium HumanMethylation450 BeadChip array (Illumina) in whole blood from 79 MZ twin pairs discordant for RA from two independent cohorts (Manchester and TwinsUK, see Fig. 1). We identified a DVP signature in the absence of a DMP signature that suggest potential roles for multiple stress response pathways and potential epigenetic disruption of RUNX3 transcription factor binding sites in RA aetiology. We also identified shared DVPs in both RA and T1D, indicating potential shared pathways for autoimmune disorders.

Methods
TwinsUK participants
Twin pairs discordant for RA were identified from the TwinsUK register [19]. RA status was assessed through questionnaires between 1997 and 2002. In addition, an advertisement was published in the National Rheumatoid Arthritis Society newsletter in spring 2013 to recruit twin volunteers with RA. All MZ twins who answered positively were phone-interviewed by a rheumatology clinical fellow to confirm the diagnosis of RA based on the American College of Rheumatology 1987 criteria ($n = 17$ RA twins). In case of unclear diagnosis of RA, participants were reviewed in clinic or were excluded. In addition, all patients willing to attend a visit were examined clinically ($n = 11$ RA twins) by a clinical fellow under the supervision of a consultant rheumatologist. Visits included detailed medical history, review of symptoms, past and present medication (NSAIDS, disease-modifying anti-rheumatic drugs (DMARDS) and/or biological agents) and joint examination. Blood samples were collected from all subjects, from which DNA and serum were extracted and stored at − 80 °C.

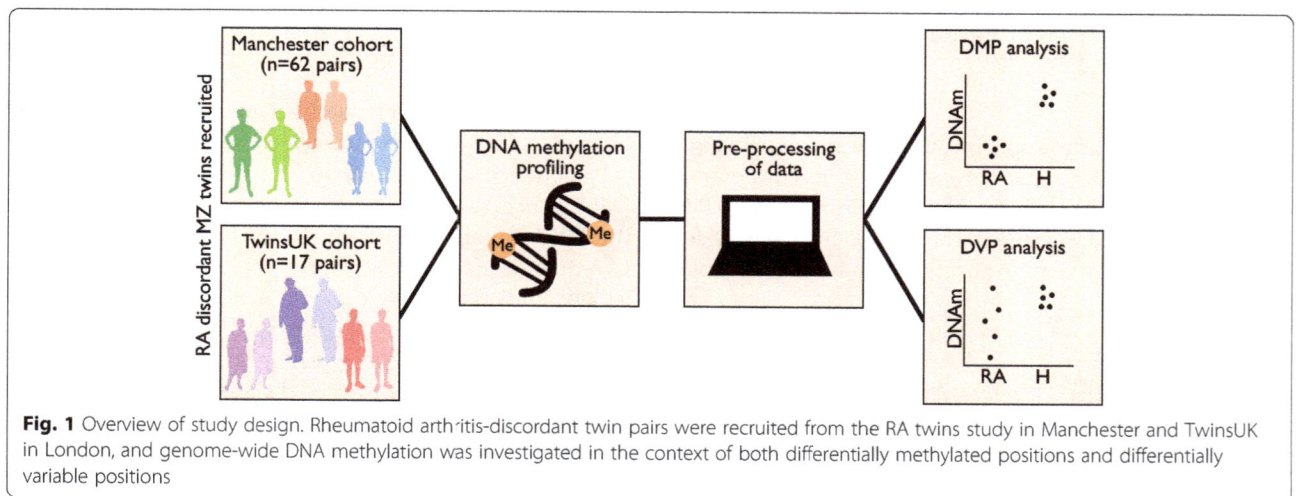

Fig. 1 Overview of study design. Rheumatoid arthritis-discordant twin pairs were recruited from the RA twins study in Manchester and TwinsUK in London, and genome-wide DNA methylation was investigated in the context of both differentially methylated positions and differentially variable positions

The healthy co-twins were also reviewed at the clinical visit. Non-RA status was supported by both clinical and immunological details, as all non-RA twins were seronegative, except one who was rheumatoid factor (RF) positive but clinically unaffected.

Manchester participants

Patients were selected from the Nationwide Rheumatoid Arthritis Twin Study based at the University of Manchester [1]. Twins were recruited in 1989 using a dual strategy: (1) all UK rheumatologists were contacted and requested to ask all of their patients with RA whether they were a twin; (2) a multimedia campaign was targeted to patients in whom RA had been diagnosed and who had a living twin. Both members of each twin pair were visited at home by trained research nurses who recorded each subject's detailed medical history and demographic characteristics and performed joint examinations. Blood samples were collected from all subjects, from which DNA and serum were extracted and stored at − 80 °C.

Measurement of genome-wide DNA methylation

For each sample, 500 ng DNA was bisulfite-converted using EZ DNA methylation kits (ZYMO Research) according to the manufacturer's amended protocol for use with the Infinium HumanMethylation450 BeadChip (Illumina). Epigenome-wide methylation was assessed using the Infinium HumanMethylation450 Assay (Illumina) and the BeadChips were then imaged using the Illumina iScan System.

Quality control and pre-processing of HumanMethylation450 data

All data analysis was performed in R 3.4.1 (R Development Core Team) using the minfi [20], ChAMP [21] and CpGassoc packages [22]. Data quality for each sample was assessed by visual inspection of kernel density plots of methylation beta values and by comparing median log2 intensities recorded in both the methylated and unmethylated channels. Probes which failed a detection p value of 0.01, probes mapping to the sex chromosomes, probes containing a SNP within two base pairs of the measured CpG site, cross reactive probes (according to Norlund, 2013) and probes with a bead count of < 3 in at least 5% of samples were removed prior to analysis. Raw beta values were logit transformed to M values following subset-quantile within array normalisation (SWAN), and principal component analysis (PCA) was performed to capture any potential technical variation. Distinct cell populations are known to have different DNA methylation signatures [23]. Therefore, to assess if cell composition differs between healthy and RA-affected twins, and whether this may confound downstream analysis, we estimated cell composition for each sample using the reference-based Houseman method to infer relative proportions of cells [24]. Differences in cell composition between groups were tested using a Welch two-sample t test. Additionally, we applied the recently developed EpiDISH algorithm to infer cell composition, which confirmed the results obtained by Houseman's algorithm (data not shown) [25].

Identification of differentially methylated positions (DMPs)

A mixed effects model was used to test for DMPs from beta values using the CpGassoc package, adjusting for sibling-pair effects as a random covariate. Factors associated with the first four principal components (PCs) were included in the model as fixed covariates. False discovery rate was calculated using the Benjamini and Hochberg method [26], and a significance threshold of 0.05 was used. Power to detect differential DNA methylation was estimated using the calculations presented in [14], with genome-wide significance threshold set to 1E–06 and the false discovery rate controlled at 0.05.

Identification of differentially variable positions (DVPs)

Differential DNA methylation variability was tested in the current study using the recently developed iEVORA algorithm [16], which employs a modified version of Bartlett's test to test for differences in variability, in combination with a standard t test to subsequently rank the identified DVPs. A significance q value threshold of 0.001 was applied for the differential variability test, while a significance p value threshold of 0.05 was applied for the differential means.

Assessment of DVP signature in an independent healthy population

In order to assess if the DVP signature identified between RA-discordant twins was present in an independent healthy cohort, methylation variability was assessed in the BIOS cohort described in [27]. Briefly, this dataset consisted of HumanMethylation450 profiles generated from three Dutch cohorts, from which 156 profiles were randomly selected to test methylation variability at the DVP sites. The variance and range of methylation values were calculated for each CpG site in the DVP signature, stratified by directionality of variability in the signature (i.e. if DVPs were hypervariable in healthy or RA twins).

Feature enrichment analysis

To investigate if DVPs identified in RA-discordant twins were enriched in particular CpG island-associated features, or in certain gene features, an enrichment analysis was performed. All CpG sites included in analysis were annotated using the HumanMethylation450 manifest. Repeated random sampling (n = 1000) of all probes that passed quality control was used to assess enrichment of features associated with DVPs [28].

Pathway analysis

Pathway analysis was performed within the MissMethyl package [29] using the gometh function. Methylation arrays have a significant bias in pathway analysis due to the differential distribution of probes across different genes [30]. For example, on the HumanMethylation450 BeadChip (Illumina), the number of probes on each gene represented on the array ranges from 1 to 1299. Consequently, during standard pathway analyses, genes with a large number of probes present on the array are more likely to be implicated in significant pathways. The MissMethyl package adjusts for such bias using a modified hypergeometric test to test for over-representation of the selected genes in each gene set. Pathways were ranked by p value for over-representation of the gene ontology terms ($p < 0.05$). False discovery rate (FDR) correction was not applied because biological pathways are not independent from each other, and the FDR procedure is only valid when tests are independent [26]. Additionally, we performed gene set enrichment analysis [31] on DVP-associated genes to corroborate top-ranked pathways.

Overlap analyses

Using a meta-analysis approach, the DVPs from the current study were compared with DVPs and DMPs identified in previously performed large-scale EWAS of various autoimmune disorders. Studies were selected that had performed a site-specific genome-wide study of DNA methylation (e.g. using methylation microarrays) in an autoimmune disease, with at least 100 individuals included in the study. The two qualifying studies focussed on T1D [15] in a discordant MZ twin approach, and RA [7] in an unrelated case-control approach. Lists of statistically significant DVPs ($q < 0.001$) and DMPs (Bonferroni corrected $p < 0.05$) respectively reported in each study were overlapped with DVPs identified in the current study. This allowed identification of DVPs which were common across different diseases and different study designs.

Results

Patient characteristics

DNA samples from 79 MZ twin pairs discordant for RA were available from the Nationwide Rheumatoid Arthritis Twin Study ($n = 62$ twin pairs) and from the TwinsUK cohort ($n = 17$ twin pairs). Patient characteristics are summarised in Table 1. There was no significant difference regarding smoking status between RA and non-RA co-twins ($p = 0.53$). Of the RA co-twins in the study, 59% were seropositive (anti-CCP and/or RF),

Table 1 Characteristics of the RA-discordant twin pairs

Characteristic	RA ($n = 79$)	Non-RA ($n = 79$)	p value
*Age (years), mean (SD)	54.2 (12.2)	54.2 (12.2)	
Female, n (%)	67 (86)	67 (86)	
*Disease duration (years), median (IQR)	9.8 (5.1, 17.2)	–	
Anti-CCP and/or RF positive, n (%)	46 (59%)	7 (9%)	
*DMARDs, n (%)	41 (52%)	–	
Smoking status			0.53
Current, n (%)	15(19)	12 (16)	
Past, n (%)	26 (33)	22(28)	
Never, n (%)	37(49)	44 (56)	
**Cell type			
CD8T	0.05	0.05	0.73
CD4T	0.24	0.19	0.16
Natural killer	0.06	0.06	0.99
B cell	0.06	0.05	0.61
Monocyte	0.08	0.07	0.15
Granulocyte	0.51	0.57	0.25

*At sampling
**Estimated from the DNA methylation data

whereas 9% of the non-RA twins were RF positive. Of the RA co-twins, 52% were taking disease-modifying anti-rheumatic drugs (DMARDs) at the time of the blood sampling, with the most prescribed being methotrexate ($n = 9$). Other commonly prescribed mono- or bi-therapy DMARDs included penicillamine ($n = 8$), gold ($n = 8$), sulphasalazine ($n = 7$) and hydroxychloroquine ($n = 5$), reflecting the prescribing practices at the time when the data was collected for the larger group of twins. Treatment with DMARDs was not associated with any of the top 20 principal components, and during assessment with multidimensional scaling of the top 1000 most variable probes, treatment with DMARDs did not separate out different groups (Additional file 1: Figure S1); therefore, it was not adjusted for in the analysis. This study had > 80% power to detect a mean methylation difference of 4% and 13% between the RA and non-RA twins, at the 5% and genome-wide significance threshold, respectively.

DMP analysis

Following stringent probe filtering, 430,780 probes were available for further analyses in the dataset. Potential confounding factors including gender, age, smoking habits, cell composition, cohort, position on array and BeadChip ID were all included as covariates in the linear regression. None of the probes investigated were significantly differentially methylated between the RA and non-RA twins following correction for multiple testing, using a false discovery rate threshold of 0.05. The mean difference in methylation between RA-discordant twins for the probes with the smallest adjusted p values ($p >$ 0.13) was less than 4% (Table 2). To assess the influence of differences in cell type composition on the epigenetic profiles, we inferred differential cell type proportions based on the DNA methylation data [24]. Proportions of each cell type were compared between the two comparison groups, and there were no significant differences ($p > 0.15$) in cellular composition between RA and healthy co-twins (Table 1, Additional file 1: Figure S2). Furthermore, adjustment for cell composition during DMP detection did not affect the results qualitatively.

Rheumatoid arthritis associated DVPs

Variability of DNA methylation has been implicated in T1D and cervical and breast cancer [15–17]. We used the recently developed iEVORA algorithm [16] to test if DNA methylation variability was significantly associated with RA status between disease-discordant MZ twins. In a group-wise test for differential variability between RA-discordant MZ twins, 1171 DVPs were identified at a stringent false discovery rate of < 0.001. An example of the six top-ranked DVPs is shown in Fig. 2 and the annotation of the top 20 DVPs is summarised in Table 3

(full list of DVPs provided in Additional file 2: Table S1). These DVPs were enriched in CpG sites that did not map to CpG islands and were enriched in the body and 3′UTR of genes (Additional file 1: Figure S3).

Of the 1171 DVPs, 763 were hypervariable in the RA twins, indicating an enrichment of methylation variability in disease-affected individuals. DVPs that were hypervariable in RA twins were enriched in the 3′UTR of genes and gene bodies, while DVPs that were hypervariable in healthy twins were enriched in gene bodies (Fig. 3). The underrepresentation of DVPs in CpG islands, particularly in DVPs that were hypervariable in healthy twins, indicates that these regions are more epigenetically stable. Of the 763 DVPs which were hypervariable in RA twins, 563 showed a trend towards hypomethylation in the RA twins, while of the 408 DVPs which were hypervariable in the healthy twins, 401 showed a trend towards hypomethylation in the healthy twins. This finding indicates that disease-associated methylation hypervariability is more commonly associated with hypomethylation.

To investigate the DNA methylation variability of RA-associated genes, DVPs were annotated and the gene associated with each DVP was compared to RA-associated genes identified during genetic studies. Meta-analysis of RA susceptibility loci has previously identified 98 genes associated with 101 genetic variants

Table 2 Top 20 differentially methylated positions between RA twins and non-RA twins. Probe names are shown, along with methylation levels, intra-pair methylation difference, unadjusted p value and probe annotation

Probe	Non-RA beta	RA beta	Diff	p value	Chr	Relationship to gene	Gene symbol
cg26547058	0.763	0.800	0.037	4.89E−07	8		
cg07693617	0.758	0.788	0.030	5.15E−07	1	Body	PRKCZ
cg07636225	0.849	0.867	0.018	9.33E−07	11	Body	RTN3
cg03517226	0.709	0.716	0.007	1.18E−06	16	5′UTR	ANKRD11
cg20666386	0.184	0.180	−0.004	1.89E−06	11	1stExon	DGKZ
cg17501210	0.766	0.740	−0.026	2.54E−06	6	Body	RPS6KA2
cg26964117	0.775	0.796	0.021	2.56E−06	19	Body	PIH1D1
cg26701826	0.396	0.419	0.023	2.71E−06	4	5′UTR	SGMS2
cg06040872	0.810	0.822	0.012	2.92E−06	17	Body	CCL18
cg25487804	0.867	0.876	0.009	3.38E−06	11	TSS1500	OSBPL5
cg06128521	0.900	0.905	0.005	3.56E−06	17		
cg16640599	0.421	0.447	0.026	3.58E−06	4	Body	SEC24D
cg02445229	0.719	0.737	0.018	3.85E−06	19		
cg01769457	0.039	0.043	0.004	3.90E−06	1		
cg15293582	0.704	0.703	−0.001	4.06E−06	10	TSS1500	PRF1
cg07090025	0.091	0.100	0.009	4.21E−06	1	TSS200	SSU72
cg06791979	0.795	0.799	0.004	4.44E−06	11	Body	RTN3
cg01934296	0.939	0.931	−0.008	4.45E−06	1	Body	
cg26272088	0.819	0.838	0.019	4.54E−06	19	Body	IRGC
cg18460107	0.674	0.679	0.005	4.71E−06	17	TSS200	SEPT9

Chr chromosome

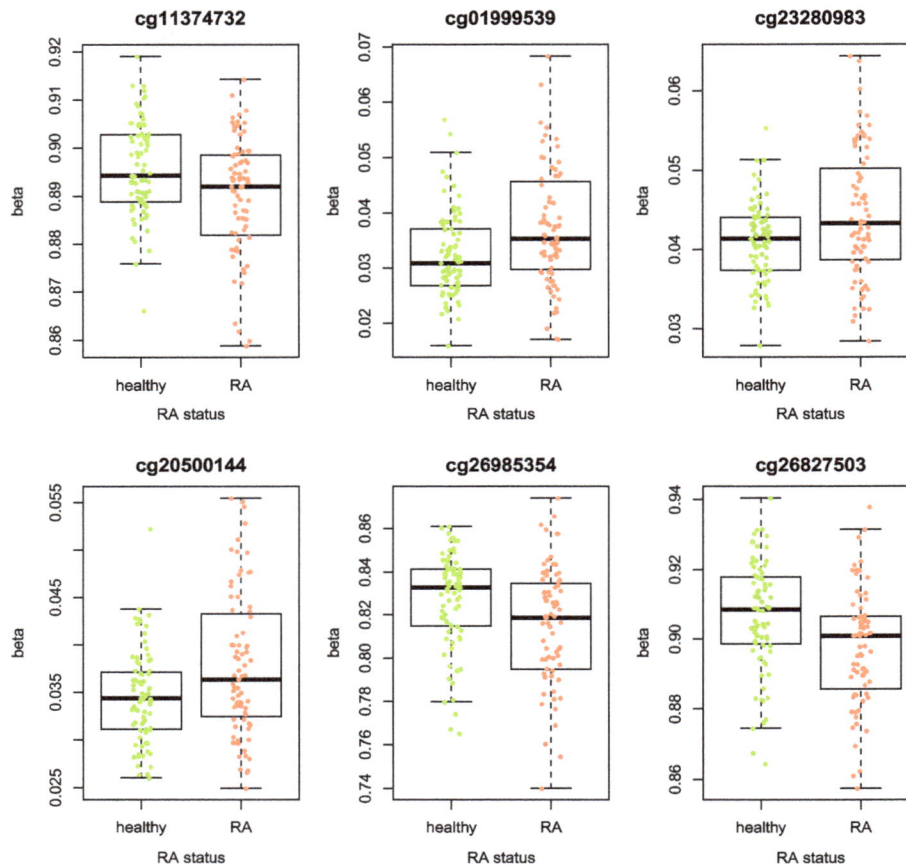

Fig. 2 CpG plots for six top ranked differentially variable positions in RA-discordant MZ twins. Cpg sites shown are cg11374732 (Bartlett's test p value = 4.09E−06), cg01999539, cg23280983, cg20500144, cg26985354 and cg26827503. Hypervariability of differentially variable positions was enriched in RA twins. Boxplots indicating the mean methylation and range of methylation values are shown overlaid with scatterplots indicating DNA methylation measurements of individual samples

[32]. Of these 98 RA-associated genes, five contained at least one DVP (*CLNK*, *JAZF1*, *ICOSLG*, *NFKBIE* and *BLK*). *JAZF1* contained two DVPs, both of which map to the body of the gene. Further, when the 377 genes with nominal association to RA from the same study were investigated, 15 genes contained at least one DVP. The presence of genetic and epigenetic variants in the same susceptibility genes indicates that disease-related changes in gene function or expression could be implemented by different mechanisms.

Functional annotation of the top ranked DVPs (ranked by *t*-statistic *p* value) showed that the second and third most highly ranked CpG sites (cg01999539 and cg23280983) overlap with the binding site of the transcription factor RUNX3. This differential variability of DNA methylation could potentially be influencing the binding of this transcription factor in multiple locations throughout the genome. Several studies have implicated RUNX3 in the development of immune-related diseases

including Crohn's disease, ankylosing spondylitis, psoriasis and ulcerative colitis (reviewed in [33]), and SNPs which disrupt RUNX binding sites have also been associated with RA [32, 34]. The disruption of the expression of RUNX3 transcription factors has also been found to alter the suppressive function of regulatory T cells in human cells and in mice, suggesting a potential functional consequence of the methylation changes observed in RUNX3 binding sites which warrants further investigation in RA [35].

Pathway analyses of rheumatoid arthritis-associated DVPs

Pathway analyses identified an enrichment of the RA-associated DVPs in pathways ($p < 0.05$) involved in response to cellular stress (Additional file 3: Table S2). A pathway involving ubiquitination of the protein K63 was also identified as enriched; this pathway has been found to modulate oxidative stress response [36] which has a role in RA pathogenesis [37]. When the pathway analysis was restricted to DVPs which are hypervariable in non-RA

Table 3 Top 20 differentially variable positions between RA-affected and non-RA twins. Probe names are shown, along with *t*-statistic *p* value, Bartlett's test for differential variability, which group was hypervariable, and probe annotation

Probe	P(tt)	P(BT)	Hypervariable group	Chr	Relationship to gene	Gene symbol
cg11374732	0.000513329	4.09E−06	RA	2	Body	INPP5D
cg01999539	0.000614047	1.50E−05	RA	6		
cg23280983	0.000689806	2.11E−05	RA	2	TSS200	C2orf42
cg20500144	0.000950244	6.82E−05	RA	3	Body	ARL6IP5
cg26985354	0.001008386	2.18E−08	RA	19	Body	SFRS16
cg26827503	0.001032395	2.68E−05	RA	4	Body	TMEM156
cg11913894	0.001053694	2.93E−06	RA	6	TSS1500	MAP3K4
cg16583193	0.001125272	4.49E−06	RA	19	Body	PIP5K1C
cg15573998	0.001139278	3.52E−05	RA	2	Body	NRXN1
cg16012388	0.001186516	5.35E−06	RA	10	Body	BICC1
cg16397722	0.00119032	9.50E−06	RA	17	Body	TP53
cg20556304	0.001192582	3.94E−11	RA	6		
cg25173129	0.00134302	2.51E−07	Healthy	17	TSS1500	EPX
cg01928104	0.001384944	3.10E−06	RA	14	TSS1500	SNORD114-7
cg06734169	0.001534366	4.20E−07	RA	3	5'UTR	LRRFIP2
cg04845047	0.00156418	4.88E−05	RA	13		
cg26788916	0.001792861	7.32E−05	RA	20		
cg00340024	0.001861004	3.01E−05	RA	1		
cg08306614	0.001980509	1.42E−05	RA	7	3'UTR	NUDCD3
cg19929189	0.001981039	3.59E−09	RA	6		

P(tt) *t*-statistic *p* value, *P(BT)* Bartlett's test *p* value, *Chr* chromosome

twins, there was an enrichment for immune-related processes in the top-ranked pathways (Additional file 4: Table S3). Two of the five top-ranked pathways were related to T cell cytokine production, a critical process in the development of RA.

Overlap with previously identified rheumatoid arthritis-associated DMPs

Changes in DNA methylation have previously been associated with RA; however, these studies were performed in unrelated case-control study designs. We hypothesised

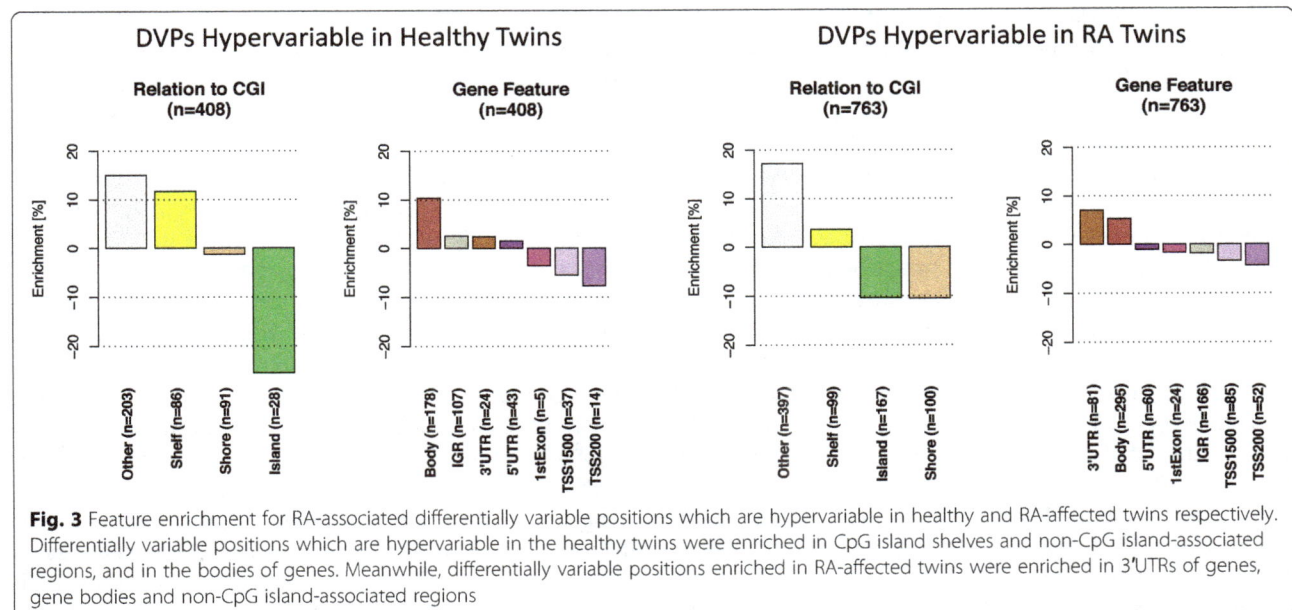

Fig. 3 Feature enrichment for RA-associated differentially variable positions which are hypervariable in healthy and RA-affected twins respectively. Differentially variable positions which are hypervariable in the healthy twins were enriched in CpG island shelves and non-CpG island-associated regions, and in the bodies of genes. Meanwhile, differentially variable positions enriched in RA-affected twins were enriched in 3'UTRs of genes, gene bodies and non-CpG island-associated regions

that the DMPs, which are found to be consistently differentially methylated across comparison groups in the analysis of unrelated individuals, may overlap with the differentially variable methylation signature identified in the current study. To test this, we overlapped the DMPs from the largest EWAS of RA to date with the DVPs identified in the current study, to assess if alternative study designs and approaches had identified common epigenetic variants.

The previous study was performed in 691 unrelated individuals ($n = 354$ RA cases and 337 unrelated controls) and identified 51,476 DMPs which were putatively associated with RA, achieving a $p < 0.05$ following Bonferroni correction [7]. Of the 1171 DVPs identified in the current study, 132 overlapped with DMPs identified in the unrelated RA EWAS. Of these, 123 DVPs were hypervariable in the RA-affected twins in the current study. In pathway analysis of these overlapping epigenetic variants, one of the top ranked pathways was associated with low-density lipoprotein receptor activity ($p = 0.003$), which associates closely with the protein produced by the *LRPAP1* gene, the methylation of which was recently reported as a potential biomarker of anti-TNF treatment response in RA patients [38].

Overlap with type 1 diabetes-associated DVPs
Genetic susceptibility loci identified in RA have also been found to confer risk for other autoimmune disorders. RA and T1D are both common autoimmune diseases with many characteristics in common, and it is possible that similarities in epigenetic profile between the two disorders may provide insight to the development of autoimmune diseases in general. To test whether epigenetic variants have commonality across different autoimmune disorders, we tested for overlap between the RA-associated DVPs identified in the current study and a set of DVPs recently identified in a T1D twin study.

A recent study of DNA methylation in T1D-discordant monozygotic twins ($n = 52$ twin pairs) identified 16,915 unique DVPs that were hypervariable in T1D across three cell types. Overlap analysis of the genes associated with these probes identified 496 genes that are associated with both RA-DVPs and T1D-DVPs, which is more than expected by chance ($p = 1.6E-29$), measured using the phyper test for hypergeometric distribution. An overlap analysis of methylation probe IDs identified 69 specific probes that overlap between RA-associated DVPs and T1D-associated DVPs. Permutation testing with 10,000 iterations indicated this overlap is more than expected by chance ($p = 0.001$). Pathway analysis of these probes identified many immune-related pathways including a pathway involved in NF-KB cascade modulation, a process that is important in inflammation and immune responses. Many of the top-ranked pathways identified were related to

embryonic development, including neural, embryonic and epithelial tube formation. The overlapping probes were enriched in 3′UTR and intergenic regions (Additional file 1: Figure S4).

Assessment of methylation variability signature in an independent healthy cohort
The DVP signature identified in RA-discordant twins was tested in an independent cohort of healthy individuals from the BIOS cohort [27] to assess if the methylation variability signature was specific to RA or can also be detected in the general population. Variance and range statistics were generated for each DVP for three comparison groups (RA co-twins, healthy co-twins and healthy BIOS individuals). The aggregated variance and range statistics for the sites were then plotted to compare distribution across the three groups, split by direction of variability. The DVPs which were hypervariable ($n = 763$) in RA-affected twins had a lower variance and a lower range of methylation values in both healthy twins and the BIOS healthy cohort when compared with RA-affected twins (Fig. 4). The DVPs that were hypervariable ($n = 408$) in the healthy co-twins were also found to have the same trend when compared with the BIOS cohort, with larger variance and range in the healthy co-twin and BIOS groups than in the RA-affected group (Additional file 1: Figure S5).

Discussion
In the largest study of DNA methylation in RA-discordant MZ twins performed to date, we have identified a significant differential variability signature in RA. Differentially methylated positions were not identified following adjustment for multiple testing in 79 pairs of disease-discordant twins. The identification of a differentially variable signature in the absence of a differentially methylated signature supports the recent findings of an EWAS of T1D-discordant monozygotic twins, which identified 10,548 DVPs in B cells, 4314 in T cells and 6508 in monocytes [15]. While the T1D study had a smaller sample size ($n = 52$ T1D-discordant twin pairs), it had increased power to detect methylation differences due to the use of individual cell types. A limitation of the current study is that it was performed in whole blood, making it more difficult to identify subtle methylation differences. However, cell estimates were imputed from the methylation data using a reference-based statistical algorithm [24] indicating that there were no significant differences in proportions of cells tested. The overlap of the RA-associated DVPs with T1D-associated DVPs identified in individual cell types is interesting as it indicates that at least a subset of DVPs identified in individual cell types can also be identified using whole blood. Another limitation of the study is that the samples were sourced from two cohorts, which inevitably confers a batch effect in the data. However, as each RA-affected individual is matched with their unaffected

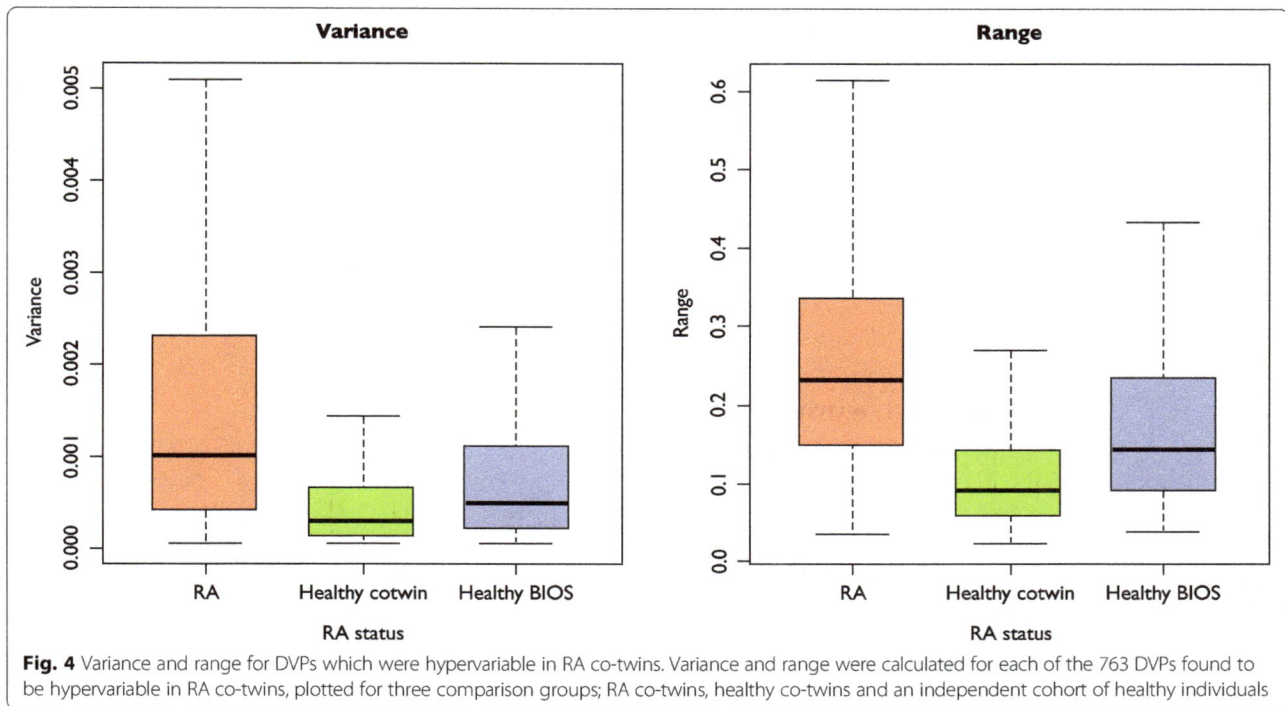

Fig. 4 Variance and range for DVPs which were hypervariable in RA co-twins. Variance and range were calculated for each of the 763 DVPs found to be hypervariable in RA co-twins, plotted for three comparison groups; RA co-twins, healthy co-twins and an independent cohort of healthy individuals

co-twin from the same study, the effect of this on the analysis is negligible. While the biological implications of DVPs are not yet fully understood, such DVPs have been found to be temporally stable over 5 years in T1D [15]. Further longitudinal studies are required to assess if this is the case in RA. It is also important to consider that the methylation variability detected may reflect either cause or consequence of the disease, which warrants further investigation into the temporal origins and functional consequences of this methylation variability signature.

RA-associated DVPs were enriched in pathways involved in the regulation of response to stress, including stress-activated kinase signalling cascades. While these pathway associations are based on bioinformatics analysis of methylation data, they have intriguing links to inflammatory pathways which warrant further functional investigation in RA. For example, stress kinases have previously been found to be induced by pro-inflammatory cytokines in RA, and the stress-activated protein kinase pathway has been shown to be active in RA synovium, while not being active in the synovium of patients with osteoarthritis [39]. These findings indicate that the inflammatory component of RA could potentially induce the observed variability of DNA methylation in stress response pathways. The variability of DNA methylation in stress response-regulating pathways might reflect the adaptation of these cells to stress-inducing conditions which are present in RA, such as increased levels of cytokines and induction of oxidative stress. These findings have lead us to propose a new working model of the development of RA (Fig. 5) illustrating

the potential role of DNA methylation variability and stress response pathways in the aetiology of disease.

The RA-associated DVPs were also enriched in a pathway controlling K63 protein ubiquitination. The ubiquitination of K63 acts as a modulator of oxidative stress response, which induces thioredoxin, a catalyst found to be overexpressed in RA patients [40]. Thioredoxin has also been found to activate the NF-KB pathway [41], which we observed to be enriched with DVPs in both RA- and T1D-affected twins.

Disease-associated epigenetic alterations have been hypothesised to be caused by chronic cellular stress, which can be induced by inflammation [42]. Accumulating evidence indicates that these stress-induced changes in the epigenetic landscape cause changes in cellular state and function, which can contribute to disease development. The enrichment of RA-associated DVPs in stress response-related pathways supports this hypothesis and suggests that, as well as altering cellular state, such epigenetic changes are also modulating the response to cellular and oxidative stress. This could be perpetuating the disease phenotype by repressing cellular stress response mechanisms in cells exposed to inflammation.

Meta-analysis of two other autoimmune EWAS studies identified a set of 496 genes that contain DVPs in both RA and T1D. This provides an intriguing possibility of common pathways in which DNA methylation is hypervariable in autoimmune disorders. These may provide novel pathways for treatment, and generate hypotheses regarding autoimmune disease pathogenesis. For example,

PREVAILING MODEL

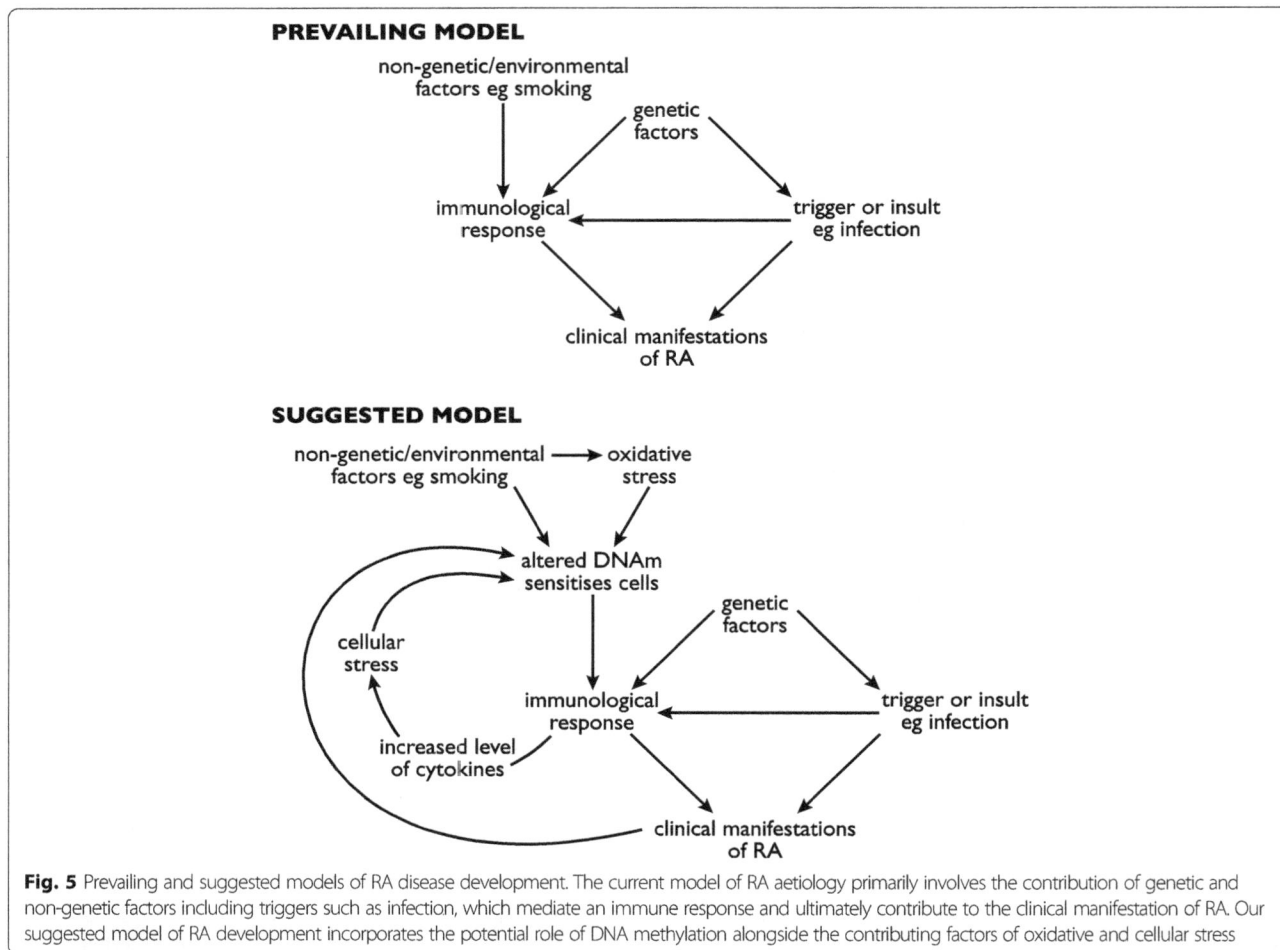

Fig. 5 Prevailing and suggested models of RA disease development. The current model of RA aetiology primarily involves the contribution of genetic and non-genetic factors including triggers such as infection, which mediate an immune response and ultimately contribute to the clinical manifestation of RA. Our suggested model of RA development incorporates the potential role of DNA methylation alongside the contributing factors of oxidative and cellular stress

one of the overlapping genes was *PRKCZ*, which was also the gene containing the second most differentially methylated probe in the current study. This gene was previously found to be hypermethylated in RA fibroblast-like synoviocyte cells [43] and has also been found to be hypomethylated in T1D monocytes and whole blood [44]. The largest RA EWAS of unrelated individuals identified 132 DMPs which were found to overlap with the DVPs identified in the current study. Pathway analysis of these sites identified a pathway associated with the *LRPAP1* gene, which was recently identified as a biomarker of treatment response in RA [38]. This overlapping signature of differential variability on methylation in two autoimmune diseases suggests that epigenetics plays a role in autoimmunity, which warrants further investigation in functional studies to elucidate its' role in autoimmune disease pathogenesis.

Conclusions

In a genome-wide investigation of DNA methylation in RA-discordant MZ twins, we have identified differential variability of DNA methylation, but no statistically significant DMPs. This supports the findings of a recent investigation of DNA methylation in T1D-discordant monozygotic twins, which identified a disease-associated DVP signature in the absence of a substantial DMP signature. Due to the influence of genetic components in establishing DNA methylation [45], our study indicates that differentially methylated positions that have previously been associated with RA [6–10] do not replicate in cohorts of disease-discordant monozygotic twins, which are less confounded by genetic heterogeneity. Furthermore, we identified a series of stress response-associated pathways which may potentially play a role in RA aetiology. These pathways interact with pro-inflammatory cytokines known to be integral in the development of RA, thus are of direct relevance to RA pathogenesis and could provide potential targets for RA therapy development. The role of stress response in RA pathology warrants further investigation to determine the downstream functional effects of this DNA methylation variability and to further characterise the role of variability of DNA methylation in complex diseases such as RA.

Additional files

Additional file 1: Figure S1. Multidimensional scaling plot of DMARD use in RA-discordant twins. **Figure S2.** Cell composition estimates for RA-discordant twins. **Figure S3.** Feature enrichment for differentially variable positions. **Figure S4.** Feature enrichment for DVPs identified in both RA and type 1 diabetes disease-discordant twins. **Figure S5.** Variance and range for DVPs which were hypervariable in healthy co-twins.

Additional file 2: Table S1. Full list of differentially variable positions ($n = 1171$) between RA-affected and non-RA twins. Probe names are shown, along with t-statistic p value, Bartlett's test for differential variability, which group was hypervariable, and probe annotation.

Additional file 3: Table S2. Pathways enriched in differentially variable positions identified in RA-discordant twins. Pathway analysis was performed using the gometh function in the MissMethyl package. Pathways are ranked by p value ($p < 0.05$).

Additional file 4: Table S3. Pathways enriched in differentially variable positions identified in RA-discordant twins, restricted to sites which were hypervariable in healthy co-twins. Pathway analysis was performed using the gometh function in the MissMethyl package. Pathways are ranked by p value ($p < 0.05$).

Abbreviations
DMARDs: Disease-modifying anti-rheumatic drugs; DMPs: Differentially methylated positions; DMR: Differentially methylated region; DVPs: Differentially variable positions; EWAS: Epigenome-wide association study; FDR: False discovery rate; MZ: Monozygotic; NF-KB: Nuclear factor kappa-light-chain-enhancer of activated B cells; PCA: Principal component analysis; PCs: Principal components; RA: Rheumatoid arthritis; RF: Rheumatoid factor; SWAN: Subset-quantile within array normalisation; T1D: Type 1 diabetes; UTR: Untranslated region

Acknowledgements
The authors thank the UCL Medical Genomics group, particularly Ismail Moghul, for their support, Andrew Teschendorff for useful conversations, and Paul Guilhamon for sharing his feature enrichment analysis method. The authors also thank Antonino Zito and Kerrin Small from TwinsUK for providing data for analysis. The authors also thank Christopher Bell and Richard Acton for their contribution to the analysis, and Tim Webster for his contribution to the figures.

Funding
This report includes independent research funded by the National Institute for Health Research Manchester Biomedical Research Centre. The views expressed in this publication are those of the author(s) and not necessarily those of the NHS, the National Institute for Health Research or the Department of Health. This work was funded by the IMI JU funded project BTCure, no 115142-2, and we thank Arthritis Research UK for their support (grant ref. 20385).
The TwinsUK study was funded by the Wellcome Trust; European Community's Seventh Framework Programme (FP7/2007–2013). The study also receives support from the National Institute for Health Research (NIHR)-funded BioResource, Clinical Research Facility and Biomedical Research Centre based at Guy's and St Thomas' NHS Foundation Trust in partnership with King's College London. APW is supported by BTCure (project no 115142–2) and the National Institute for Health Research Blood & Transplant Research Unit (NIHR-BTRU-2014-10074). SE is supported by the H2020 Project MultipleMS (693642). FZ is recipient of a fellowship from the Swiss Society of Rheumatology and SICPA foundation, Switzerland. FW is supported by Arthritis Research UK grant number 20682. AF is supported by the MRC (MR/M025411/1), the BBSRC (BB/R006172/1), Prostate Cancer UK (MA-TR15–009) and UCL BRC. The MRC/BHF Cardiovascular Epidemiology Unit is supported by the UK Medical Research Council (MR/L003120/1), British Heart Foundation (RG/13/13/30194) and NIHR Cambridge Biomedical Research Centre.

Authors' contributions
The study was conceived and designed by APW, JW and FMW. Sample collection was performed by FZ, AB, FMW and JW. Experimental work was performed by APW. Statistical analysis was performed by APW and SE with support from DP, JTB, AF, DSP and SB. The manuscript was written by APW with support from DP, SE, FZ, JTB, AF, DSP, SB, AB, FMW and JW. All authors read and approved the manuscript.

Competing interests
The authors declare that they have no competing interests.

Author details
[1]Arthritis Research UK Centre for Genetics and Genomics, Centre for Musculoskeletal Research, The University of Manchester, Manchester, UK. [2]Department of Cancer Biology, UCL Cancer Institute, University College London, London, UK. [3]NIHR Manchester Biomedical Research Centre, Manchester Academy of Health Sciences, Manchester University Foundation Trust, Manchester, UK. [4]Department of Twin Research and Genetic Epidemiology, King's College London, London, UK. [5]Division of Surgery and Interventional Science, University College London, London, UK. [6]MRC/BHF Cardiovascular Epidemiology Unit, Department of Public Health and Primary Care, University of Cambridge, Cambridge, UK.

References
1. Silman AJ, MacGregor AJ, Thomson W, Holligan S, Carthy D, Farhan A, Ollier WE. Twin concordance rates for rheumatoid arthritis: results from a nationwide study. Br J Rheumatol. 1993;32:903–7.
2. Silman AJ, Newman J, AJ MG. Cigarette smoking increases the risk of rheumatoid arthritis. Results from a nationwide study of disease-discordant twins. Arthritis Rheum. 1996;39:732–5.
3. Hoovestol RA, Mikuls TR. Environmental exposures and rheumatoid arthritis risk. Curr Rheumatol Rep. 2011;13:431–9.
4. Breitling LP, Yang R, Korn B, Burwinkel B, Brenner H. Tobacco-smoking-related differential DNA methylation: 27K discovery and replication. Am J Hum Genet. 2011;88:450–7.
5. van Steenbergen HW, Luijk R, Shoemaker R, Heijmans BT, Huizinga TW, van der Helm-van Mil AH. Differential methylation within the major histocompatibility complex region in rheumatoid arthritis: a replication study. Rheumatology (Oxford). 2014;53:2317–8.
6. Nakano K, Boyle DL, Firestein GS. Regulation of DNA methylation in rheumatoid arthritis synoviocytes. J Immunol. 2013;190:1297–303.
7. Liu Y, Aryee MJ, Padyukov L, Fallin MD, Hesselberg E, Runarsson A, Reinius L, Acevedo N, Taub M, Ronninger M, et al. Epigenome-wide association data implicate DNA methylation as an intermediary of genetic risk in rheumatoid arthritis. Nat Biotechnol. 2013;31:142–7.
8. Glossop JR, Emes RD, Nixon NB, Haworth KE, Packham JC, Dawes PT, Fryer AA, Mattey DL, Farrell WE. Genome-wide DNA methylation profiling in rheumatoid arthritis identifies disease-associated methylation changes that are distinct to individual T- and B-lymphocyte populations. Epigenetics. 2014;9:1228–37.
9. de la Rica L, Urquiza JM, Gomez-Cabrero D, Islam AB, Lopez-Bigas N, Tegner J, Toes RE, Ballestar E. Identification of novel markers in rheumatoid arthritis through integrated analysis of DNA methylation and microRNA expression. J Autoimmun. 2013;41:6–16.
10. Julia A, Absher D, Lopez-Lasanta M, Palau N, Pluma A, Waite Jones L, Glossop JR, Farrell WE, Myers RM, Marsal S. Epigenome-wide association study of rheumatoid arthritis identifies differentially methylated loci in B cells. Hum Mol Genet. 2017;26:2803–11.
11. Bell JT, Spector TD. DNA methylation studies using twins: what are they telling us? Genome Biol. 2012;13:172.
12. Javierre BM, Fernandez AF, Richter J, Al-Shahrour F, Martin-Subero JI, Rodriguez-Ubreva J, Berdasco M, Fraga MF, O'Hanlon TP, Rider LG, et al. Changes in the pattern of DNA methylation associate with twin discordance in systemic lupus erythematosus. Genome Res. 2010;20:170–9.

13. Gomez-Cabrero D, Almgren M, Sjoholm LK, Hensvold AH, Ringh MV, Tryggvadottir R, Kere J, Scheynius A, Acevedo N, Reinius L, et al. High-specificity bioinformatics framework for epigenomic profiling of discordant twins reveals specific and shared markers for ACPA and ACPA-positive rheumatoid arthritis. Genome Med. 2016;8:124.

14. Tsai PC, Bell JT. Power and sample size estimation for epigenome-wide association scans to detect differential DNA methylation. Int J Epidemiol. 2015;44(4):1429–41.

15. Paul DS, Teschendorff AE, Dang MA, Lowe R, Hawa MI, Ecker S, Beyan H, Cunningham S, Fouts AR, Ramelius A, et al. Increased DNA methylation variability in type 1 diabetes across three immune effector cell types. Nat Commun. 2016;7:13555.

16. Teschendorff AE, Gao Y, Jones A, Ruebner M, Beckmann MW, Wachter DL, Fasching PA, Widschwendter M. DNA methylation outliers in normal breast tissue identify field defects that are enriched in cancer. Nat Commun. 2016;7:10478.

17. Teschendorff AE, Widschwendter M. Differential variability improves the identification of cancer risk markers in DNA methylation studies profiling precursor cancer lesions. Bioinformatics. 2012;28:1487–94.

18. Hansen KD, Timp W, Bravo HC, Sabunciyan S, Langmead B, McDonald OG, Wen B, Wu H, Liu Y, Diep D, et al. Increased methylation variation in epigenetic domains across cancer types. Nat Genet. 2011;43:768–75.

19. Moayyeri A, Hammond CJ, Valdes AM, Spector TD. Cohort profile: TwinsUK and healthy ageing twin study. Int J Epidemiol. 2013;42:76–85.

20. Aryee MJ, Jaffe AE, Corrada-Bravo H, Ladd-Acosta C, Feinberg AP, Hansen KD, Irizarry RA. Minfi: a flexible and comprehensive bioconductor package for the analysis of Infinium DNA methylation microarrays. Bioinformatics. 2014;30:1363–9.

21. Tian Y, Morris TJ, Webster AP, Yang Z, Beck S, Feber A Teschendorff AE. ChAMP: updated methylation analysis pipeline for Illumina BeadChips. Bioinformatics. 2017;33(24):3982–4.

22. Barfield RT, Kilaru V, Smith AK, Conneely KN. CpGassoc: an R function for analysis of DNA methylation microarray data. Bioinformatics. 2012;28:1280–1.

23. Reinius LE, Acevedo N, Joerink M, Pershagen G, Dahlen SE, Greco D, Soderhall C, Scheynius A, Kere J. Differential DNA methylation in purified human blood cells: implications for cell lineage and studies on disease susceptibility. PLoS One. 2012;7:e41361.

24. Houseman EA, Accomando WP, Koestler DC, Christensen BC, Marsit CJ, Nelson HH, Wiencke JK, Kelsey KT. DNA methylation arrays as surrogate measures of cell mixture distribution. BMC Bioinformatics. 2012;13:86.

25. Teschendorff AE, Breeze CE, Zheng SC, Beck S. A comparison of reference-based algorithms for correcting cell-type heterogeneity in epigenome-wide association studies. BMC Bioinformatics. 2017;18:105.

26. Benjamini Y, Hochberg Y. Controlling the false discovery rate—a practical and powerful approach to multiple testing. J R Stat Soc Ser B Methodol. 1995;57:289–300.

27. Bonder MJ, Luijk R, Zhernakova DV, Moed M, Deelen P, Vermaat M, van Iterson M, van Dijk F, van Galen M, Bot J, et al. Disease variants alter transcription factor levels and methylation of their binding sites. Nat Genet. 2017;49:131–8.

28. Guilhamon P, Eskandarpour M, Halai D, Wilson GA, Feber A, Teschendorff AE, Gomez V, Hergovich A, Tirabosco R, Fernanda Amary M, et al. Meta-analysis of IDH-mutant cancers identifies EBF1 as an interaction partner for TET2. Nat Commun. 2013;4:2166.

29. Phipson B, Maksimovic J, Oshlack A. missMethyl: an R package for analyzing data from Illumina's HumanMethylation450 platform. Bioinformatics. 2016;32:286–8.

30. Geeleher P, Hartnett L, Egan LJ, Golden A, Raja Ali RA, Seoighe C. Gene-set analysis is severely biased when applied to genome-wide methylation data. Bioinformatics. 2013;29:1851–7.

31. Subramanian A, Tamayo P, Mootha VK, Mukherjee S, Ebert BL, Gillette MA, Paulovich A, Pomeroy SL, Golub TR, Lander ES, Mesirov JP. Gene set enrichment analysis: a knowledge-based approach for interpreting genome-wide expression profiles. Proc Natl Acad Sci U S A. 2005;102:15545–50.

32. Okada Y, Wu D, Trynka G, Raj T, Terao C, Ikari K, Kochi Y, Ohmura K, Suzuki A, Yoshida S, et al. Genetics of rheumatoid arthritis contributes to biology and drug discovery. Nature. 2014;506:376–81.

33. Lotem J, Levanon D, Negreanu V, Bauer O, Hantisteanu S, Dicken J, Groner Y. Runx3 at the interface of immunity, inflammation and cancer. Biochim Biophys Acta. 1855;2015:131–43.

34. Tokuhiro S, Yamada R, Chang X, Suzuki A, Kochi Y, Sawada T, Suzuki M, Nagasaki M, Ohtsuki M, Ono M, et al. An intronic SNP in a RUNX1 binding site of SLC22A4, encoding an organic cation transporter, is associated with rheumatoid arthritis. Nat Genet. 2003;35:341–8.

35. Klunker S, Chong MM, Mantel PY, Palomares O, Bassin C, Ziegler M, Ruckert B, Meiler F, Akdis M, Littman DR, Akdis CA. Transcription factors RUNX1 and RUNX3 in the induction and suppressive function of Foxp3+ inducible regulatory T cells. J Exp Med. 2009;206:2701–15.

36. Silva GM, Finley D, Vogel C. K63 polyubiquitination is a new modulator of the oxidative stress response. Nat Struct Mol Biol. 2015;22:116–23.

37. Quinonez-Flores CM, Gonzalez-Chavez SA, Del Rio ND, Pacheco-Tena C. Oxidative stress relevance in the pathogenesis of the rheumatoid arthritis: a systematic review. Biomed Res Int. 2016;2016:6097417.

38. Plant D, Webster A, Nair N, Oliver J, Smith SL, Eyre S, Hyrich KL, Wilson AG, Morgan AW, Isaacs JD, et al. Differential methylation as a biomarker of response to Etanercept in patients with rheumatoid arthritis. Arthritis Rheumatol. 2016;68:1353–60.

39. Schett G, Tohidast-Akrad M, Smolen JS, Schmid BJ, Steiner CW, Bitzan P, Zenz P, Redlich K, Xu Q, Steiner G. Activation, differential localization, and regulation of the stress-activated protein kinases, extracellular signal-regulated kinase, c-JUN N-terminal kinase, and p38 mitogen-activated protein kinase, in synovial tissue and cells in rheumatoid arthritis. Arthritis Rheum. 2000;43:2501–12.

40. Maurice MM, Nakamura H, Gringhuis S, Okamoto T, Yoshida S, Kullmann F, Lechner S, van der Voort EA, Leow A, Versendaal J, et al. Expression of the thioredoxin-thioredoxin reductase system in the inflamed joints of patients with rheumatoid arthritis. Arthritis Rheum. 1999;42:2430–9.

41. Yoshida S, Katoh T, Tetsuka T, Uno K, Matsui N, Okamoto T. Involvement of thioredoxin in rheumatoid arthritis: its costimulatory roles in the TNF-alpha-induced production of IL-6 and IL-8 from cultured synovial fibroblasts. J Immunol. 1999;163:351–8.

42. Johnstone SE, Baylin SB. Stress and the epigenetic landscape: a link to the pathobiology of human diseases? Nat Rev Genet. 2010;11:806–12.

43. Nakano K, Whitaker JW, Boyle DL, Wang W, Firestein GS. DNA methylome signature in rheumatoid arthritis. Ann Rheum Dis. 2013;72:110–7.

44. Chen Z, Miao F, Paterson AD, Lachin JM, Zhang L, Schones DE, Wu X, Wang J, Tompkins JD, Genuth S, et al. Epigenomic profiling reveals an association between persistence of DNA methylation and metabolic memory in the DCCT/EDIC type 1 diabetes cohort. Proc Natl Acad Sci U S A. 2016;113:E3002–11.

45. Ziller MJ, Gu H, Muller F, Donaghey J, Tsai LT, Kohlbacher O, De Jager PL, Rosen ED, Bennett DA, Bernstein BE, et al. Charting a dynamic DNA methylation landscape of the human genome. Nature. 2013;500:477–81.

6

Simple paired heavy- and light-chain antibody repertoire sequencing using endoplasmic reticulum microsomes

Praneeth Reddy Devulapally[1], Jörg Bürger[2,3], Thorsten Mielke[2], Zoltán Konthur[4], Hans Lehrach[5,6], Marie-Laure Yaspo[1,5], Jörn Glökler[7] and Hans-Jörg Warnatz[1*] (iD)

Abstract

Existing methods for paired antibody heavy- and light-chain repertoire sequencing rely on specialized equipment and are limited by their commercial availability and high costs. Here, we report a novel simple and cost-effective emulsion-based single-cell paired antibody repertoire sequencing method that employs only basic laboratory equipment. We performed a proof-of-concept using mixed mouse hybridoma cells and we also showed that our method can be used for discovery of novel antigen-specific monoclonal antibodies by sequencing human CD19+ B cell IgM and IgG repertoires isolated from peripheral whole blood before and seven days after Td (Tetanus toxoid/Diphtheria toxoid) booster immunization. We anticipate broad applicability of our method for providing insights into adaptive immune responses associated with various diseases, vaccinations, and cancer immunotherapies.

Background

High-throughput sequencing of immunoglobulin repertoires from B cells has emerged as a powerful tool to investigate repertoire changes for antibody discovery, vaccine efficacy studies, and in other healthcare applications [1–3]. Initially, antibody repertoire analysis focused on obtaining information from antibody heavy chains (HC) only [4–7], missing the native light-chain (LC) pairing information that is necessary for antibody cloning and expression. Retaining paired HC-LC data from bulk B cell populations at single-cell level remained a major obstacle for a long time. To this end, several single-cell paired sequencing technologies were reported more recently, which were initially limited by low cell numbers ($< 400–10^5$ cells) and sometimes required the use of complex microfluidic systems [8–12]; however, cellular throughput is improving through newer developments, such as droplet-based systems and the 10× Genomics platform [13, 14]. More recently, two emulsion-based methods reported paired HC-LC repertoire sequencing from $2–3 \times 10^6$ B cells at single-cell

level [15, 16]. Although substantial, the existing methods are limited by their commercial availability, high costs, and require an elaborate construction of flow-focusing or microfluidic devices and dedicated personnel for operation [17]. Here, we describe a high-throughput method which enables sequencing of paired HC-LC immunoglobulin (Ig) repertoires from millions of B cells simply by using a cooled table-top centrifuge, a magnetic stirrer, and a thermal cycler. This method makes paired Ig sequencing widely applicable even for laboratories without specialized equipment and personnel.

Methods

Cell lines

The HEK 293T cell line was obtained from the American Type Culture Collection (ATCC CRL-3216). Mouse hybridoma cell lines KT13 and KT22 were obtained from the Developmental Studies Hybridoma Bank (DSHB). Both cell lines were deposited to the DSHB by Kazumasa Takeda and Asako Sugimoto (DSHB hybridoma products KT13 and KT22). Mouse hybridoma cell line 5E4/1F1 was kindly provided by Miha Kosmač and Vladka Čurin Šerbec (University of Ljubljana). HEK 293T and hybridoma cells were grown in DMEM (Gibco) supplemented with 13% FBS (Gibco), 1× Penicillin/

* Correspondence: warnatz@molgen.mpg.de
[1]Otto Warburg Laboratory Gene Regulation and Systems Biology of Cancer, Max Planck Institute for Molecular Genetics, Berlin, Germany
Full list of author information is available at the end of the article

Streptomycin (Thermo Fisher), and 1× GlutaMAX (Gibco). Antibody HC and LC sequences from individual hybridomas were determined by reverse transcription polymerase chain reaction (RT-PCR) and capillary sequencing (Eurofins Genomics).

Cycloheximide treatment and microsome preparation

All pipetting steps were performed on ice and centrifugations were carried out at 4 °C using an Eppendorf 5810R centrifuge with fixed angle rotor F-45-30-11. Protein LoBind 1.5 mL centrifuge tubes (Eppendorf) were used to minimize cell adhesion to the tube walls. HEK 293T cells (1 million), mouse hybridoma cells (1 million of 5E4, KT13, and KT22 cells mixed in ratio 1:1:1), ARH-77 leukemia cells (ATCC CRL-1621, 1 million), or freshly isolated human $CD19^+$ B cells from pre- and post Td-booster immunization samples (1.5 million each) were resuspended in 1 mL PBS with 50 µg/mL cycloheximide and incubated for 10 min to stall ribosomes with associated messenger RNAs (mRNA) at the rough endoplasmic reticulum. The cells were pelleted with 300 g for 10 min at 4 °C and resuspended by pipetting 15× up and down in 120 µL high-density lysis buffer (25 mM HEPES-KOH pH 7.2, 110 mM potassium acetate, 5 mM magnesium acetate, 1 mM EGTA, 25% [w/w] sucrose [0.81 M], 5% [v/v] glycerol, 1 mM 1,4-dithiothreitol, 1× cOmplete EDTA-free protease inhibitor cocktail [Roche], 0.1 mg/mL cycloheximide, 0.015% digitonin, and 400 U/mL RiboLock RNase inhibitor [Thermo Fisher Scientific]). Cell and organelle lysis was completed by incubation for 10 min on ice. Each homogenate was split into two 55 µL aliquots and transferred into two fresh Protein LoBind tubes. The tubes were centrifuged at 600 g for 3 min at 4 °C to pellet nuclei and cell debris. A total of 40 µL supernatant from each tube, containing membrane fractions and cytosol, were transferred into fresh Protein LoBind tubes and the sucrose concentration was diluted to 0.37–0.40 M (12–13% w/w) by the addition of 40 µL nuclease-free water. Microsomes were then sedimented by centrifugation with 20,800 g for 120 min at 4 °C. The cytosol-containing supernatants were discarded and membrane pellets were resuspended by pipetting 10× up and down in 85 µL wash buffer (25 mM HEPES-KOH pH 7.2, 110 mM potassium acetate, 2.5 mM magnesium acetate, 1 mM EGTA, 1 mM 1,4-dithiothreitol, 1× cOmplete EDTA-free protease inhibitor cocktail, 0.1 mg/mL cycloheximide, 0.004% digitonin, and 400 U/ml RiboLock RNase inhibitor). The microsomes were sedimented again by centrifugation with 20,800 g for 60 min at 4 °C. Supernatants were discarded and the microsome pellets were resuspended in 20 µL of wash buffer and kept on ice until further use.

Transmission electron microscopy

Sample aliquots of 3.5 µL of resuspended HEK 293T microsomes were applied to freshly glow-discharged Quantifoil grids (Quantifoil, Germany) covered with an additional 2 nm carbon support film and flash-frozen in liquid ethane using a Vitrobot plunger (FEI). Samples were imaged on a Tecnai Spirit transmission electron microscope (FEI) operated at 120 kV equipped with a 2 × 2 k Eagle CCD camera (FEI). Micrographs were recorded under cryo low-dose conditions at 42,000× nominal magnification (pixel size at object scale: 5.2 Å/px) applying a defocus of − 2 to − 4 µm. Data collection was performed either manually or fully automatically using Leginon [18].

Emulsion RT-PCR assembly using mouse hybridoma microsomes

We diluted 16 µL of resuspended microsomes from mixed hybridomas 5E4, KT13, and KT22 in 184 µL RT-PCR master mix containing 1× Verso 1-Step RT-PCR master mix (Thermo Scientific), 1× Verso enzyme mix (Thermo Scientific), 0.5 µg/µL BSA, 100 µg/mL cycloheximide, and primers for reverse transcription and HC and LC assembly (0.8 µM each of primers TitA_MID1_IgM_rev and TitB_MID12_IgK_rev; 0.16 µM each of primers OE_MHV_fwd and OE_MKV_fwd). Primer sequences are shown in Additional file 1: Figure S1a. The resulting 200 µL of aqueous solution were used to form a water-in-oil emulsion by dropwise addition (13 aliquots of 15 µL in 30-s intervals) to 800 µL oil phase according to Ge et al. [19] (Mineral oil, Sigma M5904, with 4.5% [v/v] Span 80, Sigma S6760, 0.4% [v/v] Tween 80, Sigma P8074, and 0.05% [v/v] Triton X-100, Sigma T8787) during continuous stirring on a magnetic stirrer. Six aliquots of 100 µL each of the resulting emulsion were transferred into PCR tubes and subjected to thermocycling with the following conditions: reverse transcription at 50 °C for 15 min, RTase inactivation at 95 °C for 2 min, then four cycles of denaturation at 95 °C for 20 s, annealing rampdown from 60 °C to 50 °C for 50 s and extension at 72 °C for 1 min, then 16 cycles of denaturation at 95 °C for 20 s, annealing at 60 °C for 30 s and extension at 72 °C for 1 min, followed by a final extension step at 72 °C for 5 min. In parallel, an open RT-PCR control was performed by diluting 4 µL of resuspended microsomes in 46 µL RT-PCR master mix and thermocycling the reaction in parallel with the emulsion RT-PCR. PCR assembly products were extracted from the emulsion using isobutanol (2-Methyl-1-propanol, Sigma) and the Zymo DNA Clean & Concentrator-5 kit (Zymo Research) as previously published [20]. The resulting DNA and the PCR product from the open PCR control were loaded on a 1.2% TBE-agarose gel and separated with 90 V for 60 min.

Assembly products of 800–950 bp size were size-selected from the agarose gel and the products were recovered using a Zymoclean Gel DNA Recovery kit. Assembly products were eluted in 6 mM Tris-Cl pH 8 and stored at − 20 °C until further analysis.

Nested PCR amplification of mouse hybridoma assembly products

After the emulsion assembly reaction, the assembly products were further amplified with adapter primers TitA_fwd, 5′ CGT ATC GCC TCC CTC GCG CCA TCA G 3′, and TitB_rev, 5′ CTA TGC GCC TTG CCA GCC CGC TCA G 3′, using the Phusion high-fidelity DNA polymerase kit (Finnzymes) with the following thermocycling conditions: Initial denaturation at 98 °C for 30 s, then 15 cycles of denaturation at 98 °C for 7 s and annealing/extension at 72 °C for 30 s, followed by a final extension step at 72 °C for 5 min. PCR products were purified with the Zymo DNA Clean & Concentrator-5 kit. The pairing of HC and LC in the assembly products were then analyzed by PCR using nested primers specific for the three different HC and three different LC (Additional file 1: Figure S1e) using the Phusion high-fidelity DNA polymerase kit with the following thermocycling conditions: initial denaturation at 98 °C for 30 s, then 24 cycles of denaturation at 98 °C for 7 s and annealing/extension at 72 °C for 30 s, followed by a final extension step at 72 °C for 5 min. Nested PCR products were loaded on a 1.2% TBE-agarose gel and separated with 90 V for 40 min. Real-time nested PCR for quantification of cross-contamination was carried out in triplicates with the same nested primers using SYBRGreen master mix (Applied Biosystems) on a StepOne qPCR cycler (Applied Biosystems) with the following thermocycling conditions: initial denaturation at 95 °C for 10 min, followed by 40 cycles of denaturation at 95 °C for 15 s, annealing at 56 °C for 30 s and extension at 72 °C for 45 s. The initial abundances of the amplified assembly products were calculated using the $2^{(-deltaCt)}$ method and plotted as bar charts with error bars showing standard deviation from the mean.

Immunization and CD19+ B cell isolation from peripheral whole blood samples

The human peripheral whole blood samples used in this study were obtained from in.vent Diagnostica GmbH as by-products from routine diagnostic procedures. in.vent Diagnostica GmbH has written informed consent from the donor to use the by-products for research and has an ethical approval from the Freiburg Ethics Commission International (FEKI code 011/1763) for the distribution of samples. A healthy proband underwent booster immunization

with Tetanus Toxoid (TT)/Diptheria Toxoid (DT) (Td-pur®; 20 International units [IU] TT and 2 IU DT; Novartis, Basel, Switzerland). K2-EDTA peripheral whole blood derived from pre-immunization (day 0) and seven days post-Td booster immunization were used to isolate CD19+ B cells using the CD19 pluriBead Cell Separation Kit (pluriSelect GmbH, Leipzig, Germany) following the manufacturer's protocol. Isolated CD19+ B cell pellets were washed in 1 mL cold PBS and centrifuged at 300 g for 10 min at 4 °C. Cell pellets corresponding to 1.5 million B cells from both pre- and post-immunization samples were kept on ice until cycloheximide treatment and microsome preparation.

Emulsion RT-PCR assembly using human B cell microsomes

We added 2 μL of diluted microsomes prepared from frozen ARH-77 cells (as internal pairing control) to 26 μL of resuspended microsomes from B cells both pre- and post-Td immunization, so that the final fraction of ARH-77 microsomes is 0.5% (v/v). We diluted 16 μL of this microsomes suspension in 184 μL RT-PCR master mix containing 1× dART 1-step RT-PCR master buffer mix (Roboklon), 2× dART master enzyme mix (Roboklon), 0.5 μg/μL BSA, 100 μg/mL cycloheximide and primers for reverse transcription (IgM, IgG, and IgK) and heavy (VH) and light chain (VK) assembly. Primer sequences and concentrations in the RT-PCR master mix are listed in Additional file 1: Table S2. The resulting 200 μL of aqueous solution were used to form a water-in-oil emulsion by dropwise addition (13 aliquots of 15 μL in 30 s intervals) to 800 μL oil phase composed of 73% emulsion component 1, 7% emulsion component 2, and 20% emulsion component 3 of the Micellula DNA emulsion and purification kit (Roboklon) during continuous stirring on a magnetic stirrer. Six aliquots of 100 μL each of the resulting emulsion were transferred into PCR tubes and subjected to thermocycling with the following conditions: Reverse transcription at 55 °C for 30 min, initial denaturation at 95 °C for 3 min, then three cycles of denaturation at 95 °C for 20 s, annealing at 56 °C for 30 s and extension at 72 °C for 2 min, then 20 cycles of denaturation at 95 °C for 20 s, annealing at 56 °C for 30 s and extension at 72 °C for 4 min, followed by a final extension step at 72 °C for 5 min. PCR assembly products were extracted from the emulsion using isobutanol (2-Methyl-1-propanol, Sigma) and the Zymo DNA Clean & Concentrator-5 kit (Zymo Research) as previously published [20]. The resulting DNAs were loaded on a 1% TBE-agarose gel and separated with 100 V for 45 min. Assembly products of 700–800 bp were size-selected from the agarose gel, recovered using a Zymoclean Gel DNA Recovery kit, eluted in 6 mM Tris-Cl pH 8, and stored at − 20 °C until further analysis.

Nested PCR amplification of human B cell assembly products

For specific further amplification of the HC-LC assembly products, a nested PCR amplification was performed with nested primers specific for IgM, IgG, and IGK constant regions (Additional file 1: Table S2). The PCR reaction contained nested primers at 0.4 μM concentrations, 200 μM dNTP mix, 1× Q5 reaction buffer and 0.02 U/μL Q5 high-fidelity DNA Polymerase (New England Biolabs) in a reaction volume of 50 μL with 3 μL of assembled DNA. Nested PCR amplification was performed with the following thermocycling conditions: initial denaturation at 98 °C for 3 min, then 34 cycles of denaturation at 98 °C for 30 s and annealing/extension at 71 °C for 1 min, followed by a final extension step at 72 °C for 5 min. Samples were collected after three different PCR cycle numbers (28, 31, and 34 cycles). Amplified PCR products were loaded on 1% TBE-agarose gels and separated with 100 V for 60 min. The desired products of ~ 710 bp were extracted as described above, sequencing libraries were prepared following the Illumina TruSeq DNA sample preparation guide and 2 × 250 base paired-end reads were sequenced using the Illumina MiSeq platform.

Bioinformatic analysis of paired antibody heavy and light chain repertoires

Demultiplexing of 2 × 250 base paired-end reads from the MiSeq sequencing platform was performed based on adapter indices and sequencing data were obtained in fastq format. Only reads with minimum Phred quality scores of 10 over 50% of all nucleotides were retained and scanned for IgM, IgG, and IgK constant region sequences. Read pairs lacking constant region sequences or showing HC-HC or LC-LC structure were filtered out and the remaining reads were converted into fastq format and used as input for analysis with MiXCR (v1.2) [21] for alignment of reads to reference V(D)J and C gene sequences from the IMGT database [22], extraction, and clustering of CDR-H3 nucleotide (Additional file 1: Table S1). HC-CDR3 sequences containing frameshifts or stop codons and with less than two reads were filtered out. We created a HC-LC pairing statistics file to demonstrate paired VH-VK gene usage in the total paired HC-LC gene repertoires. Heat maps were generated using R and graphically displayed using ggplot2. Next, inter-individual TT-specific HC-CDR3 sequences were identified by comparing HC-CDR3 amino acid sequences obtained from the post-Td booster immunization sample to previously reported TT-specific HC-CDR3 sequences [23–26].

PCR amplification of full-length HC and LC sequences

We designed a two-step PCR-based amplification method (Additional file 1: Figure S5) to incorporate restriction digestion sites to potentially TT-specific HC and LC with complete V(D)J gene sequence. This enabled efficient cloning of HC and LC sequences into respective expression vectors as well as production of recombinant antibodies for in vitro binding studies. Briefly, we selected 14 paired HC-LC CDR3 clonotypes obtained from IgG sequencing post-Td booster immunization based on their frequency, pairing accuracy, and fold difference between top1 LC-CDR3 and top2 LC-CDR3 paired to the given HC-CDR3 sequence. We extracted total RNA from frozen B cells isolated from post-Td booster immunization using TRIzol reagent (Ambion) purification according to the manufacturer's instructions. In the first step, RT-PCR amplification for each selected HC- and LC-CDR3 clonotype was performed separately using the dART 1-step RT-PCR kit (Roboklon). The RT-PCR master mix (25 μL) contained HC and LC V gene-specific forward primers with BssHII restriction site overhangs together with individual CDR3-specific reverse primers with 18 nucleotides of FR4 region at 0.4 μM concentrations (Additional file 1: Table S3 and Figure S5), 1× dART 1-step RT-PCR master buffer mix, 1× dART master enzyme mix, and 4.5 ng total RNA. Thermocycling conditions were as follows: reverse transcription at 55 °C for 30 min, initial denaturation at 95 °C for 3 min, then 23 cycles of denaturation at 95 °C for 20 s, annealing at 56 °C for 30 s and extension at 72 °C for 90 s, followed by a final extension step at 72 °C for 5 min. RT-PCR products were purified using the Agencourt AMPure XP – PCR purification kit (Beckman Coulter) following the manufacturer's instructions and eluted in 6 mM Tris-Cl pH 8.0. In the second step, purified RT-PCR products were used as template for PCR amplification using Q5 high-fidelity DNA polymerase (New England Biolabs). The nested PCR master mix (50 μL) contained forward primers encoding a BssHII restriction site and three nucleotides of HC or LC germline gene sequence together with reverse primers containing the complete FR4 region and NheI/HindIII restriction overhangs at 0.4-μM concentrations (Additional file 1: Table S3 and Figure S5), 4 μL of purified DNA, 200 μM dNTP mix, 1× Q5 reaction buffer, and 0.02 U/μL Q5 high-fidelity DNA Polymerase (New England Biolabs). Thermocycling conditions were as follows: initial denaturation at 98 °C for 3 min, then 16 cycles of denaturation at 98 °C for 30 s, annealing at 69 °C for 30 s and extension at 72 °C for 1 min, followed by a final extension step at 72 °C for 5 min. PCR products were separated on a TBE-agarose gel, full-length HC and LC amplicons with restriction digestion sites were extracted from the gel using the Zymoclean Gel

DNA Recovery Kit (Zymo Research) and products were stored at − 20 °C until further use.

Cloning and expression of recombinant monoclonal antibodies

Restriction digestion of full length HC and LC inserts and expression vectors (pCMV-CD30-4IE3_HC and pCMV-CD30-4IE3_LC) was performed with the restriction enzymes BssHII, NheI and HindIII (New England Biolabs). The resulting products were loaded on 2% TBE-agarose gels and bands of ~ 5.9 kb for the HC vector backbone, 5.3 kb for the LC vector backbone, ~ 370 bp for HC inserts, and ~ 340 bp for LC inserts were size-selected on agarose gels and purified as described above. Ligations of the corresponding inserts and vectors for the amplified HC and LC clonotypes were performed using instant sticky-end DNA ligase (New England Biolabs) and transformed into one-shot chemically competent *E. coli* TOP10 cells (IBA) following the manufacturer's instructions. Plasmid DNAs were isolated from transformed colonies (8–16 colonies) using the QIAprep spin miniprep kit (Qiagen); similarities to the consensus sequences were confirmed using capillary Sanger sequencing. HC and LC plasmid DNA sequences that matched closest to the consensus sequences were co-transfected into human embryonic kidney cell line HEK 293 T (ATCC, CRL-11268) cells. HEK 293 T cells were cultured using rich glucose (4.5 g/L D-glucose) Dulbecco's Modified Eagle's Medium (Gibco BRL) supplemented with heat-inactivated ultra-low IgG fetal bovine serum (Thermo Fisher Scientific), 100 U/mL penicillin, and 100 μg/mL streptomycin. Purified plasmid DNAs for paired HC and LC clonotypes were co-transfected into 85–95% confluent HEK 293 T cells using PEI (polyethyleneamine, Polysciences). Culture supernatants were collected four days after transfection and TT antigen-specific clonotypes were identified by indirect ELISA.

Enzyme-linked immunosorbent assays (ELISA)

We performed indirect ELISA assays to identify mAbs derived from the immunized proband binding to TT antigen using the transfected cell culture supernatants. Nunc-Immuno MicroWell 96-well solid plates (Thermo Fisher Scientific) were coated with 100 μL of 10 μg/mL TT antigen (Statens Serum Institute, Copenhagen, Denmark) in 50 mM carbonate buffer pH 9.6, incubated overnight at 4 °C, washed three times with PBS, and blocked with 2% non-fat dried milk (Bio-Rad) in PBS for 150 min at room temperature. After blocking, 120 μL of 1:2 serially diluted transfected supernatants in PTM (PBS, 0.1% Tween-20, 2% non-fat dried milk) were added to the wells, 350 ng of mouse anti-TT mAb

(GeneTex) was applied to one well as a positive control, and plates were incubated for 1 h at room temperature. Plates were washed three times with PBS-T (0.1% Tween-20) and 50 μL of a 1:2000 dilution of goat anti-human kappa LC-HRP secondary antibody (Thermo Fisher Scientific) were added to the wells, 50 μL of a 1: 2000 dilution of goat anti-mouse IgG HC-HRP secondary antibody (Sigma #A0168) were added to the positive control well, plates were incubated for 2 min at room temperature and washed three times with PBS-T. For color development, we added 50 μL of one-step Ultra TMB-ELISA substrate (Thermo Fisher Scientific) per well, incubated the plates for 5 min at room temperature, and stopped the Ag:Ab binding reaction by addition of 50 μL 2 M H_2SO_4. The absorbance was measured at 450 nm using the GloMax Multi Detection System (Promega). ELISA assays for all clonotypes were performed in triplicates, the values were normalized to remove background signals, and errors were represented as standard deviations from the mean.

Analysis of chimeric amplicon formation during nested PCR

Four defined HC-LC amplicons were generated by amplifying the HC and LC from the respective pCMV plasmids (see above) and using a PCR assembly reaction to generate the four distinct HC-LC assemblies. HC and LC plasmid DNAs were used as templates for PCR amplification of the Top1, Top2, Top3, and Top4 clonal chain pairs using primers specific for the respective VH and VK gene families and IgG and IgK constant regions (Additional file 1: Table S2 and Figure S6a). Purified plasmid DNA (10 ng) was added to each 25 μL PCR reaction containing 0.4 μM of each primer, 200 μM dNTP mix, 1× Q5 reaction buffer, and 0.2 U/μL Q5 high-fidelity DNA Polymerase. Thermal cycling was performed with initial denaturation at 98 °C for 3 min, followed by 25 cycles of denaturation at 98 °C for 30 s, annealing/extension at 71 °C for 1 min (for HC plasmid DNA) or annealing at 64 °C for 1 min and extension at 72 °C for 1 min (for LC plasmid DNA), followed by a final extension step at 72 °C for 5 min. PCR products were loaded onto separate 1% TBE-agarose gels and separated with 100 V for 60 min. The desired DNA products of ~ 400 bp (for HC) and ~ 350 bp (for LC) were size-selected and extracted from the gel as described above. The purified HC and LC PCR products were used as templates for HC and LC assembly by overlap extension PCR (Additional file 1: Figure S6b). Briefly, 5 ng of each HC and corresponding paired LC DNA were added into each 50 μL PCR reaction containing 1× dART 1-step RT-PCR master buffer (Roboklon), 2× dART master enzyme (Roboklon), and 0.4 μM of each IgG and IgK constant region primer (Additional file 1: Table S2).

Thermal cycling was performed with RT inactivation at 95 °C for 3 min, followed by three cycles of denaturation at 95 °C for 20 s, annealing at 56 °C for 30 s and extension at 72 °C for 2 min, followed by 25 cycles of denaturation at 95 °C for 20 s, annealing at 56 °C for 30 s and extension at 72 °C for 4 min, followed by a final extension step at 72 °C for 5 min. The assembly products were loaded onto 1% TBE-agarose gels and separated with 100 V for 45 min. The assembly products of ~ 750 bp were size-selected and extracted from the agarose gel as described above. The individually assembled HC-LC clonal pairs were pooled together and used as template for nested PCR amplification with primers specific for IgG and IgK constant regions (Additional file 1: Table S2, Figure S6c). The nested PCR reaction and thermal cycling conditions were the same as described in the "Nested PCR amplification of human B cell assembly products" section except that the PCR amplification was performed for 25 cycles. PCR products were loaded onto 1% TBE-agarose gels, separated with 100 V for 60 min and desired products of ~ 720 bp were extracted as described above. Sequencing libraries from the individual assemblies and from the mixed assemblies after nested PCR were prepared following the Illumina TruSeq DNA sample preparation guide and 2 × 250 base paired-end reads were generated using the Illumina MiSeq platform.

Results

Microsome-associated mRNAs can be used to retain native antibody HC-LC pairs with high pairing accuracy

Our approach is based on the concept that each B cell contains rough endoplasmic reticulum (rER) with bound ribosomes for co-transcriptional translocation of secretory proteins. These bound ribosomes are thus associated with both Ig HC and LC mRNAs, located at translocon complexes [27], which are translated into membrane-bound or secretory antibodies. We reasoned that rER microsomes obtained after cell lysis should retain the correctly paired HC and LC mRNAs of each individual B cell and thus represent the smallest subcellular entity comprising both types of mRNAs. It is likely that several microsomes are generated from each cell which leads to a higher clonal redundancy for a more efficient library synthesis when compared to using whole cells as templates. Therefore, these microsomes can subsequently be used for clonal RT-PCR assembly of the two chains from the original single cells, providing that the derived microsomes are separated into individual reaction vessels, a step that we have carried out by using water-in-oil emulsions. The entire workflow is summarized in Fig. 1.

We developed our method using HEK 293T cells based on a protocol for preparation of microsomes from plant material [28]. To preserve the mRNAs at rER

translocon complexes, we first treated the cells with the protein synthesis inhibitor cycloheximide [29] to retain stalled ribosomes with associated mRNAs in the resulting microsomes. The cycloheximide-treated cells were incubated in a sucrose buffer containing 5% digitonin, leading to the lysis of cells and organelles during which rER sheets collapse and form multilayered structures preserving the mRNA transcripts while keeping the cell nuclei intact. The sucrose provides higher density inside the lysed microsomes. Then, cell debris, nuclei, non-secretory mRNAs, and mitochondria were removed by low-speed centrifugation (600 g). This purification step has the advantage to greatly reduce PCR artefacts due to off-target amplification by mispriming on genomic DNA and other mRNAs. The microsome-containing supernatant was diluted with water so that microsomes could subsequently be pelleted based on their higher buoyant density using high-speed centrifugation (20,800 g) in a cooled table-top centrifuge. After removal of the supernatant (cytosol), the microsomes were resuspended in wash buffer and sedimented again (20,800 g) to further enrich microsomes for downstream applications (Fig. 1b). For verification of our microsome preparation method, enriched rER-microsomes from HEK 293T cells were visualized using transmission electron microscopy (Fig. 1c). We observed that the majority of microsomes were composed of multi-lamellar vesicles of approximately spherical shape, while some others were of uni-lamellar structure. This result suggested that our method can be used to obtain stable rER microsomes, thus avoiding the use of tedious ultracentrifugation steps [28].

Next, we tested if the enriched rER microsomes could be used for clonal assembly and amplification of paired immunoglobulin HC-LC from single cells. For this, we mixed cells from three mouse hybridoma cell lines with known Ig HC and LC sequences (cell lines 5E4, KT13, and KT22) and prepared microsomes from the cell mix according to our protocol (Fig. 1a and b, Additional file 1: Figure S1). We then passed the microsomes into water-in-oil emulsion droplets containing RT-PCR assembly master mix with overlap extension primers (Fig. 1d), wherein, based on Poisson statistics, the vast majority of individual microsomes were encapsulated in separate emulsion droplets (Fig. 1e). If clonal pairing and amplification occur, the amplified sequences should be strongly enriched for the three correct chain pairs among the nine possible pairings of three different HCs and LCs (Additional file 1: Figure S1). Within the emulsion droplets, the HC and LC mRNAs from individual microsomes were reverse transcribed using isotype-specific primers (IgM and IgK), assembled by overlap extension PCR and amplified. After size selection of the assembled DNA on an agarose gel, subsequent nested PCR with hybridoma-specific primers showed that the three

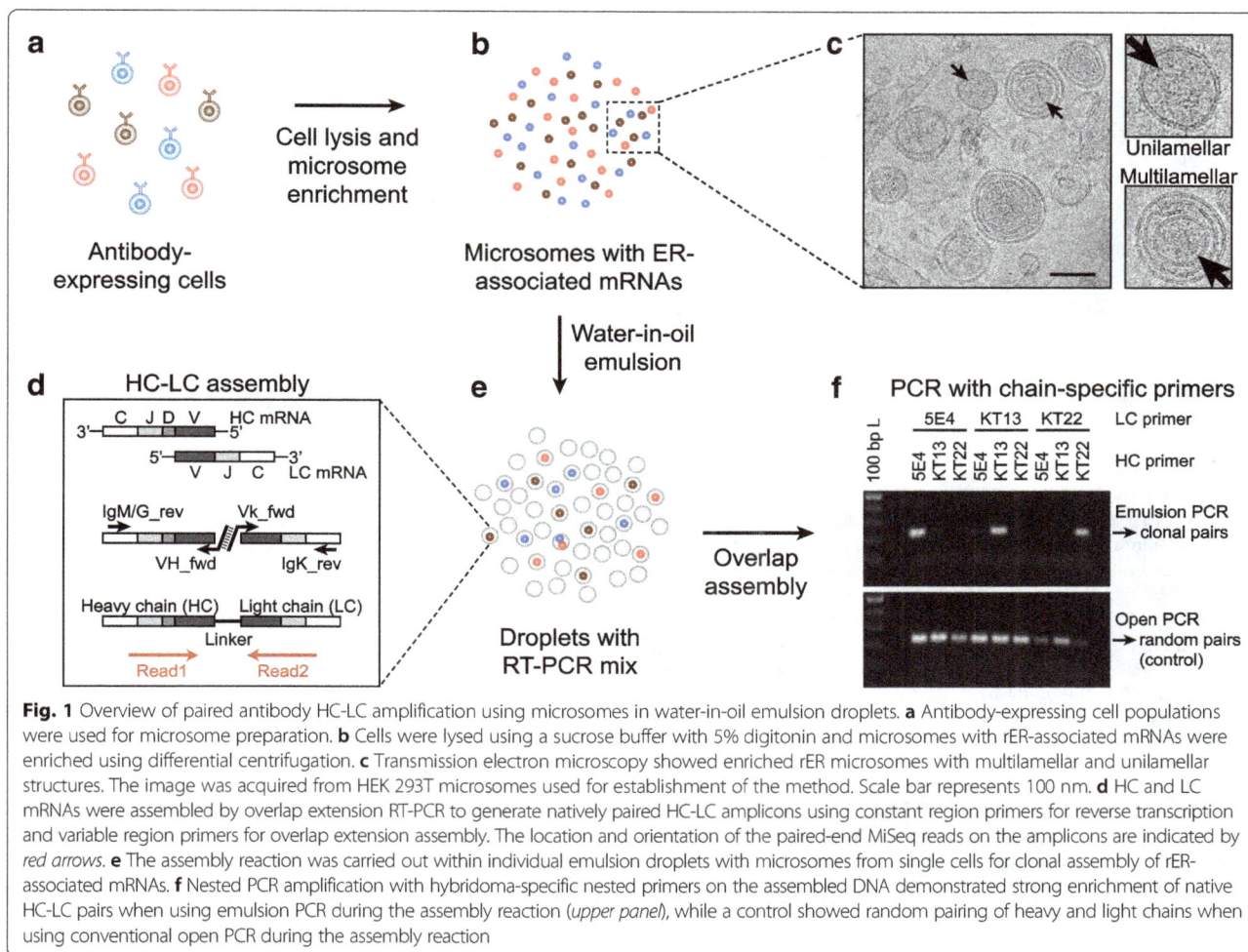

Fig. 1 Overview of paired antibody HC-LC amplification using microsomes in water-in-oil emulsion droplets. **a** Antibody-expressing cell populations were used for microsome preparation. **b** Cells were lysed using a sucrose buffer with 5% digitonin and microsomes with rER-associated mRNAs were enriched using differential centrifugation. **c** Transmission electron microscopy showed enriched rER microsomes with multilamellar and unilamellar structures. The image was acquired from HEK 293T microsomes used for establishment of the method. Scale bar represents 100 nm. **d** HC and LC mRNAs were assembled by overlap extension RT-PCR to generate natively paired HC-LC amplicons using constant region primers for reverse transcription and variable region primers for overlap extension assembly. The location and orientation of the paired-end MiSeq reads on the amplicons are indicated by *red arrows*. **e** The assembly reaction was carried out within individual emulsion droplets with microsomes from single cells for clonal assembly of rER-associated mRNAs. **f** Nested PCR amplification with hybridoma-specific nested primers on the assembled DNA demonstrated strong enrichment of native HC-LC pairs when using emulsion PCR during the assembly reaction (*upper panel*), while a control showed random pairing of heavy and light chains when using conventional open PCR during the assembly reaction

correct chain pairs were strongly enriched (> 95%) versus the nine possible permutations (Fig. 1f, upper panel, and Additional file 1: Figure S1). In contrast, we observed no enrichment of the correctly paired chains in control experiments performed in parallel where the assembly was carried out in conventional open PCR without emulsification, leading to an evenly balanced random chain assembly (Fig. 1f, lower panel). We quantified the amount of cross-contamination in the assembled DNA using real-time quantitative PCR (Additional file 1: Figure S1f) and found that cross-contamination among the distinct hybridomas was present at 0.2% frequency, while 99.8% of the chains demonstrated correct pairing. These results show that our method is suitable for clonal amplification of paired Ig HC and LC from single cells with high pairing accuracy.

A scalable high-throughput sequencing platform to retain native antibody HC-LC pairs from single B cells

We then applied our method to study immunization-induced changes in CD19+ B cell repertoires from pre- (day 0) and post- (day 7) Td booster immunization (Fig. 2). We used 1.5 million CD19+ B cells freshly isolated from peripheral whole blood samples of a healthy donor both pre- and post-Td booster immunization and prepared microsomes enriched with rER. As a control for native HC-LC pairing, we prepared microsomes from frozen ARH-77 cells expressing known IgG HC and IgK LC sequences and spiked 0.5% (v/v) of ARH-77 microsomes into B cell-derived microsomes (Additional file 1: Table S1). The microsomes were passed into water-in-oil emulsion droplets for amplification in two separate reactions with primers specific for IgM and IgG isotypes, respectively. After emulsification, overlap-extension RT-PCR, and nested PCR (Additional file 1: Figure S2), we prepared Illumina TruSeq libraries from the nested PCR amplicons and performed sequencing on the Illumina MiSeq with paired reads of 2 × 250 bases (Additional file 2: Figure S3). The raw sequencing reads were quality filtered and annotated to define the individual HC (IgM or IgG) and

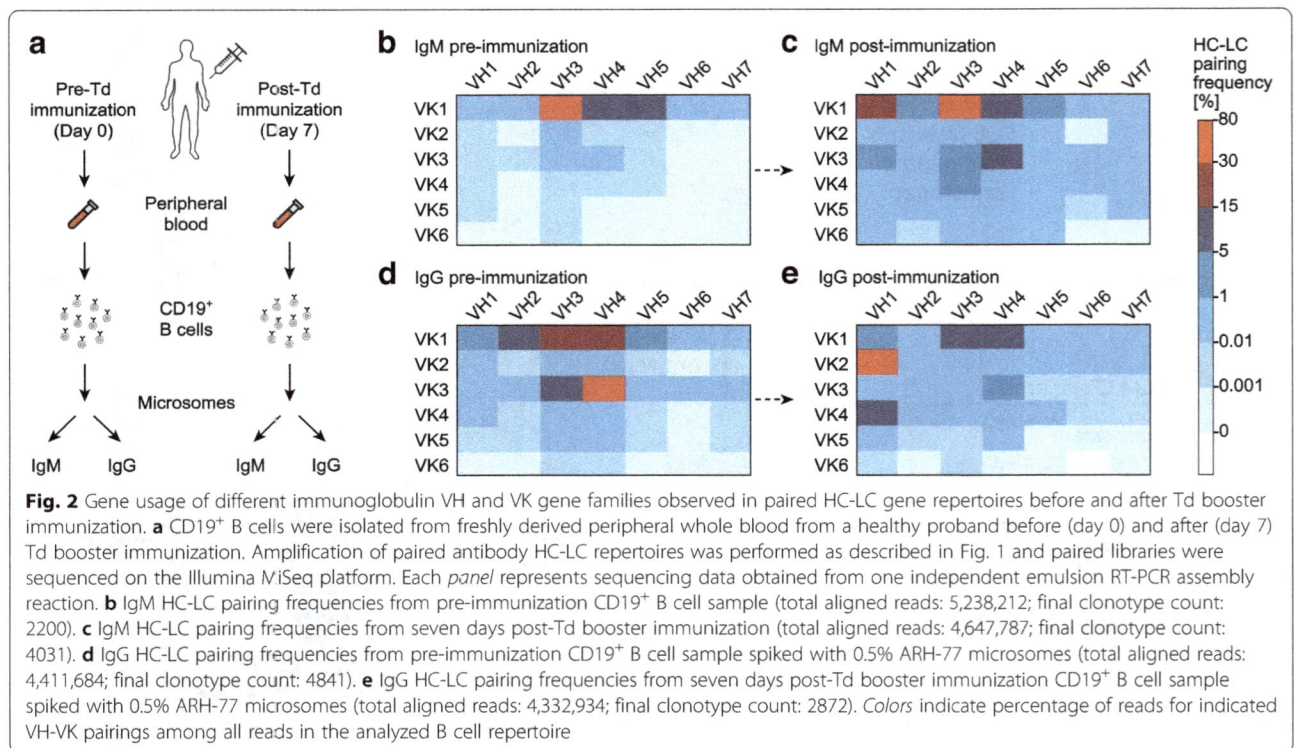

Fig. 2 Gene usage of different immunoglobulin VH and VK gene families observed in paired HC-LC gene repertoires before and after Td booster immunization. **a** CD19⁺ B cells were isolated from freshly derived peripheral whole blood from a healthy proband before (day 0) and after (day 7) Td booster immunization. Amplification of paired antibody HC-LC repertoires was performed as described in Fig. 1 and paired libraries were sequenced on the Illumina MiSeq platform. Each *panel* represents sequencing data obtained from one independent emulsion RT-PCR assembly reaction. **b** IgM HC-LC pairing frequencies from pre-immunization CD19⁺ B cell sample (total aligned reads: 5,238,212; final clonotype count: 2200). **c** IgM HC-LC pairing frequencies from seven days post-Td booster immunization (total aligned reads: 4,647,787; final clonotype count: 4031). **d** IgG HC-LC pairing frequencies from pre-immunization CD19⁺ B cell sample spiked with 0.5% ARH-77 microsomes (total aligned reads: 4,411,684; final clonotype count: 4841). **e** IgG HC-LC pairing frequencies from seven days post-Td booster immunization CD19⁺ B cell sample spiked with 0.5% ARH-77 microsomes (total aligned reads: 4,332,934; final clonotype count: 2872). *Colors* indicate percentage of reads for indicated VH-VK pairings among all reads in the analyzed B cell repertoire

LC (IgK) isotypes. The annotated reads were aligned to the human Ig germline genes (IMGT annotation [22]) and clustered using MiXCR [21] to determine the number of unique paired CDR3 clones (requiring ≥ 2 reads per pair) including correction of PCR errors. From the pre-immunization sample, we identified a total of 2200 and 4841 HC-LC pairs for IgM and IgG, respectively (Additional file 2: Data files S1 and S2). The post-Td immunization sample resulted in 4031 and 2872 HC-LC pairs for IgM and IgG, respectively (Additional file 2: Data files S3 and S4). Among these, we identified 212 (IgM) and 125 (IgG) HC-CDR3 clonotypes that were present in both the pre- and post-Td immunization samples. Of these, 50. 0% (IgM) and 60.0% (IgG) of the HC-CDR3s found in pre- and post-Td booster immunization data shared the same LC-CDR3 sequences, demonstrating the application of this technology to identify and track pre-existing B cells, possibly from the antigen-specific memory B cell compartment [30] (Additional file 2: Data files S5 and S6). The ARH-77 spike-in HC-LC pairing demonstrated preferential pairing of the known HC with the correct corresponding LC (Additional file 1: Figure S4). Of the IgM and IgG isotypes pre- and post-Td immunization, the top ten pairs constituted 57% and 49% (for IgM isotype) and 61% and 76% (for IgG isotype) of the total aligned reads, respectively, indicating a clonotype distribution that is skewed towards the most frequent HC-LC pairs.

We then generated heat maps showing the HC-LC pairing frequencies of all aligned reads and observed strong changes in VH gene family usage and expansion of certain B cell clones in response to antigen stimulation [2, 23, 30, 31]. Specifically, we found that certain VH-VK pairings (e.g. VH3-VK1, VH4-VK1, and VH4-VK3) were highly frequent (up to 78% of total reads) in the pre-immunization samples for both the IgM and IgG isotypes (Fig. 2b and d). Post Td booster immunization, other pairings such as VH1-VK1, VH1-VK2, VH3-VK1, and VH4-VK1 were predominantly observed in both IgM (Fig. 2c) and IgG (Fig. 2e) isotypes. We also identified rare HC-LC pairs (e.g. VH7-VK5 and VH7-VK6) that are generally observed at lower frequencies (Fig. 2b–e), as reported in prior studies [10, 32]. This result illustrates the sensitivity of our technique to identify rare clonal pairs.

We quantified the presence and frequency of promiscuous LC sequences (LC paired to more than one specific HC) among all identified HC-LC pairs in all four samples (Additional file 3: S1-S4). We observed that three samples (IgG pre- and post- immunization, and IgM pre-immunization) contained 15–17% promiscuous LC, while one sample (IgM post-immunization) showed a higher frequency of 38.7% promiscuous LC. These observations are in line with previous studies reporting LC promiscuity due to lower theoretical diversity of LC junctions [15, 33]. We further compared the IgG HC-

CDR3 amino acid sequences obtained from post-Td booster immunization with TT-specific HC-CDR3 sequences from previous studies [24–26, 30]. We found two previously reported TT antigen-specific HC-CDR3 sequences in our dataset (CARQADNWFDPW and CATGRTLDYW) [24, 30], suggesting the suitability of our method to track known sequences related to diseases and autoreactive antibodies [2].

Application of paired antibody HC-LC repertoire sequencing for antigen-specific mAb discovery

Finally, we demonstrated that our paired sequencing technique is suitable for the discovery of novel antigen-specific human monoclonal antibodies (mAbs) by performing antibody cloning, expression and antigen binding studies using ELISA. We selected 14 highly induced HC-LC pairs from the IgG B cell repertoire post-Td booster immunization, including the HC-LC pair for one previously reported TT-specific HC-CDR3 sequence (CARQADNWFDPW) (Fig. 3a). We used a two-step PCR strategy for incorporating restriction digestion sites to the selected HC-LC pairs (Additional file 1: Figure S5) for cloning into IgG HC and LC expression vectors. For recombinant mAb production, the HC and corresponding LC plasmids were co-transfected into HEK 293T cells (Additional file 1: Figure S5) and IgG-containing cell culture supernatants were harvested on day 4 after transfection. We performed indirect ELISA experiments with the transfected cell supernatants using plates coated with TT antigen and identified four novel TT-specific mAbs, named Top1, Top2, Top3, and Top4 here (Fig. 3b). Interestingly, the Top2, Top3, and Top4 HC-LC pairings were also present in the sequenced pre-immunization repertoire, albeit at much lower

frequencies (< 0.1% of total reads), suggesting the clonal expansion of pre-existing clonotypes after antigen exposure [30]. However, the previously reported TT-specific HC-CDR3 clonotype CARQADNWFDPW did not bind to TT antigen using our experimental setup (Fig. 3b), probably because it is a so-called public rearrangement with limited introduction of N/P nucleotides that is associated to IGHV4–39 and IGKV5–2 in our study, while similar TT-specific binders with this type of CDR3 are associated to IGHV4–30-2 and IGKV3–15. Also, the paired LC-CDR3 was different in our study (CLQHDDFPLTF) compared to the LC-CDR3 previously identified from a TT-binding memory B cell (CQQYYNWPPYTF) [26]. Our results show that almost one-third (29%) of the selected antibodies identified by our method did bind to TT antigen, thus demonstrating the applicability of this method for rapid discovery of mAbs using native Ig chain pairing information from B cells.

Immune repertoire sequencing methods can be affected by the formation of chimeric amplicons during PCR amplification [34]. To address this potential issue and to quantify the amount of chimeric amplicons generated during the second (non-emulsion) stage of our method, we generated and mixed four defined clonal HC-LC amplicons (from the Top1, Top2, Top3, and Top4 antibodies), performed the secondary PCR step and sequenced the resulting amplicons on the MiSeq platform with 2 × 250 bases (Additional file 1: Figure S6a–c). In parallel, we also sequenced the initial clonal amplicons individually as control for amplicon purity before secondary PCR. The reads generated from the initial amplicons before PCR showed > 99.6% correct HC-LC pairs (Additional file 1: Figure S6d), with < 0.4% chimeras that were probably generated during bridge

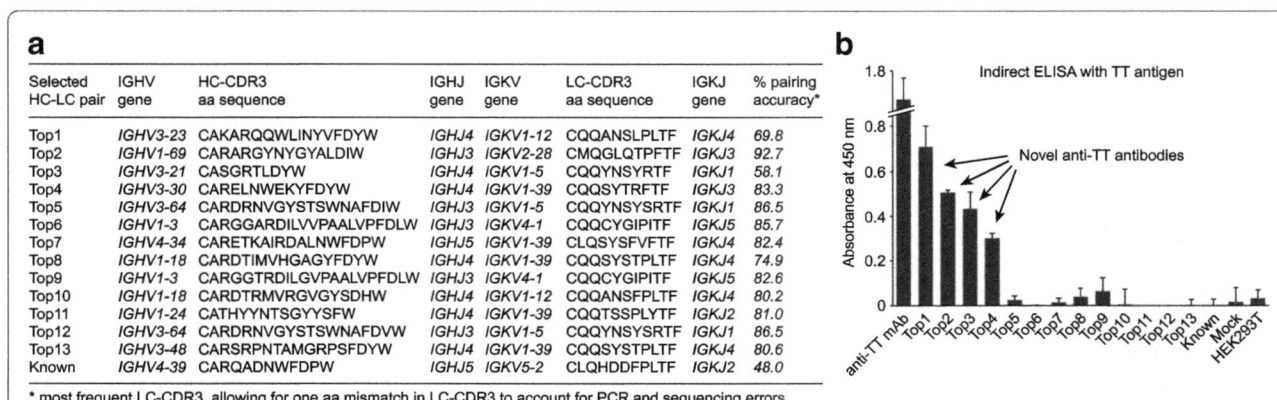

Selected HC-LC pair	IGHV gene	HC-CDR3 aa sequence	IGHJ gene	IGKV gene	LC-CDR3 aa sequence	IGKJ gene	% pairing accuracy*
Top1	IGHV3-23	CAKARQQWLINYVFDYW	IGHJ4	IGKV1-12	CQQANSLPLTF	IGKJ4	69.8
Top2	IGHV1-69	CARARGYNYGYALDIW	IGHJ3	IGKV2-28	CMQGLQTPFTF	IGKJ3	92.7
Top3	IGHV3-21	CASGRTLDYW	IGHJ4	IGKV1-5	CQQYNSYRTF	IGKJ1	58.1
Top4	IGHV3-30	CARELNWEKYFDYW	IGHJ4	IGKV1-39	CQQSYTRFTF	IGKJ3	83.3
Top5	IGHV3-64	CARDRNVGYSTSWNAFDIW	IGHJ3	IGKV1-5	CQQYNSYSRTF	IGKJ1	86.5
Top6	IGHV1-3	CARGGARDILVVPAALVPFDLW	IGHJ3	IGKV4-1	CQQCYGIPITF	IGKJ5	85.7
Top7	IGHV4-34	CARETKAIRDALNWFDPW	IGHJ5	IGKV1-39	CLQSYSFVFTF	IGKJ4	82.4
Top8	IGHV1-18	CARDTIMVHGAGYFDYW	IGHJ4	IGKV1-39	CQQSYSTPLTF	IGKJ4	74.9
Top9	IGHV1-3	CARGGTRDILGVPAALVPFDLW	IGHJ3	IGKV4-1	CQQCYGIPITF	IGKJ5	82.6
Top10	IGHV1-18	CARDTRMVRGVGYSDHW	IGHJ4	IGKV1-12	CQQANSFPLTF	IGKJ4	80.2
Top11	IGHV1-24	CATHYYNTSGYYSFW	IGHJ4	IGKV1-39	CQQTSSPLYTF	IGKJ2	81.0
Top12	IGHV3-64	CARDRNVGYSTSWNAFDVW	IGHJ3	IGKV1-5	CQQYNSYSRTF	IGKJ1	86.5
Top13	IGHV3-48	CARSRPNTAMGRPSFDYW	IGHJ4	IGKV1-39	CQQSYSTPLTF	IGKJ4	80.6
Known	IGHV4-39	CARQADNWFDPW	IGHJ5	IGKV5-2	CLQHDDFPLTF	IGKJ2	48.0

* most frequent LC-CDR3, allowing for one aa mismatch in LC-CDR3 to account for PCR and sequencing errors

Fig. 3 Binding studies of selected IgG antibodies induced in the post-Td booster immunization sample. **a** Fourteen highly induced HC-LC pairs including one known TT antigen-specific HC-CDR3 sequence were cloned into IgG HC and LC expression vectors, co-transfected, and expressed in HEK 293T cells for production of IgG mAbs. **b** Indirect ELISA using TT antigen and transfected HEK 293T cell supernatants reveals four novel anti-TT antibodies (named Top1, Top2, Top3, and Top4). A commercial TT-specific mAb used as positive control in the assays (anti-TT mAb) resulted in a strong signal while the negative controls (Mock – Mock transfection; HEK 293T – Cell culture supernatant from untransfected cells) resulted in low background signals

amplification for cluster generation on the MiSeq flow cell. Analysis of the reads from the mixed amplicons after secondary PCR showed that the PCR step indeed generated chimeric amplicons, with the extent of chimer formation depending on the sequence identity among amplicons (Additional file 1: Figure S6e). The three amplicons from the Top1, Top3, and Top4 antibodies, sharing HC V genes from the same IGHV3 superfamily, showed 10–14% chimera formation among each other, while the Top2 amplicon with IGHV1 superfamily V gene formed < 0.3% chimeras with the other three amplicons. The average amount of chimeric amplicon formation was 18.3% for the four amplicons tested here.

Discussion

We developed a simple, cost-effective, and innovative approach for high-throughput sequencing of native antibody HC-LC pairs from B cell populations. In contrast to current paired Ig repertoire sequencing technologies [9–12, 15, 35], this method does not require the physical separation of single B cells using a flow cytometer, the construction of a flow focusing apparatus, or complex microfluidic devices. Our simple method relies on preparation of rER microsomes from B cells using a table-top centrifuge, avoiding ultracentrifugation steps [28]. The use of rER microsomes to link native HC-LC pairs in emulsion droplets overcomes previously reported difficulties involving cell entrapment in emulsion droplets, cell lysis, and RNA degradation during PCR [35, 36]. Due to the removal of the bulk genomic DNA and non-secretory RNA during microsome preparation, PCR artefacts due to off-target amplification by mispriming are greatly reduced. The simplicity of this method makes it widely applicable, also for laboratories without specialized equipment.

We report that our method can efficiently capture thousands of antibody HC-LC clonal pairs (Additional file 2: Data files S1–S4) by processing over one million B cells per experiment. Our observation that the top ten HC-LC sequence pairs accounted for 49–76% of the total aligned reads indicated a skewed clonotype distribution in the sequenced repertoires. An explanation for this is that our method predominantly detects antibody mRNAs that are present in higher abundance in the analyzed B cell population. This is because this method does not use single intact B cells, but rather ER microsomes derived from B cells, for antibody chain assembly. Cells with larger secretory ER volumes, which are secreting high amounts of antibodies, contribute a larger fraction of antibody sequences to the resulting dataset. Therefore, we expect that our data does not reflect actual B cell frequencies, but instead reflects the amounts of secreted antibody molecules. Thus, the thousands of heavy-light chain pairs we detected from over one million B cells represent the

subset of cells with the highest antibody production (e.g. plasma cells), which is actually a very interesting cell subset when looking for antigen-specific antibodies. Also, we noticed preferential amplification of certain V-gene segments [8, 37], reflecting amplification biases in favor of the primers used for the VK1 and VK3 LC gene families (Fig. 2b–e), and thus the reported HC-LC pairs inadequately represent the actual clonal frequencies. However, a more accurate estimate of the human B cell repertoire using our method is possible through integrating relatively simple optimizations such as minimization of PCR primer biases by adjusting primer concentrations, limiting the amplification cycles as well as by the use of unique molecular identifiers (UMI) to reduce sequence-dependent amplification biases in the nested PCR amplification [37, 38].

We observed that the IgM repertoires obtained from CD19+ B cells demonstrated relatively low clonal diversity in the pre-immunization sample in comparison to the post-immunization sample. In contrast, the IgG clonal diversity in the post-immunization sample is lower than in the pre-immunization sample, indicating that post-immunization, the IgG repertoire was dominated by antigen-experienced clonal pairs.

We showed that our paired antibody sequencing method was adequately sensitive in detecting antigen-specific B cell clones occurring at lower frequencies. This was demonstrated by the identification of three out of four novel TT-specific antibody sequences that were also found at low frequencies in the IgG pre-immunization sample. Our method can therefore track the expansion of B cells from pre- to post-immunization [2, 24] for the discovery of antigen-specific mAbs [1–3, 10]. However, it must be noted that our method, as reported here, is dependent on highly expanded sequences post-immunization in order to identify novel antigen-specific sequences, thereby limiting the application of our method to identify antigen-specific sequences from pre-immunization samples. An improved strategy to determine antigen-specific antibody sequences from B cell repertoires before immunization would be to pre-sort or enrich B cells according to antigen specificity, so that the resulting paired antibody sequences are highly enriched for antigen-specific sequences [39].

Using a set of defined amplicons, we detected an average amount of 18.3% chimeric amplicon formation during the second (non-emulsion) stage of our method, which is below an extent that would prevent the applicability of this method for rapid discovery of mAbs. We expect that also our repertoire data from human B cells before and after immunization contains similar numbers of chimeric amplicons, which would account for the observation that the pairing accuracy is less than what would be expected from the initial experiments using mouse hybridomas. Interestingly, the mouse hybridoma sequences used for establishment of the method showed only ~ 0.2% chimeric amplicons, probably due to their very divergent V gene sequences from distant V gene superfamilies. A method-specific mitigation strategy for computational removal of chimera pairs could be based on the inclusion of short unique molecular identifier (UMI) sequences next to the overlap sequence for heavy chain assembly in the central part of the amplicons. These UMIs can be sequenced using an additional index read, which is possible on the MiSeq platform. The UMI sequences could then be used to computationally remove lower-frequency (chimeric) LC sequences for each specific combination of HC and UMI sequence, keeping only the most frequent truly paired light chains.

The whole process – from B cell isolation to sequencing paired Ig repertoires and analyzing HC-LC sequences – takes only four days. Antibody validation can be carried out within two weeks after sequencing data acquisition [10, 40]. Our approach can be combined with bioinformatic tools [41] or conventional screening technologies [42–45] to facilitate the rapid identification of antigen-specific mAbs thereby circumventing laborious large-scale screening of combinatorial B cell libraries [2, 45].

Conclusions

The presented method provides a simple, cost-effective, and scalable platform to characterize native antibody HC-LC pairs at single-cell level for rapid identification and generation of antigen-specific monoclonal antibodies with minimal costs using only common laboratory equipment. Our simple method using rER-associated mRNAs to retain paired antibody HC-LC information from single cells can be widely applicable in labs that do not have commercially available specialized equipment. We anticipate that this technology could possibly accelerate translational research towards antibody discovery for diagnostics, therapeutics, cancer immunotherapies, and investigating immune responses to vaccination, cancer neoantigens, and various aspects of immune biology research.

Abbreviations

CDR: Complementarity determining region; ELISA: Enzyme-linked immunosorbant assay; HC: Heavy chain; Ig: Immunoglobulin; IgG: Immunoglobulin G; IgK: Immunoglobulin Kappa; IgM: Immunoglobulin M; LC: Light chain; mAbs: Monoclonal antibodies; PCR: Polymerase chain reaction; qPCR: Quantitative polymerase chain reaction; rER: Rough endoplasmic reticulum; RT-PCR: Reverse transcription polymerase chain reaction; Td: Tetanus toxoid and Diphtheria toxoid; TT: Tetanus toxoid; UMI: Unique molecular identifier; V: Variable gene segment; VH: Variable heavy; VK: Variable kappa

Acknowledgements
We thank Alexander Kovacsovics and Matthias Linser for performing Illumina MiSeq sequencing and Carola Stoschek for help with ELISA experiments. We thank Vyacheslav Amstislavskiy and Sören Matzk for assistance with Perl and R scripts for bioinformatic analyses.

Funding
This research was funded by the European Union Seventh Framework Program Grant agreement no. 316655 ("VacTrain" project) to PRD and by the Max Planck Society for the Advancement of Science (MPG).

Authors' contributions
JG and HJW developed the paired antibody sequencing method using endoplasmic reticulum microsomes; PRD optimized the method for application with B cells; JB and TM performed transmission electron microscopy; PRD and HJW designed and performed the PCR and sequencing experiments; PRD and HJW carried out bioinformatics analyses and analyzed the data; PRD and ZK designed antibody cloning, expression and binding experiments, which PRD has performed; HL, MLY, and HJW supervised the project; PRD and HJW wrote the manuscript. All authors read and approved the final manuscript.

Competing interests
HL, JG, and HJW have a patent application pending (WO/2013/117591) whose value may be affected by the publication of this paper. HL is a founder of and chairman at Alacris Theranostics GmbH. MLY is a founder of and chief scientific officer at Alacris Theranostics GmbH. The remaining authors declare that they have no competing interests.

Author details
[1]Otto Warburg Laboratory Gene Regulation and Systems Biology of Cancer, Max Planck Institute for Molecular Genetics, Berlin, Germany. [2]Microscopy and Cryo-Electron Microscopy Service Group, Max Planck Institute for Molecular Genetics, Berlin, Germany. [3]Institut für Medizinische Physik und Biophysik, Charité-Universitätsmedizin, Berlin, Germany. [4]Department of Biomolecular Systems, Max Planck Institute of Colloids and Interfaces, Potsdam, Germany. [5]Alacris Theranostics GmbH, Berlin, Germany. [6]Dahlem Centre for Genome Research and Medical Systems Biology, Berlin, Germany. [7]Department of Molecular Biotechnology and Functional Genomics, Institute of Applied Biosciences, Technical University of Applied Sciences Wildau, Wildau, Brandenburg, Germany.

References

1. Reddy ST, Ge X, Miklos AE, Hughes RA, Kang SH, Hoi KH, et al. Monoclonal antibodies isolated without screening by analyzing the variable-gene repertoire of plasma cells. Nat Biotechnol. 2010;28:965–9.
2. Galson JD, Pollard AJ, Truck J, Kelly DF. Studying the antibody repertoire after vaccination: practical applications. Trends Immunol. 2014;35:319–31.
3. Georgiou G, Ippolito GC, Beausang J, Busse CE, Wardemann H, Quake SR. The promise and challenge of high-throughput sequencing of the antibody repertoire. Nat Biotechnol. 2014;32:158–68.
4. Boyd SD, Marshall EL, Merker JD, Maniar JM, Zhang LN, Sahaf B, et al. Measurement and clinical monitoring of human lymphocyte clonality by massively parallel VDJ pyrosequencing. Sci Transl Med. 2009;1:12ra23.
5. Weinstein JA, Jiang N, White RA 3rd, Fisher DS, Quake SR. High-throughput sequencing of the zebrafish antibody repertoire. Science. 2009;324:807–10.
6. Larimore K, McCormick MW, Robins HS, Greenberg PD. Shaping of human germline IgH repertoires revealed by deep sequencing. J Immunol. 2012; 189:3221–30.
7. Rubelt F, Sievert V, Knaust F, Diener C, Lim TS, Skriner K, et al. Onset of immune senescence defined by unbiased pyrosequencing of human immunoglobulin mRNA repertoires. PLoS One. 2012;7:e49774.
8. Benichou J, Ben-Hamo R, Louzoun Y, Efroni S. Rep-Seq: uncovering the immunological repertoire through next-generation sequencing. Immunology. 2012;135:183–91.
9. Sanchez-Freire V, Ebert AD, Kalisky T, Quake SR, Wu JC. Microfluidic single-cell real-time PCR for comparative analysis of gene expression patterns. Nat Protoc. 2012;7:829–38.

10. DeKosky BJ, Ippolito GC, Deschner RP, Lavinder JJ, Wine Y, Rawlings BM, et al. High-throughput sequencing of the paired human immunoglobulin heavy and light chain repertoire. Nat Biotechnol. 2013;31:166–9.

11. Busse CE, Czogiel I, Braun P, Arndt PF, Wardemann H. Single-cell based high-throughput sequencing of full-length immunoglobulin heavy and light chain genes. Eur J Immunol. 2014;44:597–603.

12. Howie B, Sherwood AM, Berkebile AD, Berka J, Emerson RO, Williamson DW, et al. High-throughput pairing of T cell receptor alpha and beta sequences. Sci Transl Med. 2015;7:301ra131.

13. Macosko EZ, Basu A, Satija R, Nemesh J, Shekhar K, Goldman M, et al. Highly parallel genome-wide expression profiling of individual cells using nanoliter droplets. Cell. 2015;161:1202–14.

14. Zheng GX, Terry JM, Belgrader P, Ryvkin P, Bent ZW, Wilson R, et al. Massively parallel digital transcriptional profiling of single cells. Nat Commun. 2017;8:14049.

15. DeKosky BJ, Kojima T, Rodin A, Charab W, Ippolito GC, Ellington AD, et al. In-depth determination and analysis of the human pa red heavy- and light-chain antibody repertoire. Nat Med. 2015;21:86–91.

16. Briggs AW GS, Timberlake S, Belmont BJ, Clouser CR, Koppstein D, Sok D, Heiden JVA, Tammien MV, Kleinstein SH, et al. Tumor-infiltrating immune repertoires captured by single-cell barcoding in emulsion. bioRxiv. 2017. https://doi.org/10.1101/134841.

17. McDaniel JR, DeKosky BJ, Tanno H, Ellington AD, Georgiou G. Ultra-high-throughput sequencing of the immune receptor repertoire from millions of lymphocytes. Nat Protoc. 2016;11:429–42.

18. Suloway C, Pulokas J, Fellmann D, Cheng A, Guerra F, Quispe J, et al. Automated molecular microscopy: the new Leginon system. J Struct Biol. 2005;151:41–60.

19. Ge Q, Liu Z, Bai Y, Zhang D, Yu P, Lu Z. Emulsion PCR-based method to detect Y chromosome microdeletions. Anal Biochem. 2007;367:173–8.

20. Schutze T, Rubelt F, Repkow J, Greiner N, Erdmann VA, Lehrach H, et al. A streamlined protocol for emulsion polymerase chain reaction and subsequent purification. Anal Biochem. 2011;410:155–7.

21. Bolotin DA, Poslavsky S, Mitrophanov I, Shugay M, Mamedov IZ, Putintseva EV, et al. MiXCR: software for comprehensive adaptive immunity profiling. Nat Methods. 2015;12:380–1.

22. Ehrenmann F, Kaas Q, Lefranc MP. IMGT/3Dstructure-DB and IMGT/DomainGapAlign: a database and a tool for immunoglobulins or antibodies, T cell receptors, MHC, IgSF and MhcSF. Nucleic Acids Res. 2010;38:D301–7.

23. Jiang N, He J, Weinstein JA, Penland L, Sasaki S, He XS, et al. Lineage structure of the human antibody repertoire in response to influenza vaccination. Sci Transl Med. 2013;5:171ra119.

24. Truck J, Ramasamy MN, Galson JD, Rance R, Parkhill J, Lunter G, et al. Identification of antigen-specific B cell receptor sequences using public repertoire analysis. J Immunol. 2015;194:252–61.

25. Lavinder JJ, Wine Y, Giesecke C, Ippolito GC, Horton AP, Lungu OI, et al. Identification and characterization of the constituent human serum antibodies elicited by vaccination. Proc Natl Acad Sci U S A. 2014;111:2259–64.

26. Franz B, May KF Jr, Dranoff G, Wucherpfennig K. Ex vivo characterization and isolation of rare memory B cells with antigen tetramers. Blood. 2011;118:348–57.

27. Lerner RS, Seiser RM, Zheng T, Lager PJ, Reedy MC, Keene JD, et al. Partitioning and translation of mRNAs encoding soluble proteins on membrane-bound ribosomes. RNA. 2003;9:1123–37.

28. Abas L, Luschnig C. Maximum yields of microsomal-type membranes from small amounts of plant material without requiring ultracentrifugation. Anal Biochem. 2010;401:217–27.

29. Schneider-Poetsch T, Ju J, Eyler DE, Dang Y, Bhat S, Merrick WC, et al. Inhibition of eukaryotic translation elongation by cycloheximide and lactimidomycin. Nat Chem Biol. 2010;6:209–17.

30. Frolich D, Giesecke C, Mei HE, Reiter K, Daridon C, Lipsky PE, et al. Secondary immunization generates clonally related antigen-specific plasma cells and memory B cells. J Immunol. 2010;185:3103–10.

31. Parameswaran P, Liu Y, Roskin KM, Jackson KK, Dixit VP, Lee JY, et al. Convergent antibody signatures in human dengue. Cell Host Microbe. 2013;13:691–700.

32. Demaison C, David D, Letourneur F, Theze J, Saragosti S, Zouali M. Analysis of human VH gene repertoire expression in peripheral CD19+ B cells. Immunogenetics. 1995;42:342–52.

33. DeKosky BJ, Lungu OI, Park D, Johnson EL, Charab W, Chrysostomou C, et al. Large-scale sequence and structural comparisons of human naive and antigen-experienced antibody repertoires. Proc Natl Acad Sci U S A. 2016;113:E2636–45.

34. Saiki RK, Gelfand DH, Stoffel S, Scharf SJ, Higuchi R, Horn GT, et al. Primer-directed enzymatic amplification of DNA with a thermostable DNA polymerase. Science. 1988;239:487–91.

35. Turchaninova MA, Britanova OV, Bolotin DA, Shugay M, Putintseva EV, Staroverov DB, et al. Pairing of T-cell receptor chains via emulsion PCR. Eur J Immunol. 2013;43:2507–15.

36. White AK, VanInsberghe M, Petriv OI, Hamidi M, Sikorski D, Marra MA, et al. High-throughput microfluidic single-cell RT-qPCR. Proc Natl Acad Sci U S A. 2011;108:13999–4004.

37. Khan TA, Friedensohn S, Gorter de Vries AR, Straszewski J, Ruscheweyh HJ, Reddy ST. Accurate and predictive antibody repertoire profiling by molecular amplification fingerprinting. Sci Adv. 2016;2:e1501371.

38. Hou XL, Wang L, Ding YL, Xie Q, Diao HY. Current status and recent advances of next generation sequencing techniques in immunological repertoire. Genes Immun. 2016;17:153–64.

39. Ouisse LH, Gautreau-Rolland L, Devilder MC, Osborn M, Moyon M, Visentin J, et al. Antigen-specific single B cell sorting and expression-cloning from immunoglobulin humanized rats: a rapid and versatile method for the generation of high affinity and discriminative human monoclonal antibodies. BMC Biotechnol. 2017;17:3.

40. Wang B, Kluwe CA, Lungu OI, DeKosky BJ, Kerr SA, Johnson EL, et al. Facile discovery of a diverse panel of anti-Ebola virus antibodies by immune repertoire mining. Sci Rep. 2015;5:13926.

41. Greiff V, Miho E, Menzel U, Reddy ST. Bioinformatic and statistical analysis of adaptive immune repertoires. Trends Immunol. 2015;36:738–49.

42. Lanzavecchia A, Corti D, Sallusto F. Human monoclonal antibodies by immortalization of memory B cells. Curr Opin Biotechnol. 2007;18:523–8.

43. Bradbury AR, Sidhu S, Dubel S, McCafferty J. Beyond natural antibodies: the power of in vitro display technologies. Nat Biotechnol. 2011;29:245–54.

44. Wardemann H, Kofer J. Expression cloning of human B cell immunoglobulins. Methods Mol Biol. 2013;971:93–111.

45. Wilson PC, Andrews SF. Tools to therapeutically harness the human antibody response. Nat Rev Immunol. 2012;12:709–19.

7

Single-cell transcriptomics reveal that PD-1 mediates immune tolerance by regulating proliferation of regulatory T cells

Cherry S. Leung[1†], Kevin Y. Yang[1†], Xisheng Li[1], Vicken W. Chan[1], Manching Ku[2], Herman Waldmann[3], Shohei Hori[4], Jason C. H. Tsang[1,5], Yuk Ming Dennis Lo[1,5] and Kathy O. Lui[1,5*] (iD)

Abstract

Background: We have previously reported an antigen-specific protocol to induce transplant tolerance and linked suppression to human embryonic stem cell (hESC)-derived tissues in immunocompetent mice through coreceptor and costimulation blockade. However, the exact mechanisms of acquired immune tolerance in this model have remained unclear.

Methods: We utilize the NOD.$Foxp3^{hCD2}$ reporter mouse line and an ablative anti-hCD2 antibody to ask if $CD4^+FOXP3^+$ regulatory T cells (Treg) are required for coreceptor and costimulation blockade-induced immune tolerance. We also perform genome-wide single-cell RNA-sequencing to interrogate Treg during immune rejection and tolerance and to indicate possible mechanisms involved in sustaining Treg function.

Results: We show that Treg are indispensable for tolerance induced by coreceptor and costimulation blockade as depletion of which with an anti-hCD2 antibody resulted in rejection of hESC-derived pancreatic islets in NOD.$Foxp3^{hCD2}$ mice. Single-cell transcriptomic profiling of 12,964 intragraft $CD4^+$ T cells derived from rejecting and tolerated grafts reveals that Treg are heterogeneous and functionally distinct in the two outcomes of transplant rejection and tolerance. Treg appear to mainly promote chemotactic and ubiquitin-dependent protein catabolism during transplant rejection while seeming to harness proliferative and immunosuppressive function during tolerance. We also demonstrate that this form of acquired transplant tolerance is associated with increased proliferation and PD-1 expression by Treg. Blocking PD-1 signaling with a neutralizing anti-PD-1 antibody leads to reduced Treg proliferation and graft rejection.

Conclusions: Our results suggest that short-term coreceptor and costimulation blockade mediates immune tolerance to hESC-derived pancreatic islets by promoting Treg proliferation through engagement of PD-1. Our findings could give new insights into clinical development of hESC-derived pancreatic tissues, combined with immunotherapies that expand intragraft Treg, as a potentially sustainable alternative treatment for T1D.

Keywords: Single-cell transcriptomics, Transplant tolerance, $CD4^+$ regulatory T cells, PD-1, Human pancreatic beta cells

Background

The global prevalence of diabetes was 8.5% in 2014 [1] and is predicted to rise due to the growing obesity epidemic. Although most type 1 (T1D) and some type 2 (T2D) diabetic patients receive insulin therapy, it does not provide a real-time glycemic control to patients compared to transplantation of glucose-sensing, insulin-secreting pancreatic islets so patients are still at risk of developing hypoglycemia and cardiovascular complications [2]. Transplantation of human cadaveric pancreatic islets has been implemented clinically [3, 4] with a majority of patients achieving insulin independence within the first year but declining rapidly afterwards [3, 4]. Any therapeutic efficacy of islet transplantation has also been largely limited by the scarcity and quality of donor islets, chronic immune rejection [3], and recurrence of autoimmunity [5].

* Correspondence: kathyolui@cuhk.edu.hk
†Cherry S. Leung and Kevin Y. Yang contributed equally to this work.
[1]Department of Chemical Pathology, Prince of Wales Hospital, The Chinese University of Hong Kong, Hong Kong, China
[5]Li Ka Shing Institute of Health Sciences, Prince of Wales Hospital, The Chinese University of Hong Kong, Hong Kong, China
Full list of author information is available at the end of the article

By virtue of their pluripotent and self-renewing properties, recent advances in human embryonic stem cell (hESC) technology have led to success in generating literally unlimited amount of human pancreatic endoderm cells or islets in vitro for transplantation, resulting in reversal of diabetes in mice [6–8]. Although transplantation of autologous induced pluripotent stem cell (iPSC) derivatives likely prevents immune rejection, T1D results from autoimmune attack so the T1D patient-specific iPSC-derived pancreatic beta cells might still harbor autoantigens to activate autoreactive memory T cells following transplantation [5]. On the other hand, direct presentation of autoantigens would be less likely with major histocompatibility complex (MHC) histoincompatible transplants. Moreover, cell therapy using derivatives of "off the shelf" hESCs is more economically and logistically feasible than hiPSCs when treating the population at large as well as patients with acute injuries [9]. Therefore, clinical trials using hESC derivatives [10, 11] and research in preventing their immune rejection still attract much attention [9, 12–14].

Transplantation of ESC-derived tissues also offers additional benefits [15–17] as they lack donor antigen-presenting cells (APCs) that elicit the direct pathway of allorecognition and are devoid of donor T cells that provoke graft-versus-host-disease (GVHD). All these features indicate that hESC-derived pancreatic tissues could be less immunogenic than human cadaveric islets for transplantation. We have previously reported that ESC-derived tissues exhibit some degree of immune privilege and can be spontaneously accepted by allogeneic recipients in conditions including disparity for a class-I MHC molecule [18].

Recently, clinical trials using encapsulated hESC-derived pancreatic endoderm cells have been approved in T1D patients [19, 20]. Cell encapsulation prevents direct contact between the transplanted cells and host immune system. Nevertheless, previous clinical studies have demonstrated that the therapeutic benefit of transplanting encapsulated human cadaveric islets into T1D patients is only temporary [21, 22]. This is likely due to the host's innate immune response reacting to the implanted capsules, resulting in fibrosis, nutrient isolation, and donor tissue necrosis [23, 24]. To ensure long-term survival of the transplanted hESC-derived pancreatic tissues, particularly in autoimmune recipients with a primed immune system, the exploitation of endogenous tolerance processes will be invaluable.

One of the mechanisms by which antigen-specific immune tolerance established in mice operates through CD4+FOXP3+ regulatory T cells (Treg). Treg are indispensable for maintaining peripheral self-tolerance [25] and are important in suppressing allogeneic responses against non-self antigens during GVHD [26] or allograft rejection [18, 27]. Following allogeneic transplantation,

Treg accumulating in tolerated grafts are immunosuppressive locally, can induce additional Treg (iTreg) from naïve T cells via infectious tolerance [27, 28], and can protect "third-party" antigens that coexist with tolerated antigens from immune rejection via linked suppression [29]. In all these situations, the mechanisms sustaining Treg survival in vivo are not yet fully understood.

Furthermore, it is unclear what Treg are doing within rejecting grafts. Are they solely bystanders, or remnants of a failed suppressive endeavor, or even contributors to the rejecting processes? We have previously reported an antigen-specific protocol to induce transplant tolerance and linked suppression to hESC-derived endothelial cells and neurons following transplantation into immunocompetent mice using coreceptor and costimulation antibody blockade [13]. Here, we demonstrate that such antibody blockade also promoted transplant tolerance to hESC-derived pancreatic islets in non-obese diabetic (NOD) mice that involved the activity of Treg. Using single-cell RNA-sequencing (scRNA-seq), we performed genome-wide characterization of 12,964 intragraft CD4+ T cells including conventional T cells and Treg of both rejecting and tolerated grafts. We show that conventional T cells found in the tolerated grafts expressed genes previously reported to support Treg function. Moreover, Treg were heterogeneous despite the beneficial transplant outcome. In contrast, there were at least two subsets of Treg in rejecting grafts that were distinct and less proliferative compared to those in tolerated grafts.

Our scRNA-seq data also show that antibody blockade augmented proliferation and PD-1 expression of Treg in tolerated grafts. Recently, immunotherapy targeting immune checkpoints including programmed cell death protein 1 (PD-1) has become a promising anti-cancer medicine. However, it has been reported that patients receiving anti-PD-1 antibodies developed T1D and other autoimmune diseases [30]. Although the role of PD-1 on conventional T cells has been well established [31], whether the PD-1 signaling can in some way affect Treg remains unclear. In this study, we observed that PD-1 blockade via a neutralizing anti-PD-1 antibody reduced proliferation of Treg and prevented tolerance induced by coreceptor and costimulation blockade. Taken together, our results suggest that coreceptor and costimulation blockade mediated transplant tolerance to hESC-derived pancreatic islets in NOD mice, at least in part, by promoting Treg proliferation via PD-1 signaling.

Methods
Human ESC cultures and pancreatic islet differentiation
The H9 hESC line (WA09, WiCell) was maintained in mTseR1 medium (Stemgent). EB induction was performed by resuspending hESCs in differentiation medium containing DMEM/F12, 10% knockout serum replacement

(KOSR), 1X non-essential amino acids, 1X glutamine, 1X penicillin/streptomycin, and 1X b-mercaptoethanol (Gibco) in hanging drop cultures overnight. Individual EBs were then transferred to suspension cultures and incubated in differentiation medium containing 1% KOSR for another 12 days before transplantation. For pancreatic islet differentiation, hESCs were differentiated by stepwise administration of growth factors as described previously [6]. Briefly, a combination of growth factors was supplemented as follows: day 1/S1: 100 ng/ml Activin A (Peprotech) + 3 μM Chir99021 (Selleck Chem); day 2/S1: 100 ng/ml Activin A; days 4 and 6/S2: 50 ng/ml KGF (Peprotech); days 7 and 8/ S3: 50 ng/ml KGF + 0.25 μM Sant1 (Sigma) + 2 μM RA (Sigma) + 200 nM LDN193189 (Sigma, on day 7 only) + 500 nM PdBU (EMD Millipore); days 9 and 11, 13/S3: 50 ng/ml KGF + 0.25 μM Sant1 + 100 nM RA; days 14 and 16/S5: 0.25 μM Sant1 + 100 nM RA + 1 μM XXI (Calbiochem) + 10 μM Alk5i II (Selleck Chem) + 1 μM T3 (EMD Millipore) + 20 ng/ml Betacellulin (Peprotech). Days 18 and 20/S5: 25 nM RA + 1 μM XXI + 10 μM Alk5i II + 1 μM T3 + 20 ng/ml Betacellulin. Days 21–35/S6 (medium changed on alternative days): 10 μM Alk5i II + 1 μM T3. In the final stage, cells were cultured in CMRL 1066 modified medium (CMRLM).

Mice

Foxp3^{hCD2} reporter mice (C57BL/6) [32] were backcrossed onto the NOD/ShiJc1 (Clea Japan. Inc) background for 12 generations. Experiments were performed with mice at 8–10 weeks old before onset of diabetes.

Kidney capsule transplantation

EBs or hESC-derived beta cell clusters were transplanted under the kidney capsule of NOD.Foxp3^{hCD2} mice as described previously [13, 18].

Administration of monoclonal antibodies

Non-depleting mAb specific for CD4 (1 mg, clone YTS 177), CD8 (1 mg, clone YTS 105), and CD40L (1 mg, clone MR1, BioXcell) were injected intraperitoneally (i.p.) on days 0, 2, and 4 following transplantation. For Treg depletion, ablative anti-hCD2 mAb (0.25 mg, clone YTH655) was injected i.p. on days 0–7 following transplantation as previously described [27]. For PD1 blockade, neutralizing anti-PD1 mAb (0.5 mg, clone RMP1-14, BioXcell) was injected i.p. on days 0, 2, 4, 6, and 8 following transplantation as previously described [33]. The hybridoma lines for making YTS177, YTS105, and YTH655 antibodies were prepared as previously described [13, 18, 34].

Immunostaining

Kidney grafts were dissected and fixed in 4% paraformaldehyde at 4 °C overnight. The fixed grafts were washed three times with PBS and equilibrated in 30% sucrose for 2 days before freezing and cryosectioning. Six-micrometer sections were blocked at 2% goat serum and then stained with the respective primary antibodies at 10 μg/ml at 4 °C overnight. Anti-human primary antibodies used are the following: PDX1 (R&D systems), NKX6.1 (R&D systems), GLUCAGON (Abcam), and C-PEPTIDE (DSHB), and the anti-mouse primary antibodies used are the following: Ki67 (eBiosciences) and FOXP3 (Cell Signaling Technology). Alexa-Fluor-488- or Alexa-Fluor-594-conjugated secondary antibodies (Invitrogen) were used at room temperature for 30 min in the dark. Slides were mounted with DAPI-containing fluorescence mounting medium (Dako), and fluorescence was detected with a confocal microscope (Leica). Some sections were also stained with hematoxylin and eosin (H&E) for histological analyses.

FACS sorting and analysis

Splenocytes were dissociated by pressing the excised spleen in PBS with a syringe plunger through a 40-μm cell strainer to obtain single cell suspension. Single blood cells were dissociated from whole blood after removal of plasma in EDTA. Single graft cells were obtained by digesting the grafts with a digestion buffer containing collagenase II (11 U/ml, Worthington), dispase (1000 U/ml, Gibco), and DNase I (10 U) at 37 °C for 20–30 min. Enzymatic action was stopped by adding 10% FBS, and the dissociated cells were washed twice with PBS. The dissociated single splenocytes, blood, or graft cells were removed from the contaminated erythrocytes by incubating with the red blood cell lysis buffer (eBiosciences) for 5 min and were then blocked with 2% heat-inactivated rabbit serum. Cells were subsequently stained with fluorochrome-conjugated antibodies against the following antigens: mCD3, mCD4, mPD1, or hCD2 (Biolegend) at a dilution of 1:100, unless specified by the manufacturer, at 4 °C for 30 min. Murine Treg were detected with the Treg staining kit according to the manufacturer's instructions (eBioscience). Cells were then washed three times with 2% FBS-containing PBS and analyzed on flow cytometer (BD FACSAria™ Fusion). Propidium iodide (PI, BD) positive dead cells were excluded for live cell analysis/sorting, and FACS data were then analyzed with the FlowJo software (Tree star).

Bulk RNA-sequencing and functional annotations

Total RNA was isolated from FACS-sorted cells using the RNeasy mini kit (Qiagen) and analyzed on the Agilent Tape station for RNA Integrity Numbers (RIN) prior to library preparation. RNA-Seq libraries were prepared using TruSeq Stranded mRNA Library Prep Kit according to manufacturer's protocol (Illumina). mRNA was isolated using poly-T oligos conjugated to magnetic beads and then fragmented and reverse-transcribed to cDNA. dUTPs were incorporated during second-strand synthesis and thus not amplified. cDNA was then undergone end-repair, ligation with indexed adapters, and PCR amplification. Nucleic acid was cleaned up after each steps using AMPure XP beads (Beckman Coulter). Libraries were then quantified, pooled, and sequenced at single-end 50 base-pair on the Illumina HiSeq platform. Libraries were sequenced at an average depth of 20 million reads per library. After trimming low-quality bases, the sequenced reads were aligned to the mouse reference genome (mm10) using STAR (v2.4.2a) with default settings [35]. Reference genome and gene model file (mm10) were obtained from HOMER [36]. The expression abundances of all genes and differentially expressed genes were calculated by HOMER (v4.7) with default parameters. The identified differentially expressed genes were further annotated with Gene Ontology (GO) using DAVID Bioinformatics Resources (v6.8) [37].

Single-cell encapsulation and library preparation
Single cells were purified by FACS sorting before library preparation, and single-cell libraries were prepared with the Chromium Single Cell 3' Reagent Kits v2 (10x Genomics) as per manufacturer's instructions. Briefly, sorted cells in suspension were first prepared as gel beads in emulsion (GEMs) on Single Cell 3' Chips v2 (10x Chromium) using the Chromium Controller (10x Genomics). Barcoded RNA transcripts in each single cell were reverse transcribed within GEM droplets. cDNA was purified with DynaBeads MyOne Silane beads (Invitrogen) and then amplified for subsequent library construction. Sequencing libraries were prepared by fragmentation, end-repair, ligation with indexed adapters, and PCR amplification using the Chromium Single Cell 3' library kit v2 (10x Genomics). Nucleic acid was cleaned up after each steps using SPRIselect beads (Beckman Coulter). Libraries were then quantified by Qubit and real-time quantitative PCR on a LightCycler 96 System (Roche).

Single-cell RNA-sequencing and functional annotations
Pooled libraries were sequenced on the Illumina NextSeq 500 platform. All single-cell libraries were sequenced with a customized paired-end dual index format (98/26/0/8 basepair) according to manufacturer's instructions. Data were processed, aligned, and quantified using the Cell Ranger Single-Cell Software Suite (v 2.0) [38]. Briefly, data were demultiplexed based on the 8 base-pair sample index, 16 base-pair Chromium barcodes, and 10 base-pair unique molecular identifiers (UMI). Two distinct groups of contaminated cells were removed as they expressed genes of the myeloid lineage. To eliminate the impact of cell number bias, data from ~ 1000 cells of each sample were randomly selected for further analysis. Cells with either very low or too high mRNA content (i.e., out of two standard deviations) or high fractions of mitochondrial encoded transcripts (> 10%) were filtered out. Data were aligned on *Mus musculus* Cell Ranger transcriptome reference (mm10-1.2.0), and analyses, including PCA, tSNE, and graph-based clustering, were performed according to Cell Ranger's pipelines with default settings. To perform differential expression analysis on each comparison, Cell Ranger's pipelines were applied with sSeq algorithm [39], which employs a negative binomial exact test to generate p values and further adjusted using Benjamini-Hochberg. To perform GO functional enrichment analysis, genes that satisfy a less stringent criterion (with at least fourfold changes) were considered to be potential targets, which were further annotated with GO using DAVID Bioinformatics Resources (v6.8) [37]. Cell cycle phase classifications were performed by scran [40] with default settings.

Statistical analysis
The data were expressed as arithmetic mean ± s.d. of biological replicates ($n = 6$, unless otherwise specified) performed under the same conditions. Statistical analysis was performed using the unpaired Student's t test with data from two groups, while data from more than two groups was performed using an ANOVA followed by Tukey's method for multiple comparisons. Significance was accepted when $P < 0.05$.

Results
Coreceptor and costimulation blockade facilitates survival and maturation of hESC-islets in NOD mice
We have previously reported that coreceptor and costimulation blockade induces transplant tolerance and linked suppression to hESC-derived progenitor cells and their differentiated progenies in immunocompetent mice [13]. To ask if the same regimen protects grafts from rejection in mice with an autoimmune background such as NOD, we transplanted surrogate hESC-derived embryoid bodies (hESC-EB) under the kidney capsule of 10-week-old NOD mice under cover of treatment with anti-CD4, anti-CD8, and anti-CD40L monoclonal antibodies (3 mAb), previously shown to allow transplants to survive for at least 3 months as previously described [13]. We found that hESC-EB survived and differentiated into three embryonic germ layers at 1 month after transplantation (Additional file 1: Figure S1), indicating that coreceptor and costimulation blockade induced graft acceptance in NOD mice. In fact, coreceptor blockade alone can reverse hyperglycemia in NOD mice as previously described [41]. Moreover, we differentiated pancreatic islets from hESCs (hESC-islets) as a surrogate tissue for transplantation (Fig. 1a) using a protocol previously demonstrated to reverse streptozotocin-induced hyperglycemia

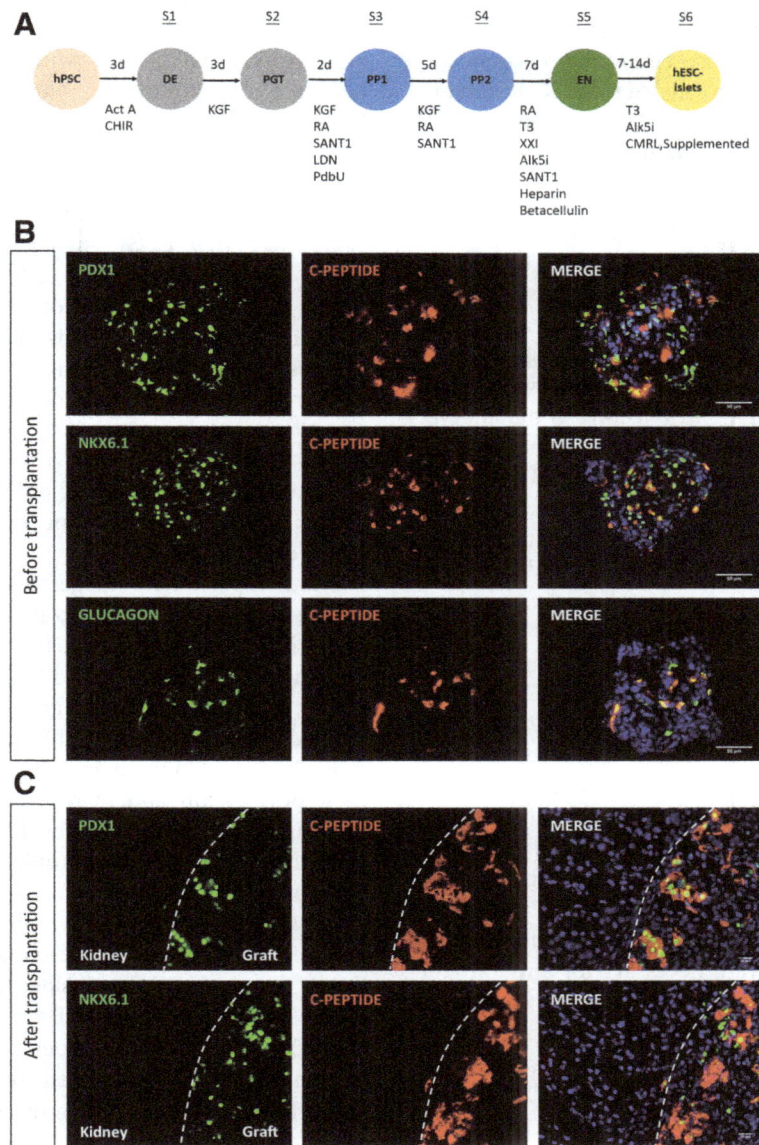

Fig. 1 Coreceptor and costimulation blockade facilitates survival and maturation of hESC-derived pancreatic islets in NOD.Foxp3[hCD2] mice. **a** A schematic diagram showing the simplified stepwise differentiation protocol to generate human pancreatic islets from hESCs. **b, c** Immunostaining for the lineage-specific markers of human pancreatic islets **b** before and **c** after 1-month transplantation of hESC-islets in NOD.*Foxp3*[hCD2] mice (*n* = 6) following treatment with coreceptor and costimulation blockade. Scale bars in **b**: 50 μm and in **c**: 20 μm

[6]. Whether the surrogate tissue reversed hyperglycemia was not the focus of this study as both the tolerance induction regimen and surrogate tissues facilitate remission of diabetes. Rather, we studied the mechanisms by which coreceptor and costimulation blockade induced transplant tolerance to hESC-derived tissues. This is why we transplanted 10-week-old NOD mice, well before the onset of diabetes, to minimize the risk that autoimmune reactions might alter analysis of mechanisms operated during induction of transplant tolerance.

Immunostaining for human PDX1, NKX6.1, or GLUCAGON with C-PEPTIDE, respectively, in stage 6 cells confirmed differentiation of hESCs into hESC-islets (Fig. 1b). We then transplanted hESC-islets under cover of treatment with 3 mAb and found that hESC-islets survived in NOD mice without teratoma formation (Fig. 1c). Moreover, immunostaining for human PDX1 or NKX6.1 with C-PEPTIDE in tolerated grafts revealed that hESC-islets matured in vivo as there were more PDX1[+]C-PEPTIDE[+] or NKX6.1[+]C-PEPTIDE[+] cells in tolerated grafts (Fig. 1c) than those before transplantation (Fig. 1b). Our results demonstrated that hESC-islets served as a surrogate tissue for downstream analysis, and coreceptor and costimulation blockade induced transplant tolerance to hESC-derived tissues not only in wildtype but also in recipients of T1D background not yet exhibiting autoimmune disease.

Coreceptor and costimulation blockade promotes transplant tolerance to hESC-derived tissues through CD4$^+$ Treg

Although Treg deficiency or dysfunction is sufficient to break self-tolerance [25], it remains unclear whether they are indispensable for maintaining transplant tolerance to hESC-derived tissues. Previously, we were unable to detect CD4$^+$FOXP3$^+$ Treg in rejecting grafts and very few were detected in tolerated grafts [13] due to cell loss through intra-nuclear immunostaining for FOXP3 and to a lack of reliable cell surface marker(s) for phenotyping of murine CD4$^+$ Treg. To examine contribution of Treg in coreceptor and costimulation blockade-mediated transplant tolerance to hESC-derived tissues, we backcrossed the $Foxp3^{hCD2}$ reporter "knockin" allele [32] onto the NOD background, which allowed us to purify Treg via their surface expression of hCD2. We first confirmed co-localization of FOXP3 and hCD2 in NOD.-$Foxp3^{hCD2}$ mice by flow cytometry (Fig. 2ba). We also detected CD4$^+$hCD2$^+$ Treg in both rejecting and tolerated hESC-derived grafts (Fig. 2), while there was no significant difference in percentage of CD4$^+$hCD2$^-$ conventional T cells (Th) of rejecting and tolerated grafts (Fig. 2c); a significantly higher percentage of CD4$^+$hCD2$^+$ Treg was found in tolerated than rejecting grafts (Fig. 2d).

To determine if Treg were necessary for antibody-mediated tolerance, we depleted them with an ablative anti-hCD2 mAb (αhCD2, Fig. 2e). On day 4 post-αhCD2 treatment, we already observed a threefold and fivefold reduction in splenic and circulatory CD4$^+$FOXP3$^+$ Treg within the CD4$^+$ population, respectively (Fig. 2f). In fact, the depletion efficiency of Treg by αhCD2 in NOD.-$Foxp3^{hCD2}$ (Fig. 2g) was comparable to that in B6.$Foxp3^{hCD2}$ as previously described [27]. We then transplanted hESC-islets in NOD.$Foxp3^{hCD2}$ and examined graft survival at 1 month following transplantation with 3 mAb or 3 mAb + αhCD2 mAb. Compared to grafts derived from 3 mAb-treated group that were 100% accepted, those from 3 mAb + αhCD2 mAb-treated group were 100% rejected (n = 6 per group, Fig. 2h). Our results indicated that Treg were indispensable for coreceptor and costimulation blockade-induced transplant tolerance.

Genome-wide transcriptomic profiling of splenic CD4$^+$ Treg during transplant rejection and tolerance

We next asked if Treg were beginning to influence transplant outcome in secondary lymphoid tissues by

purifying splenic CD4$^+$hCD2$^+$ Treg from 3 mAb + αhCD2 mAb-treated rejecting and 3 mAb-treated tolerized NOD.$Foxp3^{hCD2}$ following transplantation for bulk RNA-seq. We found 43 differentially expressed genes (Additional file 1: Figure S2), and functional annotations by GO showed that the most significantly downregulated genes in splenic Treg of tolerized compared to rejecting mice were associated with neutrophil chemotaxis (Csf3r, Ccl1, Itga1, Il1b, Ccl5), angiogenesis (Mmp9, Il1b, Lrg1, Ccl5), and regulation of T cell proliferation (Il21, Il1b, Ccl5). Even though a total of 24,020 genes were identified in splenic Treg, this paucity of differentially expressed genes might indicate that Treg were largely similar in secondary lymphoid tissues during transplant rejection and tolerance.

Genome-wide transcriptomic profiling of intragraft CD4$^+$ Th and Treg during transplant rejection and tolerance at single-cell resolution

Previous reports have suggested that Treg-mediated tolerance to allogeneic skin grafts mainly operates at the graft site [27, 42]; however, the identities and interrelationships of different CD4$^+$ T cell subsets at the graft site during transplant rejection and tolerance have not been studied. The definition of different CD4$^+$ T cell subsets is likely biased due to insufficient surface markers for their purification and manipulation. To overcome this, we sought to understand the heterogeneity of CD4$^+$ T cells through large-scale droplet-based single-cell transcriptomic profiling [38, 43]. In this system, individual cells were encapsulated in microfluidic droplets with unique nucleotide barcodes and molecule identifiers (UMI) for tagging RNAs inside the droplets. We purified about ~ 12,964 intragraft CD4$^+$ T cells by FACS including 858 CD4$^+$hCD2$^-$ helper T cells (Th) and 954 CD4$^+$hCD2$^+$ Treg from ten recipients with rejecting grafts (untreated controls) and 3654 Th and 7498 Treg from ten recipients with tolerated grafts (3 mAb treated). It is worthy of note that untreated mice were used as rejecting controls as Treg depletion via anti-hCD2 antibodies could change the T cell populations within the grafts that could interfere our heterogeneity analysis. Moreover, to eliminate the impact of cell number bias, data from ~ 1000 cells of each sample were randomly selected for further analysis (Additional file 1: Figure S3).

We defined four cell clusters according to their initial CD4 and hCD2 expression and performed unsupervised analysis that did not rely on other known CD4$^+$ T cell subset markers. From the t-distributed stochastic neighbor embedding (t-SNE) plots, we observed that CD4$^+$hCD2$^-$ Th (R-T$_H$) and CD4$^+$hCD2$^+$ Treg (R-T$_R$) of rejecting grafts mapped closely together; CD4$^+$hCD2$^-$ Th of tolerated grafts (T-T$_H$) mapped closer to R-T$_H$ and R-T$_R$ than CD4$^+$hCD2$^+$ Treg of tolerated grafts

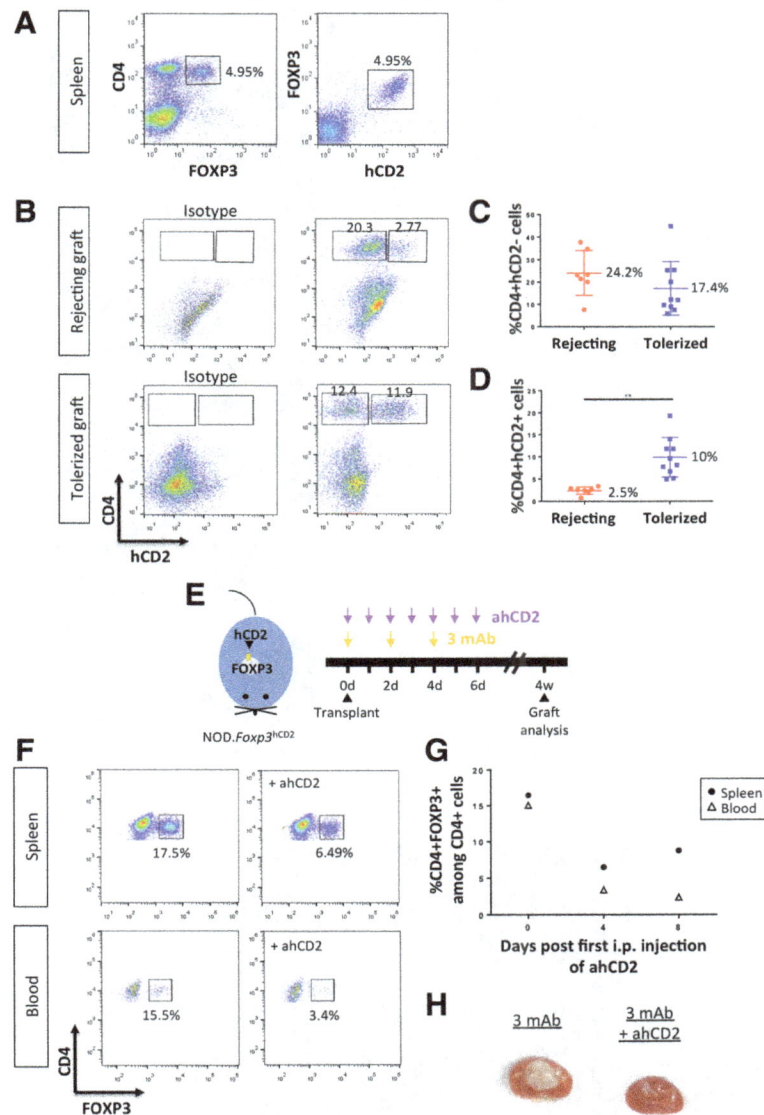

Fig. 2 Coreceptor and costimulation blockade promotes transplant tolerance to hESC-derived tissues through CD4$^+$ Treg. **a** Flow cytometric analysis showing surface expression of hCD2 by all CD4$^+$FOXP3$^+$ Treg in NOD.Foxp3^{hCD2} mice. **b** Flow cytometric analysis and **c**, **d** quantifications showing **c** comparable infiltration of CD4$^+$hCD2$^-$ conventional T cells but **d** significantly increased infiltration of CD4$^+$hCD2$^+$ Treg in tolerated ($n = 10$) than rejecting ($n = 10$) grafts at 1 month post-transplantation. ******$P < 0.01$. **e** A schematic diagram showing the protocol for antibody treatments. **f** Flow cytometric analysis and **g** time-dependent quantifications showing reduced percentage of CD4$^+$FOXP3$^+$ Treg among total CD4$^+$ T cells in the spleen and blood of NOD.Foxp3^{hCD2} mice after treatment with the ablative αhCD2 antibody. **h** Representative images showing that αhCD2 antibody abolished coreceptor and costimulation blockade-mediated tolerance to hESC-islets at 1 month following transplantation, $n = 6$ per group

(T-T$_R$); and T-T$_R$ formed a distinct population (Fig. 3a). Based on their cytokine expression profiles, we further characterized CD4$^+$ Th subsets during transplant rejection and tolerance. R-T$_H$ included *Ifng*-expressing Th1 cells, *Il4*, *Il5*, and *Il13*-expressing Th2 cells as well as Il21-expressing Th17 cells during rejection, and T-T$_H$ mainly included *Ifng*-expressing Th1 cells as well as *Il21*-expressing Th17 cells during tolerance (Additional file 1: Figure S4A).

Next, we performed pairwise analysis to identify the differentially expressed genes. Although R-T$_H$ and T-T$_H$ did not form distinct clusters on *t*-SNE (Additional file 1: Figure S5A), 392 differentially expressed genes were identified in T-T$_H$ compared to R-T$_H$ and GO functional annotations showed that the most significantly upregulated pathway was associated with negative regulation of the immune system such as expression of *Cd81* [44] and *Ccr7* [45] that support Treg function or *Tmem176a* and

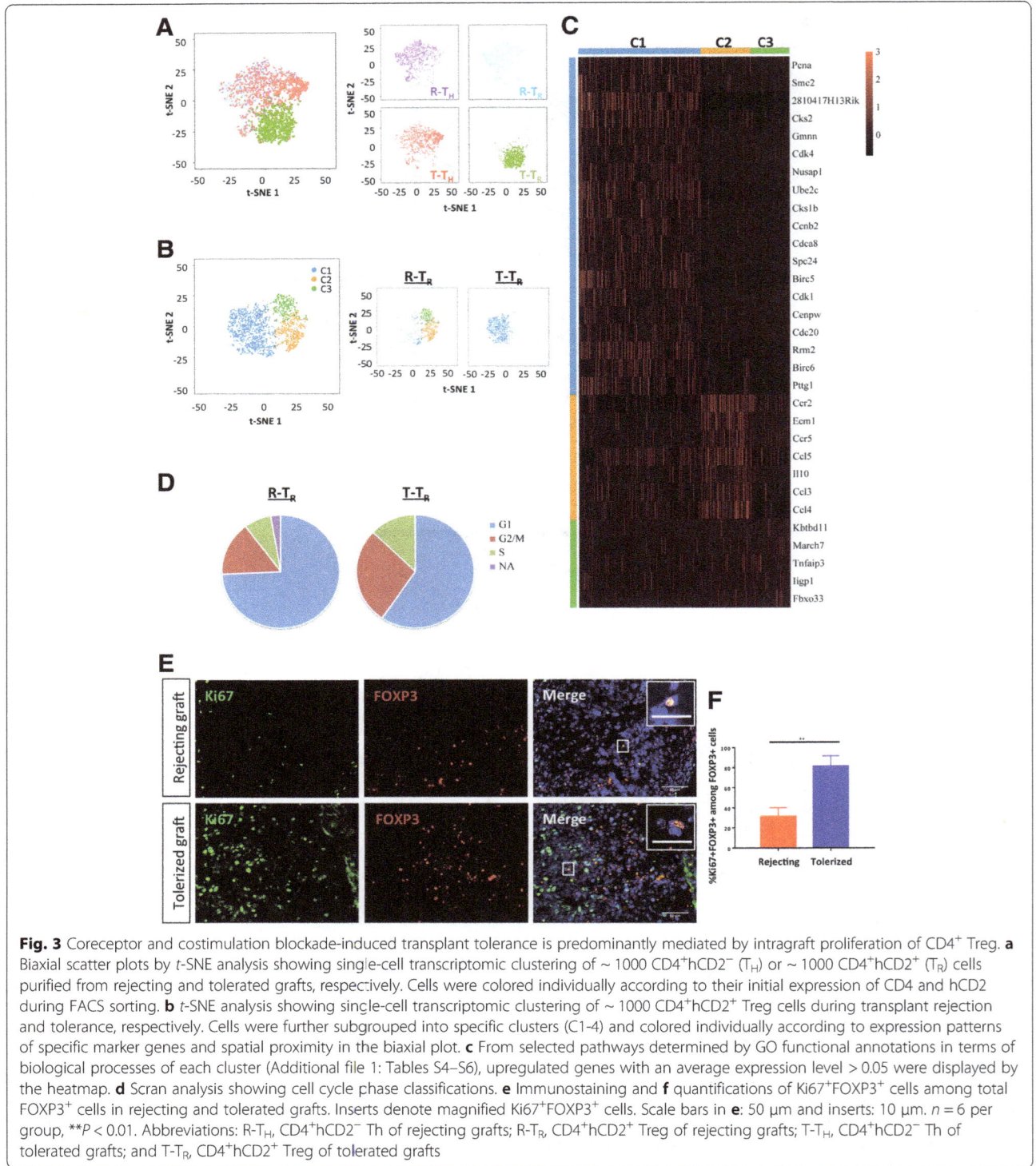

Fig. 3 Coreceptor and costimulation blockade-induced transplant tolerance is predominantly mediated by intragraft proliferation of CD4$^+$ Treg. **a** Biaxial scatter plots by *t*-SNE analysis showing single-cell transcriptomic clustering of ~ 1000 CD4$^+$hCD2$^-$ (T$_H$) or ~ 1000 CD4$^+$hCD2$^+$ (T$_R$) cells purified from rejecting and tolerated grafts, respectively. Cells were colored individually according to their initial expression of CD4 and hCD2 during FACS sorting. **b** *t*-SNE analysis showing single-cell transcriptomic clustering of ~ 1000 CD4$^+$hCD2$^+$ Treg cells during transplant rejection and tolerance, respectively. Cells were further subgrouped into specific clusters (C1-4) and colored individually according to expression patterns of specific marker genes and spatial proximity in the biaxial plot. **c** From selected pathways determined by GO functional annotations in terms of biological processes of each cluster (Additional file 1: Tables S4–S6), upregulated genes with an average expression level > 0.05 were displayed by the heatmap. **d** Scran analysis showing cell cycle phase classifications. **e** Immunostaining and **f** quantifications of Ki67$^+$FOXP3$^+$ cells among total FOXP3$^+$ cells in rejecting and tolerated grafts. Inserts denote magnified Ki67$^+$FOXP3$^+$ cells. Scale bars in **e**: 50 μm and inserts: 10 μm. $n = 6$ per group, **$P < 0.01$. Abbreviations: R-T$_H$, CD4$^+$hCD2$^-$ Th of rejecting grafts; R-T$_R$, CD4$^+$hCD2$^+$ Treg of rejecting grafts; T-T$_H$, CD4$^+$hCD2$^-$ Th of tolerated grafts; and T-T$_R$, CD4$^+$hCD2$^+$ Treg of tolerated grafts

Tmem176b that negatively regulate dendritic cell differentiation. Moreover, the most significantly down-regulated pathways were associated with responses to interferon-α/β/γ (Additional file 1: Figure S5B, gene listed in Additional file 1: Table S1). Therefore, CD4$^+$ Th

cells might, perhaps, elicit more immunomodulatory than inflammatory responses during transplant tolerance than rejection.

During transplant rejection, we found that R-T$_R$ and R-T$_H$ mapped closely together on *t*-SNE (Additional file 1:

Figure S5C). A total of 367 differentially expressed genes were identified in R-T_R compared to R-T_H, and GO functional annotations showed that the most significantly upregulated pathways were associated with negative regulation of conventional T cell function (e.g., *Cd81*, *Phlpp1*, *Foxp3*, *Sdc4*, and *Il2ra*) and the most significantly downregulated pathways were associated with adaptive immune responses (e.g., *Cd40Ig*, *Il2*, *Il4*, *Ifng*), DNA repair, and autophagy (Additional file 1: Figure S5D, gene listed in Additional file 1: Table S2). Compared to CD4$^+$ Th cells, Treg during transplant rejection could still harbor anti-inflammatory functions.

During transplant tolerance, we found that T-T_R and T-T_H formed distinct clusters on *t*-SNE (Additional file 1: Figure S5E). A total of 565 differentially expressed genes were identified in T-T_R compared to T-T_H, and GO functional annotations showed that the most significantly upregulated pathways were associated with cell proliferation and antigen presentation via MHC-II (e.g., *H2-Aa*, *Cd74*, *H2-Ab1*, *Ifi30*, *H2-Eb1*) and the most significantly downregulated pathways were associated with regulation of B cell/T cell proliferation (e.g., *Cd40Ig*, *Nckap1l*, *Tnfsf13b*, *Tnfrsf13c*, *Bcl2*, *Bmi1*, *Ccl5*, *Cd274*) and NK cell chemotaxis (e.g., *Ccl3*, *Ccl5*, *Xcl1*, Additional file 1: Figure S5F, gene listed in Additional file 1: Table S3). Compared to CD4$^+$ Th cells, Treg during transplant tolerance could replicate with immunosuppressive functions.

Intragraft CD4$^+$ Treg are phenotypically and functionally distinct during transplant rejection and tolerance

To further examine whether Treg are bystanders during transplant rejection, we identified their specific phenotypic and functional differences by comparing their transcriptomic signatures during transplant tolerance. In addition to FOXP3/hCD2, R-T_R and T-T_R also expressed other Treg markers including *Il2ra*, *Ikzf2*, *Nrp1*, and *Il10* (Additional file 1: Figure S4B). Nevertheless, they formed distinct clusters on *t*-SNE: all T-T_R but few R-T_R formed cluster C1, and a majority of R-T_R formed clusters C2 and C3 (Fig. 3b, Table 1). Comparing differentially expressed genes of these clusters by GO functional annotations, C1 was distinguished from the other clusters by upregulated cell cycle/cell division genes and downregulated inflammatory/chemotactic genes

as demonstrated by heat map (Fig. 3c) and pathway analyses (Additional file 1: Figure S6A, gene listed in Additional file 1: Table S4). Similarly, C2 was marked by upregulated chemotactic/chemokine genes and downregulated cell cycle/cell division genes (Additional file 1: Figure S6B, gene listed in Additional file 1: Table S5); C3 was characterized by upregulated genes regulating protein ubiquitination and responses to interferons and downregulated DNA/cell proliferation genes (Additional file 1: Figure S6C, gene listed in Additional file 1: Table S6). Altogether, with unbiased transcriptomic classification of FOXP3-expressing R-T_R and T-T_R, we discovered that Treg could be more heterogeneous during transplant rejection than tolerance and they skewed away from replicating, immunosuppressive C1 to less replicating, chemotactic C2 or ubiquitination-prone C3.

Coreceptor and costimulation blockade-induced transplant tolerance is associated with intragraft proliferation of CD4$^+$ Treg

We also performed cell cycle phase classification analyses with the scRNA-seq data of R-T_R and T-T_R by Scran (Fig. 3d, Table 2). Our results showed that a larger proportion of T-T_R (~40%) than R-T_R (~22%) was found in the S-G2/M phases, implying DNA/cell proliferation. Moreover, we also validated our transcriptomic results by immunostaining for the proliferation marker Ki67 (Fig. 3e). Indeed, our results revealed that significantly more Ki67$^+$FOXP3$^+$ Treg could be found in tolerated than rejecting grafts (Fig. 3f). Therefore, it is likely that Treg proliferation was a significant mechanism by which coreceptor and costimulation blockade induced transplant tolerance to hESC-derived tissues.

Proliferation of CD4$^+$ Treg in tolerated grafts requires functional PD-1 signaling

We then examined the mechanisms by which coreceptor and costimulation blockade induced tolerance through promoting intragraft Treg proliferation. From our transcriptomic profiling data, we observed that expression of *Pdcd1*/PD-1 significantly increased while expression of

Table 1 Distribution of cell number and percentage of CD4$^+$ Treg during rejection and tolerance in each cell cluster as determined by *t*-SNE

Cluster	Total cell number (#)	# R-T_R	# T-T_R	% R-T_R	% T-T_R
1	1086	134	952	14.6	99.27
2	444	441	3	48.04	0.31
3	347	343	4	37.36	0.42

R-T_R, CD4$^+$hCD2$^+$ Treg of rejecting hESC-derived grafts; *T-T_R*, CD4$^+$hCD2$^+$ Treg of tolerated hESC-derived grafts

Table 2 Distribution of cell number and percentage of CD4$^+$ Treg during rejection and tolerance in each of the cell cycle phases as determined by Scran

	# R-T_R	# T-T_R	% R-T_R	% T-T_R
Total cell number (#)	918	959		
G1	682	572	74.29	59.65
G2M	142	264	15.47	27.53
S	68	122	7.41	12.72
NA	26	1	2.83	0.1

R-T_R, CD4$^+$hCD2$^+$ Treg of rejecting hESC-derived grafts; *T-T_R*, CD4$^+$hCD2$^+$ Treg of tolerated hESC-derived grafts

other stimulatory (*Tnfrsf18*/GITR, *Icos*) and inhibitory (*Ctla4*, *Lag3*, *Havcr2*/TIM-3) checkpoint molecules remained relatively stable or significantly reduced in CD4$^+$ T cells during transplant tolerance compared to rejection (Fig. 4). We, therefore, focused on PD-1 for functional validation. We confirmed our scRNA-seq results by flow cytometry that a significantly greater percentage of PD-1$^+$CD4$^+$hCD2$^+$ population was found in tolerated than rejecting grafts, suggesting that coreceptor and costimulation blockade increased PD-1 expression by Treg during tolerance (Fig. 5a, b). Moreover, it appears that there was significantly higher PD-1 expression by CD4$^+$hCD2$^-$ than CD4$^+$hCD2$^+$ cells during rejection and vice versa during tolerance (Fig. 5b), implying that PD-1 was more predominantly expressed by the subset responsible for determining transplant outcome, i.e., more PD-1 expressed by Th during rejection and by Treg during tolerance.

With advances in immunotherapy using αPD-1 mAb in cancer patients, the inhibitory role of PD-1 signaling on conventional T cell activation has been well characterized [31]. However, whether PD-1 signaling regulates Treg proliferation and function, especially in the transplantation setting, remains elusive. To address this, we transplanted hESC-derived tissues in NOD.*Foxp3*^{hCD2} and examined graft survival in the 3 mAb- or 3 mAb + αPD-1 mAb-treated group at 1 month following transplantation (Fig. 5c). Compared to grafts derived from 3 mAb-treated group that were 100% accepted, blocking PD-1 signaling by αPD-1 mAb resulted in graft rejection ($n = 5$ per group, Fig. 5d). To investigate if PD-1 signaling regulated coreceptor and costimulation blockade-induced Treg proliferation, we performed immunostaining for Ki67 and FOXP3 in grafts derived from recipients treated with 3 mAb or 3 mAb + αPD-1 mAb (Fig. 5e). Our results revealed that

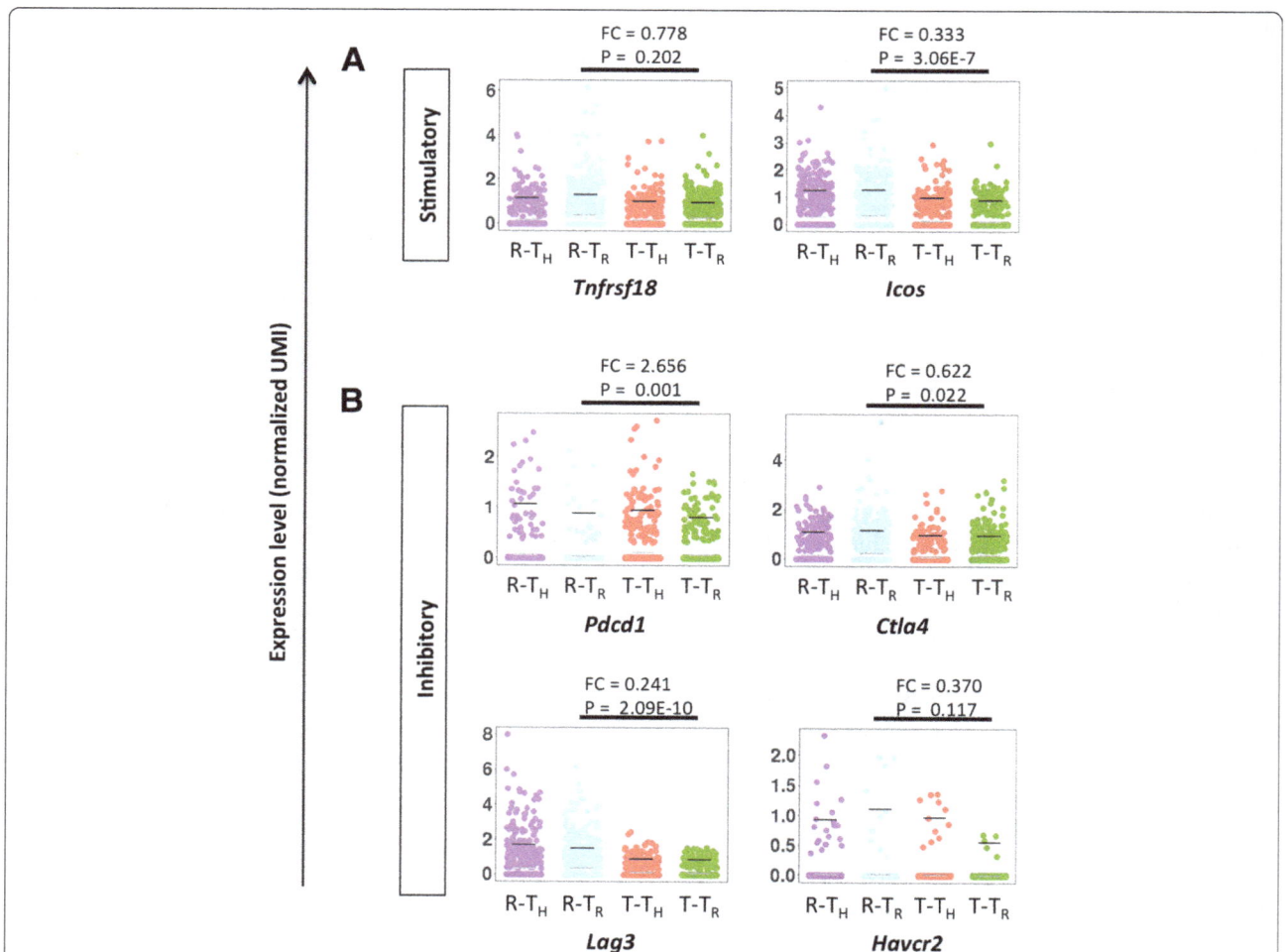

Fig. 4 Identification of immune checkpoint-specific genes expressed by CD4$^+$ T cells in rejecting and tolerated grafts. Jitter plots comparing expression levels of **a** stimulatory and **b** inhibitory immune checkpoint-specific genes expressed by CD4$^+$hCD2$^-$ Th of rejecting grafts (R-T$_H$), CD4$^+$hCD2$^+$ Treg of rejecting grafts (R-T$_R$), CD4$^+$hCD2$^-$ Th of tolerated grafts (T-T$_H$), and CD4$^+$hCD2$^+$ Treg of tolerated grafts (T-T$_R$). The fold change (FC) of T-T$_R$ over R-T$_R$ and the p value (P) by sSeq method are provided. Gray and black bars indicate the average expression level among all and expressed cells, respectively

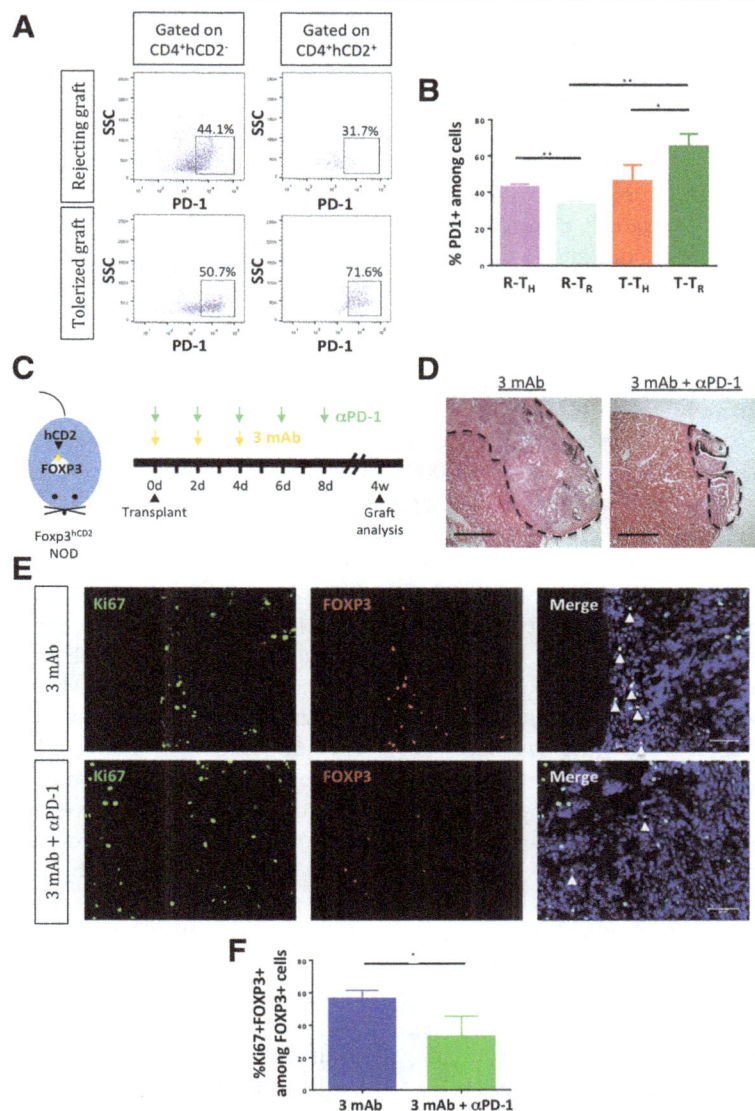

Fig. 5 Proliferation of CD4$^+$ Treg in tolerated grafts requires functional PD-1 signaling. **a** Flow cytometric analysis and **b** quantification showing expression of PD-1 in CD4$^+$hCD2$^-$ (T$_H$) or CD4$^+$hCD2$^+$ (T$_R$) cells of rejecting and tolerated grafts, respectively. **c** A schematic diagram showing the protocol for antibody treatments. **d** H&E staining showing graft rejection following treatment with αPD-1 mAb in addition to coreceptor and costimulation blockade (3 mAb). Scale bars: 1000 μm. **e** Immunostaining and **f** quantifications of Ki67$^+$FOXP3$^+$ cells among total FOXP3$^+$ cells in 3 mAb- and 3 mAb + αPD-1 mAb-treated grafts, respectively. Arrows indicate Ki67$^+$FOXP3$^+$ cells. Scale bars: 50 μm. *$P < 0.05$. (**a–f**) $n = 5$ per group

significantly less Ki67$^+$FOXP3$^+$ Treg were found in the 3 mAb + αPD-1 mAb- than 3 mAb-treated group (Fig. 5f). Therefore, our results suggested that blocking PD-1 signaling negated the effect of coreceptor and costimulation blockade on Treg proliferation for maintaining transplant tolerance.

Discussion

Despite the large body of evidence showing that CD4$^+$FOXP3$^+$ Treg play an important role in maintaining transplant tolerance, clinical studies demonstrate a correlation between intragraft CD4$^+$FOXP3$^+$ cells [46] or urinary *FOXP3* mRNA [47] and acute renal allograft rejection. Nevertheless, whether Treg mediated transplant tolerance is a numbers game or whether they are just "failed" bystanders during transplant rejection remains unknown. Since Treg determine the outcome of both autoimmunity and transplant rejection, we transplanted surrogate tissues in NOD recipients without ongoing autoimmunity in this study. We showed that Treg were indispensable for enabling coreceptor and costimulation blockade-mediated transplant tolerance to hESC-islets in NOD.*Foxp3*^{hCD2} recipients as their depletion with an ablative anti-hCD2 antibody led to graft rejection. We also found significantly more Treg resided in tolerated than rejecting grafts and showed that they were phenotypically distinct at single-cell level during transplant rejection and tolerance albeit with a common expression of the markers, CD4 and FOXP3.

Our current knowledge of Treg phenotypes is insufficient to define their cellular states correlated to transplant outcome. Recent advances in single-cell transcriptomics offer a new opportunity to discover additional subsets and cellular states of immune cells during development and disease pathogenesis at high resolution [48–50]. However, to date, there is no single-cell transcriptomic profiling data for Treg particularly in the transplantation setting. Here, we utilized the power of microfluidic scRNA-seq to establish a relatively large-scale cellular transcriptomic atlas of CD4$^+$ T cells during transplantation by profiling ∼ 13,000 cells including both conventional Th and regulator Treg from rejecting and tolerated grafts. We first analyzed data with ∼ 1000 randomly selected cells of each group to minimize the impact of cell number biases between different groups. It is noteworthy that we also observed the same conclusion by analyzing all cells (∼ 14,000 cells, Additional file 1: Figure S7). Our results offered unbiased genomic classification together with phenotypic and functional validation, leading us to revise the taxonomy of these cells in determining the transplant outcome.

Transcriptomically, we did pairwise comparisons. By comparing to Th, intragraft Treg expressed less genes that activated adaptive immunity such as B/T cell proliferation and NK cell chemotaxis during transplant tolerance. Likewise, they expressed more genes associated with negative regulation of conventional T cell function and less genes that activated adaptive immunity during transplant rejection. Since intragraft Treg still appeared to harbor immunomodulatory function, they were not bystanders during transplant rejection. So why might the grafts be rejected in the presence of Treg? We compared Treg derived from rejecting and tolerated grafts. Our data demonstrated cellular heterogeneity among Treg in the rejecting grafts: 48% Treg in C2 reflected a potential for chemotaxis of NK cells (*Ccl3, Ccl4, Ccl5, Xcl1*), monocytes (*Ccl3, Ccl4, Ccl9, Ccr2, Calca, Xcl1*), and neutrophils (*Ccl3, Ccl4, Ccl5, Ccl9, Itga1, Pde4b, Slc37a4*), and 37% Treg in C3 reflected a potential for protein ubiquitination and responses to interferons. In fact, the chemotactic genes *Ccl5* and *Itga1* were also overexpressed in splenic Treg of recipients that had rejecting grafts compared to that of the tolerated group. Furthermore, by comparing Th during rejection and tolerance, we might infer that Th negatively regulated the immune system and supported Treg function during tolerance.

Since scRNA-seq data revealed that 40% Treg of tolerated grafts were found in S-G2/M phages of the cell cycle, Treg proliferation was a possible major mechanism by which coreceptor and costimulation blockade mediated transplant tolerance. Indeed, we confirmed by immunostaining that > 80% FOXP3$^+$ cells expressed Ki67 in the tolerated grafts compared to ∼ 35% in the rejecting grafts. However, the signaling pathway driving any Treg proliferation during transplant tolerance is not clear. A previous report shows that the inhibitory checkpoint molecule PD-1 is vital in maintaining peripheral tolerance as PD-1 knockout mice spontaneously develop autoimmunity with markedly augmented proliferation of conventional T cells [51]. Since PD-L1 is found upregulated in many types of tumors, and PD-1 receptor is expressed by conventional T cells, it was hypothesized that tumors evaded immunosurveillance through the PD-L1/PD-1 pathway. Indeed, it is well characterized that signaling through PD-1 contributes to exhaustion and dysfunction of conventional T cells [31, 52], and anti-PD-1 mAb-mediated immunotherapy (e.g., Nivolumab) is currently used to treat human cancers [53]. In immune regulation, PD-1 expression on Treg is found inversely correlated to their proliferation during chronic liver inflammation [54], while in another study, PD-1 signaling promotes differentiation of CD4$^+$ naïve [55] or Th1 [56] cells into induced Treg (iTreg) with suppressive function. Such conversion can operate with [57] or without [55] TGF-β. Nevertheless, the direct role of PD-1 in survival and/or function of Treg is less clear.

Our scRNA-seq data with subsequent validation by flow cytometry revealed that a significantly greater percentage of Treg expressed PD-1 during transplant tolerance than rejection. We found that blocking PD-1 signaling via the neutralizing anti-PD-1 antibody abolished coreceptor and costimulation blockade-induced transplant tolerance, resulting in rejection of hESC-derived tissues with significantly reduced proliferation of intragraft Treg. Therefore, our results suggested that PD-1 signaling could be one of the mechanisms by which antibody blockade mediated Treg proliferation. Nevertheless, it is difficult to examine the effect of PD-1 blockade on conventional T cells in the absence of Treg in the transplantation setting, as we showed that Treg were indispensable for antibody blockade-mediated immune tolerance to hESC grafts and their absence contributed to graft rejection. Given the differential expression of PD-1 on conventional T cells and Treg during transplant rejection and tolerance, there might in principle be some differential binding and therefore efficacy of anti-PD-1 antibody on conventional T cells and Treg during the tolerance induction process. Our results suggest a therapeutic potential of PD-1 agonists in promoting transplant tolerance to hESC-derived tissues given their effect in facilitating self-renewal of Treg. Indeed, a previous report demonstrated that overexpression of PD-L1 prevents transplant rejection of mouse islets [58].

Whether the same regime could prevent rejection of human islets awaits further investigations. Although the role of therapeutic anti-PD-1 antibody on Treg has yet to be studied in cancer patients [59], our results also give new insights into the unwanted side effect of PD-1 blockade that may limit self-renewal of Treg during cancer treatment. Since Treg suppress autoreactive T cells, PD-1 blockade may cause autoimmune attack as seen in cancer patients who received anti-PD-1 antibodies and developed T1D and other autoimmune diseases [30].

Conclusions

Taken together, we have demonstrated that coreceptor and costimulation blockade induced transplant tolerance to hESC-derived pancreatic islets in NOD mouse recipients by promoting Treg proliferation via the PD-1 signaling pathway. These findings pave the way for clinical development of hESC-derived pancreatic tissues, combined with immunotherapies that expand intragraft Treg, as a potential treatment for alleviating autoimmunity in T1D. Our revised taxonomy of Treg during transplant rejection and tolerance might also enable more accurate monitoring of the outcome of solid organ transplantation.

Acknowledgements
We thank Dr. Joaquim S.L. Vong, Dr. Ji Lu, and Jiatao Li (CUHK) for their technical help throughout the study. We also thank Prof. Stephen Tsui (CUHK) for his machinery support.

Funding
This work was supported by the Research Grants Council of Hong Kong (04110515, 14111916, C4024-16W, C4026-17WF); Health and Medical Research Fund (03140346, 04152566); Croucher Foundation (Innovation Award and Start-up Allowance); Direct Grant, Faculty Innovation Award, Seed Fund from Lui Chi Woo Institute of Innovative Medicine, postdoctoral fellowship (K.Y.Y.); and postgraduate studentships (C.S.L. and X.L.) from CUHK.

Authors' contributions
CSL, XL, VWC, and MK performed the experiments. KYY performed bioinformatics analysis. CSL, XL, and KOL analyzed the experimental data. HW and SH provided the reagents. JCHT and YMDL provided support for scRNAseq platform. KOL designed the research and wrote the manuscript. All authors read and approved the final manuscript.

Competing interests
The authors declare that they have no competing interests.

Author details
[1]Department of Chemical Pathology, Prince of Wales Hospital, The Chinese University of Hong Kong, Hong Kong, China. [2]Department of Paediatrics and Adolescent Medicine, Division of Paediatric Hematology and Oncology, Faculty of Medicine, Medical Center, University of Freiburg, Freiburg im Breisgau, Germany. [3]Sir William Dunn School of Pathology, University of Oxford, Oxford, UK. [4]Laboratory of Immunology and Microbiology, Graduate School of Pharmaceutical Sciences, The University of Tokyo, Tokyo, Japan. [5]Li Ka Shing Institute of Health Sciences, Prince of Wales Hospital, The Chinese University of Hong Kong, Hong Kong, China.

References
1. Sharir R, Semo J, Shaish A, Landa-Rouben N, Entin-Meer M, Keren G, et al. Regulatory T cells influence blood flow recovery in experimental hindlimb ischaemia in an IL-10-dependent manner. Cardiovasc Res. 2014;103(4):585–96.
2. Gamble JM, Simpson SH, Eurich DT, Majumdar SR, Johnson JA. Insulin use and increased risk of mortality in type 2 diabetes: a cohort study. Diabetes Obes Metab. 2010;12(1):47–53.
3. Shapiro AM, Ricordi C, Hering BJ, Auchincloss H, Lindblad R, Robertson RP, et al. International trial of the Edmonton protocol for islet transplantation. N Engl J Med. 2006;355(13):1318–30.
4. Bellin MD, Barton FB, Heitman A, Harmon JV, Kandaswamy R, Balamurugan AN, et al. Potent induction immunotherapy promotes long-term insulin independence after islet transplantation in type 1 diabetes. Am J Transplant Off J Am Soc Transplant Am Soc Transplant Surg. 2012;12(6):1576–83.
5. Monti P, Scirpoli M, Maffi P, Ghidoli N, De Taddeo F, Bertuzzi F, et al. Islet transplantation in patients with autoimmune diabetes induces homeostatic cytokines that expand autoreactive memory T cells. J Clin Invest. 2008; 118(5):1806–14.
6. Pagliuca FW, Millman JR, Gurtler M, Segel M, Van Dervort A, Ryu JH, et al. Generation of functional human pancreatic beta cells in vitro. Cell. 2014; 159(2):428–39.
7. Rezania A, Bruin JE, Arora P, Rubin A, Batushansky I, Asadi A, et al. Reversal of diabetes with insulin-producing cells derived in vitro from human pluripotent stem cells. Nat Biotechnol. 2014;32(11):1121–33.
8. Szot GL, Yadav M, Lang J, Kroon E, Kerr J, Kadoya K, et al. Tolerance induction and reversal of diabetes in mice transplanted with human embryonic stem cell-derived pancreatic endoderm. Cell Stem Cell. 2015; 16(2):148–57.
9. Pearl JI, Lee AS, Leveson-Gower DB, Sun N, Ghosh Z, Lan F, et al. Short-term immunosuppression promotes engraftment of embryonic and induced pluripotent stem cells. Cell Stem Cell. 2011;8(3):309–17.
10. Schwartz SD, Regillo CD, Lam BL, Eliott D, Rosenfeld PJ, Gregori NZ, et al. Human embryonic stem cell-derived retinal pigment epithelium in patients with age-related macular degeneration and Stargardt's macular dystrophy: follow-up of two open-label phase 1/2 studies. Lancet. 2015; 385(9967):509–16.
11. Schwartz SD, Hubschman JP, Heilwell G, Franco-Cardenas V, Pan CK, Ostrick RM, et al. Embryonic stem cell trials for macular degeneration: a preliminary report. Lancet. 2012;379(9817):713–20.
12. Rong Z, Wang M, Hu Z, Stradner M, Zhu S, Kong H, et al. An effective approach to prevent immune rejection of human ESC-derived allografts. Cell Stem Cell. 2014;14(1):121–30.
13. Lui KO, Howie D, Ng SW, Liu S, Chien KR, Waldmann H. Tolerance induction to human stem cell transplants with extension to their differentiated progeny. Nat Commun. 2014;5:5629.
14. Vegas AJ, Veiseh O, Gurtler M, Millman JR, Pagliuca FW, Bader AR, et al. Long-term glycemic control using polymer-encapsulated human stem cell-derived beta cells in immune-competent mice. Nat Med. 2016;22(3):306–11.
15. Lui KO, Bu L, Li RA, Chan CW. Pluripotent stem cell-based heart regeneration: from the developmental and immunological perspectives. Birth Defects Res C Embryo Today. 2012;96(1):98–108.
16. Lui KO, Waldmann H, Fairchild PJ. Embryonic stem cells: overcoming the immunological barriers to cell replacement therapy. Curr Stem Cell Res Ther. 2009;4(1):70–80.
17. Lui KO, Fairchild PJ, Waldmann H. Prospects for ensuring acceptance of ES cell-derived tissues. Cambridge (MA): StemBook; 2008.
18. Lui KO, Boyd AS, Cobbold SP, Waldmann H, Fairchild PJ. A role for regulatory T cells in acceptance of ESC-derived tissues transplanted across an major histocompatibility complex barrier. Stem Cells. 2010;28(10):1905–14.

19. Schulz TC. Concise review: manufacturing of pancreatic endoderm cells for clinical trials in type 1 diabetes. Stem Cells Transl Med 2015;4(8):927–31.

20. Agulnick AD, Ambruzs DM, Moorman MA, Bhoumik A, Cesario RM, Payne JK, et al. Insulin-producing endocrine cells differentiated in vitro from human embryonic stem cells function in macroencapsulation devices in vivo. Stem Cells Transl Med. 2015;4(10):1214–22.

21. Basta G, Montanucci P, Luca G, Boselli C, Noya G, Barbaro B, et al. Long-term metabolic and immunological follow-up of nonimmunosuppressed patients with type 1 diabetes treated with microencapsulated islet allografts: four cases. Diabetes Care. 2011;34(11):2406–9.

22. Calafiore R, Basta G, Luca G, Lemmi A, Montanucci MP, Calabrese G, et al. Microencapsulated pancreatic islet allografts into nonimmunosuppressed patients with type 1 diabetes: first two cases. Diabetes Care. 2006;29(1):137–8.

23. Tuch BE, Keogh GW, Williams LJ, Wu W, Foster JL, Vaithilingam V, et al. Safety and viability of microencapsulated human islets transplanted into diabetic humans. Diabetes Care. 2009;32(10):1887–9.

24. de Groot M, Schuurs TA, van Schilfgaarde R. Causes of limited survival of microencapsulated pancreatic islet grafts. J Surg Res. 2004;121(1):141–50.

25. Brunkow ME, Jeffery EW, Hjerrild KA, Paeper B, Clark LB, Yasayko SA, et al. Disruption of a new forkhead/winged-helix protein, scurfin, results in the fatal lymphoproliferative disorder of the scurfy mouse. Nat Genet. 2001;27(1):68–73.

26. Di Ianni M, Falzetti F, Carotti A, Terenzi A, Castellino F, Bonifacio E, et al. Tregs prevent GVHD and promote immune reconstitution in HLA-haploidentical transplantation. Blood. 2011;117(14):3921–3928. https://www.ncbi.nlm.nih.gov/pubmed/21292771.

27. Kendal AR, Chen Y, Regateiro FS, Ma J, Adams E, Cobbold SP, et al. Sustained suppression by Foxp3+ regulatory T cells is vital for infectious transplantation tolerance. J Exp Med. 2011;208(10):2043–53.

28. Qin S, Cobbold SP, Pope H, Elliott J, Kioussis D, Davies J, et al. "Infectious" transplantation tolerance. Science. 1993;259(5097):974–7.

29. Davies JD, Leong LY, Mellor A, Cobbold SP, Waldmann H. T cell suppression in transplantation tolerance through linked recognition. J Immunol. 1996; 156(10):3602–7.

30. Couzin-Frankel J. Autoimmune diseases surface after cancer treatment. Science. 2017;358(6365):852.

31. Tumeh PC, Harview CL, Yearley JH, Shintaku IP, Taylor EJ, Robert L, et al. PD-1 blockade induces responses by inhibiting adaptive immune resistance. Nature. 2014;515(7528):568–71.

32. Miyao T, Floess S, Setoguchi R, Luche H, Fehling HJ, Waldmann H, et al. Plasticity of Foxp3(+) T cells reflects promiscuous Foxp3 expression in conventional T cells but not reprogramming of regulatory T cells. Immunity. 2012;36(2):262–75.

33. Baas M, Besancon A, Goncalves T, Valette F, Yagita H, Sawitzki B, et al. TGFbeta-dependent expression of PD-1 and PD-L1 controls CD8(+) T cell anergy in transplant tolerance. elife. 2016;5:e08133.

34. Leung OM, Li J, Li X, Chan VW, Yang KY, Ku M, et al. Regulatory T cells promote apelin-mediated sprouting angiogenesis in type 2 diabetes. Cell Rep. 2018;24(6):1610–26.

35. Dobin A, Davis CA, Schlesinger F, Drenkow J, Zaleski C, Jha S, et al. STAR: ultrafast universal RNA-seq aligner. Bioinformatics. 2013;29(1):15–21.

36. Heinz S, Benner C, Spann N, Bertolino E, Lin YC, Laslo P, et al. Simple combinations of lineage-determining transcription factors prime cis-regulatory elements required for macrophage and B cell identities. Mol Cell. 2010;38(4):576–89.

37. Huang da W, Sherman BT, Lempicki RA. Bioinformatics enrichment tools: paths toward the comprehensive functional analysis of large gene lists. Nucleic Acids Res. 2009;37(1):1–13.

38. Zheng GX, Terry JM, Belgrader P, Ryvkin P, Bent ZW, Wilson R, et al. Massively parallel digital transcriptional profiling of single cells. Nat Commun. 2017;8:14049.

39. Yu D, Huber W, Vitek O. Shrinkage estimation of dispersion in Negative Binomial models for RNA-seq experiments with small sample size. Bioinformatics. 2013;29(10):1275–82.

40. Lun AT, McCarthy DJ, Marioni JC. A step-by-step workflow for low-level analysis of single-cell RNA-seq data with Bioconductor. F1000Res. 2016;5:2122.

41. Yi Z, Diz R, Martin AJ, Morillon YM, Kline DE, Li L, et al. Long-term remission of diabetes in NOD mice is induced by nondepleting anti-CD4 and anti-CD8 antibodies. Diabetes. 2012;61(11):2871–80.

42. Graca L, Cobbold SP, Waldmann H. Identification of regulatory T cells in tolerated allografts. J Exp Med. 2002;195(12):1641–6.

43. Tsang JCH, Vong JSL, Ji L, Poon LCY, Jiang P, Lui KO, et al. Integrative single-cell and cell-free plasma RNA transcriptomics elucidates placental cellular dynamics. In: Proceedings of the National Academy of Sciences of the United States of America; 2017.

44. Vences-Catalan F, Rajapaksa R, Srivastava MK, Marabelle A, Kuo CC, Levy R, et al. Tetraspanin CD81 promotes tumor growth and metastasis by modulating the functions of T regulatory and myeloid-derived suppressor cells. Cancer Res. 2015;75(21):4517–26.

45. Schneider MA, Meingassner JG, Lipp M, Moore HD, Rot A. CCR7 is required for the in vivo function of CD4+ CD25+ regulatory T cells. J Exp Med. 2007;204(4):735–45.

46. Veronese F, Rotman S, Smith RN, Pelle TD, Farrell ML, Kawai T, et al. Pathological and clinical correlates of FOXP3+ cells in renal allografts during acute rejection. Am J Transplant Off J Am Soc Transplant Am Soc Transplant Surg. 2007;7(4):914–22.

47. Muthukumar T, Dadhania D, Ding R, Snopkowski C, Naqvi R, Lee JB, et al. Messenger RNA for FOXP3 in the urine of renal-allograft recipients. N Engl J Med. 2005;353(22):2342–51.

48. Lavin Y, Kobayashi S, Leader A, Amir ED, Elefant N, Bigenwald C, et al. Innate immune landscape in early lung adenocarcinoma by paired single-cell analyses. Cell. 2017;169(4):750–65 e17.

49. Proserpio V, Piccolo A, Haim-Vilmovsky L, Kar G, Lonnberg T, Svensson V, et al. Single-cell analysis of CD4+ T-cell differentiation reveals three major cell states and progressive acceleration of proliferation. Genome Biol. 2016;17:103.

50. Villani AC, Satija R, Reynolds G, Sarkizova S, Shekhar K, Fletcher J, et al. Single-cell RNA-seq reveals new types of human blood dendritic cells, monocytes, and progenitors. Science. 2017;356(6335). https://doi.org/10.1126/science.aah4573.

51. Nishimura H, Nose M, Hiai H, Minato N, Honjo T. Development of lupus-like autoimmune diseases by disruption of the PD-1 gene encoding an ITIM motif-carrying immunoreceptor. Immunity. 1999;11(2):141–51.

52. Wei F, Zhong S, Ma Z, Kong H, Medvec A, Ahmed R, et al. Strength of PD-1 signaling differentially affects T-cell effector functions. Proc Natl Acad Sci U S A. 2013;110(27):E2480–9.

53. Chen L, Han X. Anti-PD-1/PD-L1 therapy of human cancer: past, present, and future. J Clin Invest. 2015;125(9):3384–91.

54. Franceschini D, Paroli M, Francavilla V, Videtta M, Morrone S, Labbadia G, et al. PD-L1 negatively regulates CD4+CD25+Foxp3+ Tregs by limiting STAT-5 phosphorylation in patients chronically infected with HCV. J Clin Investig. 2009;119(3):551–64.

55. Francisco LM, Salinas VH, Brown KE, Vanguri VK, Freeman GJ, Kuchroo VK, et al. PD-L1 regulates the development, maintenance, and function of induced regulatory T cells. J Exp Med. 2009;206(13):3015–29.

56. Amarnath S, Mangus CW, Wang JC, Wei F, He A, Kapoor V, et al. The PDL1-PD1 axis converts human TH1 cells into regulatory T cells. Sci Transl Med. 2011;3(111):111ra20.

57. Wang L, Pino-Lagos K, de Vries VC, Guleria I, Sayegh MH, Noelle RJ. Programmed death 1 ligand signaling regulates the generation of adaptive Foxp3+CD4+ regulatory T cells. Proc Natl Acad Sci U S A. 2008;105(27):9331–6.

58. Li T, Ma R, Zhu JY, Wang FS, Huang L, Leng XS. PD-1/PD-L1 costimulatory pathway-induced mouse islet transplantation immune tolerance. Transplant Proc. 2015;47(1):165–70.

59. Tanaka A, Sakaguchi S. Regulatory T cells in cancer immunotherapy. Cell Res. 2017;27(1):109–18.

8

Comprehensive antibiotic-linked mutation assessment by resistance mutation sequencing (RM-seq)

Romain Guérillot[1], Lucy Li[1], Sarah Baines[1], Brian Howden[1]⊙, Mark B. Schultz[1,2,3], Torsten Seemann[4,2], Ian Monk[1], Sacha J. Pidot[1], Wei Gao[1], Stefano Giulieri[1], Anders Gonçalves da Silva[1,2,3], Anthony D'Agata[3], Takehiro Tomita[3], Anton Y. Peleg[5,6], Timothy P. Stinear[1,2†] and Benjamin P. Howden[1,2,3,7*†]

Abstract

Mutation acquisition is a major mechanism of bacterial antibiotic resistance that remains insufficiently characterised. Here we present RM-seq, a new amplicon-based deep sequencing workflow based on a molecular barcoding technique adapted from Low Error Amplicon sequencing (LEA-seq). RM-seq allows detection and functional assessment of mutational resistance at high throughput from mixed bacterial populations. The sensitive detection of very low-frequency resistant sub-populations permits characterisation of antibiotic-linked mutational repertoires in vitro and detection of rare resistant populations during infections. Accurate quantification of resistance mutations enables phenotypic screening of mutations conferring pleiotropic phenotypes such as in vivo persistence, collateral sensitivity or cross-resistance. RM-seq will facilitate comprehensive detection, characterisation and surveillance of resistant bacterial populations (https://github.com/rguerillot/RM-seq).

Keywords: Antibiotic resistance, Resistance mutations, Deep sequencing, *Staphylococcus aureus*, *Mycobacterium tuberculosis*, Rifampicin, Daptomycin

Background

Antimicrobial resistance is on the rise and is responsible for millions of deaths every year [1]. Bacterial populations consistently and rapidly overcome the challenge imposed by the use of a new antibiotic. Their remarkable ability to quickly develop resistance is due to their capacity to exchange genes and to their high mutation supply rate. Multidrug-resistant bacteria are therefore becoming increasingly prevalent and drug susceptibility testing (DST) is now central to avoid antibiotic misuse and minimise the risk of inducing the emergence of new resistant clones. Over recent years, genomics has become a powerful tool to understand, combat and control the rise of resistance

[2, 3]. Nevertheless, a precise definition of resistance at the genomic level is crucial to enable fast, culture-independent DST by high-throughput sequencing in the clinical context and to track and fight the spread and persistence of resistant clones globally [3, 4].

The genomic basis of resistance is relatively straightforward to establish for resistance conferred by acquisition of a specific gene. The repertoire of resistance genes (resistome) is now well defined and there are several curated databases and software prediction tools for resistance genes detection [5–7]. In contrast, comprehensive lists of mutations that confer antibiotic resistance are lacking, despite equivalent clinical relevance. Resistance to major classes of antimicrobials including quinolones, beta-lactams, rifamycins, aminoglycosides, macrolides, sulphonamides, polymyxins, glycopeptides and lipopeptides can all occur via mutations. In some species, such as *Mycobacterium tuberculosis*, resistance to all therapeutic agents is mediated by mutations [8].

Resistance mutations can be effectively selected in vitro, and so genome sequence comparisons of resistant clones

* Correspondence: bhowden@unimelb.edu.au
†Timothy P. Stinear and Benjamin P. Howden contributed equally to this work.
[1]Department of Microbiology and Immunology, The University of Melbourne at the Doherty Institute for Infection & Immunity, Melbourne, Victoria, Australia
[2]Doherty Applied Microbial Genomics, The University of Melbourne at the Peter Doherty Institute for Infection & Immunity, Melbourne, Victoria, Australia

derived from sensitive ancestral clones after antibiotic exposure have permitted the identification of numerous resistance-associated mutations [9–12]. From these studies, it is apparent that the mutational landscape for a single antibiotic combination within a specific bacterium can be broad [13–16]. Therefore, standard approaches relying on sequence comparisons of single pairs of isogenic mutants are not practical to extensively define the mutational resistome.

Resistance mutations commonly arise in genes encoding the primary drug target or central regulatory genes, such as *gyrA*, *parC*, *rpsL*, *gidB*, *rpoB*, *23S rRNA*, *rplC*, *rplD* and *walKR* (for quinolone, aminoglycoside, rifampicin, linezolid and glycopeptide resistance) [16, 17]. Because of their implications in central cell processes, such as DNA replication, translation, transcription and cell-wall metabolism regulation, mutations arising in these genes have been associated with a broad range of pleiotropic effects in addition to the antibiotic resistance that they cause [17]. An increasing body of literature shows that antibiotic resistance mutations can lead to broader negative therapeutic consequences through cross-resistance to other antimicrobials [18–20], increased biofilm formation [21], increased virulence [22–25] and enhanced immune evasion [25–28]. However, there is currently no efficient method to identify pleiotropic mutations. Comprehensively identifying mutations associated with antibiotic cross-resistance and increased risk of therapeutic failure will provide crucial information for future personalised medicine and will help to improve therapeutics guidelines through a greater understanding of the drivers and consequences of mutational resistance. At an epidemiological and evolutionary level, understanding why specific resistance mutations are preferentially selected might provide a rational basis for development of effective measures to combat the rise of resistance.

In this study, we developed an innovative workflow called resistance mutation sequencing (RM-seq) that enables the unbiased quantification of resistance alleles from complex in vitro-derived resistant clone libraries, selectable under any experimental condition, allowing identification and characterisation of mutational resistance and its consequences. Here we investigated mutational resistance in *Staphylococcus aureus* and *Mycobacterium tuberculosis* and demonstrated that complex resistant subpopulations can be effectively characterised in vitro or detected in vivo using RM-seq.

Methods
In vitro selection of rifampicin-resistant clones
All experiments were conducted with *S. aureus* USA300 strain NRS384, acquired from BEI resources. Rifampicin-resistant colonies were selected from 20 independent overnight heart infusion (HI) 10 mL broth cultures (5×10^9 CFU/mL) inoculated from single colonies. Cultures were pelleted at 10 min at 3000*g* and re-suspended in 200 μL of HI broth (2.5×10^{11} CFU/mL). These concentrated overnight cultures were then pooled and plated on HI plates supplemented with rifampicin at 0.006, 0.5, 1, and 4 mg/L. Given that the spontaneous resistance rate for rifampicin in *S. aureus* is $\sim 2 \times 10^{-8}$ [29], 20 to 30 plates inoculated with 75 μL were necessary to recover $\sim$ 10,000 resistant clones after 48-h incubation at 37 °C. All resistant colonies were recovered by scraping the plate flooded with 2 mL of phosphate buffered saline (PBS). After washing the pooled clone libraries in PBS, aliquots were used for genomic DNA extraction and RM-seq library preparation and stocked in 25% glycerol at − 80 °C.

Amplicon library preparation and deep sequencing
Genomic DNA was extracted from 1 mL aliquots adjusted to an OD_{600} of 5 in HI broth. Cells were pelleted and washed twice in PBS and genomic DNA was extracted using the DNeasy Blood & Tissue Kit (QIAGEN). Random 16 bp barcodes were introduced by performing 8 cycles of linear PCR with the primer x_rmseq_F (Additional file 1: Table S1) using the following PCR mix: 2 μL of x_rmseq_F (5 nM), 1 μL of genomic DNA (6 ng/μL), 12.5 μL Phusion® High-Fidelity PCR Master Mix (2X, New England BioLabs Inc.) and 6 μL H$_2$0. The following PCR cycle conditions were used: 30 s at 98 °C, then 8 cycles of 10 s at 98 °C, 30 s at 50 °C, 30 s 72 °C, and a 2-min elongation step at 72 °C. Following the final cycle of the linear PCR, samples were cooled to 25 °C and the nested exponential PCR were performed by immediately adding 3.5 μL of a primer mix containing 2 μL of primer x _rmseq_R (100 nM), 0.6 μL forward and 0.6 μL reverse Nextera XT Index Kit primers (10 μM), 0.3 μL H$_2$O. The PCR conditions above were then used for a further 25 cycles. The resulting amplicons comprising Illumina adaptor and indices was purified with Agencourt® AMPure® XP magnetic beads (Beckman Coulter) using beads/sample volume ratio of 0.8. Purified amplicons were then normalised at 4 nM according to expected size and measured DNA concentrations (Qubit™ dsDNA HS Assay Kit). Amplicons with different indices were pooled and the sequencing library was diluted to 15 pM with 10% *phiX* control spike and sequenced on Illumina Miseq or Nextseq using Reagent Kit v3 to produce 300 bp or 150 bp paired-end reads. Sequencing reads of RM-seq experiments are available from NCBI/ENA/DDBJ under BioProject number PRJNA399605.

Bioinformatics analysis pipeline
The RM-seq pipeline processes raw reads after demultiplexing by the Illumina sequencing instrument. The pipeline uses *bwa mem* read aligner (0.7.15-r1140) [30] to map

reads to a reference locus (*rpoB*) and *samtools* (v1.3) [31] to remove unmapped and low-quality reads from the read sets. Then *pear* (v0.9.10) [32] is used to merge paired reads. Merged reads sharing identical barcodes are aligned using *Clustal Omega* (v1.2.1) [33]. Cons from the EMBOSS suite (v6.6.0.0) [34] is used to collapse the alignments into single error-corrected consensus reads. To speed-up processing, read alignment and consensus sequence generation tasks are executed in parallel using *GNU parallel* [35]. Unique consensus DNA sequences are identified via clustering using the *cd-hit-est* module of the *CD-HIT* (v4.7) software [36]. Resultant unique representative consensus sequences are translated to amino acids using *getorf* and annotated at the protein and nucleotide level using *diffseq*, both modules of the EMBOSS suite. The annotated effect of mutation is then re-associated to each barcode in the final output table. The RM-seq bioinformatics pipeline is available from Github (https://github.com/rguerillot/RM-seq).

Construction of *rpoB* mutants by allelic exchange

Allelic exchange experiments were performed using shuttle vector pIMAY-Z [37] with some modifications. Full-length *rpoB* sequences corresponding to the 19 different *rpoB* alleles reconstructed by allelic exchange in the *S. aureus* NRS384 strain were obtained by performing PCR overlap extension with Phusion High-Fidelity DNA Polymerase (New England Biolabs) and introducing *rpoB* codon mutations to the primer tails (Additional file 1: Table S1). Gel-purified *rpoB* amplicons were then joined with pIMAY-Z using Seamless Ligation Cloning Extract (SLiCE) cloning [38] and transformed into *Escherichia coli* strain IM08B [37] to allow CC8-like methylation of the plasmid and bypass the *S. aureus* restriction barrier. The presence of a cloned *rpoB* insert in pIMAY-Z plasmid was then confirmed by colony PCR using primers pIMAY-Z-MCSF and pIMAY-Z-MCSR. Purified plasmid was then electroporated into *S. aureus* and plated on HI supplemented with chloramphenicol at 10 mg/L and X-gal (5-bromo-4-chloro-3-indolyl-β-d-galactopyranoside; Melford) at 100 mg/L and grown 48 h at 30 °C. Blue colonies were picked and grown in HI broth at 37 °C without Cm selection pressure overnight to allow loss of the pIMAY-Z thermosensitive plasmid. Double cross-overs leading to allelic replacement of the wild type with the desired rifampicin-resistant *rpoB* alleles were directly selected by plating cultures on HI plates supplemented with 0.06 mg/L of rifampicin. Rifampicin-resistant and chloramphenicol-sensitive colonies arising at a frequency higher than 10^{-3} were considered as potentially positive clones for allelic exchange as spontaneous rifampicin resistance arises at a much lower frequency of ~ 2×10^{-8} (resistant clones per culture) [29] in the wild-type strain. Clones were then colony purified on HI plates before glycerol storage and extraction of

genomic DNA. To validate the allelic exchange procedure, the whole genome sequence of all reconstructed strains was determined with the Illumina Miseq or Nextseq 500 platforms, using Nextera XT paired-end libraries (2 × 300 bp or 2 × 150 bp respectively). To ensure that no additional mutations were introduced during the allelic exchange procedure, reads of all mutant strains were mapped to the reference NRS384 genome [37] using Snippy (v 2.9) (https://github.com/tseemann/snippy). The results of the SNP/indel calling of the reconstructed mutants were then compared with our NRS384 WT reference isolate. The SNP/indel profile for each mutant is presented in Additional file 1: Table S2 and sequence reads have been deposited under BioProject numbers PRJNA360176 and PRJNA399605.

Antibiotic susceptibility testing and time kill assays

Rifampicin and daptomycin MIC were measured using E-tests (BioMérieux) on Mueller-Hinton plates supplemented with 50 mg/L Ca^{2+} following the manufacturer's instructions. For daptomycin time kill assays, 10 mL of brain heart infusion (BHI) broth supplemented with 8 mg/L daptomycin and 50 mg/L Ca^{2+} was inoculated with 10^6 CFU/mL of an overnight culture. Cultures were incubated at 37 °C with constant shaking, and samples were collected at 3, 6 and 24 h time points. Cell survival after daptomycin exposure was assessed by calculating the ratio of the CFU at 3, 6 and 24 h on the CFU of the initial inoculum (10^6 CFU/mL) and taking the average colony counts of duplicate BHI agar plates. All daptomycin time kill assays were performed in biological triplicate.

Mutant differential abundance analysis after daptomycin selection

Three replicates of daptomycin selection were performed on a rifampicin selected population (in vitro 1 population selected with rifampicin at 0.06 mg/L). A high initial inoculum of 5×10^8 CFU/mL was used to recover a sufficient amount of bacterial DNA from surviving cells after daptomycin exposure. After 3 h or 24 h of exposure to daptomycin at 8 mg/L, surviving bacterial populations were pelleted and washed. To remove extracellular DNA resulting from daptomycin-induced cell death, cell pellets were incubated 45 min at 37 °C with 1 μL of Amplification Grade DNase I (1 U/μL Invitrogen) in 5 μL of 10X DNase I reaction buffer and 44 μL laboratory grade H_2O. Then, DNase I was inactivated with 5 μL of 25 mM EDTA (pH 8.0) and 10 min incubation at 65 °C. Genomic DNA was extracted, and *rpoB* mutant abundance was assessed by RM-seq as described above. Differential abundance analysis of the mutant before and after daptomycin exposure was performed with the R *DESeq2* (1.10.1) package [39], using the count of mutation calculated from table output of the RM-seq data processing pipeline. DESeq2 analysis was performed with all mutations count superior to 1 using default parameters and Cooks cut-off set to false. The Wald statistical test performed by *DESeq2* to estimate the significance of the changes in mutation abundance after exposure to daptomycin was used to screen *rpoB* mutations that were associated with increased or decreased tolerance to daptomycin. The detailed explanation of this test is described in [39]. Wald test *P* values were adjusted for multiple testing using the procedure of Benjamini and Hochberg [40].

Mouse infection model

Wild-type 6-week-old female BALB/c mice were injected via the tail vein with approximately 2×10^6 colony-forming units (CFU) in a volume of 100 μL PBS. The mice were monitored every 8 h until completion of the experiment and were euthanized after 1 day or 7 days post-infection. Bacteria from the liver, kidney, and spleen were recovered by mechanical homogenisation in 1 mL of phosphate buffered saline (PBS), serially diluted and plated on BHI plates. Colonies forming after overnight incubation at 37 °C were pooled and assessed by RM-seq.

Detection of resistant sub-populations of *M. tuberculosis* from sputum samples

DNA was extracted from isolates cultured from sputum specimens as previously described [41]. RM-seq libraries were prepared as described above using the *rmseq* primers specific to *pncA*, *ethA*, and *rpoB* resistance determining regions (Additional file 1: Table S1). Deep sequencing was performed on a Nextseq 500 platform using Reagent Kit v3 to produce 150 bp overlapping paired-end reads and analyses were performed using the RM-seq bioinformatics analysis pipeline. Primary *M. tuberculosis* culture and phenotypic susceptibility testing was performed using the radiometric BACTEC 460TB system (Becton Dickinson).

Results

The RM-seq workflow

RM-seq is an amplicon-based, deep sequencing technique founded on the single molecule barcoding method [42]. Here we have adapted the LEA-seq barcoding method first described for unbiased detection of 16S rRNA gene alleles, in order to identify and quantify at high-throughput, mutations that confer resistance to a given antibiotic [42, 43]. RM-seq can take advantage of the ability of bacteria to quickly develop resistance in vitro to identify and functionally characterise resistance-associated mutations at high throughput. A large and genetically diverse population of resistant clones that encompass the mutational landscape of resistance is selected (Fig. 1a). In order to maximise the genetic diversity, a large number of resistant

clones (~ 10,000) are pooled from multiple independent culture and genomic DNA of the mixed resistant population is extracted and the mutational repertoire interrogated by amplicon deep sequencing.

The high sensitivity and the accurate quantification of the frequency of all the selected mutations in a given genetic locus, enabled screening of complex, mixed libraries of resistant clones. In theory, genetic interactions can be tracked and associated with any selectable pleiotropic phenotype of interest (e.g. cross-resistance to other antimicrobials, immune evasion) by measuring the relative abundance of resistant clones before and after selection. Specific mutations that favour the growth or survival under in vitro or in vivo test condition will increase in frequency within the population and be readily detected by RM-seq.

Unbiased allele quantification and a low error rate are enabled by single-molecule barcoding during the PCR amplicon library preparation (Fig. 1b). Sequencing reads sharing identical barcodes are grouped to create consensus sequences of the genetic variants initially present in the population. The single-molecule barcoding step has two major advantages. Firstly, it allows error correction of the sequenced DNA and thus high confidence in calling of resistance-associated mutations that might occur at a frequency well below the inherent error rate (~ 1% [44]) of the sequencer. Secondly, it permits accurate quantification of allele frequencies by correcting for the amplification bias introduced during the exponential PCR step. The RM-seq bioinformatics pipeline takes as input the raw reads and outputs a table of all annotated substitutions, insertions and deletions identified in the selected population given the original sequence (the target locus sequence before selection). A diagram of the steps in the data analysis pipeline is presented in Fig. 1c (RM-seq analysis tool is available from https://github.com/rguerillot/RM-seq).

Sensitive and quantitative detection of single-nucleotide variants in complex bacterial populations

To assess the capability of the RM-seq protocol to detect and quantify rare genetic variants from mixed populations of resistant bacteria, we first evaluated its error correction efficiency. We sequenced at high depth a 270 bp region comprising the rifampicin resistance-determining region (RRDR) of a *S. aureus* rifampicin susceptible isolate (wild-type strain NRS384). By counting incorrect nucleotide calls at each position after aligning raw reads to the WT sequence, we found an average error rate per position of $2.8 \times 10^{-2} \pm 1.7 \times 10^{-2}$ (standard deviation [SD]), which is commonly observed for the Miseq instrument [44]. Merging forward and reverse reads replaces the lower quality score bases from one read by the higher quality score of the paired read and

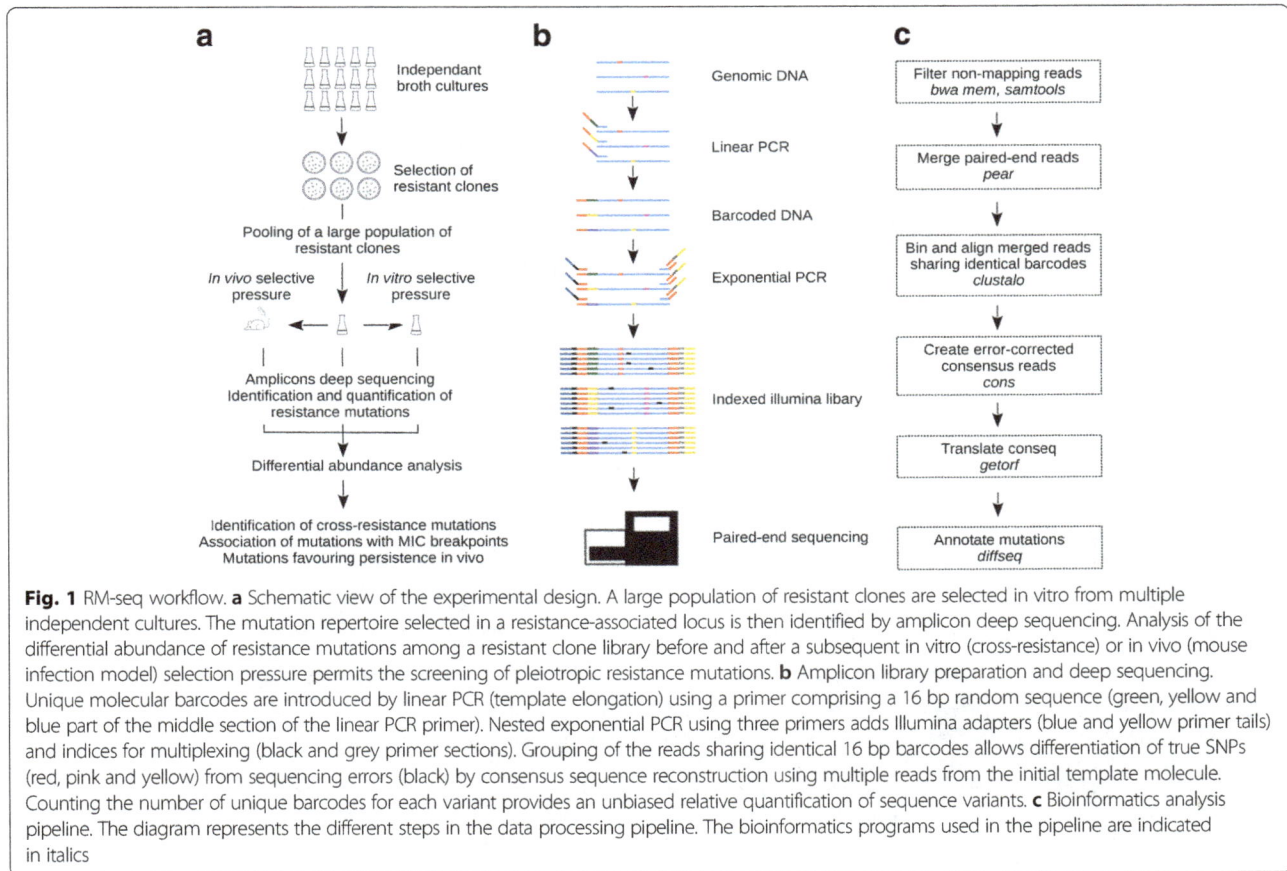

Fig. 1 RM-seq workflow. **a** Schematic view of the experimental design. A large population of resistant clones are selected in vitro from multiple independent cultures. The mutation repertoire selected in a resistance-associated locus is then identified by amplicon deep sequencing. Analysis of the differential abundance of resistance mutations among a resistant clone library before and after a subsequent in vitro (cross-resistance) or in vivo (mouse infection model) selection pressure permits the screening of pleiotropic resistance mutations. **b** Amplicon library preparation and deep sequencing. Unique molecular barcodes are introduced by linear PCR (template elongation) using a primer comprising a 16 bp random sequence (green, yellow and blue part of the middle section of the linear PCR primer). Nested exponential PCR using three primers adds Illumina adapters (blue and yellow primer tails) and indices for multiplexing (black and grey primer sections). Grouping of the reads sharing identical 16 bp barcodes allows differentiation of true SNPs (red, pink and yellow) from sequencing errors (black) by consensus sequence reconstruction using multiple reads from the initial template molecule. Counting the number of unique barcodes for each variant provides an unbiased relative quantification of sequence variants. **c** Bioinformatics analysis pipeline. The diagram represents the different steps in the data processing pipeline. The bioinformatics programs used in the pipeline are indicated in italics

reduced the error rate by an order of magnitude to $5.6 \times 10^{-3} \pm 4.4 \times 10^{-3}$ (SD). By reconstructing consensus reads supported by at least 10 reads, the RM-seq further reduced the error rate by three orders of magnitude to $1.16 \times 10^{-5} \pm 3.1 \times 10^{-5}$ (SD) (Fig. 2a). At the protein level no further mutations were observed among the 16,516 consensus reads generated (error rate $< 6 \times 10^{-5}$).

We then tested the performance of RM-seq genetic variant quantification on a defined population of genetically reconstructed rifampicin-resistant clones. Six different double or single nucleotide variants (SNV) representing different rifampicin-resistant *rpoB* mutants were mixed at a relative CFU frequency of 0.9, 0.09, 0.009, up to 0.000009. We applied RM-seq protocol three times independently from three different genomic DNA extractions obtained from this mock community. After library preparation and sequencing on the Illumina MiSeq platform, we obtained 1.8–2.2 million raw reads per library, which yielded between 32,433 and 35,496 error-corrected consensus reads, supported by 10 reads or more. At this sequencing depth, the mutants ranging from a relative frequency of ~ 1 to 10^{-4} were readily identified in all three replicates. The normalised count of the different mutants showed little variation between the replicate experiments

(Fig. 2b) and we observed a very good correlation between the expected mutant frequencies and the observed frequencies after RM-seq (Fig. 2c). We also assessed the technical variability of the detection and quantification of RM-seq by independently processing three times the same complex population of in vitro selected resistant clones (~ 10,000 colonies). The relative standard error (RSE) of variant quantification ranged from 0.3% for the most frequent to 38% for rarest variants and the median RSE was 11% (Fig. 2d).

High-throughput identification of rifampicin resistance mutations

In order to comprehensively characterise the mutational repertoire associated with rifampicin resistance, we applied RM-seq on the RRDR of three independent pools of ~ 10,000 colonies capable of growing on agar supplemented with 0.06 mg/L of rifampicin (European Committee on Antimicrobial Susceptibility Testing [EUCAST] non-susceptibility clinical breakpoint). In total, we identified 72 different predicted protein variants; among these, 34 were identified in the three independent resistant populations, 17 variants were identified among two resistant populations, and 21 were identified in a single selection

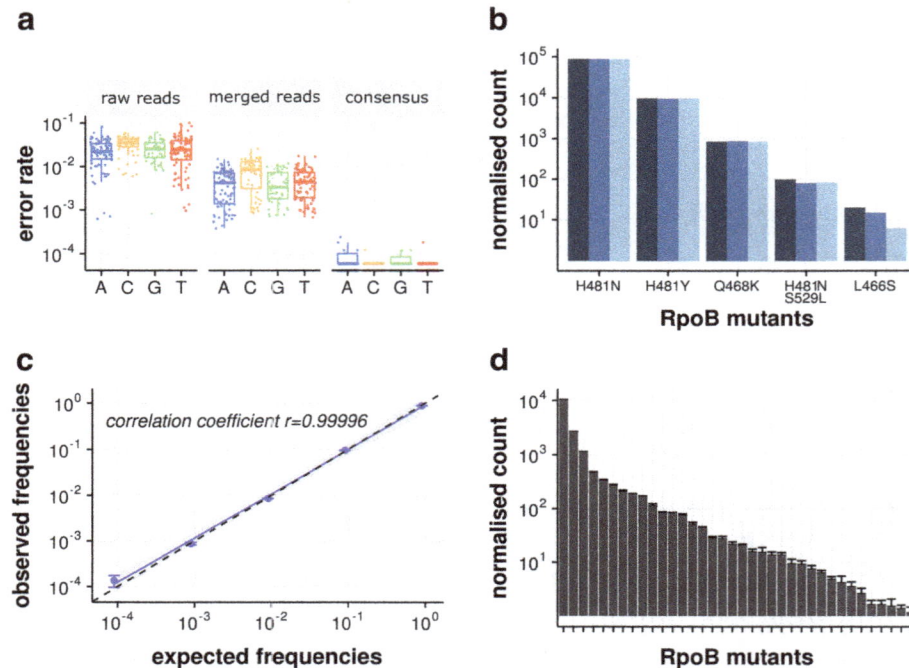

Fig. 2 Assessments of the RM-seq protocol. **a** Error correction evaluation. RM-seq error correction combining merging of paired-end reads with consensus sequence determination from grouped reads sharing identical barcode allows a three order of magnitude reduction in false SNP calling when compared with raw reads calling for the different base. **b** Quantification of populations of *S. aureus rpoB* mutants. Three independent assessments of *rpoB* mutants from three independent genomic DNA preparations originating from a defined population are presented by the different blue bars (technical replicates). **c** Correlation of observed versus expected SNV frequencies. Blue points represent means and error bars represent SEM of three technical replicates. The blue line represents the linear regression of the frequencies measured by RM-seq and the dashed line represent the perfect correlation between expected and observed frequencies. **d** Quantification of *S. aureus rpoB* mutants from a complex population of in vitro selected rifampicin-resistant mutants. Columns represent mean normalised counts of the different *rpoB* mutations that were observed among all triplicates, and error bars represent SEM

experiment (Fig. 3). According to our recent extensive literature review of the alleles previously associated with rifampicin resistance [45], 30 mutations were previously associated with rifampicin non-susceptibility and 42 alleles identified by RM-seq represent new associations.

By looking at the different mutated positions, 21 amino acid positions were repeatedly affected along the RRDR with a similar pattern of mutation frequency at these positions. We observed that 11 different amino acid positions have never previously been associated with rifampicin resistance. The 3D structure modelling of *S. aureus* RpoB protein from *Escherichia coli* RpoB-rifampicin structure showed that the mutated positions were all in close proximity (≤ 10 Å) to the rifampicin binding pocket of the beta-subunit of the RNA polymerase (Additional file 2: Figure S1). Therefore, amino acid sequence alteration at these positions are likely to reduce the rifampicin-RNA polymerase affinity and thus to promote resistance. Interestingly, several residues in close proximity to the rifampicin binding pocket were never affected, suggesting that amino acid substitution at these locations do not impair rifampicin binding or that functional constraints make changes to these positions lethal for *S. aureus*. The vast

majority of the variants led to amino acid substitutions and several positions, such as 471 and 481, were found to be affected by a high number of different substitutions (11 and 12, respectively). We also observed one complex insertion (S464QF) and eight different deletions. Positions 485 and 487 represented deletion hotspots, as they were affected by single, triple and quadruple residue deletions (L485., LSA485., LSAL485.) and single and double deletions (A487. and AL487.), respectively.

We used allelic exchange and site-directed mutagenesis in the WT susceptible background (rifampicin MIC 0.012 mg/L) to reconstruct 19 different *rpoB* alleles that were identified by RM-seq. After whole genome sequencing was used to ensure no secondary non-synonymous mutations or insertion/deletion were introduced (Additional file 1: Table S2), we confirmed that all these mutations resulted in rifampicin non-susceptibility or resistance with rifampicin MICs above 0.095 mg/L (Additional file 1: Table S3).

High-throughput genotype to phenotype associations of resistance mutations with clinical breakpoints
To test if RM-seq could be applied to link a repertoire of resistance mutations to a particular resistance threshold, we

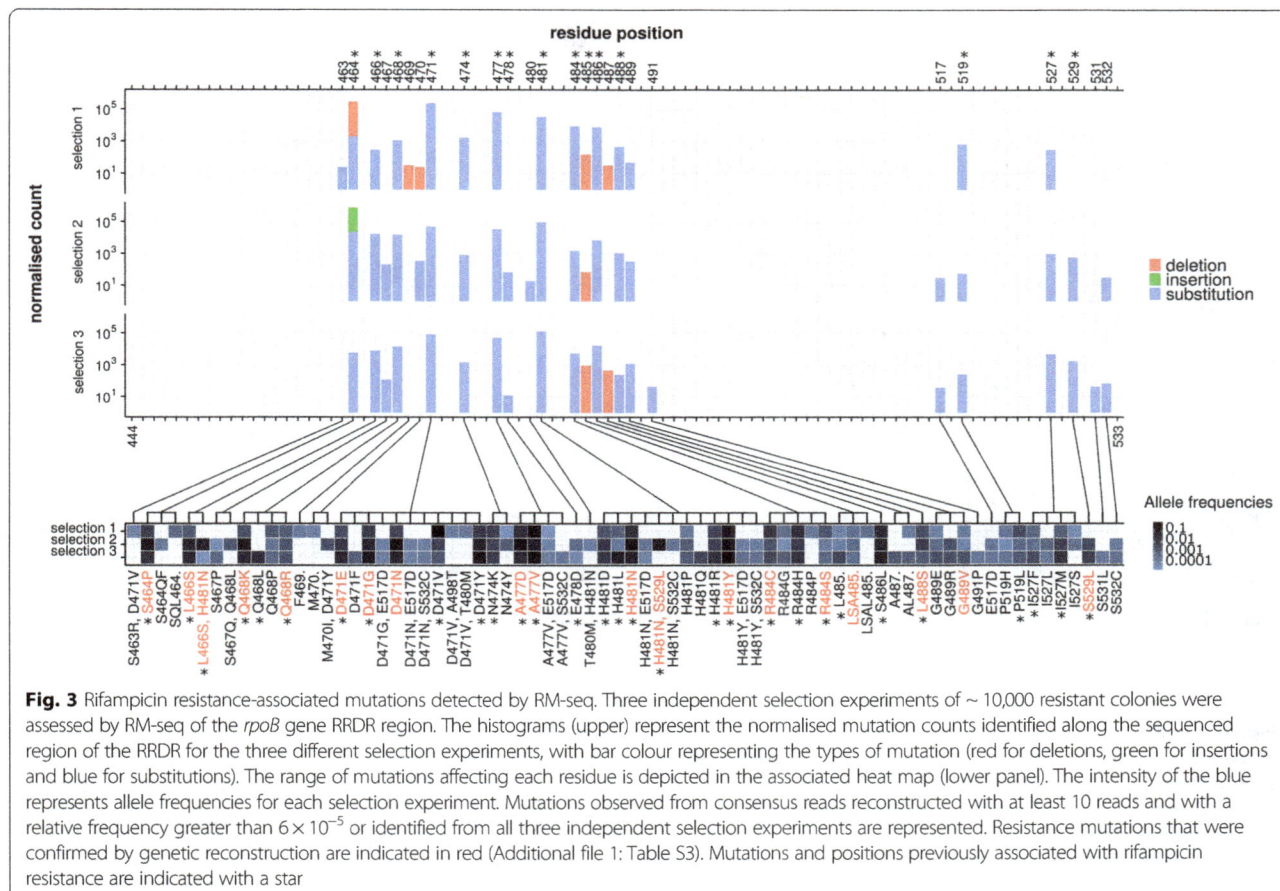

Fig. 3 Rifampicin resistance-associated mutations detected by RM-seq. Three independent selection experiments of ~ 10,000 resistant colonies were assessed by RM-seq of the *rpoB* gene RRDR region. The histograms (upper) represent the normalised mutation counts identified along the sequenced region of the RRDR for the three different selection experiments, with bar colour representing the types of mutation (red for deletions, green for insertions and blue for substitutions). The range of mutations affecting each residue is depicted in the associated heat map (lower panel). The intensity of the blue represents allele frequencies for each selection experiment. Mutations observed from consensus reads reconstructed with at least 10 reads and with a relative frequency greater than 6×10^{-5} or identified from all three independent selection experiments are represented. Resistance mutations that were confirmed by genetic reconstruction are indicated in red (Additional file 1: Table S3). Mutations and positions previously associated with rifampicin resistance are indicated with a star

selected rifampicin-resistant clones, grown on plates supplemented with different concentrations of antibiotic (in this case, rifampicin). To select resistant sub-populations, we used the most widely used clinical resistance breakpoints from the guidelines of the European Committee on Antimicrobial Susceptibility Testing (EUCAST) and the Clinical & Laboratory Standards Institute (CLSI) [46, 47]. Therefore, we selected sub-populations growing on plates supplemented with rifampicin at concentrations of 0.06 mg/L (EUCAST non-susceptibility), 0.5 mg/L (EUCAST resistance), 1 mg/L (CLSI non-susceptibility) and 4 mg/L (CLSI resistance). The result of resistant sub-population detection and quantification by RM-seq associated with the different antibiotic concentration thresholds is presented in Fig. 4. Among 43 mutations, 24 mutations were detected at all antibiotic concentration thresholds and therefore would be classified as resistance-conferring mutations by both guidelines. Among the 19 other mutations detected, four were associated with resistance levels ranging from 1 to 4 mg/L, three with resistance ranging from 0.5 to 1 mg/L and the remaining 12 with resistance ranging from 0.006 to 0.5 mg/L. Interestingly, *S. aureus* with any of these last 12 alleles, selected only at low antibiotic concentrations, would be classified as non-susceptible by EUCAST and susceptible by CLSI.

Similarly, *S. aureus* with three mutations associated with resistance by EUCAST would be classified as susceptible by CLSI (Fig. 4).

We used mutants reconstructed by allelic-exchange to verify that the resistance level predicted by RM-seq matched the MIC conferred by a particular allele. Among 17 reconstructed mutants tested, 16 showed MICs in complete accord with the RM-seq prediction (Additional file 1: Table S3). One mutant (D471G) with a borderline measured MIC of 0.5 mg/L was predicted to have an MIC superior to 0.5 and inferior or equal to 1 despite showing clear reduction in abundance on 0.5 mg/L plate by RM-seq (Fig. 4).

High-throughput screening of resistance mutations associated with antimicrobial cross-resistance or collateral sensitivity

In order to evaluate if RM-seq can be used to characterise pleiotropic resistance mutations that confer an increased or decreased susceptibility to a second antibiotic (cross-resistance or collateral sensitivity respectively), we followed the differential abundance of resistance mutations of a complex rifampicin-resistant population after selection with a second antibiotic, daptomycin. We

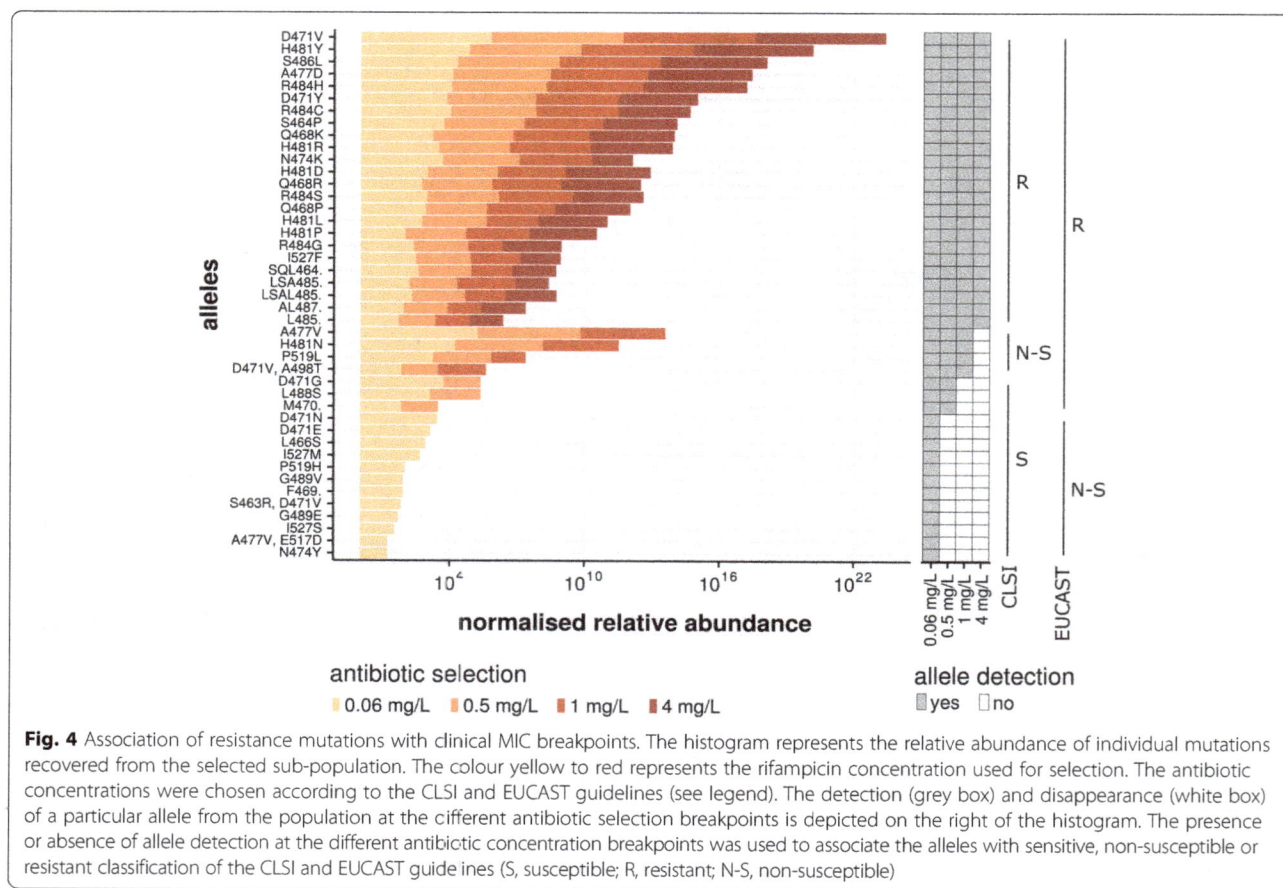

Fig. 4 Association of resistance mutations with clinical MIC breakpoints. The histogram represents the relative abundance of individual mutations recovered from the selected sub-population. The colour yellow to red represents the rifampicin concentration used for selection. The antibiotic concentrations were chosen according to the CLSI and EUCAST guidelines (see legend). The detection (grey box) and disappearance (white box) of a particular allele from the population at the different antibiotic selection breakpoints is depicted on the right of the histogram. The presence or absence of allele detection at the different antibiotic concentration breakpoints was used to associate the alleles with sensitive, non-susceptible or resistant classification of the CLSI and EUCAST guidelines (S, susceptible; R, resistant; N-S, non-susceptible)

chose daptomycin because it is a last-line antibiotic used against multidrug-resistant *S. aureus*, commonly deployed in combination therapy with rifampicin to treat complicated infections [48–50]. Furthermore, some *rpoB* mutations have been previously associated with subtle changes in daptomycin MIC [51, 52]. We screened for pleiotropic effects on daptomycin resistance by performing three independent time killing experiments using a large in vitro-derived population of rifampicin-resistant clones. Daptomycin concentrations of 8 mg/L corresponding to the minimal plasma concentration commonly reached during standard antibiotic therapy were used [53]. Survival of the rifampicin-resistant population at 3 h represented 1.6% ($\pm$ 0.1 SEM) of the initial inoculum and bacterial regrowth was observed to 8.8% ($\pm$ 6.9 SEM) at 24 h (Fig. 5a). The abundance of all rifampicin resistance mutations were then quantified by RM-seq for the initial bacterial population (the inoculum) and the surviving population at 3 h and 24 h after daptomycin exposure for the three independent killing experiments (Fig. 5b).

We tested for significant differential abundance of all the different mutations detected (Fig. 5c). After 3 h of daptomycin treatment, one mutation appeared to

increase in frequency (Q468K) and another decreased (P519L) but the null hypothesis (no change) could not be rejected ($p > 0.05$ after correction for multiple testing [Wald test]). At 24 h of daptomycin selection, differential abundance of these two mutations increased, together with 10 other rifampicin resistance mutations when compared with the mutant abundance in the initial population (Fig. 5d). All the rifampicin resistance mutations that were previously identified as conferring decreased susceptibility to daptomycin ($n = 6$) were found enriched after daptomycin selection, and four mutations had significant fold changes at the 24-h time point ($p < 0.05$, Wald test). These experiments show that changes in relative allele abundance as measured by RM-seq are concordant with changes in daptomycin susceptibility [52, 54].

In order to validate the use of RM-seq as a screening method to identify new mutations that confer cross-resistance or collateral sensitivity, we introduced in the wild-type strain by allelic exchange seven rifampicin-resistant mutations that were significantly enriched and three mutations that were significantly rarefied after daptomycin selection. Among these mutations, MIC testing validated six of the seven rifampicin

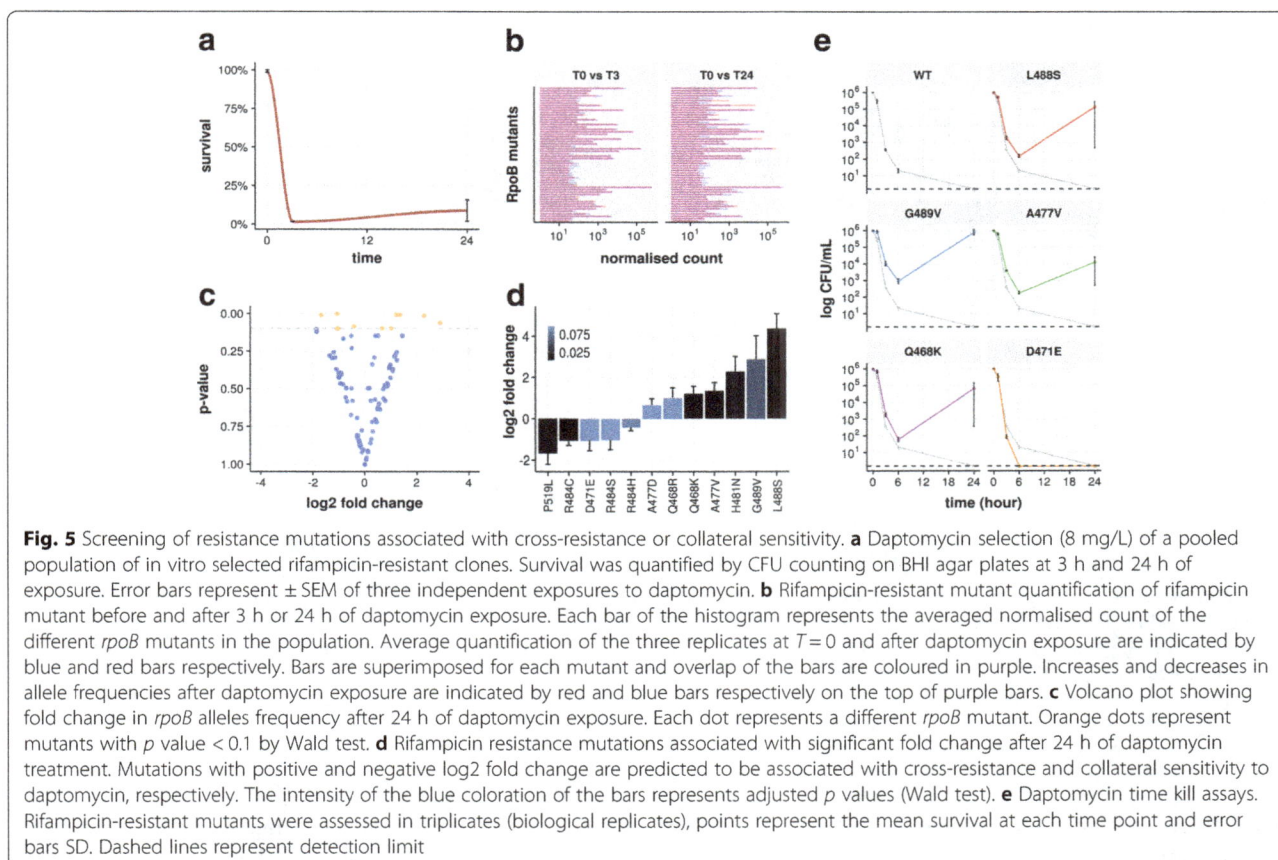

Fig. 5 Screening of resistance mutations associated with cross-resistance or collateral sensitivity. **a** Daptomycin selection (8 mg/L) of a pooled population of in vitro selected rifampicin-resistant clones. Survival was quantified by CFU counting on BHI agar plates at 3 h and 24 h of exposure. Error bars represent ± SEM of three independent exposures to daptomycin. **b** Rifampicin-resistant mutant quantification of rifampicin mutant before and after 3 h or 24 h of daptomycin exposure. Each bar of the histogram represents the averaged normalised count of the different *rpoB* mutants in the population. Average quantification of the three replicates at $T = 0$ and after daptomycin exposure are indicated by blue and red bars respectively. Bars are superimposed for each mutant and overlap of the bars are coloured in purple. Increases and decreases in allele frequencies after daptomycin exposure are indicated by red and blue bars respectively on the top of purple bars. **c** Volcano plot showing fold change in *rpoB* alleles frequency after 24 h of daptomycin exposure. Each dot represents a different *rpoB* mutant. Orange dots represent mutants with *p* value < 0.1 by Wald test. **d** Rifampicin resistance mutations associated with significant fold change after 24 h of daptomycin treatment. Mutations with positive and negative log2 fold change are predicted to be associated with cross-resistance and collateral sensitivity to daptomycin, respectively. The intensity of the blue coloration of the bars represents adjusted *p* values (Wald test). **e** Daptomycin time kill assays. Rifampicin-resistant mutants were assessed in triplicates (biological replicates), points represent the mean survival at each time point and error bars SD. Dashed lines represent detection limit

resistance mutations as decreasing susceptibility to daptomycin and one mutation as increasing the daptomycin susceptibility (Additional file 1: Table S3). We then performed daptomycin time kill assays and found that even though the D471E mutation did not show a decreased MIC to daptomycin (Additional file 1: Table S3), this mutant was less tolerant to daptomycin (Fig. 5e), concordant with the RM-seq prediction which demonstrated reduced abundance of this mutation after daptomycin exposure (Fig. 5d). Similarly, rifampicin resistance mutations L488S, G489V, A477V and Q468K were clearly associated with increased tolerance to daptomycin killing (Fig. 5e).

Taken together, our data demonstrate that RM-seq can identify pleiotropic resistance mutations conferring changes in susceptibility to a secondary antibiotic from large pool of resistant clone selected in vitro after exposure to a primary antibiotic.

Tracking-resistant clones in vivo in a mouse infection model

The relationship between resistance selection, in vivo fitness cost and pathogenicity has been a long standing research topic [24, 27, 55–57]. In a proof-of-principle experiment to investigate the dynamics and fitness of

resistance mutations in vivo, we followed the abundance of rifampicin resistance mutation by RM-seq in a mouse model of persistent infection. Six-week-old BALB/c mice were injected via the tail vein with a complex, in vitro-derived population of rifampicin-resistant mutants that also included susceptible WT clones. We then quantified the abundance of RpoB mutants in the inoculum and at 1 and 7 days post-infection in the kidney, liver and spleen of the mice (Fig. 6). At 24-h post-infection, we recovered a diverse set of RpoB mutants with different relative abundances in the two mice tested. The diversity of mutants appeared to be reduced when compared with the inoculum in the different organs and several initially abundant mutants were not recovered showing a rapid clearance of several inoculated clones. Interestingly, at 7 days post-infection, we observed a drastic reduction in resistant clone diversity with only a small number of clones dominating. This result supports the concept that the establishment of *S. aureus* infection in the mouse is highly clonal, following a "bottleneck" in which very few bacterial cells establish infectious foci or abscesses in invaded organs [58]. Despite the intravenous inoculum containing a diversity of resistant clone, we observed that within a given mouse different organs were infected with the same clones.

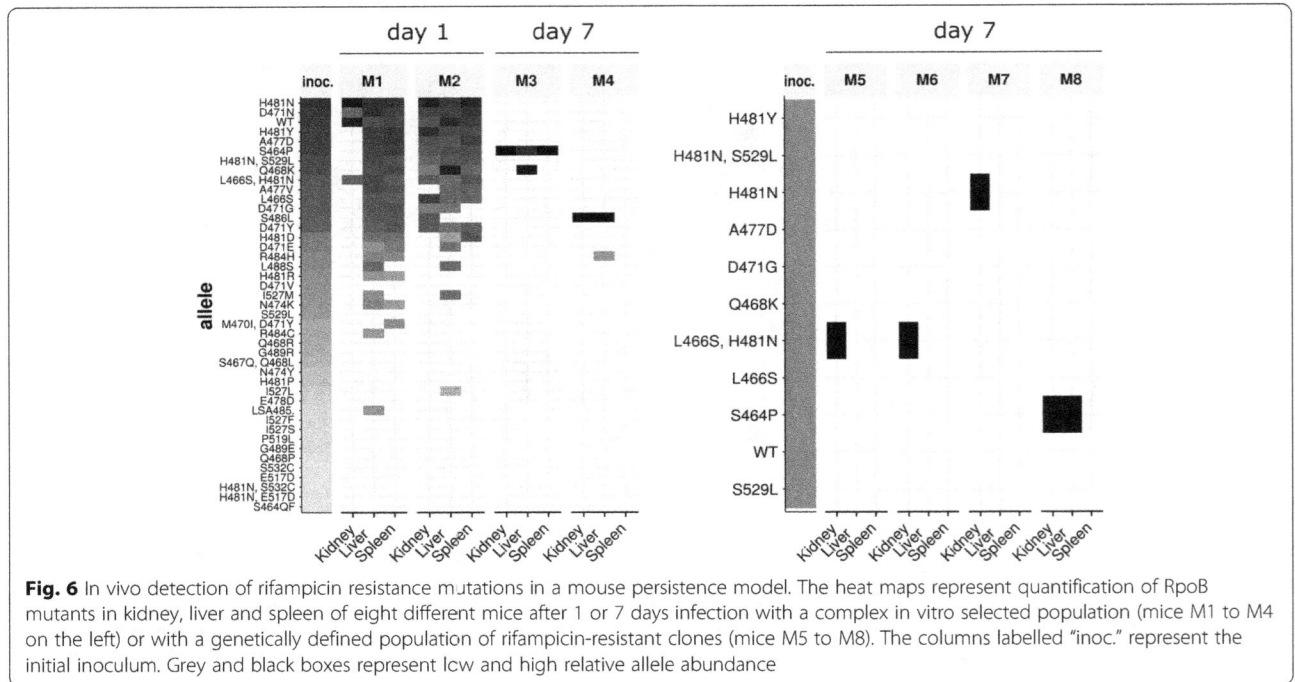

Fig. 6 In vivo detection of rifampicin resistance mutations in a mouse persistence model. The heat maps represent quantification of RpoB mutants in kidney, liver and spleen of eight different mice after 1 or 7 days infection with a complex in vitro selected population (mice M1 to M4 on the left) or with a genetically defined population of rifampicin-resistant clones (mice M5 to M8). The columns labelled "inoc." represent the initial inoculum. Grey and black boxes represent low and high relative allele abundance

We then infected mice with an inoculum comprising an equal amount of 10 reconstructed RpoB mutants together with the wild-type-susceptible strain. After 7 days of infection, four mice were analysed for RpoB mutant abundance by RM-seq. As observed in the previous experiment, the wild-type allele did not persist after 7 days, showing that resistant clones are not outcompeted by the wild-type clone for persistence in the mouse model; even without antibiotic selective pressure (Fig. 6). Three out of four mice were infected with clones encoding the H481N mutation, which has been found to be the most frequent mutation among sequenced *S. aureus* human isolates [45], two had the L466S, H481N double mutation and one had H481N only. Intriguingly, because the mice were infected simultaneously with 11 different clones, the probability is low that at least two mice would become infected with the L466S, H481N by chance ($p = 0.043$). The probability is also low that at least three mice would become randomly infected by a clone encoding the H481N mutation ($p = 0.057$). Given the relatively small number of mice investigated here, no conclusions can be drawn on the potential competitive advantage of specific resistance mutations in vivo. Nevertheless, we show here that RM-seq can be used to follow the dynamics of complex populations of clones in a mouse infection model and that the design of complex multi-clone competition assays in vivo is achievable with RM-seq.

Detection of low-frequency resistant sub-populations of *M. tuberculosis* from sputum samples

A primary motivation for developing RM-seq is to reduce inappropriate antimicrobial therapy by allowing the early detection of low-frequency drug-resistant sub-populations that can arise during antimicrobial therapy. Treatment of tuberculosis, caused by infection with *M. tuberculosis*, could be significantly improved by an accurate and sensitive amplicon sequencing method. This is because phenotypic testing of resistance take weeks to obtain a result and current rapid molecular diagnostic methods only detect a handful of commonly occurring mutations and have low sensitivity for the detection of resistant sub-populations [59]. To assess the potential applicability of RM-seq for clinical detection of resistant sub-population, we retrospectively applied RM-seq on genomic DNA extracted from cultured sputum sample of a previously reported example of chronic pulmonary multidrug-resistant tuberculosis that had been investigated by whole genome sequencing [60]. Here we investigated the emergence of resistance mutations from two samples (sampling interval of 11 years) of three different loci in the genes *rpoB*, *pncA* and *ethA* associated with resistance to rifampicin, pyrazinamide and ethionamide. The multiple changes that were made to the treatment regimen are summarised in Fig. 7. Using RM-seq, we found four other low frequencies of *rpoB* mutants in addition to the dominant *rpoB*-S450L

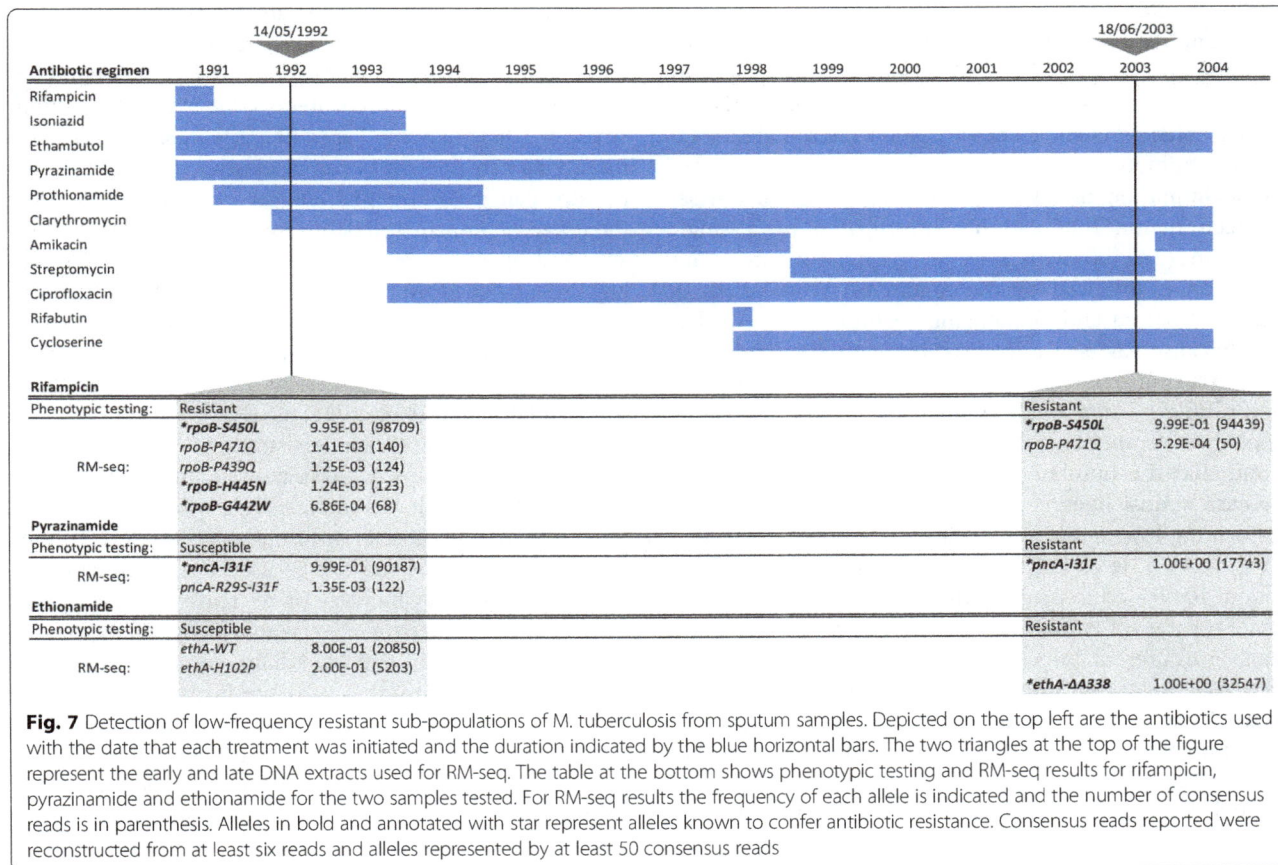

Antibiotic regimen timeline (1991–2004) with treatment durations indicated by blue horizontal bars. Two triangles mark the early (14/05/1992) and late (18/06/2003) DNA extracts used for RM-seq.

Antibiotics listed: Rifampicin, Isoniazid, Ethambutol, Pyrazinamide, Prothionamide, Clarythromycin, Amikacin, Streptomycin, Ciprofloxacin, Rifabutin, Cycloserine

Rifampicin

	Early sample		Late sample	
Phenotypic testing:	Resistant		Resistant	
RM-seq:	*rpoB-S450L	9.95E-01 (98709)	*rpoB-S450L	9.99E-01 (94439)
	rpoB-P471Q	1.41E-03 (140)	rpoB-P471Q	5.29E-04 (50)
	rpoB-P439Q	1.25E-03 (124)		
	*rpoB-H445N	1.24E-03 (123)		
	*rpoB-G442W	6.86E-04 (68)		

Pyrazinamide

	Early sample		Late sample	
Phenotypic testing:	Susceptible		Resistant	
RM-seq:	*pncA-I31F	9.99E-01 (90187)	*pncA-I31F	1.00E+00 (17743)
	pncA-R29S-I31F	1.35E-03 (122)		

Ethionamide

	Early sample		Late sample	
Phenotypic testing:	Susceptible		Resistant	
RM-seq:	ethA-WT	8.00E-01 (20850)		
	ethA-H102P	2.00E-01 (5203)		
			*ethA-ΔA338	1.00E+00 (32547)

Fig. 7 Detection of low-frequency resistant sub-populations of M. tuberculosis from sputum samples. Depicted on the top left are the antibiotics used with the date that each treatment was initiated and the duration indicated by the blue horizontal bars. The two triangles at the top of the figure represent the early and late DNA extracts used for RM-seq. The table at the bottom shows phenotypic testing and RM-seq results for rifampicin, pyrazinamide and ethionamide for the two samples tested. For RM-seq results the frequency of each allele is indicated and the number of consensus reads is in parenthesis. Alleles in bold and annotated with star represent alleles known to confer antibiotic resistance. Consensus reads reported were reconstructed from at least six reads and alleles represented by at least 50 consensus reads

alleles previously associated with rifampicin resistance in this case (Fig. 7) [61]. Among those, rpoB-H445N (frequency of 1.24×10^{-3}) and rpoB-G442W (frequency of 6.86×10^{-4}) represent known rifampicin resistance-conferring alleles [62, 63]. In the later sputum samples collected 12 years after the end of rifampicin treatment, these low frequency sub-populations of rifampicin-resistant clones were not detected but the dominant rifampicin-resistant population harbouring mutation rpoB-S450L persisted together with a low-frequency population harbouring the rpoB-P471Q allele. In association with pyrazinamide resistance the resistant allele pncA-I31F dominated the population after a year and half of treatment together with a low frequency of double mutant sub-population represented by the allele pncA-R29S-I31F. The resistant mutant pncA-I31F was also detected on the later isolate. Surprisingly, early samples were susceptible to pyrazinamide as established by phenotypic testing despite a high prevalence of the pncA-I31F-resistant allele. For ethionamide resistance, the wild-type version of the gene ethA was initially dominant in the population (frequency of 8×10^{-1}) together with a low-frequency allele not associated with resistance ethA-H102P (frequency of 2×10^{-1}). The ethionamide

resistance mutation ethA-ΔA338 causing a frameshift in the gene was readily detected in accordance with phenotypic testing in the later sputum sample. Thus, RM-seq was able to identify low-frequency sub-populations of antibiotic-resistant M. tuberculosis.

Discussion

In this study, we designed and validated a new high-throughput workflow call RM-seq that enables fast and comprehensive characterisation of antibiotic resistance mutations. We show that a straightforward molecular PCR-based barcoding step coupled with high-throughput sequencing significantly reduces background sequencing noise and permits accurate identification and quantification of rare resistance mutations in complex bacterial populations. By applying RM-seq on large pools of in vitro selected rifampicin-resistant S. aureus clones, we demonstrate that the mutational resistome of a resistance locus can be defined. We found that the range of rifampicin resistance mutations in S. aureus is broader than previously understood, highlighting the inadequacy of our understanding of the genetic basis of resistance. Here, 72 mutations were associated with rifampicin resistance in S. aureus. In comparison, the Comprehensive

Antibiotic Resistance Database (CARD) only contains six rifampicin resistance mutations [5]. As the RM-seq protocol can be applied on any combination of microorganisms and resistance, its use has the potential to greatly enhance current knowledge on microbial adaptation to antibiotic exposure.

One limitation of RM-seq is the size limit of the sequenced region that can be interrogated by a single amplicon (270 bp with fully overlapping reads). This limitation is imposed by the maximum read length of Illumina® paired-end sequencing technology. Nevertheless, because RM-seq is compatible with standard Nextera® indexing primers, up to 384 resistance targets can be multiplexed in a single sequencing run. Furthermore, when performing read sub-sampling simulation, we found that the number of high-quality consensus reads increase almost linearly with the number of reads when performing low-depth sequencing (Additional file 2: Figure S2). As little as 140,000 reads would be sufficient to obtain 10,000 consensus reads supported by 10 reads. Theoretically, all resistance variants arising among more than 350 different targeted regions of 270 bp would be accurately identified from a mixed population 1000 bacterial clones using a single MiSeq run (94,500 bp, ~ 86 different genes). This kind of experimental design would be valuable to characterise the genetic basis of poorly defined resistance mechanisms or to determine all the resistance mutation arising in a particular gene. During the preparation of this manuscript, we scanned the full genes *mprF* (2523 bp) and *cls2* (1482 bp) for mutations conferring daptomycin resistance in *S. aureus* by sequencing 10 and six amplicons respectively (manuscript in preparation). For the development of diagnostic tool, multiple resistance hotspots could be assessed by RM-seq using a similar design.

RM-seq trades sequencing depth with accuracy of detection and require a relatively high-sequencing depth (Additional file 1: Table S4) to be effective. Compared with widely used PCR deep sequencing approaches, the method repeatedly sequences the same template DNA molecule to allow consensus-based sequence error correction. This permits accurate detection and quantification of sequence variants that occur at a frequency below 10%. When mutations are expected to occur at a frequency above 10%, then barcoded amplicon deep sequencing is not necessary (see error correction comparison of Fig. 2a).

The application of RM-seq is not restricted to the high-throughput identification of resistance mutations and can also be used to characterise the phenotypic impact of specific resistance mutations. We demonstrate here that differential mutation abundance analysis can be performed to link subsets of mutations with clinical resistance breakpoints and to identify resistance mutations that favour survival or multiplication in particular conditions.

Comparisons of allele frequencies in mixed populations before and after exposure to a second antibiotic permitted the identification of specific resistance mutations that confer cross-resistance and collateral sensitivity. The demonstration that several specific rifampicin resistance mutations can prevent bacterial clearance by daptomycin in vitro can have potential clinical implication regarding the usage rifampicin and daptomycin in combination therapy. A deeper understanding of how evolution of microbial resistance towards a given antibiotic influences susceptibility or resistance to other drugs would have profound impact as it could be exploited to fight resistance rise through combination therapy or by the temporal cycling of different antibiotics [18, 64, 65].

We also showed that the persistence of resistance alleles can be followed during experimental infection (murine blood stream infection model). As it is known that specific resistance mutations can favour pathogenesis and immune evasion [24–26], RM-seq can be used to screen for resistance mutations that increase or decrease survival against ex vivo selective pressures (e.g. whole blood killing, phagocytosis, antimicrobial peptide killing, complement killing) or that favour colonisation or tissue invasion (e.g. biofilm formation, cell attachment, intracellular persistence). A better characterisation of critical resistance mutations that confer cross-resistance or that impact pathogenesis would permit both improving antibiotic resistance surveillance and drug management if a higher therapeutic risk is confirmed.

Fast and culture-independent molecular diagnostic tools have revolutionised pathogen identification and resistance typing in clinical settings. We show here that RM-seq can be used to detect very low frequency sub-population of resistant clones from patients infected by *M. tuberculosis*. The development of diagnostic tools based on the combination of PCR-based barcoding and massively parallel sequencing represents a promising approach for the next generation of genetic-based diagnostics. RM-seq has potential advantages over standard quantitative and molecular probe-based diagnostic tests. For instance, RM-seq would be more sensitive than the current best practice platform for rifampicin resistance detection in *M. tuberculosis*, GeneXpert, as this platform fails to identify sub-populations of rifampicin-resistant strains representing less than 10% of the population [59] and digital PCR and qPCR assays that have been validated for rare mutations with frequencies-of-occurrence not lower than 0.1% [66]. This property of RM-seq may have important clinical implications as similarly to molecular test, most phenotypic tests fail to detect heterogeneous resistance with resistance allele frequency below 1%, and lower frequency of resistance have been frequently described [2, 13, 67]. RM-seq detection is not conditional on the affinity of short DNA probes;

therefore, all sensitive and resistant variant can be detected and differentiated at the sequence level. Nevertheless, like all PCR-based sequence assays, RM-seq variant detection and quantification assumes that the primers bind equally efficiently in all alleles in the population and consequently primers should be designed outside potentially variable regions. Taken together, diagnostic tools based on molecular barcoding and deep sequencing have the potential to perform better than current state of the art diagnostic tests by accurately detecting pre-existing rare resistant sub-population as well as uncommon resistance mutations.

Conclusions

We expect that RM-seq will be a valuable tool for the comprehensive characterisation of the mutational resistance repertoire. A deeper understanding of resistance at the DNA level will be the basis for improved genomic surveillance of antibiotic-resistant pathogens, optimised antibiotic treatment regimens, and can ultimately lead to precision medicine approaches for treating microbial infections.

Abbreviations

BHI: Brain heart infusion; CFU: Colony-forming unit; CLSI: Clinical & Laboratory Standards Institute; E. coli: Escherichia coli; EUCAST: European committee on antimicrobial susceptibility testing; M. tuberculosis: Mycobacterium tuberculosis; PBS: Phosphate buffered saline; RM-seq: Resistance mutation sequencing; S. aureus: Staphylococcus aureus; SLiCE: Seamless ligation cloning extract; WT: Wild type

Funding

This work was supported by the National Health and Medical Research Council (NHMRC), Australia project grant (GNT1066791) and Research Fellowship to TPS (GNT1008549) and Practitioner Fellowship to BPH (GNT1105905). Doherty Applied Microbial Genomics is funded by the Department of Microbiology and Immunology at The University of Melbourne.

Authors' contributions

RG, TPS and BPH designed and planned the project. RG, LL, SB, BH, WG, AD and TT designed and performed the laboratory experiments. RG, TT, IM, SP, SG, AG, MBS, TS, AYP, TPS and BPH provided intellectual input and analysed the data. The manuscript was drafted by RG, TPS and BPH. All authors reviewed and contributed to the final manuscript.

Competing interests

The authors declare that they have no competing interests.

Author details

[1]Department of Microbiology and Immunology, The University of Melbourne at the Doherty Institute for Infection & Immunity, Melbourne, Victoria, Australia. [2]Doherty Applied Microbial Genomics, The University of Melbourne at the Peter Doherty Institute for Infection & Immunity, Melbourne, Victoria, Australia. [3]Microbiological Diagnostic Unit Public Health Laboratory, The University of Melbourne at the Peter Doherty Institute for Infection & Immunity, Melbourne, Victoria, Australia. [4]Melbourne Bioinformatics, The University of Melbourne, Melbourne, Victoria, Australia. [5]Department of Infectious Diseases, The Alfred Hospital and Central Clinical School, Monash University, Melbourne, Victoria, Australia. [6]Infection and Immunity Theme, Monash Biomedicine Discovery Institute, Department of Microbiology, Monash University, Clayton, Victoria, Australia. [7]Infectious Diseases Department, Austin Health, Heidelberg, Victoria, Australia.

References

1. World Health Organization. Antimicrobial resistance: global report on surveillance 2014: World Health Organization; 2014. http://www.who.int/drugresistance/documents/surveillancereport/en/. Accessed 27 July 2018.
2. Köser CU, Ellington MJ, Peacock SJ. Whole-genome sequencing to control antimicrobial resistance. Trends in Genetics. 2014;30(9):401–7.
3. Schürch AC, van Schaik W. Challenges and opportunities for whole-genome sequencing based surveillance of antibiotic resistance. Ann N Y Acad Sci. 2017;1388:108–20.
4. Van Belkum A, Dunne WM. Next generation antimicrobial susceptibility testing. Journal of clinical microbiology. 2013:JCM–00313. https://doi.org/10.1128/JCM.00313-13.
5. McArthur AG, Waglechner N, Nizam F, Yan A, Azad MA, Baylay AJ, et al. The comprehensive antibiotic resistance database. Antimicrob Agents Chemother. 2013;57:3348–57.
6. de Man, Tom JB, and Brandi M. Limbago. SSTAR, a stand-alone easy-to-use antimicrobial resistance gene predictor. mSphere 2016;1.1:e00050–15.
7. Liu B, Pop M. ARDB - antibiotic resistance genes database. Nucleic Acids Res. 2009;37(Database issue):D443–7.
8. Smith T, Wolff KA, Nguyen L. Molecular biology of drug resistance in Mycobacterium tuberculosis. Curr Top Microbiol Immunol. 2013;374:53–80.
9. Feng J, Lupien A, Gingras H, Wasserscheid J, Dewar K, Légaré D, et al. Genome sequencing of linezolid-resistant Streptococcus pneumoniae mutants reveals novel mechanisms of resistance. Genome Res. 2009;19:1214–23.
10. Livermore DM, Warner M, Jamrozy D, Mushtaq S, Nichols WW, Mustafa N, et al. In vitro selection of ceftazidime-avibactam resistance in enterobacteriaceae with KPC-3 carbapenemase. Antimicrob Agents Chemother. 2015;59:5324–30.
11. Chen CJ, Lin MH, Shu JC, Lu JJ. Reduced susceptibility to vancomycin in isogenic Staphylococcus aureus strains of sequence type 59: tracking evolution and identifying mutations by whole-genome sequencing. J Antimicrob Chemother. 2014;69:349–54.
12. Mwangi MM, Wu SW, Zhou Y, Sieradzki K, de Lencastre H, Richardson P, et al. Tracking the in vivo evolution of multidrug resistance in Staphylococcus aureus by whole-genome sequencing. Proc Natl Acad Sci U S A. 2007;104:9451–6.
13. Howden BP, Peleg AY, Stinear TP. The evolution of vancomycin intermediate Staphylococcus aureus (VISA) and heterogenous-VISA. Infect Genet Evol. 2014;21:575–82.
14. Barbosa C, Trebosc V, Kemmer C, Rosenstiel P, Beardmore R, Schulenburg H, Jansen G. Alternative evolutionary paths to bacterial antibiotic resistance cause distinct collateral effects. Molecular biology and evolution. 2017;34(9):2229–44.
15. Howden BP, Davies JK, Johnson PDR, Stinear TP, Grayson ML. Reduced vancomycin susceptibility in Staphylococcus aureus, including vancomycin-intermediate and heterogeneous vancomycin-intermediate strains: Resistance mechanisms, laboratory detection, and clinical implications. Clin Microbiol Rev. 2010;23:99–139.
16. Händel N, Schuurmans JM, Feng Y, Brul S, Ter Kuile BH. Interaction between mutations and regulation of gene expression during development of de novo antibiotic resistance. Antimicrob Agents Chemother. 2014;58:4371–9.
17. Hershberg R. Antibiotic-independent adaptive effects of antibiotic resistance mutations. Trends Genet. 2017;33(8):521–8.
18. Rodriguez De Evgrafov M, Gumpert H, Munck C, Thomsen TT, Sommer MO. Collateral resistance and sensitivity modulate evolution of high-level resistance to drug combination treatment in Staphylococcus aureus. Mol Biol Evol. 2015;32:1175–85.

19. Jugheli L, Bzekalava N, de Rijk P, Fissette K, Portaels F, Rigouts L. High level of cross-resistance between kanamycin, amikacin, and capreomycin among *Mycobacterium tuberculosis* isolates from Georgia and a close relation with mutations in the rrs gene. Antimicrob Agents Chemother. 2009;53:5064–8.

20. Sacco E, Cortes M, Josseaume N, Bouchier C, Dubée V, Hugonnet J-E, et al. Mutation landscape of acquired cross-resistance to glycopeptide and β-lactam antibiotics in *Enterococcus faecium*. Antimicrob Agents Chemother. 2015;59:5306–15.

21. Yu J, Wu J, Francis KP, Purchio TF, Kadurugamuwa JL. Monitoring in vivo fitness of rifampicin-resistant *Staphylococcus aureus* mutants in a mouse biofilm infection model. J Antimicrob Chemother. 2005;55:528–34.

22. Helms M, Simonsen J, Mølbak K. Quinolone resistance is associated with increased risk of invasive illness or death during infection with *Salmonella* serotype typhimurium. J Infect Dis. 2004;190:1652–4.

23. Smani Y, López-Rojas R, Domínguez-Herrera J, Docobo-Pérez F, Martí S, Vila J, et al. In vitro and in vivo reduced fitness and virulence in ciprofloxacin-resistant *Acinetobacter baumannii*. Clin Microbiol Infect. 2012;18(1):E1–4.

24. Beceiro A, Tomás M, Bou G. Antimicrobial resistance and virulence: a successful or deleterious association in the bacterial world? Clin Microbiol Rev. 2013;26:185–230.

25. Gao W, Cameron DR, Davies JK, Kostoulias X, Stepnell J, Tuck KL, et al. The RpoB H481Y rifampicin resistance mutation and an active stringent response reduce virulence and increase resistance to innate immune responses in *Staphylococcus aureus*. J Infect Dis. 2013;207:929–39.

26. Bæk KT, Thøgersen L, Mogenssen RG, Mellergaard M, Thomsen LE, Petersen A, et al. Stepwise decrease in daptomycin susceptibility in clinical *Staphylococcus aureus* isolates associated with an initial mutation in *rpoB* and a compensatory inactivation of the *clpX* gene. Antimicrob Agents Chemother. 2015;59:6983–91.

27. Cameron DR, Howden BP, Peleg AY. The interface between antibiotic resistance and virulence in *Staphylococcus aureus* and its impact upon clinical outcomes. Clin Infect Dis. 2011;53:576–82.

28. Miskinyte M, Gordo I. Increased survival of antibiotic-resistant *Escherichia coli* inside macrophages. Antimicrob Agents Chemother. 2013;57:189–95.

29. O'Neill AJ, Cove JH, Chopra I. Mutation frequencies for resistance to fusidic acid and rifampicin in *Staphylococcus aureus*. J Antimicrob Chemother. 2001; 47:647–50.

30. Li H. Aligning sequence reads, clone sequences and assembly contigs with BWA-MEM. arXiv. 2013;0:3.

31. Li H, Handsaker B, Wysoker A, Fennell T, Ruan J, Homer N, et al. The sequence alignment/map format and SAMtools. Bioinformatics. 2009;25:2078–9.

32. Zhang J, Kobert K, Flouri T, Stamatakis A. PEAR: a fast and accurate Illumina paired-end reAd mergeR. Bioinformatics. 2014;30:614–20.

33. Sievers F, Higgins DG. Clustal Omega. Curr Protoc Bioinforma. 2014;48:3.13. 1–16.

34. Rice P, Longden I, Bleasby A. EMBOSS: the European molecular biology open software suite. Trends Genet. 2000;16:276–7.

35. Tange O. GNU parallel: the command-line power tool. USENIX Mag. 2011;36: 42–7.

36. Fu L, Niu B, Zhu Z, Wu S, Li W. CD-HIT: accelerated for clustering the next-generation sequencing data. Bioinformatics. 2012;28:3150–2.

37. Monk IR, Tree JJ, Howden BP, Stinear TP, Foster TJ. Complete bypass of restriction systems for major *Staphylococcus aureus* lineages. MBio. 2015;6: e00308–15.

38. Zhang Y, Werling U, Edelmann W. SLiCE: a novel bacterial cell extract-based DNA cloning method. Nucleic Acids Res. 2012;40(8):e55.

39. Love MI, Huber W, Anders S, Lönnstedt I, Speed T, Robinson M, et al. Moderated estimation of fold change and dispersion for RNA-seq data with DESeq2. Genome Biol. 2014;15:550.

40. Benjamini Y, Hochberg Y. Controlling the false discovery rate: a practical and powerful approach to multiple testing. Journal of the royal statistical society. Series B (Methodological). 1995;1:289–300.

41. Ross BC, Raios K, Jackson K, Sievers A, Dwyer B. Differentiation of *Mycobacterium tuberculosis* strains by use of a nonradioactive southern blot hybridization method. J Infect Dis. 1991;163:904–7.

42. Faith JJ, Guruge JL, Charbonneau M, Subramanian S, Seedorf H, Goodman AL, et al. The long-term stability of the human gut microbiota. Science. 2013;341:1237439.

43. Kivioja T, Vähärautio A, Karlsson K, Bonke M, Enge M, Linnarsson S, et al. Counting absolute numbers of molecules using unique molecular identifiers. Nat Methods. 2011;9:72–4.

44. Schirmer M, Ijaz UZ, D'Amore R, Hall N, Sloan WT, Quince C. Insight into biases and sequencing errors for amplicon sequencing with the Illumina MiSeq platform. Nucleic Acids Res. 2015;43:e37.

45. Guérillot R, da Silva AG, Monk I, Giulieri S, Tomita T, Alison E, Porter J, Pidot S, Gao W, Peleg AY, Seemann T. Convergent Evolution Driven by Rifampin Exacerbates the Global Burden of Drug-Resistant *Staphylococcus aureus*. mSphere. 2018;3(1):e00550–17.

46. EUCAST. Antimicrobial susceptibility testing for bacteria: EUCAST; 2015. http://www.eucast.org/ast_of_bacteria/. Accessed 27 July 2018.

47. CLSI. Performance standards for antimicrobial susceptibility testing. CLSI supplement M100S. CLSI Suppl. M100S. Wayne: Clin. Lab. Stand. Inst; 2016.

48. Forrest GN, Tamura K. Rifampin combination therapy for nonmycobacterial infections. Clin. Microbiol. Rev. 2010;23(1):14–34.

49. Saleh-Mghir A, Muller-Serieys C, Dinh A, Massias L, Crémieux AC. Adjunctive rifampin is crucial to optimizing daptomycin efficacy against rabbit prosthetic joint infection due to methicillin-resistant *Staphylococcus aureus*. Antimicrob Agents Chemother. 2011;55:4589–93.

50. Garrigós C, Murillo O, Euba G, Verdaguer R, Tubau F, Cabellos C, et al. Efficacy of usual and high doses of daptomycin in combination with rifampin versus alternative therapies in experimental foreign-body infection by methicillin-resistant *Staphylococcus aureus*. Antimicrob Agents Chemother. 2010;54:5251–6.

51. Cui L, Isii T, Fukuda M, Ochiai T, Neoh HM, Da Cunha Camargo ILB, et al. An RpoB mutation confers dual heteroresistance to daptomycin and vancomycin in *Staphylococcus aureus*. Antimicrob Agents Chemother. 2010; 54:5222–33.

52. Aiba Y, Katayama Y, Hishinuma T, Murakami-Kuroda H, Cui L, Hiramatsu K. Mutation of RNA polymerase β-subunit gene promotes heterogeneous-to-homogeneous conversion of β-lactam resistance in methicillin-resistant *Staphylococcus aureus*. Antimicrob Agents Chemother. 2013;57:4861–71.

53. Reiber C, Senn O, Muller D, Kullak-Ublick G, Corti N. Therapeutic drug monitoring of daptomycin: a retrospective monocentric analysis. Ther Drug Monit. 2015;37:634–40.

54. Berti AD, Baines SL, Howden BP, Sakoulas G, Nizet V, Proctor RA, et al. Heterogeneity of genetic pathways toward daptomycin nonsusceptibility in *Staphylococcus aureus* determined by adjunctive antibiotics. Antimicrob Agents Chemother. 2015;59:2799–806.

55. Holmes NE, Turnidge JD, Munckhof WJ, Robinson JO, Korman TM, O'Sullivan MVN, et al. Antibiotic choice may not explain poorer outcomes in patients with *Staphylococcus aureus* bacteremia and high vancomycin minimum inhibitory concentrations. J Infect Dis. 2011;204:340–7.

56. Gao W, Chua K, Davies JK, Newton HJ, Seemann T, Harrison PF, et al. Two novel point mutations in clinical *Staphylococcus aureus* reduce linezolid susceptibility and switch on the stringent response to promote persistent infection. PLoS Pathog. 2010;6:e1000944.

57. Beceiro A, Tomás M, Bou G. Antimicrobial resistance and virulence: a beneficial relationship for the microbial world? Enferm Infecc Microbiol Clin. 2012;30:492–9.

58. McVicker G, Prajsnar TK, Williams A, Wagner NL, Boots M, Renshaw SA, et al. Clonal expansion during *Staphylococcus aureus* infection dynamics reveals the effect of antibiotic intervention. PLoS Pathog. 2014;10:e1003959.

59. Zetola NM, Shin SS, Tumedi KA, Moeti K, Ncube R, Nicol M, et al. Mixed *Mycobacterium tuberculosis* complex infections and false-negative results for rifampin resistance by genexpert MTB/RIF associated with poor clinical outcomes. J Clin Microbiol. 2014;52:2422–9.

60. Meumann EM, Globan M, Fyfe JAM, Leslie D, Porter JL, Seemann T, et al. Genome sequence comparisons of serial multi-drug-resistant *Mycobacterium tuberculosis* isolates over 21 years of infection in a single patient. Microb genomics. 2015;1:e000037.

61. Donnabella V, Martiniuk F, Kinney D, Bacerdo M, Bonk S, Hanna B, et al. Isolation of the gene for the beta subunit of RNA polymerase from rifampicin-resistant *Mycobacterium tuberculosis* and identification of new mutations. Am J Respir Cell Mol Biol. 1994;11:639–43.

62. Ramaswamy SV, Dou S, Rendon A, Yang Z, Cave MD, Graviss EA. Genotypic analysis of multidrug-resistant *Mycobacterium tuberculosis* isolates from Monterrey, Mexico. J Med Microbiol. 2004;53:107–13.

63. Pozzi G, Meloni M, Iona E, Orrù G, Thoresen OF, Ricci ML, et al. *rpoB* Mutations in multidrug-resistant strains of *Mycobacterium tuberculosis* isolated in Italy. J Clin Microbiol. 1999;37:1197–9.

9

Genotype effects contribute to variation in longitudinal methylome patterns in older people

Qian Zhang[1*] (iD), Riccardo E Marioni[2,3], Matthew R Robinson[1], Jon Higham[4], Duncan Sproul[4,5], Naomi R Wray[1,6], Ian J Deary[2,7†], Allan F McRae[1†] and Peter M Visscher[1,6†]

Abstract

Background: DNA methylation levels change along with age, but few studies have examined the variation in the rate of such changes between individuals.

Methods: We performed a longitudinal analysis to quantify the variation in the rate of change of DNA methylation between individuals using whole blood DNA methylation array profiles collected at 2–4 time points ($N = 2894$) in 954 individuals (67–90 years).

Results: After stringent quality control, we identified 1507 DNA methylation CpG sites (rsCpGs) with statistically significant variation in the rate of change (random slope) of DNA methylation among individuals in a mixed linear model analysis. Genes in the vicinity of these rsCpGs were found to be enriched in Homeobox transcription factors and the Wnt signalling pathway, both of which are related to ageing processes. Furthermore, we investigated the SNP effect on the random slope. We found that 4 out of 1507 rsCpGs had one significant ($P < 5 \times 10^{-8}/1507$) SNP effect and 343 rsCpGs had at least one SNP effect (436 SNP-probe pairs) reaching genome-wide significance ($P < 5 \times 10^{-8}$). Ninety-five percent of the significant ($P < 5 \times 10^{-8}$) SNPs are on different chromosomes from their corresponding probes.

Conclusions: We identified CpG sites that have variability in the rate of change of DNA methylation between individuals, and our results suggest a genetic basis of this variation. Genes around these CpG sites have been reported to be involved in the ageing process.

Keywords: DNA methylation, Longitudinal analysis, Methylation change, G by AGE

Background

DNA methylation is a widely studied epigenetic modification with a role in the regulation of gene expression [1]. Local levels of DNA methylation differ within and between individuals. This variation in local methylation is associated with both genetic and environmental factors [2–5]. The majority of DNA methylation studies in human are based on cross-sectional cohorts. Such studies have reported that methylation levels at many CpG sites in the genome correlate with age [6–10]. Therefore, age is frequently treated as a covariate and adjusted for in a

linear regression framework in which differences of DNA methylation between cell types, tissues and diseases are tested [11–13]. One implicit assumption behind this correction is that the rate of change at a methylation CpG site across time is constant between individuals, which may not be true. Several studies have revealed that there is a potential change in variability of DNA methylation with age [14, 15], indicating that the rate of change of DNA methylation is different between individuals.

Estimation of the variation in such trajectories of DNA methylation with age between individuals is possible in a longitudinal analysis. Previous longitudinal analyses have investigated the relationship between SNPs and longitudinal DNA methylation [16, 17]. Other studies focused on the association between DNA methylation and a phenotype measured on the same individual [18–20]. Differences

* Correspondence: q.zhang@uq.edu.au
†Ian J Deary, Allan F McRae and Peter M Visscher contributed equally to this work.
[1]Institute for Molecular Bioscience, The University of Queensland, Brisbane, QLD 4072, Australia
Full list of author information is available at the end of the article

between individuals in the pattern of change of DNA methylation over time were not considered in these studies. Here, we estimate the variation in trajectories of DNA methylation change among individuals in a longitudinal analysis. This approach may elucidate how epigenetic marks change differently between individuals and whether this variation is associated with genetic factors and biological function.

In this study, we estimated between-individual variation in the rate of change of DNA methylation at 344,000 loci in a longitudinal sample of older people from the Lothian Birth Cohorts 1921 and 1936. For each CpG site, we estimated the variation in the rate of change in each individual. Furthermore, the identification of such probes facilitates the estimation and partitioning of the variation underlying DNA methylation changes, for example, the contribution of genetic factors. We identified genetic loci that are associated with differences in the longitudinal changes in DNA methylation across individuals.

Methods
Methylation data
DNA was extracted from whole blood samples in Lothian Birth Cohort 1921 (LBC1921) at MRC Technology, Western General Hospital, Edinburgh (LBC1921), and the Wellcome Trust Clinical Research Facility (WTCRF), Western General Hospital, Edinburgh (LBC1936), using standard methods. Methylation typing of 485,512 probes was performed at the WTCRF. Bisulphite converted HD Methylation protocol and Tecan robotics (Illumina). Raw intensity data were background-corrected and normalized using internal controls, and methylation M values were generated using the R minfi package [21]. Detailed further quality control steps are given in Additional file 1.

Batch and covariate adjustment
Our analysis was based on the M value of DNA methylation. We regularized the M value by constraining it to be in the interval between − 9.96 and 9.96 (corresponding to the interval 0.001 to 0.999 of the beta-value). Furthermore, for each probe, we removed individuals with DNA methylation three standard deviations above and below the mean M value to exclude outliers. On average, 34 (out of 2894 samples, 1.2%) outliers were removed for each probe. DNA methylation (M value) in most (79.5%) of these outliers is in the range between − 6.6 and 6.6 (corresponding to the interval 0.01 to 0.99 of the beta-value), suggesting the "abnormal" DNA methylation values in the majority of outliers are not extreme values caused by the transformation from beta-value to M value. Covariates including sex, age and cell counts (CC), and batch effects including position in array (PIA), hybridization date (HD), set ID (SI), plate ID (PI) and array ID (AI, both PI and AI were regarded as random effects), were corrected for each

probe. We used the residuals after this adjustment for further analysis. If y_j is the DNA methylation value for probe j, then we used the residuals from the model

$$y_j \sim \text{sex} + \text{age} + \text{CC} + \text{PIA} + \text{HD} + \text{SI} + \text{PI} + \text{AI} + e_j.$$

LBC genotype and imputation
Individuals from LBC1921 and LBC1936 were genotyped on Illumina 610-Quad Beadchip arrays. Full details of genotyping procedures are given elsewhere [22]. Standard QC filters were applied, and remaining genotyped SNPs were phased using HAPI-UR [23] and imputed using 1000 Genomes Phase I Version 3 [24] with Impute V2 [25]. Raw imputed SNPs were filtered to remove any SNPs with low imputation quality as defined by an $R^2 < 0.8$. Subsequent quality control removed SNPs with MAF < 0.01, those with HWE $P < 1 \times 10^{-6}$ and a missing rate > 10%. After filtering, 7,760,689 SNPs remained for further analysis.

Estimation of random slope effects
For each probe, we fitted a mean level and a rate of change of DNA methylation for each individual and tested whether the variance due to these random effects was significantly larger than zero, using the mixed model

$$y_{ij} = u_1 + u_2 \times t_{ij} + a_i + b_i \times t_{ij} + e_{ij}$$

$$\begin{bmatrix} a_i \\ b_i \end{bmatrix} \sim N(0, \Omega) \text{ with } \Omega = \begin{bmatrix} \sigma_a^2 & \sigma_{ab} \\ \sigma_{ab} & \sigma_b^2 \end{bmatrix} \text{ and } e_{ij} \sim N(0, \sigma_e^2).$$

where y_{ij} is the methylation residual after QC steps, i is the ith individual, j represents the jth observation in individual i, u_1 is the mean effect, u_2 is the mean age effect, a_i and b_i are the random intercept (mean level of DNA methylation in each individual) and random slope, t_{ij} represents standardized age (mean = 0 and variance = 1) and e_{ij} is the random error. The random effects of e_{ij}, a_i and b_i are assumed to follow a normal distribution. σ_a^2 and σ_b^2 are the variances of a_i and b_i, respectively. σ_{ab} is the covariance between a_i and b_i, it was set to be zero under the assumption of independence between a_i and b_i. The likelihood ratio test (LRT) was used to test if σ_a^2 and σ_b^2 are equal to zero.

We obtained a P value from the LRT using a $\chi^2(1)$ distribution and then dividing the P value by two. This can be justified since under the null hypothesis, in 50% of cases, the test statistic is zero (or, follows a $\chi^2(0)$), and in 50% of cases it follows a $\chi^2(1)$ [26]. Probes with a P value smaller than 1.5×10^{-7} (0.05/344,000) for the random slope are defined as rsCpG.

Covariance between a_i and b_i

We applied an extended model that included the covariance σ_{ab} between the random intercept and random slope to quantify the effect of covariance on the estimation of random effects. We calculated the Pearson corrections between the estimated random slope effects before and after incorporating the covariance term. All correlations were larger than 0.7 in the 1507 rsCpGs (mean correlation = 0.93). These results indicated that the introduction of the covariance term did not alter the results substantially.

Quadratic effect

We investigated the effect of modelling a quadratic average trajectory by adding a squared term for age (t^2) in the model $y_{ij} = u_1 + u_2 \times t_{ij} + a_i + b_i \times t_{ij} + t_{ij}^2 + e_{ij}$. All the correlations of the probes with and without fitting this additional term were found to be larger than 0.98 in 1507 rsCpGs.

Estimating the confidence interval of the correlation based on bootstrapping

Considering the background correlation of DNA methylation between CpG sites, we used bootstrapping to calculate the 95% confidence interval of the correlation (of the estimated variances) between two groups of individuals. We resampled 344,000 pairs of variances with replacement from the original data and estimated the correlation based on these pairs. We repeated this step 30,000 times to calculate the 95% confidence interval of the correlation.

GWAS on random effects

Based on the random effects estimated from the above mixed linear model, we performed a series of genome-wide association studies by using the random effects as the dependent variables with the software PLINK2 [27]. All QC-ed SNPs were used, and P value threshold for the significance was Bonferroni corrected ($P < 5 \times 10^{-8}/1507$).

Permutation analysis of the random slope test statistics

The mean and median test statistic across CpG sites for the effect of the random slope was very large, with a λ inflation value (mean test statistic) of 11.0. To verify if the results are inflated under the null hypothesis, we permuted ages across individuals and waves 500 times. For each round, we re-fitted the full model on the permuted data, and the mean chi-square among the probes was calculated. The mean of this distribution was around 0.73 (SD = 0.32), which shows no significant difference ($P = 0.48$) with the expected value of 0.5 under the null hypothesis. This indicates the statistical significance of the estimated effects of a random slope is not caused by the violations of the assumptions of the distribution of the test statistic under the null hypothesis.

Mapping CpG Islands and differently methylated region (DMR)

Genomic positions of the CpG island were obtained from the UCSC Genome Browser [28]. Annotation information of the differently methylated region (DMR) was from the Illumina DNA methylation annotation file (GEO ID GPL13534). The significance of enrichment analysis was assessed by permutation.

PANTHER over-representation test

We used all 25,537 genes that are adjacent to the QC-ed 344,000 probes as the background. Eighteen thousand six hundred seven of the genes overlapped with the gene list in the PANTHER database. Ten thousand twenty out of 1235 rsCpG nearby genes were in the PANTHER database. The enrichment test was based on Fisher's exact test, and protein classes with a false discovery rate (FDR) smaller than 0.05 were selected.

Heritability of probes

We utilized the heritability of the significant probes estimated in the Brisbane Systems Genetics Study (BSGS) cohort [29, 30] to validate the genetic contribution to these probes. The significance of the difference from the null distribution of the mean heritability was estimated based on the average heritability of 1507 randomly selected probes from 30,000 permutation tests.

SNP by age effect on DNA methylation

The SNP effect on random slope can be defined as slope$_i$ = $\beta_k \times d_{ik} + e_i$, i is the ith individual, β_k is the effect size of SNP k on random slope, and d_{ik} is the dosage of SNP k in individual i. Since the DNA methylation of individual i at time point t_{ij} is y_{ij} = slope$_i \times t_{ij} + e_{ij} = (\beta_k \times d_{ik} + e_i) \times t_{ij} + e_{ij}$ = $\beta_k \times d_{ik} \times t_{ij} + e_i \times t_{ij} + e_{ij}$ (main effects are ignored here), the SNP effect on random slope can be interpreted as SNP by age effect on DNA methylation. To compare the power in detecting these two effects, we simulated 3000 individuals, each with three age points sampled at round 60, 70 and 80 years old. DNA methylation of individual i at time point t_{ij} was simulated by using $y_{ij} = (\beta_k \times d_{ik} + e_i) \times t_{ij} + e_{ij}$. d_{ik} was sampled from (0,1,2) assuming Hardy–Weinberg equilibrium, the minor allele frequency of the SNP ranges from 0.05 to 0.5, the random error e_{ij} and random slope e_i (not explained by SNP) are assumed to follow a standard normal distribution. The effect size β_k of the SNP on the random slope was simulated in two ways: (1) β_k was sampled from a uniform distribution in the range of -0.1 to 0.1 and (2) β_k was set to zero. For each type of data, we obtained P values in three ways: (1) from association between the SNP and the estimated random slope from a mixed linear model, (2) from association between DNA methylation and a SNP by age effect and (3) from association between DNA methylation and a SNP by age effect with random slope fitted as a covariate. We repeated this simulation 300,000 times and compared P values and median chi-square (λ_{median}) between these associations. Based on the simulated data with no SNP effect on the random slope ($\beta_k = 0$), we found the P values from the second analysis method were inflated ($\lambda_{\text{median}} = 2.01$). P values from the other two ways were not inflated ($\lambda_{\text{median}} = 1.00$), and no difference in the detecting power was identified between these two ways based on the simulated data with SNP effect on the random slope ($\beta_k \sim U(-0.1, 0.1)$).

Linkage disequilibrium (LD) clumping

We applied LD clumping on the GWAS significant SNPs using PLINK2 [27], and imputed LBC genotype data was used as the reference. For each significant ($P < 5 \times 10^{-8}$) SNP, LD (R^2) between this SNP and other significant ($P < 5 \times 10^{-8}$) SNPs within 1 Mbp distance were calculated and SNPs with LD larger than 0.1 were defined as a clump. Within each clump, only the SNP with smallest P value would be selected during LD clumping.

All analysis was performed by using R package, version 3.2.2 [31]. Figures were generated using ggplot2 [32].

Results

Data

DNA methylation was measured on individuals from Lothian Birth Cohort 1921 (LBC1921) and Lothian Birth Cohort 1936 (LBC1936) [33, 34] using Illumina Infinium HumanMethylation450K BeadChip arrays. There were 3471 samples across all waves of data collection (Additional file 1: Table S1), and 344,000 DNA methylation probes remained after removing probes encompassing SNPs annotated by Illumina (GEO ID GPL13534) and probes identified as potentially cross-hybridizing [35] (see details of quality control steps in Additional file 1). Only individuals with DNA methylation measured at two or more different time points were considered, and samples with inconsistent measurements (match rate < 0.8) of control probes within individuals were removed (Additional file 2: Figure S1), leaving 2894 samples from 954 individuals (Table 1). Among them, 283 individuals had DNA methylation measured at two time points, and 356 and 315 individuals were measured at three and four time points, respectively. The effects of covariates (sex, age and cell counts) and batches (position in the array, hybridization date, set ID, plate ID and array ID) on DNA methylation were removed before further analysis ('Methods', Additional file 1: Figures S2 and S3).

Table 1 Description of the DNA methylation samples in the LBC cohorts, for individuals with DNA methylation measured in at least two waves

Cohort wave	Mean age (SD)	Age range	Female	Male	Total
LBC1921W1	79.1 (0.6)	(77.9,80.6)	77	63	140
LBC1921W3	86.6 (0.4)	(85.8,87.5)	82	71	153
LBC1921W4	90.2 (0.1)	(90,90.6)	42	36	78
LBC1936W1	69.6 (0.8)	(67.7,71.3)	326	359	685
LBC1936W2	72.5 (0.7)	(70.9,74.2)	353	399	752
LBC1936W3	76.3 (0.7)	(74.7,77.7)	284	312	596
LBC1936W4	79.3 (0.6)	(78.0,80.9)	240	250	490

Identification of CpG sites with a random slope in methylation

For each CpG site, we estimated the variance of the rate of change (random slope) between individuals in a mixed linear model ('Methods'). A non-zero variance indicates the existence of individual differences in the rate of change in DNA methylation across time. Forty-two thousand two hundred fifty-three probes were found to have a statistically significant random slope (likelihood ratio test, $P < 0.05/344,000$, Bonferroni corrected) based on 2894 samples. Permutation test analyses indicated that the statistical significance of the estimated effects of the random slope is not caused by the violations of the assumptions of the test statistic ('Methods', Additional file 2: Figures S4 and S5). Moreover, no substantial impact on the estimation of random effects was found by introducing a covariance ('Methods', Additional file 2: Figure S6A) between the random slope and the mean level of DNA methylation in each individual into the model, or the inclusion of additional corrections for age effects such as a quadratic term ('Methods', Additional file 2: Figure S6B). To obtain a robust set of CpG sites with a statistically significant variation in the rate of change, we divided the individuals into two groups according to the number of time points for which they have a measurement. One group contains individuals with two or three time points, and the other group has individuals with four time points. We applied the mixed linear model on each of these two groups and found that the estimated variances of random slopes for each CpG site were correlated between these independent groups ($R = 0.41$, 95% bootstrap CI 0.40–0.42, bootstrapping was repeated 30,000 times, 'Methods', Fig. 1a). One thousand five hundred seven CpG sites were identified to have a statistically significant ($p < 0.05/344,000$) variation in the rate of change of DNA methylation in both groups (rsCpGs, Fig. 1b, Additional file 3: Table S2). The overlap is statistically significant (odds ratio = 4.9, $P < 3.3 \times 10^{-5}$, permutation test, 30,000 times), and these 1507 rsCpGs were used for further analysis. A summary of chi-square statistics for the variance of the random slope is presented in Table 2.

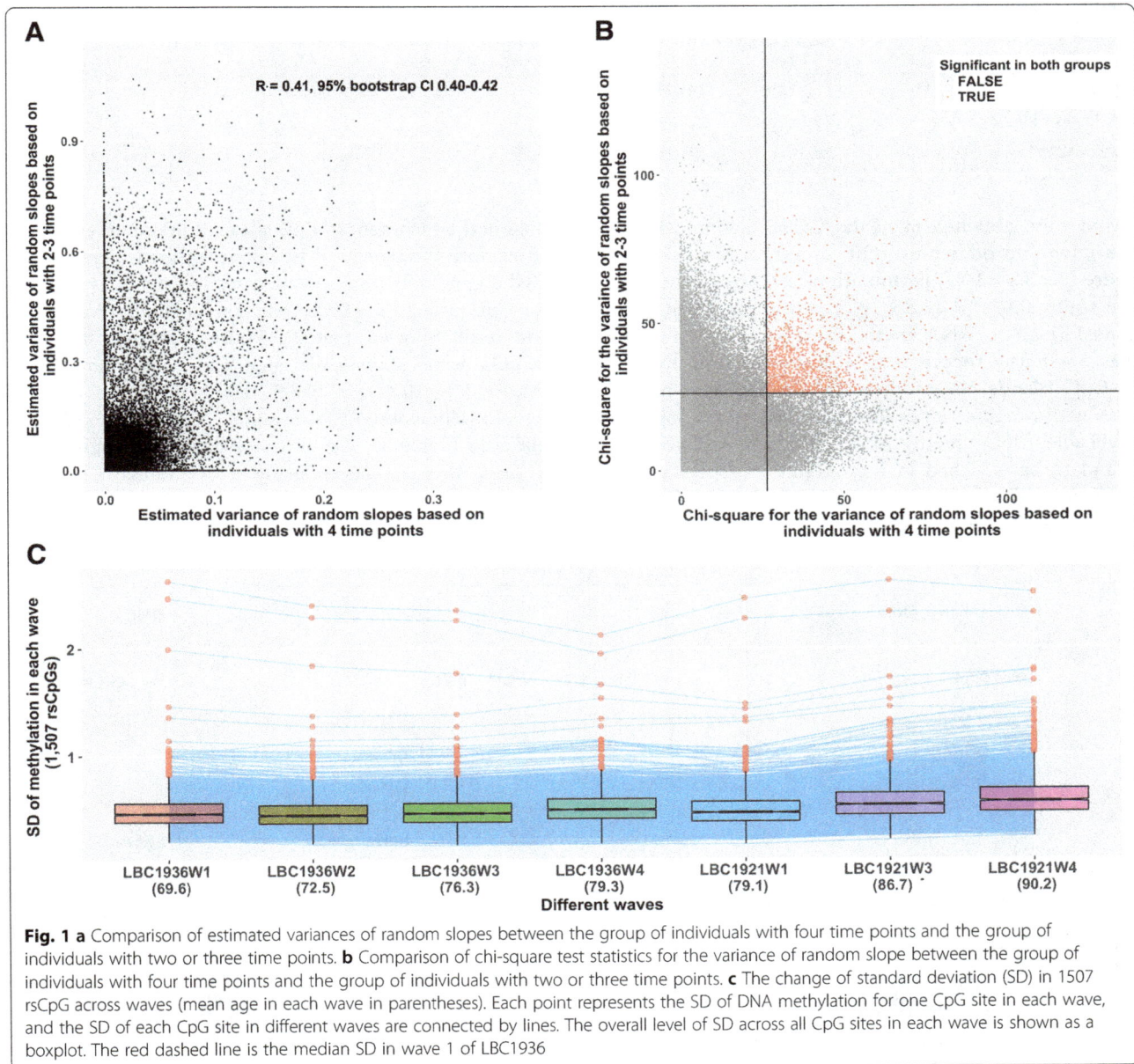

Fig. 1 a Comparison of estimated variances of random slopes between the group of individuals with four time points and the group of individuals with two or three time points. **b** Comparison of chi-square test statistics for the variance of random slope between the group of individuals with four time points and the group of individuals with two or three time points. **c** The change of standard deviation (SD) in 1507 rsCpG across waves (mean age in each wave in parentheses). Each point represents the SD of DNA methylation for one CpG site in each wave, and the SD of each CpG site in different waves are connected by lines. The overall level of SD across all CpG sites in each wave is shown as a boxplot. The red dashed line is the median SD in wave 1 of LBC1936

We observed a larger variation in DNA methylation of rsCpGs compared to randomly selected probes in each wave (Additional file 2: Figure S7). Moreover, an increase in the variability of DNA methylation with age can be identified in most of these rsCpGs (Fig. 1c). These rsCpGs overlapped with probes identified by Slieker and colleagues [14]. Based on a cross-sectional study, Slieker et al. identified 6366 positions that showed changes in variably of methylation with age using 3295 whole blood DNA methylation profiles. Among those positions, 540 probes overlap with the 1507 rsCpGs in our study. This highly significant overlap (odds ratio = 45.9, $P < 3.3 \times 10^{-5}$,

permutation test, 30,000 times) provides an independent confirmation of our results.

Genomic locations of CpG sites with random effects

The dynamicity of DNA methylation varies across the human genome [36, 37]. To investigate whether the rsCpGs locate in the more variable genomic regions, we mapped these CpG sites to the genome and applied an enrichment test on these probes ('Methods'). We observed an enrichment of rsCpGs in the Shore region of CpG islands (regions within 2 kb upstream or downstream of a CpG island are called north shore and south shore, respectively). Genomic positions of the CpG

Table 2 The summary of chi-square statistics for the variance of random slope in different groups of individuals

	$\lambda_{mean}/\lambda_{median}$	Number of probes with significant random slopes	Largest χ^2	Proportion of zero χ^2 ($\chi^2 < 10^{-5}$) (%)	$\lambda_{mean}/\lambda_{median}$ of non-zero χ^2
All individuals	11.0/13.9	42,253	206.2	21.3	14.0/22.1
Individuals with 2 or 3 time points	7.9/9.6	20,291	139.1	21.3	10.0/15.5
Individuals with 4 time points	3.8/1.9	6729	128.2	30.6	5.4/5.9

island were obtained from the UCSC Genome Browser [28]), with an odds ratio (OR) of 2.0 for both the north shore ($p < 3.3 \times 10^{-5}$, permutation test, 30,000 times) and the south shore ($P < 3.3 \times 10^{-5}$, permutation test, 30,000 times) (Fig. 2). DNA methylation in the shore region was previously reported to be more dynamic than that in CpG islands [36], and our results indicate that CpG sites with random slopes locate in the regions with more malleable DNA methylation. Similarly, rsCpGs were found to be enriched in reprogramming-specific differently methylated regions (RDMR, regions differentially methylated in the reprogramming process) [37].

Biological enrichment of CpG sites with random effects

To explore the biological function of the rsCpGs, we applied a gene over-representation test on the nearest genes of rsCpGs using PANTHER (version 13.1) [38] ('Methods'). The result showed that 1235 genes around the 1507 rsCpGs were statistically significantly (Fisher's exact test, $P = 3.7 \times 10^{-10}$, FDR = 3.9×10^{-8}) enriched in Homeodomain (Homeobox) transcription factor (PC00119) protein class (Table 3). We also investigated the significance of these protein classes using a permutation test and found they remained significant (100 repeats). Furthermore, we performed Gene Ontology (GO) analysis on

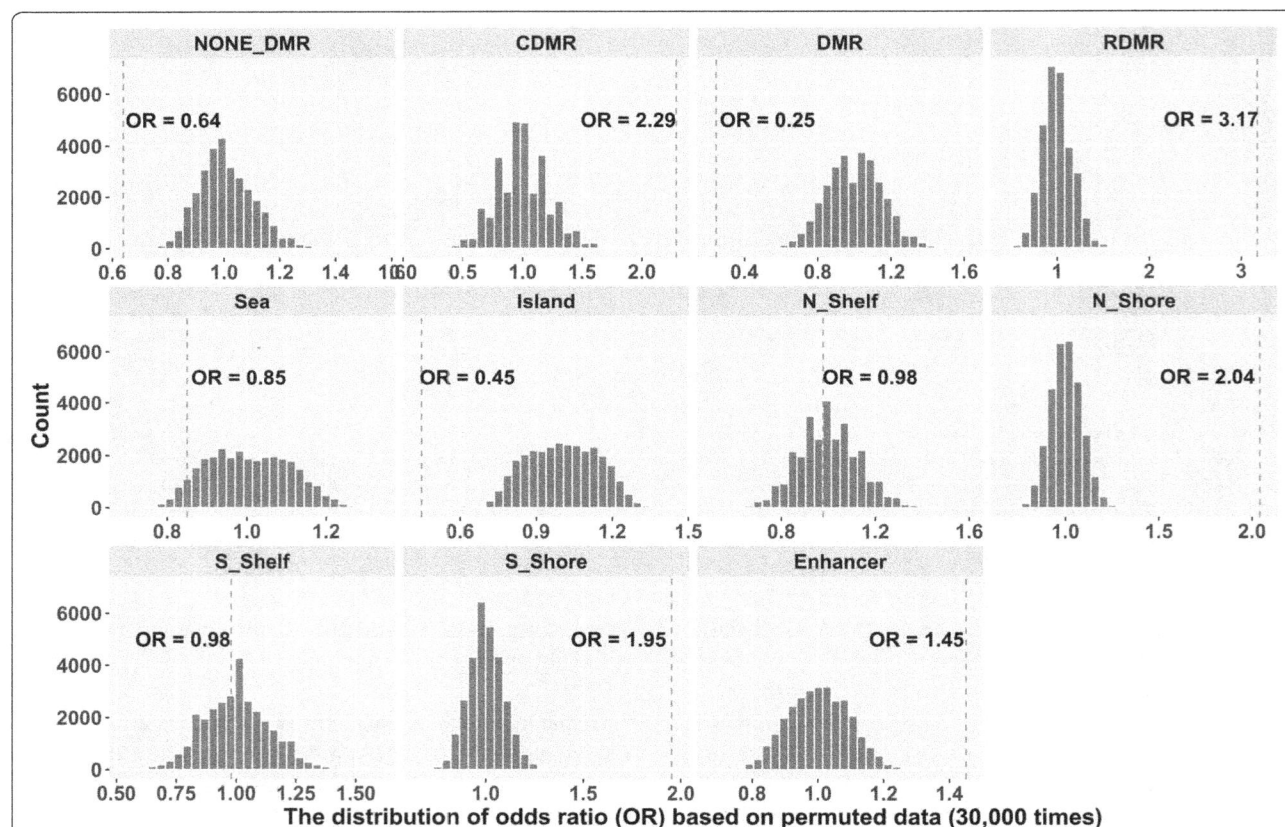

Fig. 2 Enrichment analysis of rsCpGs in different CpG regions based on the permutation test. For each CpG region, the distribution of odds ratio based on permuted data (30,000 times) and the odds ratio based on the original data (red dashed line) are presented. DMR: differentially methylated region; CDMR: cancer-specific DMR; RDMR: reprogramming-specific DMR; NONE_DMR other CpGs not in DMR. Island: CpG island provided by UCSC [28]; N_Shore: 0–2 Kb upstream of CpG island; S_Shore: 0–2 Kb downstream of CpG island; N_Shelf: 2–4 Kb upstream of CpG island; S_Shelf: 2–4 Kb downstream of CpG island; Sea: 4 Kb away from CpG island. Enhancer: Predicted enhancer elements determined by ENCODE Consortium [46]

Table 3 Gene enrichment test on the 1235 genes around the 1507 rsCpGs. Only protein classes with FDR smaller than 0.05 are listed

	Reference genes (18607)	Test genes	Expected genes	Over/ under	Fold enrichment	Raw P value	FDR
PANTHER protein class							
Homeodomain transcription factor (PC00119)	101	27	5.5	+	4.9	3.7×10^{-11}	3.9×10^{-8}
Basic helix-loop-helix transcription factor (PC00055)	76	13	4.2	+	3.1	6.7×10^{-4}	2.4×10^{-2}
Helix-turn-helix transcription factor (PC00116)	176	36	9.7	+	3.7	3.1×10^{-10}	6.6×10^{-8}
G-protein coupled receptor (PC00021)	250	31	13.7	+	2.3	1.0×10^{-4}	4.5×10^{-3}
Receptor (PC00197)	644	71	35.3	+	2.0	1.7×10^{-7}	1.2×10^{-5}
Transcription factor (PC00218)	1073	95	58.8	+	1.6	1.2×10^{-5}	6.6×10^{-4}
PANTHER pathway							
Cadherin signalling pathway (P00012)	157	27	8.6	+	3.1	1.0×10^{-6}	1.7×10^{-4}
Wnt signalling pathway (P00057)	307	39	16.8	+	2.3	6.3×10^{-6}	5.2×10^{-4}
Heterotrimeric G-protein signalling pathway-Gq alpha and Go alpha-mediated pathway (P00027)	123	18	6.7	+	2.7	3.8×10^{-4}	1.6×10^{-2}

these genes and found that ectoderm development (GO 0007398, $P = 5.9 \times 10^{-18}$, FDR $= 1.5 \times 10^{-15}$) and developmental process (GO 0032502, $P = 1.8 \times 10^{-17}$, FDR $= 2.2 \times 10^{-15}$) were the most significantly over-represented biological processes (Additional file 4: Table S3). Cadherin signalling pathway (P00012), Wnt signalling pathway (P00057) and Heterotrimeric G-protein signalling pathway-Gq alpha and Go alpha-mediated pathway (P00027) were found to be significantly enriched pathways for genes around rsCpGs in a PANTHER pathway analysis (Table 3). Since there are only 177 primarily signalling pathways in PANTHER database [38], we further performed the pathway analysis in an integrated pathway database ConsensusPathDB (version 33) [39]. This analysis on the same gene sets showed that the most significant pathway for rsCpGs was "Neuronal System" ($P = 1.4 \times 10^{-9}$). Full details of significant pathway results are given in the Additional file 5: Table S4.

Genetic effects on the random slope

rsCpGs were found to be enriched in the CpG sites with large heritability ($p < 3.3 \times 10^{-5}$, permutation test, 30,000 times, 'Methods', Fig. 3a), indicating a substantial genetic component to their variation. To examine the genetic contribution on the random effects of rsCpGs, we performed genome-wide association studies (GWASs) using PLINK2 [27], fitting the predicted random slope for each person (obtained from the mixed model analysis) as the dependent trait ('Methods'). Results showed that there were four significant SNP-probe pairs in total ($P < 5 \times 10^{-8}/1507$, after linkage disequilibrium (LD) clumping, 'Methods'), three of them are *cis* (in same chromosome) (Table 4, Fig. 3b). In addition, 343 rsCpGs were identified to have at least one genome-wide significant ($P < 5 \times 10^{-8}$, after LD clumping) SNP effect (436 SNP-probe pairs).

Ninety-five percent of the SNPs are on different chromosomes from their corresponding probes (Fig. 4, Additional file 6: Table S5). The SNP effect on the random slope can also be interpreted as the SNP by age effect on DNA methylation ('Methods', Additional file 2: Figure S8). Van Dongen et al. reported 71,894 CpG sites to have an interaction between genetic effects and age ($P < 0.05$) on DNA methylation [5], and the 343 rsCpGs with a significant SNP effect on the random slope from our analyses were enriched ($P < 3.3 \times 10^{-5}$, permutation test, 30,000 times) in these probes (Additional file 2: Figure S9). This provides an independent confirmation of our results.

Relationship between rate of DNA methylation change and covariates

To detect a possible contribution of the covariates in estimating the random slope of DNA methylation, we investigated two covariates that were previously identified to have a change of variation with ageing: body mass index (BMI) and walking speed (the time to walk 6 m) [20, 40]. We fitted each of the covariates in the full model and re-estimated the significance of the variance of random slope. No significant changes were observed (Additional file 2: Figure S10), implying no contribution of these two covariates to variation of the random slope.

Discussion

We estimated the variation in the rate of change of DNA methylation for each probe by implementing a mixed linear model in a longitudinal analysis. One thousand five hundred seven probes (rsCpGs) were found to have statistically significant variation in the rate of change between individuals. These rsCpGs were enriched in the shore region of CpG island, which is

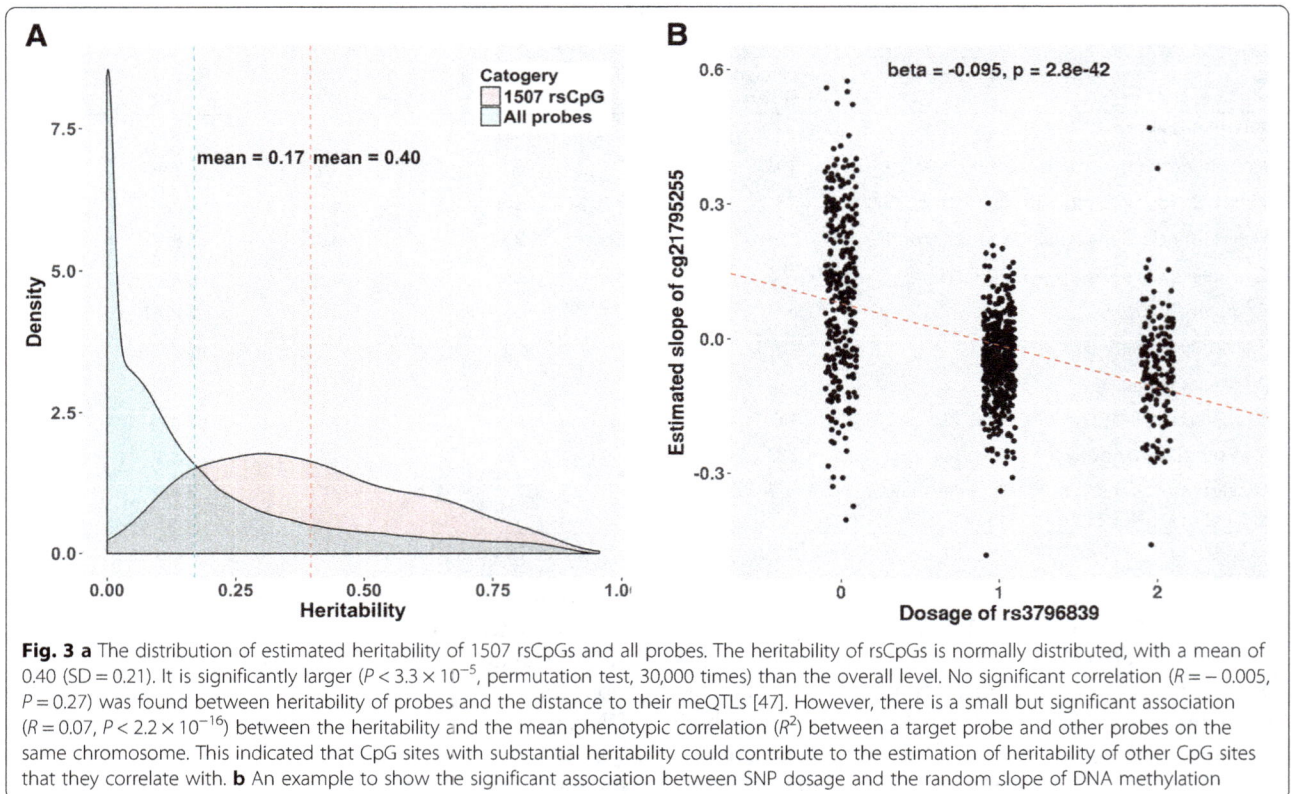

Fig. 3 a The distribution of estimated heritability of 1507 rsCpGs and all probes. The heritability of rsCpGs is normally distributed, with a mean of 0.40 (SD = 0.21). It is significantly larger ($P < 3.3 \times 10^{-5}$, permutation test, 30,000 times) than the overall level. No significant correlation ($R = -0.005$, $P = 0.27$) was found between heritability of probes and the distance to their meQTLs [47]. However, there is a small but significant association ($R = 0.07$, $P < 2.2 \times 10^{-16}$) between the heritability and the mean phenotypic correlation (R^2) between a target probe and other probes on the same chromosome. This indicated that CpG sites with substantial heritability could contribute to the estimation of heritability of other CpG sites that they correlate with. **b** An example to show the significant association between SNP dosage and the random slope of DNA methylation

consistent with more dynamicity of DNA methylation in CpG island shore region than the CpG island itself [37].

We found that the closest genes of rsCpGs were enriched in the Homeobox gene cluster, which was also reported in Slieker et al. to be associated with age-related variably methylated positions (aVMP) in *cis* [14]. The Homeobox gene cluster is involved in the process of cell development [41], and recent evidence showed that it is related to ageing [42, 43]. Pathway analysis on these genes in PANTHER database indicated they were enriched in Wnt signalling pathway (P00057), which was also reported to be related to the ageing process [44, 45]. One of the most significantly over-represented Gene Ontology (GO) category in these genes was the developmental process (GO 0032502), which was discovered to be significant for the probes that consistently drift among twins over time [16]. These results indicate the rsCpGs may be involved in the developmental process (such as ageing) by regulating their nearby genes.

There is a significant higher heritability of the 1507 rsCpGs compared to the overall level. GWAS results on the random slope identified 436 SNP-probe pairs (343 rsCpGs) with a genome-wide significant association ($P < 5 \times 10^{-8}$), suggesting a SNP by age effect on the CpG sites. Among them, 95% of the SNPs were on different chromosomes from their probes, which (in the absence of non-identified confounders) indicated a potential major *trans* SNP by age effect on DNA methylation of rsCpGs.

Our study has several limitations. Although the permutation test indicates our results will not be inflated by the violations of the assumptions of the distribution of the test statistic under the null hypothesis, our results could be inflated by unknown confounding factors. We adjusted for known possible confounders, including the chronological age at which the samples were taken, but cannot exclude the possibility of unknown confounders that have effects on the mean or variance of the measured DNA

Table 4 Four SNPs with significant ($P < 5 \times 10^{-8}/1507$) effects on the random slope

SNP ID	SNP CHR	SNP POS	Probe ID	Probe CHR	Probe POS	Beta	SE	P value
rs3796839	4	10009917	cg21795255	4	10009916	−0.095	0.0066	2.8×10^{-42}
rs10948674	6	51978145	cg26820259	6	51953096	0.081	0.0067	3.2×10^{-31}
rs190148485	20	4776083	cg24804768	12	754911	0.089	0.013	1.5×10^{-11}
rs8015861	14	22372304	cg12819537	14	22372304	0.046	0.0053	4.6×10^{-18}

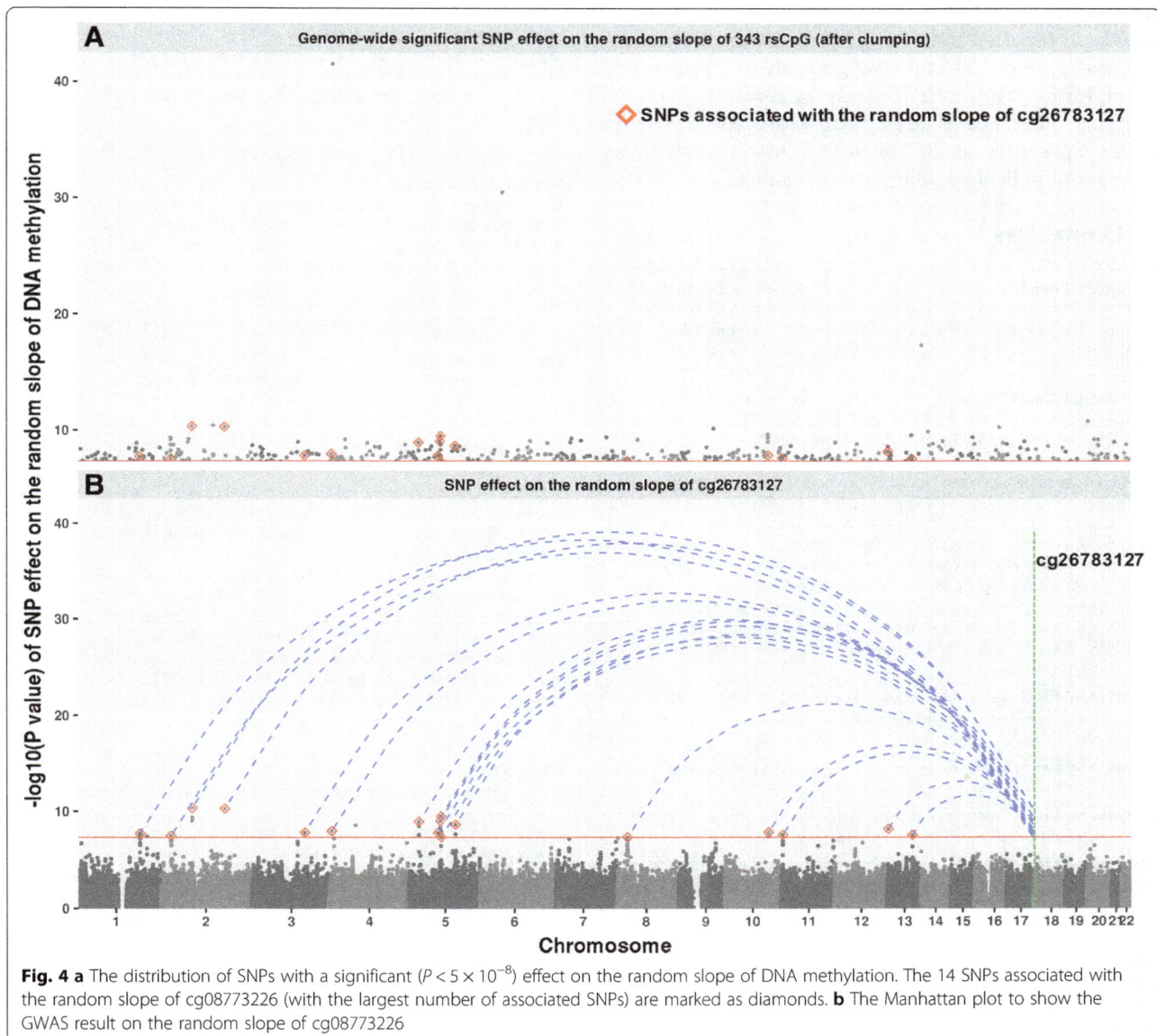

Fig. 4 a The distribution of SNPs with a significant ($P < 5 \times 10^{-8}$) effect on the random slope of DNA methylation. The 14 SNPs associated with the random slope of cg08773226 (with the largest number of associated SNPs) are marked as diamonds. **b** The Manhattan plot to show the GWAS result on the random slope of cg08773226

methylation. The effects of covariates including age, sex and cell counts were adjusted in our quality control steps, and we further confirmed that BMI and walking speed have no effects on the rate of change in DNA methylation. However, other exposures, like medication, smoking status and disease status may potentially contribute to this variation, which can influence the estimation of random effects. Nevertheless, the 1507 rsCpGs that have a statistically significant random slope in two separate groups of individuals indicate that these results should be robust. There was no gene expression data on the same individuals available, and we simply assume that the expression of a gene can be regulated by its closest

DNA methylation CpG site, which may not be true. Finally, our results are based on older individuals and may not apply to different age ranges.

Conclusions

Ageing is strongly correlated with changes in DNA methylation, and the rates of change over time at one CpG site can differ between individuals. We detected CpG sites with different changing rates (random slope) using a mixed linear model and found 1507 CpG sites that have a statistically significant rate of change in methylation between individuals, and that these different rates of change can be partially explained by genetic effect. Genes around rsCpGs were enriched in Homeobox gene clusters and Wnt signalling pathway, both of which have been reported to be involved in the ageing process. Our results imply that the changing rate of DNA methylation varies between individuals at several CpG sites, and this difference is associated with genetic factors. These CpG sites might be useful markers to better understand individual differences in ageing.

Additional files

Additional file 1: Quality control steps for DNA methylation. **Table S1.** Summary information for the age of all samples. **Figure S2.** Comparison of mean DNA methylation for duplicates between sets. **Figure S3.** Comparison of mean adjusted DNA methylation for duplicates between sets.

Additional file 2: Figure S1. The distribution of match rates of control probes between and within individuals. **Figure S4.** Q-Q plot for P values from the detection of the random slope. **Figure S5.** The distribution of λ_{mean} from 500 permutation tests. **Figure S6.** Quantifying the effect of t^2 and covariance between the random slope and random intercept on the estimation of random effects. **Figure S7.** The comparison of standard deviation (SD) of DNA methylation between 1507 rsCpGs and 1507 randomly selected CpG sites in each wave. **Figure S8.** Power comparison between two methods in detecting associations between SNP and DNA methylation change. **Figure S9.** The distribution of P value of the interaction effect between age and genetic effects from Van Dongen et al. [5] of two probe sets. **Figure S10.** The comparison of the significance of the variation of DNA methylation rate of change before and after fitting BMI and walking in the model.

Additional file 3: Table S2. Probes with a significant random slope in two groups of different individuals. Probe id, chi-square and P value were provided.

Additional file 4: Table S3. Gene Ontology analysis on the genes around the 1507 rsCpGs.

Additional file 5: Table S4. Pathway analysis on the genes around the 1507 rsCpGs in ConsensusPathDB database.

Additional file 6: Table S5. Four hundred thirty-six SNPs with genome-wide significant ($P < 5 \times 10^{-8}$) effects on the random slope of 343 rsCpGs.

Abbreviations

BMI: Body mass index; BSGS: Brisbane Systems Genetics Study; DMR: Differently methylated region; FDR: False discovery rate; GEO: Gene Expression Omnibus; GO: Gene Ontology; GWAS: Genome-wide association study; LBC: Lothian Birth Cohort; LD: Linkage disequilibrium; LRT: Likelihood ratio test; SNP: Single nucleotide polymorphism

Acknowledgements

Phenotype collection in the Lothian Birth Cohort 1921 was supported by the UK's Biotechnology and Biological Sciences Research Council (BBSRC), The Royal Society and The Chief Scientist Office of the Scottish Government. Phenotype collection in the Lothian Birth Cohort 1936 was supported by the Age UK (The Disconnected Mind project). Methylation typing was supported by the Centre for Cognitive Ageing and Cognitive Epidemiology (Pilot Fund award), Age UK, The Wellcome Trust Institutional Strategic Support Fund, the Gertrude Winifred Gear Fund, The University of Edinburgh and The University of Queensland.

Funding

This research was supported by the Australian National Health and Medical Research Council (grants 1010374, 1046880 and 1113400) and by the Australian Research Council (DP160102400). PMV, NRW and AFM are supported by the NHMRC Fellowship Scheme (1078037, 1078901 and 1083656). REM and IJD conducted the research in The University of Edinburgh Centre for Cognitive Ageing and Cognitive Epidemiology (CCACE), part of the cross-council Lifelong Health and Wellbeing

Initiative (MR/K026992/1); funding from the Biotechnology and Biological Sciences Research Council (BBSRC) and Medical Research Council (MRC) is gratefully acknowledged. D.S. is a Cancer Research UK Career Development Fellow (reference C47648/A20837), and the work in his laboratory is also supported by a Medical Research Council University grant to the MRC Human Genetics Unit.

Authors' contributions

AMcR, PMV and IJD conceived and designed the experiments. QZ performed all statistical analyses. QZ, AMcR and PMV wrote the paper. REM, MRR and NWR advised on statistical methodology, and JH and DS contributed to analyses and interpretation of results. All authors read and approved the final manuscript.

Competing interests

The authors declare that they have no competing interests.

Author details

^{1}Institute for Molecular Bioscience, The University of Queensland, Brisbane, QLD 4072, Australia. ^{2}Centre for Cognitive Ageing and Cognitive Epidemiology, University of Edinburgh, Edinburgh EH8 9JZ, UK. ^{3}Medical Genetics Section, Centre for Genomic and Experimental Medicine, Institute of Genetics & Molecular Medicine, University of Edinburgh, Edinburgh EH4 2XU, UK. ^{4}Medical Research Council Human Genetics Unit, Medical Research Council Institute of Genetics and Molecular Medicine, University of Edinburgh, Edinburgh EH4 2XU, UK. ^{5}Edinburgh Cancer Research Centre, Medical Research Council Institute of Genetics and Molecular Medicine, University of Edinburgh, Edinburgh EH4 2XU, UK. ^{6}The Queensland Brain Institute, The University of Queensland, St Lucia, QLD 4072, Australia. ^{7}Department of Psychology, University of Edinburgh, Edinburgh EH8 9JZ, UK.

References

1. Robertson KD. DNA methylation and human disease. Nat Rev Genet. 2005;6: 597–610.
2. Feinberg AP, Fallin MD. Epigenetics at the crossroads of genes and the environment. Jama. 2015;314:1129–30.
3. Feil R, Fraga MF. Epigenetics and the environment: emerging patterns and implications. Nat Rev Genet. 2012;13:97–109.
4. Jirtle RL, Skinner MK. Environmental epigenomics and disease susceptibility. Nat Rev Genet. 2007;8:253–62.
5. van Dongen J, Nivard MG, Willemsen G, Hottenga JJ, Helmer Q, Dolan CV, Ehli EA, Davies GE, van Iterson M, Breeze CE, et al. Genetic and environmental influences interact with age and sex in shaping the human methylome. Nat Commun. 2016;7:11115.
6. Richardson B. Impact of aging on DNA methylation. Ageing Res Rev. 2003;2:245–61.
7. Hernandez DG, Nalls MA, Gibbs JR, Arepalli S, van der Brug M, Chong S, Moore M, Longo DL, Cookson MR, Traynor BJ. Distinct DNA methylation changes highly correlated with chronological age in the human brain. Hum Mol Genet. 2011;20:1164–72.
8. Suzuki MM, Bird A. DNA methylation landscapes: provocative insights from epigenomics. Nat Rev Genet. 2008;9:465–76.
9. Bell JT, Tsai P-C, Yang T-P, Pidsley R, Nisbet J, Glass D, Mangino M, Zhai G, Zhang F, Valdes A. Epigenome-wide scans identify differentially methylated regions for age and age-related phenotypes in a healthy ageing population. PLoS Genet. 2012;8:e1002629.
10. Florath I, Butterbach K, Müller H, Bewerunge-Hudler M, Brenner H. Cross-sectional and longitudinal changes in DNA methylation with age: an epigenome-wide analysis revealing over 60 novel age-associated CpG sites. Hum Mol Genet. 2013;23:1186–201.
11. Shah S, McRae AF, Marioni RE, Harris SE, Gibson J, Henders AK, Redmond P, Cox SR, Pattie A, Corley J. Genetic and environmental exposures constrain epigenetic drift over the human life course. Genome Res. 2014;24:1725–33.
12. Wockner L, Noble E, Lawford B, Young RM, Morris C, Whitehall V, Voisey J. Genome-wide DNA methylation analysis of human brain tissue from schizophrenia patients. Transl Psychiatry. 2014;4:e339.

13. Dick KJ, Nelson CP, Tsaprouni L, Sandling JK, Aïssi D, Wahl S, Meduri E, Morange P-E, Gagnon F, Grallert H. DNA methylation and body-mass index: a genome-wide analysis. Lancet. 2014;383:1990–8.

14. Slieker RC, van Iterson M, Luijk R, Beekman M, Zhernakova DV, Moed MH, Mei H, Van Galen M, Deelen P, Bonder MJ. Age-related accrual of methylomic variability is linked to fundamental ageing mechanisms. Genome Biol. 2016;17:191.

15. Talens RP, Christensen K, Putter H, Willemsen G, Christiansen L, Kremer D, Suchiman HED, Slagboom PE, Boomsma DI, Heijmans BT. Epigenetic variation during the adult lifespan: cross-sectional and longitudinal data on monozygotic twin pairs. Aging Cell. 2012;11:694–703.

16. Martino D, Loke YJ, Gordon L, Ollikainen M, Cruickshank MN, Saffery R, Craig JM. Longitudinal, genome-scale analysis of DNA methylation in twins from birth to 18 months of age reveals rapid epigenetic change in early life and pair-specific effects of discordance. Genome Biol. 2013;14:R42.

17. Gaunt TR, Shihab HA, Hemani G, Min JL, Woodward G, Lyttleton O, Zheng J, Duggirala A, McArdle WL, Ho K. Systematic identification of genetic influences on methylation across the human life course. Genome Biol. 2016;17:61.

18. Simpkin AJ, Suderman M, Gaunt TR, Lyttleton O, McArdle WL, Ring SM, Tilling K, Smith GD, Relton CL. Longitudinal analysis of DNA methylation associated with birth weight and gestational age. Hum Mol Genet. 2015;24:3752–63.

19. Christiansen L, Lenart A, Tan Q, Vaupel JW, Aviv A, McGue M, Christensen K. DNA methylation age is associated with mortality in a longitudinal Danish twin study. Aging Cell. 2016;15:149–54.

20. Marioni RE, Shah S, McRae AF, Ritchie SJ, Muniz-Terrera G, Harris SE, Gibson J, Redmond P, Cox SR, Pattie A. The epigenetic clock is correlated with physical and cognitive fitness in the Lothian Birth Cohort 1936. Int J Epidemiol. 2015;44:1388–96.

21. Aryee MJ, Jaffe AE, Corrada-Bravo H, Ladd-Acosta C, Feinberg AP, Hansen KD, Irizarry RA. Minfi: a flexible and comprehensive Bioconductor package for the analysis of Infinium DNA methylation microarrays. Bioinformatics. 2014;30:1363–9.

22. Medland SE, Nyholt DR, Painter JN, McEvoy BP, McRae AF, Zhu G, Gordon SD, Ferreira MA, Wright MJ, Henders AK. Common variants in the trichohyalin gene are associated with straight hair in Europeans. Am J Hum Genet. 2009;85:750–5.

23. Williams AL, Patterson N, Glessner J, Hakonarson H, Reich D. Phasing of many thousands of genotyped samples. Am J Hum Genet. 2012;91:238–51.

24. Consortium GP. An integrated map of genetic variation from 1,092 human genomes. Nature. 2012;491:56.

25. Howie B, Fuchsberger C, Stephens M, Marchini J, Abecasis GR. Fast and accurate genotype imputation in genome-wide association studies through pre-phasing. Nat Genet. 2012;44:955.

26. Visscher PM. A note on the asymptotic distribution of likelihood ratio tests to test variance components. Twin Res Hum Genet. 2006;9:490–5.

27. Chang CC, Chow CC, Tellier LC, Vattikuti S, Purcell SM, Lee JJ. Second-generation PLINK: rising to the challenge of larger and richer datasets. Gigascience. 2015;4:7.

28. Casper J, Zweig AS, Villarreal C, Tyner C, Speir ML, Rosenbloom KR, Raney BJ, Lee CM, Lee BT, Karolchik D, et al. The UCSC genome browser database: 2018 update. Nucleic Acids Res. 2018;46:D762–9.

29. McRae AF, Powell JE, Henders AK, Bowdler L, Hemani G, Shah S, Painter JN, Martin NG, Visscher PM, Montgomery GW. Contribution of genetic variation to transgenerational inheritance of DNA methylation. Genome Biol. 2014;15:R73.

30. Powell JE, Henders AK, McRae AF, Caracella A, Smith S, Wright MJ, Whitfield JB, Dermitzakis ET, Martin NG, Visscher PM. The Brisbane Systems Genetics Study: genetical genomics meets complex trait genetics. PLoS One. 2012;7:e35430.

31. Team RC. R: a language and environment for statistical computing. 2013.

32. Wickham H. ggplot2: Elegant Graphics for Data Analysis. New York: Springer-Verlag; 2016. https://cran.r-project.org/web/packages/ggplot2/citation.html.

33. Deary IJ, Gow AJ, Pattie A, Starr JM. Cohort profile: the Lothian Birth Cohorts of 1921 and 1936. Int J Epidemiol. 2011;41:1576–84.

34. Deary IJ, Gow AJ, Taylor MD, Corley J, Brett C, Wilson V, Campbell H, Whalley LJ, Visscher PM, Porteous DJ. The Lothian Birth Cohort 1936: a study to examine influences on cognitive ageing from age 11 to age 70 and beyond. BMC Geriatr. 2007;7:28.

35. Price EM, Cotton AM, Lam LL, Farré P, Emberly E, Brown CJ, Robinson WP, Kobor MS. Additional annotation enhances potential for biologically-relevant analysis of the Illumina Infinium HumanMethylation450 BeadChip array. Epigenetics Chromatin. 2013;6(1):1756–8935.

36. Ziller MJ, Gu H, Muller F, Donaghey J, Tsai LT, Kohlbacher O, De Jager PL, Rosen ED, Bennett DA, Bernstein BE, et al. Charting a dynamic DNA methylation landscape of the human genome. Nature. 2013;500:477–81.

37. Doi A, Park I-H, Wen B, Murakami P, Aryee MJ, Irizarry R, Herb B, Ladd-Acosta C, Rho J, Loewer S. Differential methylation of tissue-and cancer-specific CpG island shores distinguishes human induced pluripotent stem cells, embryonic stem cells and fibroblasts. Nat Genet. 2009;41:1350–3.

38. Mi H, Huang X, Muruganujan A, Tang H, Mills C, Kang D, Thomas PD. PANTHER version 11: expanded annotation data from Gene Ontology and Reactome pathways, and data analysis tool enhancements. Nucleic Acids Res. 2016;45:D183–9.

39. Kamburov A, Stelzl U, Lehrach H, Herwig R. The ConsensusPathDB interaction database: 2013 update. Nucleic Acids Res. 2012;41:D793–800.

40. Block JP, Subramanian SV, Christakis NA, O'Malley AJ. Population trends and variation in body mass index from 1971 to 2008 in the Framingham Heart Study Offspring Cohort. PLoS One. 2013;8:e63217.

41. Pearson JC, Lemons D, McGinnis W. Modulating Hox gene functions during animal body patterning. Nat Rev Genet. 2005;6:893–904.

42. McClay JL, Aberg KA, Clark SL, Nerella S, Kumar G, Xie LY, Hudson AD, Harada A, Hultman CM, Magnusson PKE. A methylome-wide study of aging using massively parallel sequencing of the methyl-CpG-enriched genomic fraction from blood in over 700 subjects. Hum Mol Genet. 2014;23:1175–85.

43. Bork S, Pfister S, Witt H, Horn P, Korn B, Ho AD, Wagner W. DNA methylation pattern changes upon long-term culture and aging of human mesenchymal stromal cells. Aging Cell. 2010;9:54–63.

44. Lezzerini M, Budovskaya Y. A dual role of the Wnt signaling pathway during aging in Caenorhabditis elegans. Aging Cell. 2014;13:8–18.

45. White BD, Nguyen NK, Moon RT. Wnt signaling: it gets more humorous with age. Curr Biol. 2007;17:R923–5.

46. Siggens L, Ekwall K. Epigenetics, chromatin and genome organization: recent advances from the ENCODE project. J Intern Med. 2014;276:201–14.

47. McRae A, Marioni RE, Shah S, Yang J, Powell JE, Harris SE, Gibson J, Henders AK, Bowdler L, Painter JN, et al. Identification of 55,000 replicated DNA methylation QTL. bioRxiv. 2017.

10

Integrative omics analyses broaden treatment targets in human cancer

Sohini Sengupta[1,2†], Sam Q. Sun[1,2†], Kuan-lin Huang[1,2], Clara Oh[1,2], Matthew H. Bailey[1,2], Rajees Varghese[3], Matthew A. Wyczalkowski[1,2], Jie Ning[3], Piyush Tripathi[3], Joshua F. McMichael[2], Kimberly J. Johnson[4], Cyriac Kandoth[5], John Welch[1], Cynthia Ma[1,7], Michael C. Wendl[1,2,6,7], Samuel H. Payne[8], David Fenyö[9,10], Reid R. Townsend[1,11], John F. Dipersio[1,11], Feng Chen[3,7*] and Li Ding[1,2,7,11*] [ID]

Abstract

Background: Although large-scale, next-generation sequencing (NGS) studies of cancers hold promise for enabling precision oncology, challenges remain in integrating NGS with clinically validated biomarkers.

Methods: To overcome such challenges, we utilized the Database of Evidence for Precision Oncology (DEPO) to link druggability to genomic, transcriptomic, and proteomic biomarkers. Using a pan-cancer cohort of 6570 tumors, we identified tumors with potentially druggable biomarkers consisting of drug-associated mutations, mRNA expression outliers, and protein/phosphoprotein expression outliers identified by DEPO.

Results: Within the pan-cancer cohort of 6570 tumors, we found that 3% are druggable based on FDA-approved drug-mutation interactions in specific cancer types. However, mRNA/phosphoprotein/protein expression outliers and drug repurposing across cancer types suggest potential druggability in up to 16% of tumors. The percentage of potential drug-associated tumors can increase to 48% if we consider preclinical evidence. Further, our analyses showed co-occurring potentially druggable multi-omics alterations in 32% of tumors, indicating a role for individualized combinational therapy, with evidence supporting mTOR/PI3K/ESR1 co-inhibition and BRAF/AKT co-inhibition in 1.6 and 0.8% of tumors, respectively. We experimentally validated a subset of putative druggable mutations in BRAF identified by a protein structure-based computational tool. Finally, analysis of a large-scale drug screening dataset lent further evidence supporting repurposing of drugs across cancer types and the use of expression outliers for inferring druggability.

Conclusions: Our results suggest that an integrated analysis platform can nominate multi-omics alterations as biomarkers of druggability and aid ongoing efforts to bring precision oncology to patients.

Keywords: Cancer genomics, Multi-omics, Proteogenomics, Precision medicine, Cancer and druggability

Background

With the development of novel therapeutics and next-generation sequencing (NGS), medicine is entering an era in which cancer treatment can be tailored to the tumor molecular profile of the individual patient. While an increasing number of FDA-approved cancer drugs are paired with a companion diagnostic for mutational

[1–3] or protein expression abnormalities [4], a given drug is often only considered for the cancer type (breast carcinoma, etc.) for which it was approved. Pan-cancer analyses have identified significantly mutated genes shared across cancer type subsets [5–7], suggesting the potential for treating patients based on the genetic profile of their tumor, regardless of cancer type. Efforts are underway to implement NGS in the clinical setting [8–11], and several studies have examined practical aspects of NGS implementation, such as use of FFPE tumor samples [12–14], concordance between NGS and other diagnostic platforms [15, 16], and quality assurance of variant calls [12–16] (Additional file 1). However, using tumor molecular

---

* Correspondence: fchen@wustl.edu; lding@wustl.edu
†Sohini Sengupta and Sam Q. Sun contributed equally to this work.
3Division of Nephrology, Department of Medicine, Washington University, St. Louis, MO 63108, USA
1Division of Oncology, Department of Medicine, Washington University, St. Louis, MO 63108, USA
Full list of author information is available at the end of the article

profiles from NGS and other platforms to infer druggability is an ongoing challenge [12, 17, 18]. In particular, no systematic pan-cancer analysis has yet been conducted to explore the potential impact of comprehensive multi-omics for informing cancer therapy.

The Cancer Genome Atlas (TCGA), the Clinical Proteomic Tumor Analysis Consortium (CPTAC) [19], and other large-scale sequencing data sets represent an opportunity to identify "druggable" variants, i.e., variants that render a cancer type susceptible to a drug. A recent study quantified the percentages and types of cancers that may benefit from therapies traditionally used for other indications [17]. Although the general approach is promising and has important implications for clinical practice [20, 21], these efforts primarily use gene/drug interactions rather than mutation/drug interactions to infer druggability [12, 15, 17, 22]. None leverage transcriptomic and proteomic data in tandem with genomic profiles generated through TCGA. Moreover, none leverage the compendium of known mutation/drug interactions to either discover or validate putative mutation/drug interactions.

Here, we present an analysis of the full spectrum of putatively druggable alterations in 6570 TCGA tumors based on integrative omics approaches. We utilized known variant/drug interactions from several data sources with each variant associated with sensitivity or resistance to a drug in preclinical or clinical studies [20, 23–25] (Sun et al. [26], in revision, http://dinglab.wustl.edu/depo). We identified tumors with drug-associated mutations and found considerable opportunity for repurposing of drugs across cancer types. We used a structure-based computational tool [27–29] to identify putative druggable mutations based on proximity to known druggable mutations and experimentally validated a subset of putative druggable mutations in BRAF. We then analyzed druggability based on mRNA, protein, and phosphosite expression levels. To identify opportunities for combinational therapy, we examined co-occurring potentially druggable alterations across multiple data types in tumors. Finally, we used a large-scale drug screen to validate our approach for inferring druggability across human cancers. By applying and validating novel approaches for inferring druggability, this report shows that more tumors than previously thought may be susceptible to targeted therapy and provides a concrete path for using integrative omics analyses to guide precision cancer therapy.

Methods
Construction of Database of Evidence for Precision Oncology (DEPO)
DEPO (Sun et al. [26], in revision, http://dinglab.wustl.edu/depo) was created as an information knowledgebase to facilitate downstream analyses in our study. Druggable variants in DEPO were filtered such that each

variant corresponded to one of several categories: single nucleotide polymorphisms or SNPs (missense, frameshift, and nonsense mutations), in-frame insertions and deletions (indels), copy number variations (CNVs), or expression changes. The vast majority of SNPs and in-frame indels in DEPO are unambiguous, e.g., BRAF V600E. To accommodate looser categories of genomic events, DEPO allows missense mutations for which the substituted base is not specified (e.g., BRAF V600). Similarly, for SNPs and in-frame indels in a given exon (e.g., EGFR exon 19 in-frame deletion), we used Ensembl to convert to a codon-mapped nomenclature (e.g., EGFR p.729-761 in-frame deletion) [30].

Each variant/drug entry in DEPO was paired with several annotations of potential interest to oncologists. These annotations were generally derived from DEPO's source databases, then standardized to the nomenclature discussed here. *Tumor type* is included for each variant/drug entry because, with infrequent exception, a variant's effect on a tumor's response to a given drug has only been rigorously studied in one or only a few cancer type(s). For a variant/drug entry based on preclinical data, tumor type was either inferred from the xenograft or cell line, or left unspecified. As indicated previously, *variant* can be annotated in several ways for SNPs and indels. It could be either a specific mutation, a specific amino acid position with no specified amino acid change, or a range of amino acid/genomic positions. Copy number amplifications (CNA) and losses (CNL), high expression outliers in oncogenes, low expression outliers in tumor suppressors, and fusions that may lead to druggability are also included. *Effect* describes whether a variant correlates with increased sensitivity of a tumor to a drug or increased resistance of a tumor to a drug. *Level of evidence* describes the quality of data supporting a given variant/drug entry: preclinical, case reports, clinical trials, and FDA approved. Some of this information was mined from clinicaltrials.gov. *Drug class* was determined using a look-up table that was generated manually from DrugBank/NIHClasses (Additional file 2: Table S1). A given drug entry in DEPO could be associated with multiple drug families to allow for the possibility of combining therapies (e.g., dabrafenib [B-Raf inhibitor] and trametinib [MEK inhibitor] for BRAF V600E/K-mutant melanoma) and multi-targeted tyrosine kinase inhibitors (e.g., afatinib as a dual HER2 and EGFR inhibitor). Finally, each entry in DEPO is linked to a *PubMed ID*, which was used to manually curate any missing annotations.

If two variant/drug entries had identical annotations for tumor type and effect, the entry with the highest level of evidence was used in DEPO. Otherwise, if two variant/drug entries had non-identical annotations, both were included. DEPO is available as a web portal (http://

dinglab.wustl.edu/depo), through which users can search for variant entries to obtain therapeutic information. The version used for this analysis was from February 2017.

Pan-cancer cohort and cancer types

We conducted analyses of druggability across a pan-cancer cohort of 6570 TCGA tumor samples from 22 cancer types [31]. These cancer types consisted of adrenocortical carcinoma (ACC), bladder urothelial carcinoma (BLCA), breast adenocarcinoma (BRCA), cervical squamous cell carcinoma and endocervical adenocarcinoma (CESC), colon and rectal carcinoma (COADREAD), glioblastoma multiforme (GBM), head and neck squamous cell carcinoma (HNSC), kidney chromophobe (KICH), kidney renal clear cell carcinoma (KIRC), kidney renal papillary cell carcinoma (KIRP), acute myeloid leukemia (AML/LAML), low-grade glioma (LGG), liver hepatocellular carcinoma (LIHC), lung adenocarcinoma (LUAD), lung squamous cell carcinoma (LUSC), ovarian serous carcinoma (OV), prostate adenocarcinoma (PRAD), skin cutaneous melanoma (SKCM), stomach adenocarcinoma (STAD), thyroid carcinoma (THCA), uterine corpus endometrial carcinoma (UCEC), and uterine carcinosarcoma (UCS).

Collection of mutations in pan-cancer cohort

Variant calls were obtained from the TCGA Genome Data Analysis Centers (GDAC), Data Coordinating Center (DCC), and previously published TCGA marker papers until the end of 2014 (https://cancergenome.nih.gov/publications). Variant calls were excluded if metastases or recurrent samples were present for samples that already had a primary tumor in the mutation annotation file (MAF). When necessary, we used UCSC's liftOver with an Ensemble chain file to convert variants from NCBI36 to GRCh37. Annotation was done by VEP v77 on Gencode Basic v19 transcripts, using vcf2maf (https://github.com/mskcc/vcf2maf) to a single canonical isoform per gene. We followed strict quality control processes and excluded variants without both nucleotide changes and genomic positions and variants whose MAF genotypes did not match VCF genotypes after accounting for matched strand. We filtered large indels (> 100 bp) and complex indels, which are not supported by the MAF specification. To remove duplicate samples, we excluded samples with > 60% variant concordance with another sample, unless both samples had five or fewer total variants. Furthermore, we filtered common variants, defined as minor allele frequency > 0.05% in the Exome Variant Server or 1000G [32, 33] cohort that were not pathogenic or deleterious/damaging according to Clinvar [34] and SIFT/Polyphen [35, 36].

Drug-associated mutations in pan-cancer cohort

We identified tumors in our pan-cancer cohort that harbored one or more drug-associated SNP or indel.

Iterating through a mutation annotation format (MAF) file containing all variants in our pan-cancer cohort, we performed two actions for each entry in the MAF. First, we queried a hash table containing all druggable, unambiguous mutations in DEPO (e.g., BRAF V600E) and a separate hash table containing all druggable, ambiguous, single-residue mutations in DEPO (e.g., BRAF V600). Second, we queried several classes of mutations that occur in a specific exon or segment of a gene (EGFR exon 19 in-frame deletion). All mutation entries in the MAF (Synapse ID, syn12618789) that map onto an entry in DEPO are stored, along with the corresponding TCGA tumor ID and tumor type (Additional file 2: Table S2).

In some cases, DEPO contains multiple entries per gene/mutation pair to reflect possible druggability of a gene/mutation pair in more than one tumor type, or that it may confer an effect (e.g., sensitivity or resistance) that depends on tumor type or other therapeutic context. Multiple DEPO entries per variant were used to generate visualizations of druggability. For example, when visualizing "drug repurposing" across tumor types, a given mutation could be associated with > 1 "cancer-type-specific" tumor type, if a given gene/mutation pair had druggability information in DEPO in multiple tumor types at the same level of evidence. For each unique gene/mutation pair, the cancer types that had the highest levels of evidence for a drug were considered cancer type specific. All other cancer types are considered non-specific for a gene/mutation pair. For example, DEPO indicates that BRAF V600E-mutated THCA is sensitive to BRAF inhibitor; however, because a higher level of evidence exists for BRAF V600E druggability in SKCM, THCA is "off-label" or "cancer type non-specific." When considering potential druggable events in the cancer-type-non-specific setting, the drug with the highest level of evidence found across all tumor types was used for a specific variant (Additional file 2: Table S3). For downstream analyses (i.e., protein structure-based clustering, co-occurring mutation analysis, and integration analysis), variant/drug interactions were considered in this cancer-type-non-specific setting. If any sensitive interaction for a variant was found regardless of the tumor type and level, it was considered a "druggable" event for these analyses. Additionally, if there was evidence for both resistant and sensitive drug interactions for a specific variant, the sensitive interaction was utilized.

Proximity-based clustering of drug-associated mutations with pan-cancer cohort

HotSpot3D [27] was used to spatially cluster "known" drug-associated mutations in DEPO with putative druggable mutations in our pan-cancer cohort. In brief, pairwise distances between all amino acids are calculated to give a background distribution. We assigned a P value to the pairwise distance and defined it as the proportion of all pairwise amino acid 3D distances that are less than or equal to the distance between the pair of amino acids in question. After this, we only performed clustering on significant pairs having $p < 0.05$ and distance less than 5 Å.

Single-link agglomerative clustering forms initial clusters from the significant proximal pairs by iteratively adding new mutations to a cluster if they are significantly paired with a mutation already in the cluster. To prevent a cluster with unbounded size, we applied a limit to the physical extent of the clusters. If the initial cluster is modeled as an undirected graph $G = (V, E)$, where V is the set of all mutations in the initial cluster and E is the set of 3D distances of all proximal pairs in V, we can calculate the shortest path from each vertex to all other vertices. We identify a centroid of the cluster to be the mutation that is found more frequently in patient samples as well as the one found in close proximity to highly recurrent mutations. The clusters are then focused according to a specified graph radius limit from the centroid.

The original clustering approach for HotSpot3D was improved upon in this analysis by using recursive clustering. Briefly, setting a maximum radius limit could lead to potentially functional regions being ignored. To bypass this problem, instead of discarding mutations outside of the radius limit, we performed clustering on the remaining mutations in the initial cluster. We continued to do this until no more clusters could be found. For this analysis, a radius limit of 5 Å was used in order to limit clusters to a relatively conservative size. We did not use a linear distance limit in order to detect all mutations that cluster closely to drug-associated mutations, regardless of position on amino acid sequence.

Druggable expression outliers in pan-cancer cohort

RNA expression data (TCGA level 3, normalized) were downloaded from firehose (October 17, 2014). We log$_2$--transformed the RNA-seq by expectation-maximization (RSEM) values of RNA expression data for outlier analysis. RPPA data (level 4, normalized) were downloaded from The Cancer Protein Atlas (TCPA) and were normalized across batches using replicates-based normalization (RBN) as previously described [37].

To discover expression outliers, we utilized a strategy incorporating multiple steps. First, we limited our search to genes in DEPO whose overexpression or copy number amplification is associated with drug sensitivity; these tended to be proto-oncogenes. We then narrowed down the list to genes that are observed in at least 10 tumor samples in the dataset under investigation. Additionally, we did not include AML in our expression analysis. Outlier expressions were defined as values that are

greater than 1.5 interquartile ranges (IQRs) above the third quartile (Q3), or below the first quartile (Q1) across the pan-cancer cohort. To rank order outlier expression for each gene, we calculated an outlier score defined as:

$$\text{Outlier score} = (x - Q3)/IQR$$
$$\text{or}$$
$$\text{Outlier score} = (Q1 - x)/IQR$$

By definition, genes with outlier score greater than 1.5 are considered as expression outliers. Outlier score for each gene were ranked within each tumor sample to select the most promising "druggable" targets.

Only RNA-seq and RPPA data was utilized for all subsequent analysis and calculating potential druggable targets for transcriptomic and proteomic expression outliers.

Fusion analysis

Fusions were obtained from a prior publication [31] that identified fusion transcripts in 4366 tumors. We restricted our analysis to the intersection between the 4366 tumors in Yoshihara et al. and the 6570 tumors assessed in the present study. Only fusion transcripts corresponding to a druggable fusion gene in DEPO were considered in constructing Additional file 3: Figure S1. To correlate fusion transcripts and expression, we identified RNA and phosphoprotein expression levels (outlier scores) for druggable fusion genes (Additional file 3: Figure S1).

Proteomic analysis with CPTAC mass spectrometry data

The 251 Clinical Proteome Tumor Analysis Consortium (CPTAC) tumors used in our analysis included 77 breast cancer tumors [38], 90 colorectal cancer tumors [39], and 84 ovarian cancer tumors (from PNNL only) [40]. Proteomic data were processed using the Common Data Analysis Pipeline [41]. Analysis was conducted with this data to reveal potential druggable proteomic outliers in the three cancer types (Additional file 1, Additional file 3: Figure S2); however, these numbers were not included in our subsequent analyses or our summative assessment of pan-cancer druggability.

Cell line-based validation

Cell line data was downloaded from the Genomics of Drug Sensitivity in Cancer (GDSC) database (http://www.cancerrxgene.org/downloads). Specifically, the data of interest were the screened compounds (Additional file 2: Table S4), log(IC50) and AUC values, the expression array data for cell lines, and the WES data for cell lines. The first step was to convert DEPO drug names into the drug IDs provided in the screened compounds. We were inclusive in terms of matching drugs from the cell line data to

DEPO, so that we would have enough statistical power and data points to study trends. The drug ID for the screened compound was included for a DEPO drug if one of the following were satisfied: (1) drug name in DEPO matched exactly the drug name or synonym in screened compounds from the cell line data and (2) the gene target of the drug class/drug in DEPO matches the gene target of the drug in screened compounds. Additionally, the list was refined through manual manipulation.

For mutation analysis, cell lines that contained mutations in DEPO were analyzed for their LN(IC50) values. These mutations were separated into cancer-type-specific and non-specific if the cancer type of the cell line did not have the highest level of evidence in DEPO for a specific mutation (Additional file 2: Table S5). Similar to our mutation analysis of TCGA data, the drug with the highest level of evidence for a particular mutation was used (Additional file 2: Table S3). The distribution of LN(IC50) values of cell lines with DEPO mutations (both sensitive and resistant) for both the cancer-type-specific and non-specific settings were compared to a background distribution using the Mann-Whitney U test. The background distribution consists of all LN(IC50) values from every drug-cell line combination whether they have a DEPO mutation or not. In addition to comparing overall distributions, we also compared distributions of LN(IC50) for cell lines with a specific sensitive mutation to the distribution of LN(IC50) values across all cell lines for the particular drug in question (Additional file 2: Table S6). This was done in both the cancer-type-specific and non-specific settings. We required that there be at least five cell lines that contain the specific sensitive mutation A tested against drug B in order to deem significance of the drug-mutation combination.

For expression analysis, Affymetrix Human Genome U219 array data from ArrayExpress (E-MTAB-3610) were used. The expression data were in the form of an Affymetrix *CEL* Data File, which required conversion to a gene expression matrix in order to run through the expression outlier analysis pipeline. This was done using Bioconductor in R and the "affy" Library. The file was then annotated with genes using an annotation package (hgu219.db) through Bioconductor. The resulting matrix was run through the outlier expression pipeline detailed above. Genes that were known to confer drug sensitivity through expression based on DEPO were analyzed. Each gene could have multiple probes, and all probes were included in downstream analysis. To test whether gene expression is correlated with drug sensitivity, we conducted linear regressions on all probe-drug combinations in the form of $y_i = Bx_i + a$, where x_i is the gene expression outlier score for a specific gene probe in cell line i and y_i is the LN(IC50) value for a drug associated with the gene in cell line i. There were 496

probe-drug combinations with sufficient sample size, at least five samples, to conduct regression analysis (Additional file 2: Table S7). Probe-drug combinations that had $P < 0.05$ and $B < 0$ were considered to have a significant correlation between gene expression and drug sensitivity.

In reporting potential druggability across the TCGA cohort, we considered all tumors with mutational evidence; however, we only considered tumors with mRNA and protein/phosphoprotein outliers for genes that could be validated against GDSC data regardless of level of approval. A gene was considered to be "validated" if at least one of its probes had a significant P value for the regression between gene outlier score and LN(IC50) and these two variables were negatively correlated.

Experimental validation

HEK293T cells were authenticated by DNA finger printing targeting short tandem repeat (STR) profiles through Genetica Cell Line Testing. They are negative for mycoplasma as determined by the absence of extranuclear signals in DAPI staining. Cells were cultured in DMEM (Corning) supplemented with 5% fetal bovine serum (FBS) (Thermo Fisher). Constructions expressing BRAF variants were generated from a plasmid expressing a wild-type BRAF (Addgene, #40775) with an N-terminal Flag tag using Q5 site-directed mutagenesis (New England BioLabs). All constructs were confirmed by sequencing. Cells were transiently transfected with wild-type or mutant BRAF constructs using Lipofectamine 2000 reagent (Life Technologies) in six-well plates. Twenty-four hours after transfection, cells were switched to medium containing 0.5% FBS for 24 h before the initiation of 6 h of treatment with Dabrafenib (0–1 uM). Cells were lysed in buffer containing 20 mM Tris-HCl (pH 7.5), 150 mM NaCl, 1 mM Na2EDTA, 1 mM EGTA, 1% NP-40, 1% sodium deoxycholate, 2.5 mM sodium pyrophosphate, 1 mM β-glycerophosphate, 1 mM sodium orthovanadate, and 1 μg/ml leupeptin (Cell Signaling Technology). Protease and phosphatase inhibitors (Roche) were added immediately before use. Samples (15 μg/lane) were boiled in standard commercial SDS-gel loading buffer and run on SDS 10% polyacrylamide gels. Immunoblotting was performed on Immobilon-P PVDF membrane (Millipore). The following antibodies were used for immunoblotting: rabbit polyclonal anti-phosphor-MEK1/2 (Ser217/221) antibodies (Cell Signaling #9121, at 1:1000 dilution), mouse monoclonal anti-MEK1/2 antibodies (Santa Cruz, sc-81504, at 1:500 dilution), mouse monoclonal anti-Flag antibodies (Sigma-Aldrich F1804, 1:1000), and rabbit polyclonal anti-GAPDH antibodies (Cell Signaling, #5174, at 1:1000 dilution). Appropriate secondary antibodies with infrared dyes (LI-COR) were used. Protein bands were visualized using the Odyssey Infrared Imaging System (LI-COR) and further quantified by ImageJ.

Integrative omics analysis of druggability

To analyze and visualize druggability based on multi-omics information, we first identified tumors whose druggability is implicated by two or more variant types (genomic, transcriptomic, proteomic). Drug-associated genomic variants include both known mutations in DEPO and putative mutations identified using protein structure-based clustering. Transcriptomic and proteomic variants include mRNAs and phosphoproteins/proteins with expression outliers based on RNA-seq and RPPA data, respectively. For each tumor, we mapped its "druggable" variants against one or more drugs, which were then mapped to one or more drug classes (Additional file 2: Table S8). For each variant, we used the drug that had the highest level of evidence in DEPO regardless of cancer type (Additional file 2: Table S3). For the purposes of visualization, we only considered ten FDA-approved drug classes (Additional file 2: Table S9) mapping to the largest number of variants across our pan-cancer cohort (Additional file 2: Table S10).

Druggability and demographics

We assessed differences in druggability as a function of demographics (sex, race) (Additional file 1, Additional file 2: Table S11, Additional file 3: Figure S4). We limited our analyses to cancer types for which at least 20 tumors are represented for each demographic category (e.g., ≥ 20 Caucasians with BRCA, ≥ 20 Asians with BRCA). For the sex analysis, this excluded certain cancer types (BRCA, CESC, PRAD, OV, UCEC, and UCS). Next, we determined the most commonly druggable genes at the mutational, RNA, and phosphoprotein levels; to merit inclusion, a druggable gene must be observed in ≥ 40 tumors and ≥ 150 tumors for the race and sex analyses, respectively. A matrix was then generated of cancer types and druggable genes, with each matrix value corresponding to the log-odds ratio between druggability and traits:

$$\log_2 \left(\frac{\text{druggable trait A patients/trait A patients}}{\text{druggable trait B patients/trait B patients}} \right)$$

for a specific cancer type (e.g., BRCA) and a specific druggable gene (e.g., elevated ERBB2 phosphoprotein expression). If fewer than 10 tumors contain a specific druggable gene in a specific cancer type, no matrix value was calculated. For the purposes of graphical visualization, matrix values of $+\infty$ and $-\infty$ are set to $+ 3$ and $- 3$, respectively.

To determine whether a specific druggable gene is statistically more prevalent in a given demographic group, Fisher exact tests were performed. FDR correction to p values was applied with a cutoff of 0.05.

Results

Database of Evidence for Precision Oncology

We utilized a repository of known variant/drug interactions, which we refer to as "Database of Evidence for Precision Oncology" or DEPO (Sun et al.[26], in revision), containing data from publically available datasets and papers [20, 23–25] (Fig. 1a).

In aggregate, 609 unique variants with known drug interactions currently reside in DEPO, and account for a total of ~ 800 unique variant/drug interactions (Fig. 1b). Approximately 70% of known variant/drug interactions result in increased sensitivity to therapy. Further, a substantial number (~ 25%) of sensitive variant/drug interactions are approved by the FDA for a particular cancer type or are based on late-stage clinical studies. Several genes account for a large proportion of variant/drug interactions (e.g., EGFR, KIT, ERBB2, BRCA1, PDGFRA), reflecting interest in therapeutically exploiting a relatively limited number of cancer driver genes [5] (Fig. 1c). Altogether, 168 genes are represented in the current version of DEPO.

Drug-associated mutations in pan-cancer cohort

We leveraged the genomic sequence data of 6570 tumor samples from TCGA representing 22 adult cancer types (Synapse ID, syn12618789). Mutations associated with drug sensitivity in DEPO were matched against the TCGA cohort. Our analysis reveals 2364 mutations across 2114 tumors that are associated with sensitivity to one or more drugs (mean = 1.12/tumor) (Additional file 2: Table S2). Three hundred sixty-two distinct mutations are represented across 40 genes. The low fraction of drug-associated mutations likely reflects the large number of passengers in cancer [42, 43]. Thirty-two percent of tumors had at least one drug-associated mutation, a percentage that is consistent with the 28% of screened patients that could be matched with a targeted therapy or trial [44].

Initially, we analyzed the percentage of potentially druggable tumors in a cancer-type-specific setting (Fig. 2), that is, tumors with mutations associated with a known drug response in the cancer type with the highest level of evidence. Only 3.3% of the samples contain a druggable mutation known to be FDA approved; however, if we consider less mature evidence: clinical trials, preclinical, and case reports, we could potentially increase the percentage of tumors with drug-associated mutations to 8.2, 8.5, and 10.5%, respectively. Here, skin cutaneous melanoma (SKCM) is the cancer type with the largest fraction of drug-associated mutations (78%). SKCM with a BRAF V600E/K mutation (40% of patients)

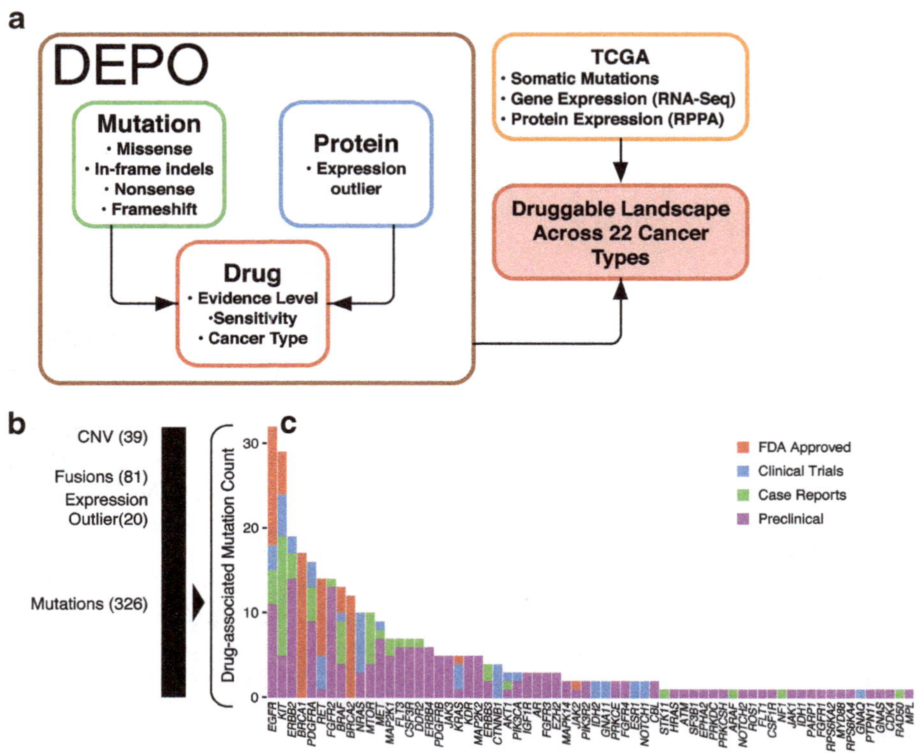

Fig. 1 DEPO database. **a** The methodology supporting curation of the drug-variant depository, which we refer to as DEPO, or *Database of Evidence for Precision Oncology*, and its use in determining the "druggable" landscape of TCGA tumors. **b** The composition of sensitive variants in DEPO by variant type. For each variant type, only unique variants were counted even if a given variant is associated with multiple levels of evidence, multiple drugs, and/or multiple cancer types. "CNV" (copy number variation) corresponds to "CNA" (copy number amplification) and "CNL" (copy number loss) entries in DEPO; this includes genes for which CNA or CNL is associated with drug response, respectively. "Expression" refers to genes whose elevated and reduced expression is associated with drug response. "Mutations" refers to missense, nonsense, in-frame indels, and frameshift mutations. **c** Number of uniquely drug-associated mutations in DEPO by gene, sorted by evidence level: FDA approved, clinical trials, case reports, and preclinical

can be treated with BRAF and MEK inhibitors based on FDA approval. The NRAS Q61 mutations found in 12% of SKCM patients are more challenging to treat, as is any RAS-mutant cancer due to activation of multiple signaling pathways. Early generation MEK-exclusive inhibition proved to be ineffective, with multiple failed clinical trials prompting exploration of newer generation MEK inhibitors and MEK inhibitor combinations with downstream targets of NRAS [45]. In colon and rectal carcinoma (COAD-READ), glioblastoma multiforme (GBM), and lung adenocarcinoma (LUAD), 21, 14, and 40% of their respective tumors contain a drug-associated mutation in a cancer-type-specific setting. In COADREAD, drug-associated variants PIK3CA E542K, E545K, and H1047R are present in 2.1, 5.2, and 1.8% of tumors, respectively, and are associated with sensitivity to PI3K/AKT/mTOR pathway inhibitors in early-stage trials [46] and aspirin in observational studies [47, 48]. PIK3CA-mutant cancers are also an ongoing challenge to treat clinically; co-occurring drugs targeting the PI3K pathway have been more effective than single-agent PI3K inhibition in

treating PIK3CA-mutant cancers, but efficacy varies with mutation profile [46]. In GBM, the EGFR extracellular mutations (A289V, G598V, and R108K) and *IDH1* mutation R132H are present in 10 and 4.5% of tumors, respectively, and are associated with drug response based on preclinical data [49]. In non-small cell lung cancer, EGFR inhibitors (e.g., erlotinib) are FDA approved for tumors with activating EGFR mutations, which are present at 10 and 1% in our LUAD and lung squamous cell carcinoma (LUSC) cohorts, respectively.

Despite the promise of targeted therapy, only 10.5% of this pan-cancer cohort contains potential drug-associated mutations in a cancer-type-specific setting. With drug repurposing across cancer types, in which a drug used primarily in cancer type A with mutation X is repurposed for cancer type B with mutation X, we find that an additional 5.4% of patients may be treated with a FDA-approved drug-variant interaction (Figs. 2 and 3, Additional file 2: Table S12). This number can be increased to 22.8% if we consider repurposing of lower tier drug-variant pairs to other cancer types; however, these interactions will require

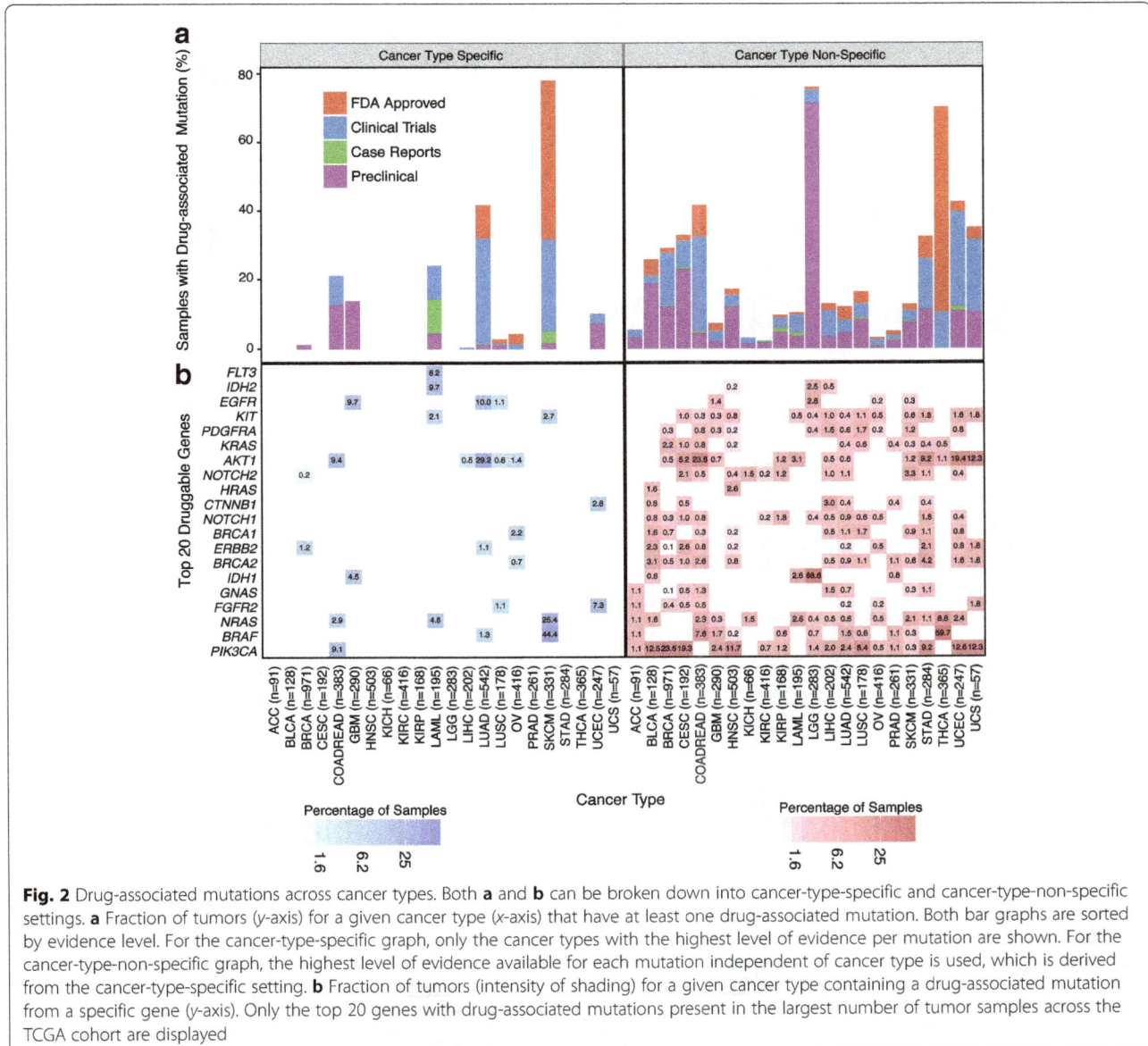

Fig. 2 Drug-associated mutations across cancer types. Both **a** and **b** can be broken down into cancer-type-specific and cancer-type-non-specific settings. **a** Fraction of tumors (y-axis) for a given cancer type (x-axis) that have at least one drug-associated mutation. Both bar graphs are sorted by evidence level. For the cancer-type-specific graph, only the cancer types with the highest level of evidence per mutation are shown. For the cancer-type-non-specific graph, the highest level of evidence available for each mutation independent of cancer type is used, which is derived from the cancer-type-specific setting. **b** Fraction of tumors (intensity of shading) for a given cancer type containing a drug-associated mutation from a specific gene (y-axis). Only the top 20 genes with drug-associated mutations present in the largest number of tumor samples across the TCGA cohort are displayed

clinical validation to be considered truly druggable. In this cancer-type-non-specific setting, cancer types in which at least 40% of tumors have drug-associated mutations include low-grade glioma (LGG, 76%), thyroid carcinoma (THCA, 70%), and colorectal adenocarcinoma (COAD-READ, 42%). A small number of drug-associated mutations occur at high frequency in these cancer types. For example, in THCA, the BRAF V600E variant is found in 60% of tumors. Clinical trials have investigated the use of BRAF inhibitors combined with MEK inhibitors in THCA. However, *BRAF* V600E also occurs at a lower frequency in HNSC, KIRP, LGG, and GBM, indicating significant repurposing potential for BRAF inhibitors [50, 51] (Fig. 3).

COADREAD may also have potential for therapeutic intervention via repurposing (Fig. 2a). However, COAD-READ has been difficult to treat due to a large presence of KRAS and BRAF mutations; EGFR inhibition as monotherapy is used for COADREAD, but only in tumors with wild-type KRAS [52, 53]. Repurposing drugs that inhibit downstream effectors of KRAS (e.g., MEK) is an alternative therapeutic strategy for KRAS-mutant COADREAD (23.8% of patients). The efficacy of MEK inhibition in combination with sorafenib has been tested in clinical trials for KRAS- or NRAS-mutant liver hepatocellular carcinoma (LIHC) [54] and has shown positive results. Co-targeting of MEK and AKT signaling showed some durable response in a phase I study [55], and most

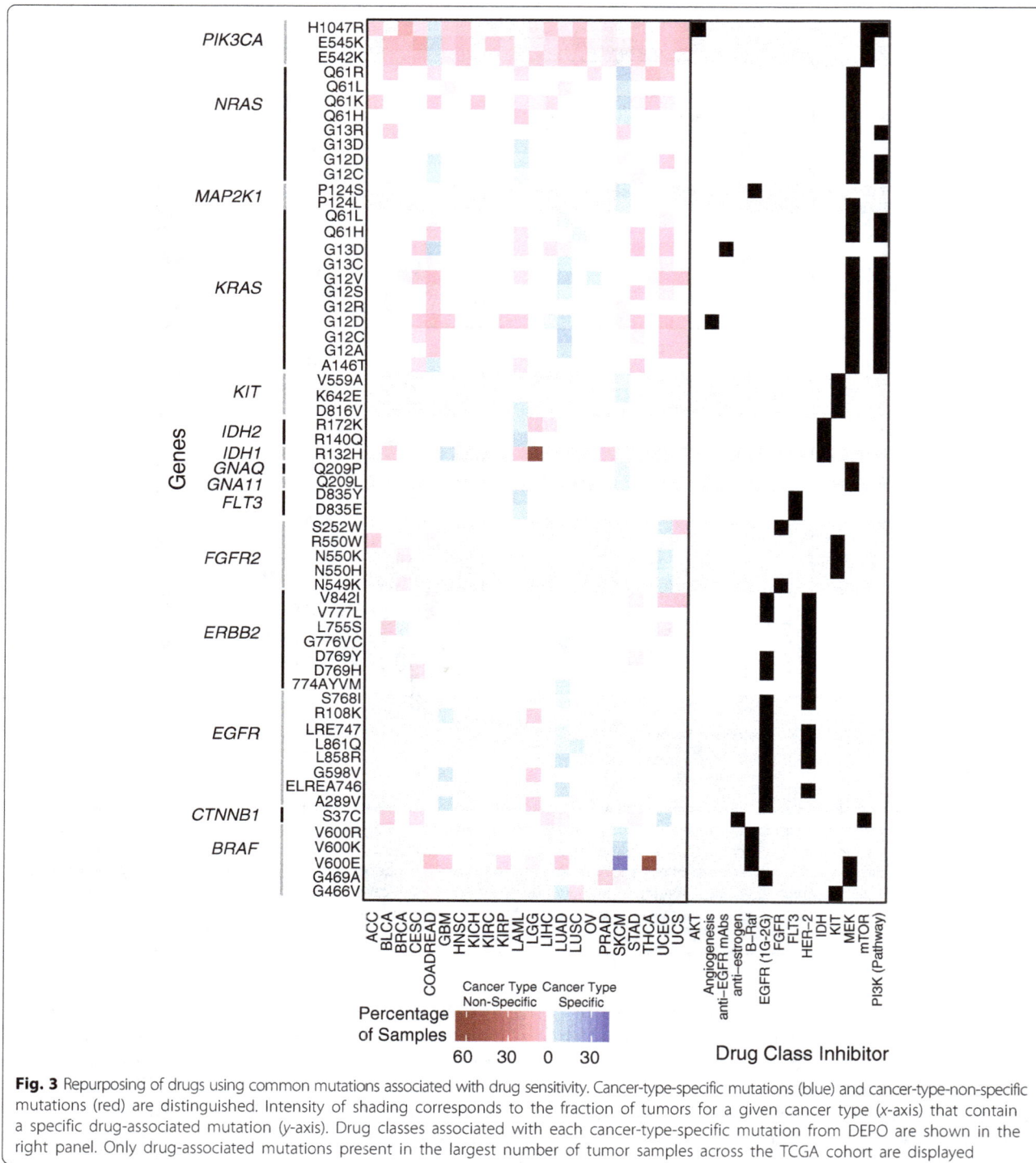

Fig. 3 Repurposing of drugs using common mutations associated with drug sensitivity. Cancer-type-specific mutations (blue) and cancer-type-non-specific mutations (red) are distinguished. Intensity of shading corresponds to the fraction of tumors for a given cancer type (x-axis) that contain a specific drug-associated mutation (y-axis). Drug classes associated with each cancer-type-specific mutation from DEPO are shown in the right panel. Only drug-associated mutations present in the largest number of tumor samples across the TCGA cohort are displayed

recently, a small trial showed some success combining an investigational MEK inhibitor with a CDK4/6 inhibitor in non-small cell lung cancer (NSCLC) (trial NCT number NCT02022982). COADREAD or other cancer types having RAS mutations, such as cervical squamous cell carcinoma and endocervical adenocarcinoma (CESC),

acute myeloid leukemia (AML), stomach adenocarcinoma (STAD), and uterine corpus endometrial carcinoma (UCEC), could benefit from further exploration of combinatorial therapies targeting downstream targets of KRAS (Fig. 2b). BRAF-mutant COADREAD (7.6% of patients) presents a similar problem in that BRAF inhibitor monotherapy is ineffective unlike in BRAF-mutant melanoma and that triple drug combination targeting the EGFR, MAPK, and PI3K pathway has shown more positive results. Numerous clinical trials are underway to find the best combination therapies with BRAF inhibitors, including new drugs that are Wnt pathway and cyclin-dependent kinase inhibitors [56]. Together, cancer-type-specific and non-specific mutational analyses identified potential therapeutic targets in 2114 tumors (32%), some of which will be considered druggable only with further clinical development and FDA approval.

Protein structure-based clustering of drug-associated mutations

We applied a structure-based clustering tool, HotSpot3D [27], to the pan-cancer dataset to reveal putative functional mutations (Additional file 2: Table S13). HotSpot3D's utility in predicting functional mutations is supported by experimental evidence using cell lines expressing one of several EGFR-mutant proteins [36]. HotSpot3D identifies mutations that, by clustering in

protein space with mutations from DEPO associated with drug sensitivity or resistance, may themselves affect drug binding affinity and response. Out of 160 "sensitive" mutations from DEPO that mapped onto protein structures, we identified 134 "sensitive" mutations in HotSpot3D clusters, which in turn were clustered with 214 putative sensitive mutations that were not catalogued in DEPO. These mutations were found in 55 clusters from 24 genes (Fig. 4a). Among all genes in our analysis, EGFR contains the highest number of putative sensitive mutations, with 36 mutations that clustered with 19 mutations in DEPO from seven different clusters (Fig. 4a). This clustering analysis helps winnow down the mutation list to candidates likely to affect drug response and provides context for further experimental testing, but does not necessarily indicate the direction of drug response; in total, HotSpot3D analysis identified potential therapeutic targets in 458 tumors (7%).

We identified putative resistant mutations as those that clustered with "resistant" mutations from DEPO; further, to prevent contradictory annotation of putative

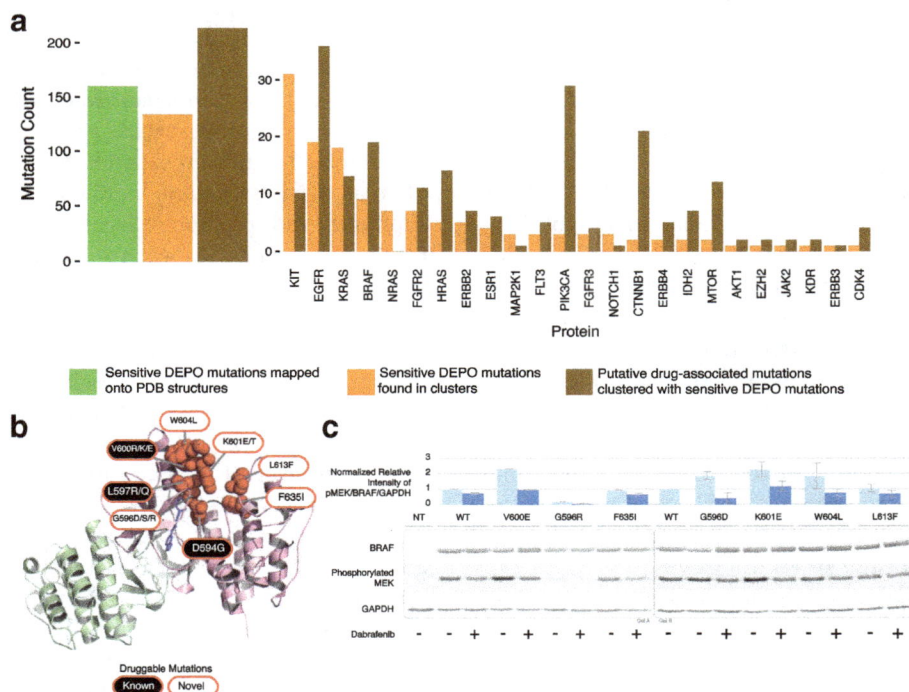

Fig. 4 Protein structure-based analysis of drug-associated mutations. **a** The number of known drug-associated mutations that can be mapped onto PDB structures, the number of known drug-associated mutations that are found in HotSpot3D clusters, and the number of putative druggable mutations are shown, both in aggregate and for specific genes (x-axis). **b** Protein structure views of one HotSpot3D cluster in BRAF (PDB: 4MBJ). Known and putative druggable mutations are distinguished by different colors in mutation labels. A drug molecule in the binding pocket is indicated in blue. **c** Western blot for BRAF mutation cluster found in **b**. HEK293T cells were transiently transfected with wild-type (WT) or mutant BRAF constructs and were cultured in 0.5% calf serum for 24 h before treatment with Dabrafenib (0–1uM) for 6 h. BRAF activity was analyzed by quantifying phosphorylation changes in MEK1/2. To normalize for transfection and loading variations, pMEK levels were divided by BRAF levels and then by GAPDH levels to produce the normalized relative intensities of pMEK/BRAF/GAPDH. This was then normalized to the WT sample without drug treatment that was set as 1. The error bars represent biological replicates

mutations as both "sensitive" and "resistant," we limited our analysis of clusters containing "resistant" mutations to those that did not overlap with clusters containing sensitive mutations. This procedure yielded four different clusters with a "resistant" mutation in AKT1, MAP2K1, and *RAC1*; these four clusters contained 14 putative resistant mutations clustering with four known resistant mutations (Additional file 2: Table S13). RAC1 yielded the largest cluster, with RAC1 P29S mediating resistance to BRAF inhibitors in BRAF-mutant SKCM [57]. Other mutations in this cluster that may affect binding affinity of BRAF inhibitors (or that may mediate resistance to BRAF inhibitors) are C18Y, E31D, A159V, P29L/T, and P34S.

To provide evidence in support of mutation clustering as a method for identifying putative druggable mutations, we first show that known drug-associated mutations in DEPO that affect binding affinity of drugs in the same drug class cluster spatially. Most clusters contain more than one known drug-associated mutation. For example, KIT has multiple clusters with known mutations; one of which has three known mutations (E490D, Y494C, S476G) in the same cluster, which are FDA approved as sensitive to combined therapy of imatinib, sunitinib, and regorafenib (KIT and angiogenesis inhibitor). In addition, this cluster contains two other unique mutations (D439H, I438L) not in DEPO that, based on our analysis using HotSpot3D, could also affect binding affinity and potentially tumor sensitivity to KIT combined with angiogenesis inhibitors (Additional file 2: Table S13). Second, we experimentally validated HotSpot3D as a tool for identifying functional mutations associated with drug response. To do this, we assessed the activity and drug sensitivity of a set of six BRAF mutations (F635I, G596D, K601E, W604L, L613F, G596R) in close spatial proximity to the well-studied V600E pathogenic mutation (Fig. 4b). A key function of BRAF is phosphorylating MEK1/2. Therefore, we transfected BRAF mutations, along with wild-type BRAF and BRAF V600E, into HEK293T cells in the presence or absence of BRAF inhibitor dabrafenib, and used phosphorylation changes in MEK1/2 as an indicator of BRAF activity. The undetectable level of endogenous BRAF in HEK293T cells eliminates potential ambiguity in interpreting the effects of transfected BRAF mutations. As expected, BRAF V600E caused drastically increased phosphorylation in MEK1/2 that is reduced by dabrafenib (Fig. 4c). Three (G596D, K601E, and W604L) out of six other transfected BRAF mutations also showed higher levels of MEK1/2 phosphorylation and sensitivity to dabrafenib than wild-type BRAF, suggesting that a high percentage of mutations identified by Hotspot3D in close spatial proximity to V600E are activated and similarly sensitive to dabrafenib. Notably, BRAF G596R-transfected cells appeared to have

a much lower level of MEK1/2 phosphorylation when compared to those transfected with wild-type BRAF, supporting prior findings that G596R results in BRAF loss of function [58]. Our ongoing development of comprehensive computational tools combining spatial proximity with considerations of specific amino acid substitutions and other structural features will further improve the accuracy of identifying functional mutations. Overall, HotSpot3D, combined with experimental assays, can help identify functional mutations that are candidates for inclusion in DEPO and worth further clinical exploration.

Druggable gene and protein expression outliers in pan-cancer cohort

In addition to driver mutations in oncogenes, elevated expression of genes or gene products can also be used to select tumors for targeted therapy [59–61]. For example, in the case of breast cancer, elevated mRNA expression and copy number amplification of ESR1 correlate with elevated protein expression of ER [62, 63], as well as with sensitivity to hormonal therapy with tamoxifen [62, 64]. In general, tumors with elevated protein expression may respond to drugs that activate antibody-dependent cell-mediated cytotoxicity [65], suppress signaling pathways essential for tumor survival [66], or deliver cytotoxic agents via tumor-specific antigens [67].

Therefore, to further expand the set of tumors with potential drug-associated biomarkers, we sought transcriptomic and proteomic evidence of elevated gene/protein expression. For each gene in DEPO whose expression is associated with drug response, tumors with outliers were identified using the pan-cancer cohort as a reference. We defined outliers as expression values exceeding 1.5 interquartile ranges (IQR) above the third quartile of the cohort [68]. We applied this outlier detection strategy across mRNA, protein, and protein phosphorylation levels. RNA-seq and protein RPPA data are available for 5286 and 3877 tumors out of 6570 tumors in the TCGA cohort, respectively (Additional file 2: Table S14). DEPO has 50 genes whose expression is associated with drug response, 39 of which are associated with drug sensitivity. We identified elevated expression of druggable genes with drug sensitivity in 16 and 30% of the pan-cancer cohort of 6570 TCGA tumors at the mRNA and protein/phosphoprotein levels, respectively (Fig. 5). Interestingly, tumors with "druggable" gene fusions tend to express elevated levels of the corresponding druggable gene (Additional file 2: Table S15, Additional file 3: Figure S1) [69], suggesting that fusions may be one of several drivers of gene and protein expression.

To determine mRNA expression outliers in tumor samples, we used RNA-seq data from TCGA (Fig. 5a).

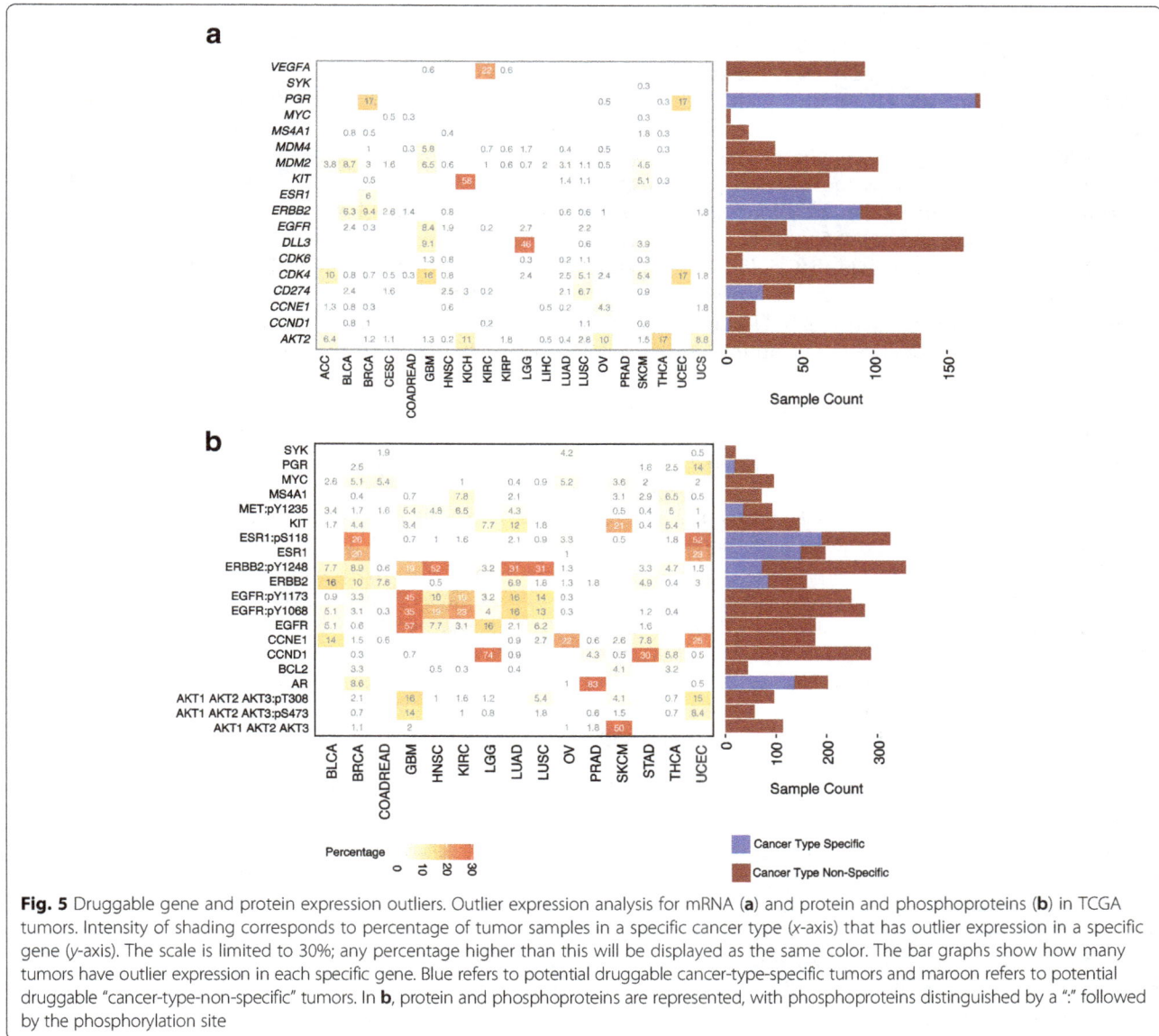

Fig. 5 Druggable gene and protein expression outliers. Outlier expression analysis for mRNA (**a**) and protein and phosphoproteins (**b**) in TCGA tumors. Intensity of shading corresponds to percentage of tumor samples in a specific cancer type (x-axis) that has outlier expression in a specific gene (y-axis). The scale is limited to 30%; any percentage higher than this will be displayed as the same color. The bar graphs show how many tumors have outlier expression in each specific gene. Blue refers to potential druggable cancer-type-specific tumors and maroon refers to potential druggable "cancer-type-non-specific" tumors. In **b**, protein and phosphoproteins are represented, with phosphoproteins distinguished by a ":" followed by the phosphorylation site

Elevated DLL3 expression was identified in 161 tumors, including LGG, GBM, and SKCM tumors. DLL3 contributes to neuroendocrine tumorigenesis by inhibiting the Notch signaling pathway, whose role is to suppress tumor growth. A DLL3-targeted antibody-drug conjugate in phase II clinical trials effectively targets DLL3-expressing cells in high-grade pulmonary neuroendocrine tumors [70, 71]. This same therapy could potentially benefit GBM, LGG, and SKCM via repurposing due to shared levels of high DLL3 expression. Seventeen percent of BRCA and UCEC express PGR and 9.4% of BRCA express ERBB2 in our cohort, reflecting the FDA-approved use of anti-estrogen hormone therapy and HER-2 inhibitors, respectively, in these cancer types. ERBB2 is expressed in other cancer types, such as BLCA and CESC, which could benefit from repurposing and further exploration of HER2-inhibition; HER-2 inhibitors for COADREAD are currently being explored in late-stage clinical trials.

To examine tumors with potential drug-associated biomarkers based on protein expression and phosphosite levels, we used TCGA reverse phase protein array (RPPA) data (Fig. 5b). Compared to the pan-cancer cohort, 83% of prostate adenocarcinoma (PRAD) express elevated AR, reflecting their tissue of origin. Elevated AR is also present in 9% of breast adenocarcinoma (BRCA). These 9% of BRCA express higher levels of AR than 17% of PRAD, suggesting that androgen-deprivation therapy can potentially be repurposed for AR-positive BRCA [72] (Additional file 2: Table S16). Similarly, 26 and

52% of BRCA and UCEC, respectively, show elevated activity at ESR1's p.S118 phosphosite. These only represent a fraction of druggable BRCA, as 77% of tumors in a large breast cancer registry are ER positive [73]. Elevated expression and activity of EGFR protein and its phosphosites across cancer types suggest that phosphoproteome analysis may inform treatment response. EGFR phosphosites p.Y1068 and p.Y1173 are active in GBM, head and neck squamous cell carcinoma (HNSC), KIRC, LUAD, and LUSC. Some evidence has shown that HNSC, LUAD, and LUSC are responsive to EGFR tyrosine kinase inhibitors (TKIs) [74, 75], perhaps because EGFR TKIs inhibit autophosphorylation rather than elevated protein expression [76]. In KIRC, EGFR inhibitors have negligible activity [77–79] despite active phosphosites in our analysis, possibly because EGFR is one of many growth factors expressed in KIRC or because EGFR inhibition is ineffective in the absence of functioning VHL [80].

Altogether, our results suggest that protein outlier analysis may require integration with mutational and/or mRNA expression analyses to better predict response to therapy. Additionally, mass spectrometry for protein expression can be valuable in validating RNA-seq and RPPA data as well as capturing new putative druggable events (Additional file 1, Additional file 3: Figure S2). mRNA and phosphoprotein expression outlier analysis identified potential therapeutic targets in 2559 tumors (39%).

Integrative omics analysis of druggability

Assessing alterations in multiple levels of data across genes may improve predictions of druggability. For example, with trastuzumab, a single testing method or biomarker (CNV, mRNA expression, protein expression, etc.) can be insufficient for stratifying patients into responders and non-responders [59]. Therefore, we assessed druggability using comprehensive mutational, RNA-seq, and RPPA data in 3121 tumors. Of these, 1003 tumors (32%) are potentially druggable based on two or more data types (genomic, transcriptomic, proteomic) (Fig. 6a, Additional file 2: Table S8), affording an opportunity for clinical or mechanistic analyses connecting drug-associated mutations with transcriptomic/proteomic expression events. Figure 6b and Additional file 2: Table S10 depict tumors with multiple levels of alterations associated with sensitivity to one of ten categories of FDA-approved cancer drugs (Additional file 2: Table S9). Seventy-two tumors had elevated mRNA and protein expression of HER2; these may be expected to have greater or more uniform sensitivity to HER2 inhibition than tumors with elevated mRNA or protein expression alone. Identifying mutations associated with drug resistance may further improve predictions of druggability. RAC1 P29S co-occurs with mutations in BRAF and MEK1 in four

SKCM tumors (Additional file 2: Table S17, Additional file 3: Figure S3). RAC1 P29S renders SKCM resistant to BRAF/MEK inhibition [57]; testing for RAC1 P29S may identify patients with BRAF V600E SKCM unlikely to benefit from BRAF/MEK inhibitor. In this case, the single-gene paradigm of existing companion diagnostics may be insufficient to determine best treatment options; rather, comprehensive mutational profiling should be considered.

Multi-omics profiling also reveals opportunities for combinatorial therapy. AKT1 E17K co-occurs with BRAF V600E in five tumors (Additional file 2: Table S17, Additional file 3: Figure S3). Combining an AKT inhibitor with the current standard of treatment for BRAF V600E-positive SKCM (BRAF/MEK co-inhibition) may delay drug resistance [81]. Transcriptomic and proteomic expression profiling reveals 48 additional tumors with BRAF V600E/K and elevated AKT (AKT1/2/3) expression at the mRNA or protein/phosphoprotein levels; these may also benefit from BRAF/AKT inhibition (Fig. 6b, Additional file 2: Table S10). Similarly, Fig. 6b shows that 38 tumors contain biomarkers of response (i.e., mutational or expression based) for both EGFR and CDK inhibitors. Though both therapies are FDA approved, no clinical trials to date have examined combinatorial therapy with EGFR and CDK dual inhibition. Additionally, 105 tumors contain activating PIK3CA mutations co-occurring with elevated mRNA or protein expression of ESR1 or PGR. Given the success of mTOR and anti-estrogen therapy in ER-positive breast cancer [82], this combination may be useful in other cancer types that are dependent on hormonal or PI3K/mTOR signaling. By identifying tumors with biomarkers of response to multiple drugs, and by identifying variations in biomarkers across gender and ethnicity (Additional file 1, Additional file 2: Table S11, Additional file 3: Figure S4), multi-omics profiling can facilitate the rational design of clinical trials for combinatorial therapy.

Validation of druggability analyses with large-scale drug screening

We sought to provide support for our two hypotheses that our approaches relied upon: (1) a drug with evidence supporting use in a given cancer type can be repurposed to other cancer types that contain a shared genetic alteration; (2) gene/protein expression outlier score is a predictor of drug sensitivity. To test these hypotheses, we utilized the Genomics of Drug Sensitivity in Cancer (GDSC) database, which contains drug sensitivity data for around 75,000 experiments of 138 anticancer drugs (Additional file 2: Table S4) across 700 cancer cell lines [83]. We extracted tissue type, the mutational landscape (missense mutations and in-frame indels), gene expression, and drug sensitivity information for each cell line.

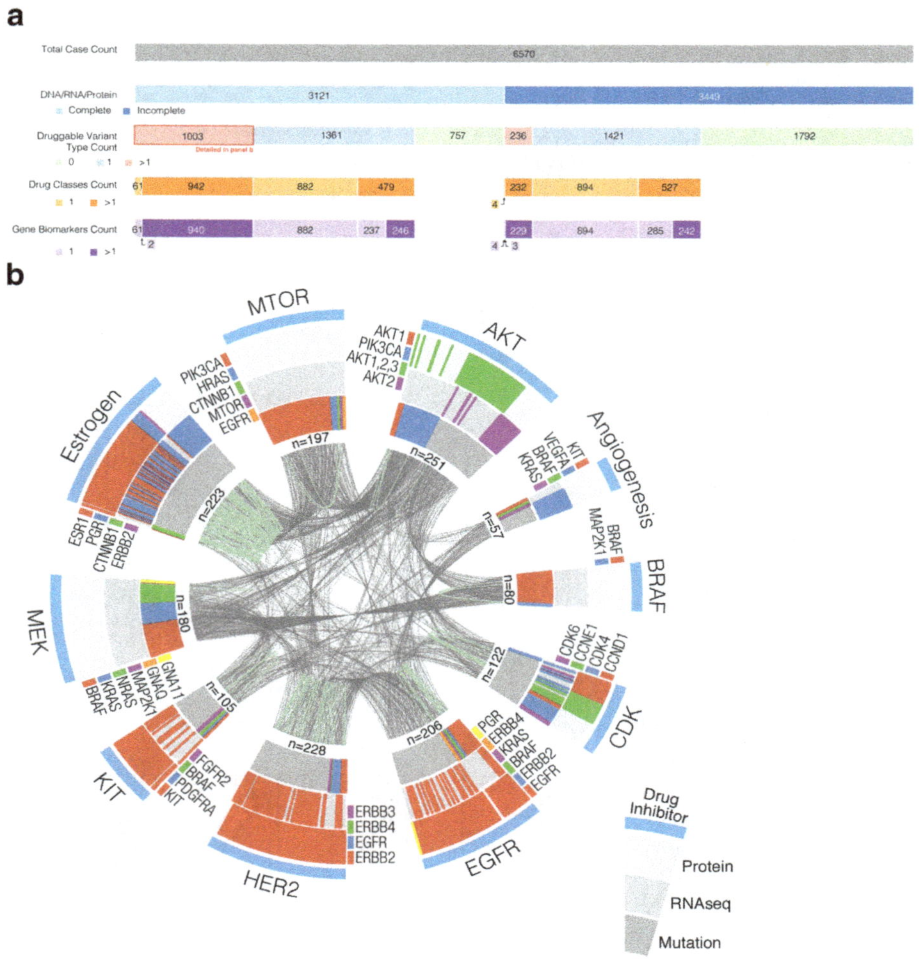

Fig. 6 Integrative omics analysis of druggability. **a** TCGA tumor samples are sorted by completeness of DNA/RNA/protein profiling, number of variant types supporting druggability, number of drug classes, and number of druggable genes. Of the 3121 tumor samples with complete profiling, 1003 are potentially druggable based on > 1 variant types (mutational, RNA expression, protein expression) and are represented in **b**. **b** Multi-drug and multi-omic relationships within tumor samples. Ten outer sectors separate samples according to biomarkers associated with sensitivity to one of ten FDA-approved drug classes. Each outer sector consists of three tracks: DNA mutation (inner), RNA expression (middle), and protein expression (outer). Different colored bands within these tracks represent different genes whose variants implicate druggability in a single tumor sample. The genes represented in each sector vary according to drug class; adjacent to each sector is a legend indicating represented genes. The total number of unique samples is labeled under each sector. A gray link (between wedges) represents a single tumor with biomarkers associated with sensitivity to multiple drug classes. A green link (within a wedge) represents a single tumor with multiple biomarkers of the same variant type associated with sensitivity to a single drug class (e.g., a single tumor with RNA expression in *ESR1* and *PGR*)

Twenty-six sensitive mutations from DEPO are found in GDSC cell lines paired with 44 drugs (Additional file 2: Table S5). BRAF V600E, PIK3CA H1047R, and KRAS G12D occur most frequently in GDSC cell lines. Overall, the mean $LN(IC_{50})$ for cell lines that contain a sensitive mutation from DEPO was significantly lower than background $LN(IC_{50})$ in both the cancer-type-specific and non-specific setting (Mann-Whitney U test, $P = 1.1e-96$ and $P = 1.3e-109$, respectively) (Fig. 7a). Individual variant/drug combinations from DEPO also performed well; 39 variant/drug combinations in the cell line data occurred in sufficient samples in both the cancer-type-specific and

non-specific settings for statistical analysis (Additional file 2: Table S6). This represented 6 of 26 sensitive mutations. In both the cancer-type-specific and non-specific settings, 19 variant/drug combinations had significantly lower mean $LN(IC_{50})$ than background $LN(IC_{50})$ for the corresponding drug. Based on these 19 drug-variant combinations, 4 out of 6 sensitive mutations in DEPO (KRAS G12V, BRAF V600E, NRAS Q61K, and KRAS G12D) were significantly associated with sensitivity to at least one of their paired drugs in both the cancer-type-specific and non-specific settings. For example, cell lines with BRAF V600E were associated with sensitivity to BRAF inhibitors PLX4720 (1),

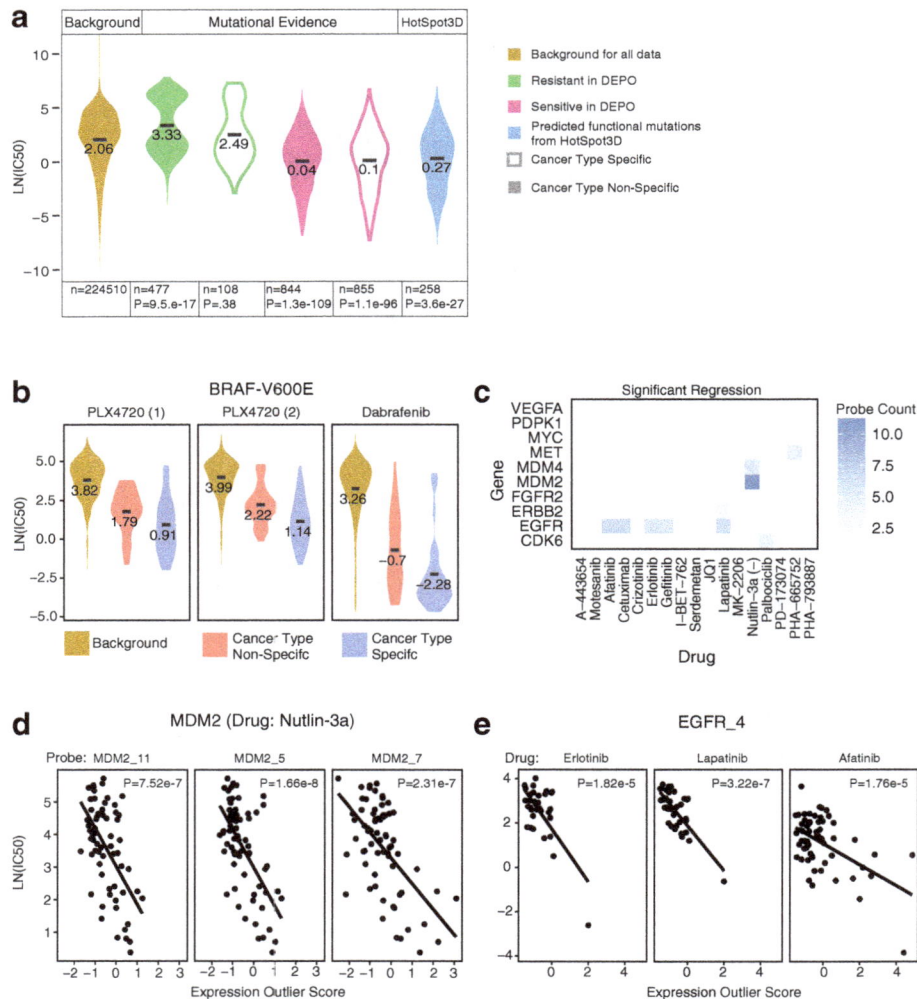

Fig. 7 Cell line-based validation. **a** Violin plots show the distribution of drug response (y-axis) of cell lines with drug-associated mutations compared to the background distribution (dark yellow). The type of distribution is indicated in the top gray bar of the panel with distributions of the background, cell lines with mutations in DEPO (Mutational Evidence), and cell lines with putative functional mutations as predicted by HotSpot3D (HotSpot3D). Sensitive and resistant mutations in DEPO are indicated by a green and pink fill color, respectively. Violin plots outlined in a bold black color indicate the cancer-type-specific distribution. The bottom gray bar indicates sample size and P value (Mann-Whitney U test) for the distribution when compared to the background. **b** The distribution of drug response (y-axis) for three BRAF inhibitors (PLX4720 (1), PLX4720 (2), and dabrafenib) are shown. For each drug, the background distribution and drug response for cell lines with the BRAF V600E mutation in the cancer-type-specific setting and non-specific setting are shown. **c** Expression outlier scores for genes (y-axis) with significant negative correlation with a paired drug (x-axis) are shown. The intensity of shading corresponds to the number of probes that registered as significant for a gene-drug pair. **d** Scatter plots of the drug response (y-axis) of Nutlin-3a and expression outlier scores (x-axis) are shown for three different probes of MDM2. The best fit line and P values for the linear regression are also shown. **e** Scatter plots of the drug response (y-axis) to three different drugs (erlotinib, lapatinib, and afatinib) and expression outlier scores (x-axis) are shown for 1 probe of EGFR. The best fit line and P values for the linear regression are also shown

PLX4720 (2), and dabrafenib in both the cancer-type-specific (SKCM) and non-specific settings (BRCA, COADREAD, GBM, LGG, LIHC, and THCA) (Fig. 7b). Two out of six mutations (PIK3CA H1047R and KRAS G12C) was associated with sensitivity in either the cancer-type-specific or the non-specific setting. Cell lines with PIK3CA H1047R had a significantly lower mean $LN(IC_{50})$ in the cancer-type-non-specific setting; however, this category encompassed several cancer types, including BRCA, HNSC, and ovarian serous carcinoma (OV). Similarly, cell lines with KRAS G12C had a significant lower mean $LN(IC_{50})$ in the cancer-type-specific setting, encompassing LIHC, LUAD, LUSC, and pancreatic adenocarcinoma (PAAD). Overall, our analyses provide some evidence to support our hypothesis that drugs can potentially be repurposed across several cancer types using shared mutational biomarkers of druggability. It must be noted, however, that sensitivity to drug response in cell lines does not necessarily translate over to clinical efficacy, and RAS- and PIK3CA-mutant cancers continue to be controversial.

To verify that gene expression outlier score was correlated with drug response, we conducted linear regression analysis for gene probe/drug combinations (Additional file 2: Table S18) using 116 different probes for 22 genes in DEPO. Forty-two probe/drug combinations corresponding to 10 genes had significant negative correlation ($P < 0.05$) between $LN(IC_{50})$ and gene expression outlier score (Fig. 7c, Additional file 2: Table S7). For example, MDM2 expression correlates with sensitivity to nutlin-3a and EGFR expression correlates with sensitivity to erlotinib, lapatinib, and gefitinib (Fig. 7d, e). Similar trends are observed in CDK6 with palbociclib (PD-0332991: CDK4/6 inhibitor) and ERBB2 with lapatinib (Additional file 2: Table S7). Though cell line-based validation does not guarantee 100% drug response in patients, our analysis demonstrates that expression in 10 of 22 genes correlates with drug sensitivity in GDSC. Expression in other genes such as AKT2 and KIT did not correlate with drug sensitivity (Additional file 2: Table S7). However, this does not rule out the clinical utility of expression assays for these genes given that, for instance, KIT protein expression is an FDA-approved companion diagnostic for imatinib use. Overall, our analysis suggests that using gene expression outliers is a reasonable approach for predicting druggability in

human cancers; however, some of these interactions still need to be validated in a clinical setting.

Discussion

This study presents a pan-cancer analysis of multi-omics-driven prescription of targeted therapy across 6570 TCGA patients. Using DEPO, a curated database of variant/drug interactions with clinically relevant annotations, we investigated the frequency of potential druggable multi-omics alterations based on various levels of evidence to help guide future clinical trials. After adjusting the percentages of potentially druggable tumors based on our validation strategy, we found that mutational, mRNA expression outliers, and phosphoprotein/protein expression outliers implicate druggability of 5% of tumors, respectively based on FDA-approved interactions only. However, up to 15.6% of the cohort could benefit if repurposing of these FDA-approved interactions to other cancer types are further explored; this percentage could increase to 33.9, 34.4, 44.6, and 48.4% of tumor samples based on clinical trials, case reports, preclinical evidence, and HotSpot3D evidence, respectively should these drug-variant interactions be approved clinically in their respective cancer types (Fig. 8, Additional file 2: Table S19, Additional file 3: Figure S5).

Our analysis illustrates the potential of a "precision oncology" approach to prescribe targeted therapy to a pan-cancer cohort of patients. Compared to prior work [17], our study offers four novel advancements. First,

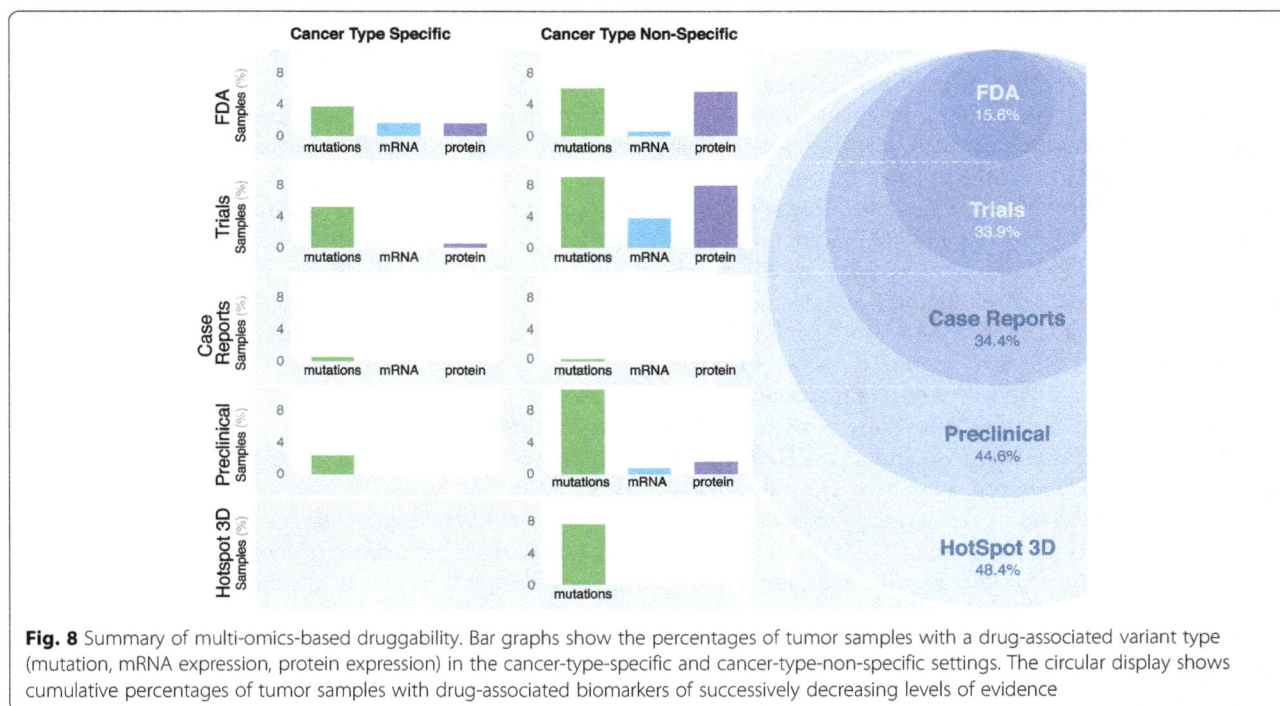

Fig. 8 Summary of multi-omics-based druggability. Bar graphs show the percentages of tumor samples with a drug-associated variant type (mutation, mRNA expression, protein expression) in the cancer-type-specific and cancer-type-non-specific settings. The circular display shows cumulative percentages of tumor samples with drug-associated biomarkers of successively decreasing levels of evidence

with DEPO, our analysis of druggability in a given tumor is exclusively based on mutation/drug interactions rather than gene/drug interactions, with variants including both predefined mutations (e.g., BRAF V600E) and categories of mutations (e.g., EGFR exon 19 deletions). The most comprehensive prior study assessing prescription of anticancer drugs included fewer than 10 mutations associated with drug sensitivity [17] (http://www.intogen.org/downloads); in comparison, the present study includes 362 mutations associated with drug sensitivity. Second, while prior studies exclusively used genomic data to infer druggability [12, 17], ours is comprehensive in its use of genomic, transcriptomic, *and* proteomic data types, specifically leveraging mRNA expression and phosphoproteomic expression data to further define tumors with potential drug-associated biomarkers. It further demonstrates that integrating data types can allow novel, personalized combinatorial therapy. Third, it uses an analytic tool to create a set of putative druggable mutations, of which a subset occurring in BRAF were tested and validated in vitro. Finally, we used a large-scale drug screening dataset (GDSC) to support our predictions of druggability based on repurposing across cancer types and expression outlier analysis. GDSC and other drug screening datasets have been used to identify biomarkers of drug sensitivity in hypothesis-free analyses [18, 84, 85], but our study is unique in using GDSC as orthogonal validation of putative biomarkers from clinical trials, case reports, and preclinical studies.

Though our study and prior studies [12, 15, 17] implicate large percentages of tumors as potentially druggable (48% and 94%/76%/73%, respectively), prior studies made several assumptions regarding off-variant and off-target drug activity that may not be clinically feasible. For example, using the more stringent prescription guidelines of the present study (variant/drug prescription with no off-variant or off-target effects), only 12.3% of tumors in Rubio-Perez et al. would be druggable. Furthermore, ongoing clinical trials [86, 87] argue that more accurate druggability annotations require specifying alterations at the variant level, as the present study does, but which Frampton et al. [15] and Van Allen et al. [12] do not. Realistically, only a fraction of the 48% of tumors with potential drug-associated omics alterations will be clinically druggable because the mere presence of a shared genetic biomarker (mutation, mRNA/protein expression outlier) does not guarantee clinical efficacy across cancer types, nor does it guarantee acceptable clinical toxicity. Not all preclinical drug-biomarker pairs, including those predicted with HotSpot3D, will advance to clinical trials. Further, we recognize that our computational survey of the landscape of potential drug-associated omics alterations may include some controversial drug/biomarker relationships (e.g.,

PI3K inhibitors in PIK3CA-mutant cancers), some of which have either failed clinical trials and/or are still being actively developed in clinical trials. Nonetheless, our study is important in identifying which drug-biomarker pairs, repurposing events, and combinatorial therapies are worth exploring and provides a robust platform for both design and analysis of clinical trials.

Our analysis has several limitations. First, TCGA tumor samples are treatment naïve. Given that targeted therapy is often used once other therapeutic options (e.g., cytotoxic chemotherapy, radiotherapy) have been exhausted, tumors treated in the clinical setting may have different genomic profiles than those in this study. Second, our analysis does not account for clonal heterogeneity, which is not unreasonable given that therapies targeting genomic alterations with high variant allele frequencies can induce substantial tumor regression [88]. However, we acknowledge that for clonally heterogeneous cancer types such as GBM, even if the dominant clone is sensitive to therapy, one or more subclones lacking a druggable genomic event may escape [89]. Third, some potential expression outliers may be missed since we do not compute cancer-specific expression outliers; therefore, outliers in cancer types with low overall expression may not be identified, and only high confidence outliers that are most likely targetable are reported. Additionally, some outliers may represent cancer lineage markers or non-cancer cells within tumors and not necessarily a somatically altered pathway, such as the 58% of KICH expressing KIT (Fig. 5a). Future studies can determine which kinase expression outliers are contributing to a somatically altered pathway by checking phosphorylation and/or expression of downstream substrates. Fourth, our analysis does not consider germline mutations that sensitize a tumor to targeted therapy, nor does it attempt to use integrative omics data to predict sensitivity to immune checkpoint inhibitors. Finally, our analysis ignores therapeutic toxicity. In particular, toxicity is often a limiting factor for combination therapy [90, 91], though rationally designed combinations can reduce toxicity [92].

Conclusions

This study is the first to comprehensively profile the druggability of cancer types using integrative omics TCGA data. While multi-omics-driven prescription of anticancer drugs is a powerful concept [17], the efficacy of each drug still requires testing within the context of clinical trials. By describing the landscape of potentially druggable alterations across cancer types, our study serves as a roadmap for the interpretation and design of clinical trials in precision oncology.

Additional files

Additional file 1: Supplementary Materials and Methods.

Additional file 2: Table S1. Drug classes in DEPO (database of evidence for precision oncology). **Table S2.** Sensitive druggable mutations in 6570 TCGA tumors. **Table S3.** Highest level of evidence present per variant for both resistant and sensitive. **Table S4.** Drugs represented in the GDSC Cell Line Data. **Table S5.** Cell lines that contain a sensitive mutation in DEPO. **Table S6.** Mann-Whitney *U* test of distribution of Ln(IC50) values in cell lines with DEPO sensitive mutations against background distribution for each drug. **Table S7.** Linear regression statistics for probe-drug pairs. **Table S8.** TCGA tumors (out of 3121) that are druggable based on two or more variant types (genomic, transcriptomic, proteomic). **Table S9.** Ten FDA-approved drug classes. **Table S10.** TCGA tumors that are druggable with one of ten classes of FDA-approved cancer drugs based on two or more variant types (genomic, transcriptomic, proteomic). **Table S11.** Druggability and demographics. **Table S12.** Cancer types responsible for the levels of evidence in the cancer type non-specific setting for Fig. 2a. **Table S13.** Novel druggable mutations clustering with known druggable mutations identified using HotSpot3D, a proximity-based clustering tool. **Table S14.** RNA-seq data and protein RPPA data for 6366 and 3877 TCGA tumors, respectively. **Table S15.** Druggable fusions in TCGA samples. **Table S16.** Evidence to support repurposing of proteogenomic alterations across cancer types. **Table S17.** Co-occurring druggable mutations. **Table S18.** Gene expression outlier scores and drug response for all cell lines. **Table S19.** TCGA tumors (out of 6570) that are druggable based on atleast one variant (genomic, transcriptomic, proteomic). (.xlsx 2.1 MB)

Additional file 3: Figure S1. Fusions in the TCGA cohort. **Figure S2.** Druggable protein expression outliers using mass spectrometry. **Figure S3.** Co-occurring druggable mutations represent opportunities for combinational and alternative therapy. **Figure S4.** Druggability and Demographics. **Figure S5.** Potential Druggability by Cancer Type.

Abbreviations

ACC: Adrenocortical carcinoma; AML/LAML: Acute myeloid leukemia; BLCA: Bladder urothelial carcinoma; BRCA: Breast adenocarcinoma; CESC: Cervical squamous cell carcinoma and endocervical adenocarcinoma; CNA: Copy number amplification; CNL: Copy number loss; CNV: Copy number variation; COADREAD: Colon and rectal carcinoma; CPTAC: Clinical Proteomic Tumor Analysis Consortium; DCC: Data Coordinating Center; DEPO: Database of Evidence for Precision Oncology; FBS: Fetal bovine serum; FDA: Food and Drug Administration; FFPE: Formalin-fixed, paraffin-embedded; GBM: Glioblastoma multiforme; GDAC: Genome Data Analysis Centers; GDSC: Genomics of Drug Sensitivity in Cancer; HNSC: Head and neck squamous cell carcinoma; IQR: Interquartile range; KICH: Kidney chromophobe; KIRC: Kidney renal clear cell carcinoma; KIRP: Kidney renal papillary cell carcinoma; LGG: Low-grade glioma; LIHC: Liver hepatocellular carcinoma; LUAD: Lung adenocarcinoma; LUSC: Lung squamous cell carcinoma; MAF: Mutation annotation file; NGS: Next-generation sequencing; NSCLC: Non-small cell lung cancer; OV: Ovarian serous carcinoma; PNNL: Pacific Northwest National Laboratory; PRAD: Prostate adenocarcinoma; RBN: Replicates-based normalization; RPPA: Reverse phase protein array; SKCM: Skin cutaneous melanoma; SNP: Single nucleotide polymorphism; STAD: Stomach adenocarcinoma; STR: Short tandem repeat; TCGA: The Cancer Genome Atlas; TCPA: The Cancer Protein Atlas; THCA: Thyroid carcinoma; TKI: Tyrosine kinase inhibitor; UCEC: Uterine corpus endometrial carcinoma; UCS: Uterine carcinosarcoma; VCF: Variant call format

Acknowledgements
We acknowledge the support of computational resources from McDonnell Genome Institute and appreciate the valuable discussions with members of the TCGA Research Network.

Funding
This work was supported by the National Cancer Institute grants R01CA178383 and R01CA180006 to L.D.; U24CA210972 to D.F, L.D., and S.P; U24CA211006 to L.D.; and National Human Genome Research Institute grant U01HG006517 to L.D. F.C. is supported by National Institute of Diabetes and Digestive and Kidney Diseases grant R01DK087960.

Authors' contributions

LD designed and supervised the research. FC guided the experimental and biological evaluations. SS, SQS, KH, MHB, and ADS analyzed the data. SS, SQS, KH, MHB, MAW, and JFM prepared the figures and tables. SQS and PB constructed the DEPO. CO, SS, MHB, JN, RV, and PT conducted the experiments. SQS, SS, and LD wrote the manuscript. SS, SQS, CM, JW, RRT, JFD, KJJ, MCW, FC, CK, SP, DF, and LD revised the manuscript. All authors read and approved the final manuscript.

Competing interests

The authors declare that they have no competing interests.

Author details
[1]Division of Oncology, Department of Medicine, Washington University, St. Louis, MO 63108, USA. [2]McDonnell Genome Institute, Washington University, St. Louis, MO 63108, USA. [3]Division of Nephrology, Department of Medicine, Washington University, St. Louis, MO 63108, USA. [4]Brown School, Washington University, St. Louis, MO 63105, USA. [5]Marie-Josée and Henry R. Kravis Center for Molecular Oncology, Memorial Sloan Kettering Cancer Center, New York, NY, USA. [6]Department of Mathematics, Washington University, St. Louis, MO 63108, USA. [7]Department of Genetics, Washington University, St. Louis, MO 63108, USA. [8]Biological Sciences Division, Pacific Northwest National Laboratory, Richland, WA 99352, USA. [9]Department of Biochemistry and Molecular Pharmacology, New York University Langone School of Medicine, New York, NY 10016, USA. [10]Institute for Systems Genetics, New York University Langone School of Medicine, New York, NY 10016, USA. [11]Siteman Cancer Center, Washington University, St. Louis, MO 63108, USA.

References
1. Hudis CA. Trastuzumab—mechanism of action and use in clinical practice. N Engl J Med. 2007;357:39–51.
2. Bollag G, et al. Clinical efficacy of a RAF inhibitor needs broad target blockade in BRAF-mutant melanoma. Nature. 2010;467:596–9.
3. Roper N, Stensland KD, Hendricks R, Galsky MD. The landscape of precision cancer medicine clinical trials in the United States. Cancer Treat Rev. 2015; 41(5):385–90.
4. Fridlyand J, et al. Considerations for the successful co-development of targeted cancer therapies and companion diagnostics. Nat Rev Drug Discov. 2013;12:743–55.
5. Kandoth C, et al. Mutational landscape and significance across 12 major cancer types. Nature. 2013;502:333–9.
6. Vogelstein B, et al. Cancer genome landscapes. science. 2013;339:1546–58.
7. Lawrence MS, et al. Discovery and saturation analysis of cancer genes across 21 tumour types. Nature. 2014;505:495–501.
8. Roychowdhury S, et al. Personalized oncology through integrative high-throughput sequencing: a pilot study. Sci Transl Med. 2011;3(111):111ra121.
9. André F, et al. Comparative genomic hybridisation array and DNA sequencing to direct treatment of metastatic breast cancer: a multicentre, prospective trial (SAFIR01/UNICANCER). Lancet Oncol. 2014;15:267–74.
10. LoRusso PM, et al. Pilot trial of selecting molecularly-guided therapy for patients with non-V600 BRAF mutant metastatic melanoma: experience of the SU2C/MRA melanoma dream team. Mol Cancer Ther. 2015;0153:2015.
11. Govindan R, et al. Genomic landscape of non-small cell lung cancer in smokers and never-smokers. Cell. 2012;150:1121–34.
12. Van Allen EM, et al. Whole-exome sequencing and clinical interpretation of formalin-fixed, paraffin-embedded tumor samples to guide precision cancer medicine. Nat Med. 2014;20:682–8.
13. Chen K, et al. Clinical actionability enhanced through deep targeted sequencing of solid tumors. Clin Chem. 2015;61:544–53.

14. Beltran H, et al. Whole-exome sequencing of metastatic cancer and biomarkers of treatment response. JAMA Oncol. 2015;´:466–74.

15. Frampton GM, et al. Development and validation of a clinical cancer genomic profiling test based on massively parallel DNA sequencing. Nat Biotechnol. 2013;31:1023–31.

16. Wagle N, et al. High-throughput detection of actionable genomic alterations in clinical tumor samples by targeted, massively parallel sequencing. Cancer Discov. 2012;2:82–93.

17. Rubio-Perez C, et al. In silico prescription of anticancer drugs to cohorts of 28 tumor types reveals targeting opportunities. Cancer Cell. 2015;27:382–96.

18. Iorio F, et al. A landscape of pharmacogenomic interactions in cancer. Cell. 2016;166:740–54.

19. Ellis MJ, et al. Connecting genomic alterations to cancer biology with proteomics: the NCI clinical proteomic tumor analysis consortium. Cancer Discov. 2013;3:1108–12.

20. Johnson A; et al. The right drugs at the right time for the right patient: the MD Anderson precision oncology decision support platform. Drug Discov Today. 2015;20(12):1433–8.

21. Le Tourneau C, et al. Treatment algorithms based on tumor molecular profiling: the essence of precision medicine trials. J Natl Cancer Inst. 2016; 108(4).

22. Griffith M, et al. DGIdb: mining the druggable genome. Nat Methods. 2013; 10:1209–10.

23. Dienstmann R, Jang IS, Bot B, Friend S, Guinney J. Database of genomic biomarkers for cancer drugs and clinical targetability in solid tumors. Cancer Discov. 2015;5:118–23.

24. Swanton C. My Cancer Genome: a unified genomics and clinical trial portal. Lancet Oncol. 2012;13:668–9.

25. Kumar R, et al. CancerDR: cancer drug resistance database. Sci Rep. 2013;3:1445.

26. Sun SQ, et al. Database of Evidence for Precision Oncology Portal. Bioinformatics. 2018.

27. Niu B, et al. Protein-structure-guided discovery of functional mutations across 19 cancer types. Nat Genet. 2016;48(8):827–37.

28. Kamburov A, et al. Comprehensive assessment of cancer missense mutation clustering in protein structures. Proc Natl Acad Sci. 2015;112:E5486–95.

29. Zhao J, Cheng F, Wang Y, Arteaga CL, Zhao Z. Systematic prioritization of druggable mutations in ~5000 genomes across 16 cancer types using a structural genomics-based approach. Mol Cell Proteomics. 2016;15:642–56.

30. Hubbard T, et al. The Ensembl genome database project. Nucleic Acids Res. 2002;30:38–41.

31. Yoshihara K, et al. The landscape and therapeutic relevance of cancer-associated transcript fusions. Oncogene. 2014; 34(37):4845-54.

32. Project NGES. NHLBI Exome Sequencing Project (ESP). Exome Variant Server. Seattle, WA. University of Washington: Seattle, GO, 20´3 (updated 7 June 2013; v.0.0.20 (Exome Variant Server). http://evs.gs.washington.edu/EVS/. Accessed Jan 2015.

33. Consortium GP. An integrated map of genetic variation from 1,092 human genomes. Nature. 2012;491:56–65.

34. Landrum MJ, et al. ClinVar: public archive of relationships among sequence variation and human phenotype. Nucleic Acids Res. 2014;42:D980–5.

35. Adzhubei IA, et al. A method and server for predicting damaging missense mutations. Nat Methods. 2010;7:248–9.

36. Ng PC, Henikoff S. SIFT: predicting amino acid changes that affect protein function. Nucleic Acids Res. 2003;31:3812–4.

37. Li J, et al. TCPA: a resource for cancer functional proteomics data. Nat Methods. 2013;10:1046–7.

38. Mertins P, et al. Proteogenomics connects somatic mutations to signalling in breast cancer. Nature. 2016;534:55–62.

39. Zhang B, et al. Proteogenomic characterization of human colon and rectal cancer. Nature. 2014;513:382–7.

40. Zhang H, et al. Integrated proteogenomic characterization of human high-grade serous ovarian cancer. Cell. 2016;166:755–65.

41. Rudnick PA, et al. A description of the clinical proteomic tumor analysis consortium (CPTAC) common data analysis pipeline. J Proteome Res. 2016;15:1023–32.

42. Tomasetti C, Vogelstein B, Parmigiani G. Half or more of the somatic mutations in cancers of self-renewing tissues originate prior to tumor initiation. Proc Natl Acad Sci. 2013;110:1999–2004.

43. Welch JS, et al. The origin and evolution of mutations in acute myeloid leukemia. Cell. 2012;150:264–78.

44. Kris MG, et al. Using multiplexed assays of oncogenic drivers in lung cancers to select targeted drugs. JAMA. 2014;311:1998–2006.

45. Munoz-Couselo E, Adelantado EZ, Ortiz C, Garcia JS, Perez-Garcia J. NRAS-mutant melanoma: current challenges and future prospect. Onco Targets Ther. 2017;10:3941–7.

46. Janku F, et al. PIK3CA mutation H1047R is associated with response to PI3K/AKT/mTOR signaling pathway inhibitors in early-phase clinical trials. Cancer Res. 2013;73:276–84.

47. Liao X, et al. Aspirin use, tumor PIK3CA mutation, and colorectal-cancer survival. N Engl J Med. 2012;367:1596–606.

48. Ye X, Wang J, Shi W, He J. Relationship between aspirin use after diagnosis of colorectal cancer and patient survival: a meta-analysis of observational studies. Br J Cancer. 2014;111:2172–9.

49. Lee JC, et al. Epidermal growth factor receptor activation in glioblastoma through novel missense mutations in the extracellular domain. PLoS Med. 2006;3:e485.

50. Peters S, Michielin O, Zimmermann S. Dramatic response induced by vemurafenib in a BRAF V600E-mutated lung adenocarcinoma. J Clin Oncol. 2013;31:e341–4.

51. Planchard D, et al. ASCO annual meeting proceedings, Vol. 31; 2013. p. 8009.

52. Amado RG, et al. Wild-type KRAS is required for panitumumab efficacy in patients with metastatic colorectal cancer. J Clin Oncol. 2008;26:1626–34.

53. Douillard J-Y, et al. Panitumumab–FOLFOX4 treatment and RAS mutations in colorectal cancer. N Engl J Med. 2013;369:1023–34.

54. Lim HY, et al. A phase II study of the efficacy and safety of the combination therapy of the MEK inhibitor refametinib (BAY 86-9766) plus sorafenib for Asian patients with unresectable hepatocellular carcinoma. Clin Cancer Res. 2014;20:5976–85.

55. Tolcher AW, et al. Antitumor activity in RAS-driven tumors by blocking AKT and MEK. Clin Cancer Res. 2015;21:739–48.

56. Sanz-Garcia E, Argiles G, Elez E, Tabernero J. BRAF mutant colorectal cancer: prognosis, treatment, and new perspectives. Ann Oncol. 2017;28:2648–57.

57. Watson IR, et al. The RAC1 P29S hotspot mutation in melanoma confers resistance to pharmacological inhibition of RAF. Cancer Res. 2014;74:4845–52.

58. Noeparast A, et al. Non-V600 BRAF mutations recurrently found in lung cancer predict sensitivity to the combination of Trametinib and Dabrafenib. Oncotarget. 2016;8(36):60094-108.

59. Paik S, Kim C, Wolmark N. HER2 status and benefit from adjuvant trastuzumab in breast cancer. N Engl J Med. 2008;358:1409–11.

60. Drebin JA, Link VC, Stern DF, Weinberg RA, Greene MI. Down-modulation of an oncogene protein product and reversion of the transformed phenotype by monoclonal antibodies. Cell. 1985;41:695–706.

61. Carter P, et al. Humanization of an anti-p185HER2 antibody for human cancer therapy. Proc Natl Acad Sci. 1992;89:4285–9.

62. Holst F, et al. Estrogen receptor alpha (ESR1) gene amplification is frequent in breast cancer. Nat Genet. 2007;39:655–60.

63. Badve SS, et al. Estrogen-and progesterone-receptor status in ECOG 2197: comparison of immunohistochemistry by local and central laboratories and quantitative reverse transcription polymerase chain reaction by central laboratory. J Clin Oncol. 2008;26:2473–81.

64. Kim C, et al. Estrogen receptor (ESR1) mRNA expression and benefit from tamoxifen in the treatment and prevention of estrogen receptor–positive breast cancer. J Clin Oncol. 2011;29:4160–7.

65. Clynes RA, Towers TL, Presta LG, Ravetch JV. Inhibitory Fc receptors modulate in vivo cytoxicity against tumor targets. Nat Med. 2000;6:443–6.

66. Hynes NE, Lane HA. ERBB receptors and cancer: the complexity of targeted inhibitors. Nat Rev Cancer. 2005;5:341–54.

67. Hayashi T, et al. Targeting HER2 with T-DM1, an antibody cytotoxic drug conjugate, is effective in HER2 over expressing bladder cancer. J Urol. 2015; 194:1120–31.

68. McGill R, Tukey JW, Larsen WA. Variations of box plots. Am Stat. 1978; 32:12–6.

69. Zhang X, et al. Fusion of EML4 and ALK is associated with development of lung adenocarcinomas lacking EGFR and KRAS mutations and is correlated with ALK expression. Mol Cancer. 2010;9:188.

70. Saunders LR, et al. A DLL3-targeted antibody-drug conjugate eradicates high-grade pulmonary neuroendocrine tumor-initiating cells in vivo. Sci Transl Med. 2015;7(302):302ra136.

71. Pietanza, M. et al. in European Journal of Cancer, Vol. 51 S712-S712 (Elsevier SCI Ltd the boulevard, Langford Lane, Kidlington, Oxford OX5 1GB, OXON, England, 2015).
72. Gucalp A, et al. Phase II trial of bicalutamide in patients with androgen receptor–positive, estrogen receptor–negative metastatic breast cancer. Clin Cancer Res. 2013;19:5505–12.
73. Li CI, Daling JR, Malone KE. Incidence of invasive breast cancer by hormone receptor status from 1992 to 1998. J Clin Oncol. 2003;21:28–34.
74. Bonner JA, et al. Radiotherapy plus cetuximab for squamous-cell carcinoma of the head and neck. N Engl J Med. 2006;354:567–78.
75. Kris MG, et al. Efficacy of gefitinib, an inhibitor of the epidermal growth factor receptor tyrosine kinase, in symptomatic patients with non–small cell lung cancer: a randomized trial. JAMA. 2003;290:2149–58.
76. Wakeling AE, et al. ZD1839 (Iressa) an orally active inhibitor of epidermal growth factor signaling with potential for cancer therapy. Cancer Res. 2002;62:5749–54.
77. Bukowski RM, et al. Randomized phase II study of erlotinib combined with bevacizumab compared with bevacizumab alone in metastatic renal cell cancer. J Clin Oncol. 2007;25:4536–41.
78. Dawson NA, et al. A phase II trial of gefitinib (Iressa, ZD1839) in stage IV and recurrent renal cell carcinoma. Clin Cancer Res. 2004;10:7812–9.
79. Rowinsky EK, et al. Safety, pharmacokinetics, and activity of ABX-EGF, a fully human anti–epidermal growth factor receptor monoclonal antibody in patients with metastatic renal cell cancer. J Clin Oncol. 2004;22:3003–15.
80. Dancey JE. Epidermal growth factor receptor and epidermal growth factor receptor therapies in renal cell carcinoma: do we need a better mouse trap? J Clin Oncol. 2004;22:2975–7.
81. Hechtman JF, et al. AKT1 E17K in colorectal carcinoma is associated with BRAF V600E but not MSI-H status: a clinicopathologic comparison to PIK3CA helical and kinase domain mutants. Mol Cancer Res. 2015;2015:0062.
82. Baselga J, et al. Everolimus in postmenopausal hormone-receptor–positive advanced breast cancer. N Engl J Med. 2012;366:520–9.
83. Yang W, et al. Genomics of Drug Sensitivity in Cancer (GDSC): a resource for therapeutic biomarker discovery in cancer cells. Nucleic Acids Res. 2013;41:D955–61.
84. Garnett MJ, et al. Systematic identification of genomic markers of drug sensitivity in cancer cells. Nature. 2012;483:570–5.
85. Barretina J, et al. The Cancer Cell Line Encyclopedia enables predictive modelling of anticancer drug sensitivity. Nature. 2012;483:603–7.
86. Janku F, et al. Assessing PIK3CA and PTEN in early-phase trials with PI3K/AKT/mTOR inhibitors. Cell Rep. 2014;6:377–87.
87. De Roock W, et al. Association of KRAS p. G13D mutation with outcome in patients with chemotherapy-refractory metastatic colorectal cancer treated with cetuximab. JAMA. 2010;304:1812–20.
88. Alizadeh AA, et al. Toward understanding and exploiting tumor heterogeneity. Nat Med. 2015;21:846–53.
89. Sottoriva A, et al. Intratumor heterogeneity in human glioblastoma reflects cancer evolutionary dynamics. Proc Natl Acad Sci. 2013;110:4009–14.
90. Gelmon KA, et al. Lapatinib or trastuzumab plus taxane therapy for human epidermal growth factor receptor 2-positive advanced breast cancer: final results of NCIC CTG MA. 31. J Clin Oncol. 2015;33:1574–83.
91. Azad NS, et al. Combination targeted therapy with sorafenib and bevacizumab results in enhanced toxicity and antitumor activity. J Clin Oncol. 2008;26:3709–14.
92. Long GV, et al. Combined BRAF and MEK inhibition versus BRAF inhibition alone in melanoma. N Engl J Med. 2014;371:1877–88.

11

Enabling multiplexed testing of pooled donor cells through whole-genome sequencing

Yingleong Chan[1,2]* (iD), Ying Kai Chan[1,2], Daniel B. Goodman[1,2,3], Xiaoge Guo[1,2], Alejandro Chavez[4], Elaine T. Lim[1,2] and George M. Church[1,2]*

Abstract

We describe a method that enables the multiplex screening of a pool of many different donor cell lines. Our method accurately predicts each donor proportion from the pool without requiring the use of unique DNA barcodes as markers of donor identity. Instead, we take advantage of common single nucleotide polymorphisms, whole-genome sequencing, and an algorithm to calculate the proportions from the sequencing data. By testing using simulated and real data, we showed that our method robustly predicts the individual proportions from a mixed-pool of numerous donors, thus enabling the multiplexed testing of diverse donor cells *en masse*.

Keywords: Multiplexed testing, Barcode free method, Single nucleotide polymorphisms, Expectation maximization algorithm, Next-generation sequencing, Personal Genome Project

Background

The screening of many cell lines for specific phenotypes is commonly performed to discover factors that confer donor cell specific effects. For example, several studies have employed the screening of multiple cancer cell lines for identifying cell type specific essential genes [1–3]. Other studies have also used primary cells from different donors to identify genetic variants associated with various cellular phenotypes. In one study, the authors reported six loci associated with immune response to pathogens by measuring cytokine production in peripheral blood mononuclear cells from hundreds of different donors [4]. Other groups measured the transcriptional response to pathogenic stimulus in primary monocytes obtained from many African and European individuals [5, 6]. In these studies, the experiments were performed on cells from each individual donor separately. However, with increasing numbers of donors, generating data from cells from more donors would require more research effort and time. As such, it would be advantageous to multiplex these assays by performing a single experiment on a pool of all donor cells and simultaneously retrieve phenotypic data from each donor.

To achieve this, one would require a method to accurately estimate the individual proportion of each donor from a pool of cells containing multiple donors. With such a method, one can perform a selection assay or perform fluorescence-activated cell sorting (FACS) to sort the pool of cells based on criteria of interest (e.g. response to pathogen, drug resistance, protein expression) and identify the proportion of every individual donor within this new pool (case group). A similar experiment can be performed for the control group, to identify the donor proportion either at baseline or from cells sorted with different criteria. The phenotype for an individual donor is then measured by comparing the difference in proportion between case and control groups (Fig. 1). A recent study aimed at discovering genotype-specific effects in a mixture of cancer cells reported a method (PRISM) that achieved this [7]. Briefly, PRISM uses a unique 24-nt barcode that was integrated into each donor cell line by lentiviral delivery before pooling. To obtain individual donor proportions, the barcodes were

---

* Correspondence: ychan@genetics.med.harvard.edu;
gchurch@genetics.med.harvard.edu
[1]Wyss Institute for Biologically Inspired Engineering, Harvard University, Boston, MA 02115, USA
Full list of author information is available at the end of the article

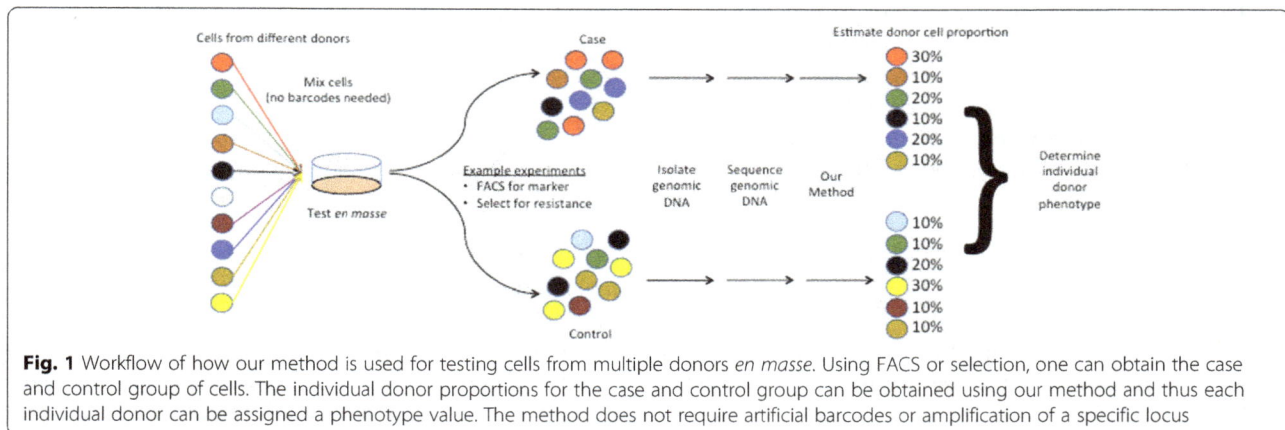

Fig. 1 Workflow of how our method is used for testing cells from multiple donors *en masse*. Using FACS or selection, one can obtain the case and control group of cells. The individual donor proportions for the case and control group can be obtained using our method and thus each individual donor can be assigned a phenotype value. The method does not require artificial barcodes or amplification of a specific locus

amplified using polymerase chain reaction (PCR) and sequenced by next-generation sequencing. Each individual donor proportion is then estimated by calculating the proportion of their corresponding barcodes from the sequenced reads. However, the PRISM method requires the barcoding of individual donor cells using lentiviral delivery, which is a tedious process because each lentiviral barcode has to be generated, applied to the donor cells, and selected for separately. Furthermore, primary cells, non-dividing cells, and cells with limited ability to be passaged in vitro cannot be effectively barcoded in this manner. Here, we describe a method that can accurately estimate each donor proportion in a mixed pool without the use of exogenous barcodes or amplification of a specific locus using PCR.

Our method harnesses the presence of millions of common single nucleotide polymorphisms (SNPs) within the human genome. These SNPs, which are usually bi-allelic, can be exploited as a natural barcode and are distributed throughout the entire genome. These SNPs are spaced relatively far apart, with approximately one common SNP for every 1000 base pairs in the human genome [8]. The genotypes of these SNPs for each donor are pre-determined before executing the method. These SNP genotypes can be easily acquired using whole-genome genotyping arrays or by performing whole-genome sequencing for each donor. While each individual SNP is not unique, the combination of SNPs throughout the genome is unique to each donor. However, PCR amplification and sequencing of any genomic locus is not adequate enough to cover enough SNPs to uniquely identify an individual donor. As such, our method overcomes this problem by using all the SNPs distributed throughout the host genome. Using the standard process of sequencing a human genome from a library of short DNA fragments, many of the short sequencing reads (200–300 bp) generated will cover a SNP in the human population [9]. Our method works

by first extracting genomic DNA from the mixed pool of cells and sequencing it. The method then employs an expectation–maximization (EM) algorithm that takes the genotypes for all the donors as well as the sequencing reads from the mixed pool as input to calculate the individual donor proportion. Using an iterative process, the algorithm determines the donor proportion that best matches the expected allelic fraction with the observed allelic fraction for all the SNPs analyzed.

In this study, we demonstrated the feasibility of our approach by designing simulation experiments to determine how well our method can accurately predict donor proportion. From simulation experiments, we tested a number of scenarios by varying the number of donors, number of SNPs as well as the sequencing read-depth per SNP. We found that in most cases, our method accurately predicts the donor proportion even at the lowest possible read-depth (1X) as long as a sufficient number of SNPs were analyzed (> 500,000 SNPs). Finally, we empirically tested our method by sequencing a mixed pool of human donor cells and demonstrate that our approach can accurately predict donor proportion within the mixed population.

Methods
EM algorithm for estimating proportion of individual donors within the pool
We first define θ as the probability or proportion of any individual donor, which is the probability that we are trying to estimate, i.e.

$$\theta = (P_1, P_2, P_3, ..., P_N)$$
$$\theta_n = P_n$$

where P_n is the probability or proportion of donor n within the pool of N donors, the sum of which is 1.

Next, we assume that we only analyze sequenced reads from autosomes and only at SNP positions that are known to be bi-allelic, i.e. having only two alleles, Reference (R) or Alternate (A), although the algorithm can be amended to consider X and/or Y chromosomes as well as also incorporating multiallelic polymorphisms. Given this, we define *Reads* as the number of sequence reads (read-depth) for each allele for each SNP, i.e.

$Reads_{m,R} = No.of\ observed\ reads\ with\ allele\ R\ at\ SNP\ position\ m$

$Reads_{m,A} = No.of\ observed\ reads\ with\ allele\ A\ at\ SNP\ position\ m$

where m is the index defining the SNP at that position.

Next, we assume that the genotypes for all bi-allelic SNPs analyzed for every donor is accurately known. As such, the genotype for each donor for each SNP can only be one of the following states: *RR*, *RA*, or *AA*, i.e.

$SNP_{m,\ n}$= genotype of donor n at SNP m *(RR, RA, or AA)*.

To estimate θ, we employ an EM algorithm and initialized the values of θ so that each donor has the same starting proportion or probability [10], i.e.

$$\theta_n^0 = 1\big/N$$

where θ_n^0 is the proportion or probability estimate of individual n at iteration *0*.

Next, we calculate the *Total* function for each SNP given θ, which is the expected number of R and A alleles given the current estimate of θ, i.e.

$$Total_{m,R} = \sum_{n=1}^{N} \begin{cases} \theta_n^t & if\ SNP_{m,n} = RR \\ 0.5 * \theta_n^t & if\ SNP_{m,n} = RA \\ 0 & if\ SNP_{m,n} = AA \end{cases}$$

$$Total_{m,A} = \sum_{n=1}^{N} \begin{cases} 0 & if\ SNP_{m,n} = RR \\ 0.5 * \theta_n^t & if\ SNP_{m,n} = RA \\ \theta_n^t & if\ SNP_{m,n} = AA \end{cases}$$

where m is the index for each SNP, R and A represent the respective alleles, and θ_n^t represents the current estimate of θ for individual n at the current iteration t.

Next, we calculate the likelihood function L for each individual given the current estimate of θ by going through all the SNPs (M being the total number of SNPs), i.e.

Finally, we re-estimate θ for each donor for the next iteration, i.e.

$$\theta_n^{t+1} = \frac{L_n}{\sum_{n=1}^{N} L_n}$$

This procedure is repeated until θ converges to a stable estimate, $t = 2000$. The final value of t can be adjusted depending on the number of donors and SNPs analyzed. For a sample size of ten donors, we used $t = 500$ as the last iteration. To help explain the algorithm, we provide a working example of estimating the proportion of a mixed pool of five donors (Additional file 1: Note S1). We also included a short description of how our method would be used in a real experimental setting by comparing our method against the lentiviral barcoding method (PRISM) used in Yu et al. [7] (Additional file 1: Note S2).

Simulating individual donors in a mixed pool and estimating their proportions using the EM algorithm

Individuals were simulated by first defining the value of several variables, namely,

1) N, the total number of individual donors;
2) M, the total number of SNPs;
3) X, the read-depth (coverage) for every SNP.

First, a total of M SNPs were simulated by randomly assigning a minor allele frequency (MAF) by drawing from a uniform distribution in the range of 5–50%.

$MAF_m = random\ number\ between\ 5\%\ and\ 50\%$

Next, genotypes for each SNP were randomly assigned according to their MAF to each of the N donors, i.e. for any donor at any SNP with a MAF of f, the probability of having a genotype of *RR*, *RA*, and *AA* is f^2, $2f(1-f)$, and $(1-f)^2$, respectively.

Next, each individual was randomly assigned a copy-number count ($Donor_n$) by drawing from a uniform distribution in the range of 1–10,000 to represent the true number of copies of that donor.

$$L_n = \sum_{m=1}^{M} \begin{cases} \dfrac{\theta_n^t}{Total_{m,R}} * Reads_{m,R} & if\ SNP_{m,n} = RR \\[3ex] 0.5\left(\dfrac{\theta_n^t}{Total_{m,R}} * Reads_{m,R} + \dfrac{\theta_n^t}{Total_{m,A}} * Reads_{m,A}\right) & if\ SNP_{m,n} = RA \\[3ex] \dfrac{\theta_n^t}{Total_{m,A}} * Reads_{m,A} & if\ SNP_{m,n} = AA \end{cases}$$

$Donor_n = random\ number\ between\ 1\ and\ 10,000$

The true proportion for each donor (θ_n) was then calculated by taking their copy-number count divided by the sum of all the copy-number for all donors.

$$\theta_n = \frac{Donor_n}{\sum\limits_{n=1}^{N} Donor_n}$$

The sequencing-reads were then simulated by randomly drawing X number of alleles from a binomial distribution where the probability of drawing the R allele for that SNP ($P_{m,R}$) is the sum of the true proportion multiplied by the likelihood for drawing the R allele given the genotype for that individual, i.e.

$$P_{m,R} = \sum_{n=1}^{N} \begin{cases} \theta_n & if\ SNP_{m,n} = RR \\ 0.5 * \theta_n & if\ SNP_{m,n} = RA \\ 0 & if\ SNP_{m,n} = AA \end{cases}$$

The simulation can also be done with regards to the A allele by changing the above equation or subtracting from 1 the probability of drawing the R allele.

$$P_{m,A} = 1 - P_{m,R}$$

Nonetheless, if the random draw for the read fails to draw the R allele, it will be assigned the A allele and vice versa. The simulated alleles and SNP genotypes for all N individuals are then used as inputs to the EM algorithm to estimate the individual donor proportion. The estimated proportion is then compared to the true proportion and the accuracy of the prediction is evaluated using the Pearson correlation coefficient (represented as R).

Pooling B-lymphocytes from Personal Genome Project samples

B-lymphocytes from the Harvard Personal Genome Project (PGP) were obtained from the NIGMS Human Genetic Cell Repository at the Coriell Institute for Medical Research (https://www.coriell.org). To create the initial pool of donor cells, we used five distinct pools of B-lymphocytes previously mixed together at approximately equal numbers (Invitrogen Countess) and kept cryopreserved in liquid nitrogen. The five pools of frozen cells were resuscitated and grown overnight separately in upright T25 flasks in a standard incubator at 37 °C with 15 mL of growth media upright (Thermofisher, RPMI 1640 Medium, GlutaMAX™ Supplement, HEPES + 10% fetal bovine serum + 1% Penicillin-Streptomycin [10,000 U/mL]). The pools of cells were counted (Invitrogen Countess) and cells were taken from Pool 1, Pool 2, Pool 3, Pool 4, and Pool 5 at increments of 100,000 cells, i.e. 100,000 cells were taken from Pool 1, 200,000 cells were taken from Pool 2, ... and 500,000 cells were taken from Pool 5. The cells were mixed together to form the final pool. To create the subsequent (more accurate) pool of donor cells, a different set of 50 donor cells were resuscitated and cultured for five days separately in 24-well plates in a standard incubator at 37 °C with 0.5 mL of growth media (Thermofisher, RPMI 1640 Medium, GlutaMAX™ Supplement, HEPES + 10% fetal bovine serum + 1% Penicillin-Streptomycin [10,000 U/mL]). On the day of cell sorting, each donor cell was collected in 1.5-mL micro-centrifuge tubes and resuspended in 0.5 mL of Dulbecco's Phosphate Buffered Saline (DPBS) solution. The donor cells were then sorted into a single 15-mL conical centrifuge tube containing 5 mL of DPBS (Sony SH800S Cell Sorter). Ten different donors were selected for each of the five pools and 10,000, 20,000, 30,000, 40,000, and 50,000 events were used to sort donors representing pools 1, 2, 3, 4, and 5, respectively.

DNA extraction, library preparation, and sequencing

Genomic DNA of the initial pool was extracted using the QIAamp DNA FFPE Tissue Kit (QIAGEN). Genomic DNA of the subsequent pool was extracted using the AccuPrep Genomic DNA extraction kit (BioNEER). The extracted genomic DNA of both pools were submitted to Biopolymers facility at Harvard Medical School (https://genome.med.harvard.edu/) for genomic DNA library preparation (Genomic-Seq Wafergen) and subsequent next-generation sequencing using Illumina MiSeq. The DNA from the initial pool resulted in 5,112,179 paired sequencing reads while the DNA from the subsequent pool resulted in 13,111,543 paired sequencing reads that mapped to the human genome. The reads were aligned to the human genome reference sequence (GRCh37/hg19) using bwa (version 0.7.8-r566) [11].

SNP identification

Whole-genome sequencing information was available for all 102 PGP samples (Complete Genomics) and the genotypes of all bi-allelic SNPs within the autosomes were recorded. We compared the sequencing reads with the recorded SNPs to determine the allele for each SNP sequenced. The final alignment of the sequencing reads for the initial pool resulted in the sequencing of 1,425,723 SNPs at 1.16X coverage while the subsequent pool resulted in the sequencing of 1,988,295 SNPs at 1.23X coverage.

Results

An algorithm that accurately predicts the proportion of individuals within a simulated mixed pool

To test the efficacy of our algorithm, we designed and implemented a simulation program to generate simulated data for testing the robustness of the prediction given the number of donors, number of SNPs as well as sequencing read-depth. Taking these parameters as input, the program first randomly simulates the true proportion for each donor within the mixed pool. Next, it generates genotypes for all SNPs and donors by simulating SNPs with MAF randomly selected in the range of 5–50%. Finally, for each SNP, it stochastically samples the number of each of the alleles under a probabilistic model that reflects the true donor proportion according to the assigned read-depth. The program then applies our algorithm on the simulated data to determine how accurately it can predict the individual donor proportion (see "Methods").

Using our program, we first simulated two sets of ten diploid individuals with similar proportions, the first (set A) having genotypes from 500 SNPs with sequencing read-depth (coverage) of 1000X while the second (set B) having genotypes from 500,000 SNPs but with sequencing read-depth of only 1X (Additional file 2: Table S1). We ran the algorithm to estimate the individual proportions given the simulated sequencing reads and genotypes of the individuals for both sets and found that the prediction converges to a fixed estimate (Fig. 2a, b) and accurately predicted the real simulated proportion for

both set A and set B (Fig. 2c, Additional file 2: Table S2). This result shows that the algorithm is as effective on high coverage sequencing data across a small number of SNPs compared with low-coverage sequencing data across a much larger number of SNPs.

Testing the algorithm on simulated mixed pools by varying the sample size, number of SNPs, and sequencing read-depth

To test how the number of SNPs and read-depth (coverage) would scale with increased sample size, we perform simulations on pools of 100, 500, and 1000 different donors, using 500,000 SNPs with 1X, 10X, and 30X coverage. For a pool of 100 donors, we obtained Pearson correlation coefficients of 0.956, 0.994, and 0.998 for 1X, 10X, and 30X coverage respectively, demonstrating that under these circumstances, low-coverage sequencing data would be sufficient to accurately predict individual donor proportion (Fig. 3a–c, Additional file 2: Table S3). With a pool of 500 donors, the algorithm produced Pearson correlation coefficients of 0.511, 0.877, and 0. 947 for 1X, 10X, and 30X coverage, respectively, indicating a drop in prediction accuracy with increased sample size (Fig. 3d–f). Finally, when the number of donors was

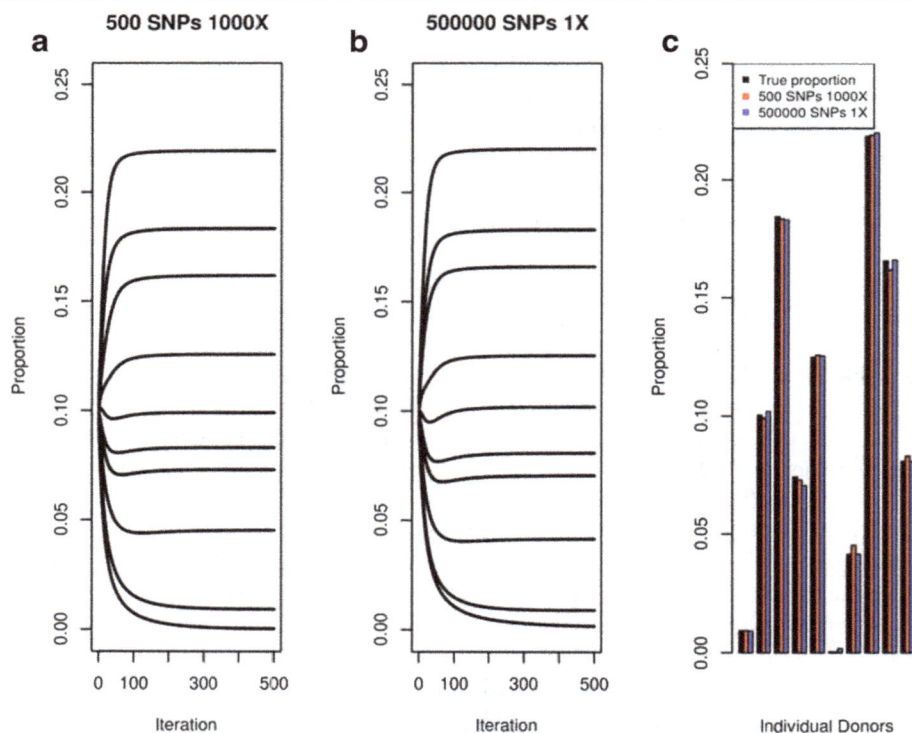

Fig. 2 Estimating the proportions of ten simulated donor individuals. Showing the results of simulating (**a**) deep-coverage sequencing (1000X) on a small number (500) of SNPs and (**b**) low-coverage sequencing (1X) on many (500,000) SNPs. Both graph shows the estimated proportion (*y-axis*) by the algorithm at every iteration (*x-axis*). **c** *Bar plot* comparing the estimated proportion against the true proportion for both set A and set B after 500 iterations. The *black bars* represent the true proportion for each simulated donor, while the *red* and *blue* bars represent the estimated proportion of set A and set B, respectively

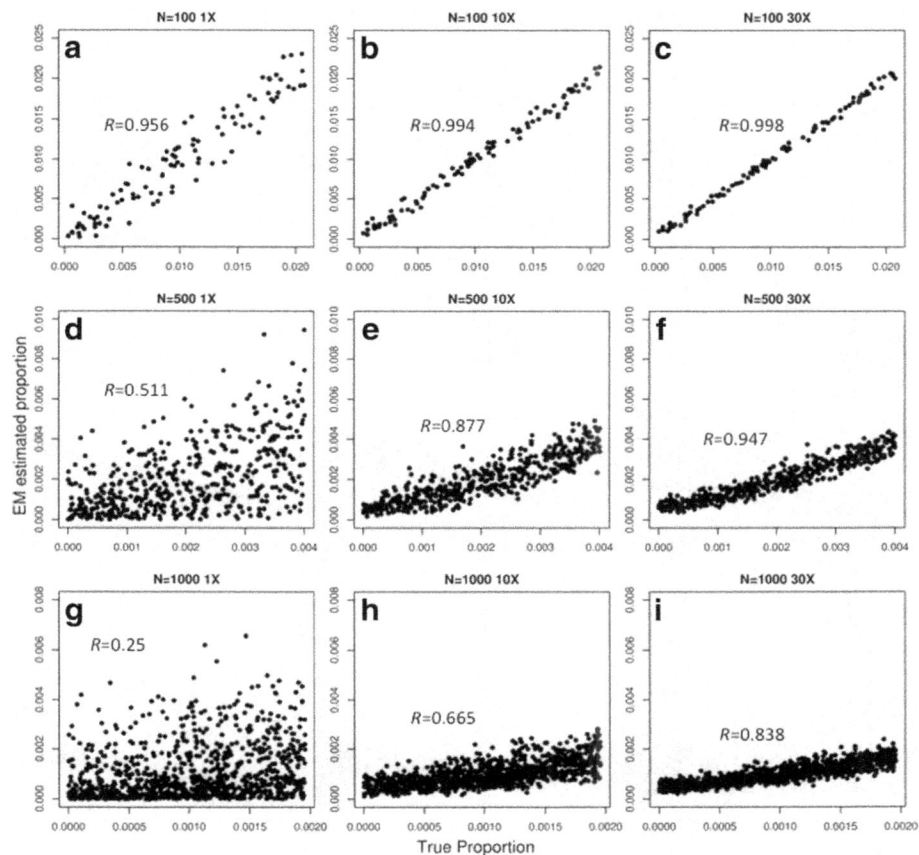

Fig. 3 Comparing the true proportions with the estimated proportions of varying number of simulated donor individuals by simulating 500,000 SNPs at varying coverage. The x-axis represents the true simulated proportion while the y-axis represents the estimated proportion by our algorithm (EM estimated proportion). **a** 100 donors at 1X coverage. **b** 100 donors at 10X coverage. **c** 100 donors at 30X coverage. **d** 500 donors at 1X coverage. **e** 500 donors at 10X coverage. **f** 500 donors at 30X coverage. **g** 1000 donors at 1X coverage. **h** 1000 donors at 10X coverage. **i** 1000 donors at 30X coverage. R represents the Pearson-correlation coefficient of comparing the true proportions with the estimated proportions

increased to 1000, the accuracy further declined for 1X, 10X, and 30X coverage (R = 0.25, 0.665, and 0.838, respectively) (Fig. 3g–i). These results show that by analyzing 500,000 SNPs positions, the algorithm can accurately estimate pools of 100 different donors at any read-depth but higher read-depths would be required to accurately estimate donor proportion for pools with substantially more donors.

To determine if the accuracy of the algorithm increases with the use of more SNPs in the analysis, we repeated the simulation experiments using 1,000,000 SNPs. Indeed, when we doubled the number of SNPs, the accuracy for all the simulation experiments increased when compared to their previous counterpart (Fig. 4, Additional file 2: Table S4). This suggests that even for a pool of > 100 donors, sequencing more SNPs in general increases the accuracy of the prediction. Based on these results, we tabulated the minimal read-depth required to obtain an accurate prediction with Pearson correlation coefficient ≥ 0.9 (Table 1).

The method accurately predicts the donor proportions of a mixed pool of actual human donor cells

To test if our method can accurately estimate the proportions of actual human donor samples, we set up a system using a pool of immortalized B-lymphocytes from the Harvard PGP [12–14]. We combined five pools of PGP B-lymphocytes with ten individuals per pool at 1X, 2X, 3X, 4X, and 5X concentration, respectively (see "Methods"). We extracted genomic DNA from the pool of B-lymphocytes and subjected the DNA to low-coverage whole-genome sequencing which resulted in the sequencing of 1,425,723 SNPs at 1.16X coverage. Using our method, we estimated the individual proportion of donors within the pool of 102 PGP individuals, including 52 donors that were not part of the combined pool and acted as negative controls. We found that the method predicted the proportion of the individuals within the pool (Fig. 5, Additional file 2: Table S5). The results showed that pool 0, which consists of the 52 individuals not part of the combined pool, had very low

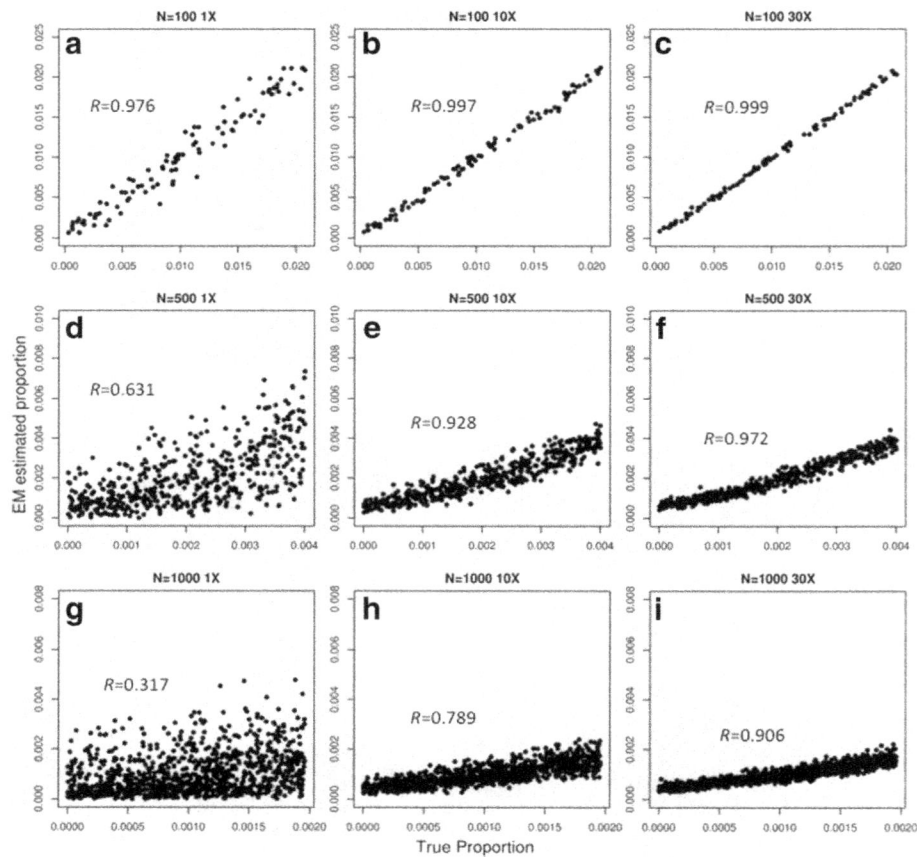

Fig. 4 Comparing the true proportions with the estimated proportions of varying number of simulated donor individuals by simulating 1,000,000 SNPs at varying coverage. The x-axis represents the true simulated proportion while the y-axis represents the estimated proportion by our algorithm (EM estimated proportion). **a** 100 donors at 1X coverage. **b** 100 donors at 10X coverage. **c** 100 donors at 30X coverage. **d** 500 donors at 1X coverage. **e** 500 donors at 10X coverage. **f** 500 donors at 30X coverage. **g** 1000 donors at 1X coverage. **h** 1000 donors at 10X coverage. **i** 1000 donors at 30X coverage. R represents the Pearson-correlation coefficient of comparing the true proportions with the estimated proportions

estimated proportions, with a mean proportion of 0.07% and none of the 52 samples had proportions > 0.18%. In contrast, pools 1–5 gave mean estimated proportions of 0.57%, 1.08%, 1.87%, 2.8%, and 3.35%, respectively, which accurately reflected the expected proportions (expected proportions being 0.67%, 1.33%, 2%, 2.67%, and 3.33%, respectively).

The initial pools had undergone a few rounds of passaging and they were created using a relatively inaccurate method for counting cells (Invitrogen Countess).

Table 1 Minimal read-depth required for accurate prediction of donor proportion

	500,000 SNPs	1,000,000 SNPs
100 donors	1X	1X
500 donors	30X	10X
1000 donors	>30X	30X

The read-depth necessary to obtain an accurate prediction of donor proportion with Pearson correlation coefficient > 0.9 for a mix pool of 100, 500, and 1000 unique donors when 500,000 and 1,000,000 SNPs are analyzed with our method

Because of this, it is expected that the predicted individual proportions within each pool will vary greatly. We decided to repeat the experiment but with a more accurate way of determining the actual donor proportion before sequencing. Instead of using the pre-pooled cells, we chose a different set of 50 different donor cell lines to culture individually. We then sorted each donor cells using a cell sorter by assigning the number of live cell events (either 10,000, 20,000, 30,000, 40,000, or 50,000) for each donor to create the new pools (pools 1–5) (see "Methods"). Although there was a single outlier in pool 4 (hu52F345), we found that our method accurately predicted the proportion of the individuals within the pool (Fig. 6, Additional file 2: Table S6). The ranges of proportions for the different pools are as follows: pool 0 (0.00–0.16%); pool 1 (0.41–1%); pool 2 (1.11–1.4%); pool 3 (1.75–2.19%); pool 4 (2.41–3.99%); pool 5 (2.87–3.26%) (Additional file 2: Table S6). We observed that pools 0–5 gave mean estimated proportions of 0.03%, 0.6%, 1.29%, 1.99%, 2.84%, and 3.08%, respectively, which

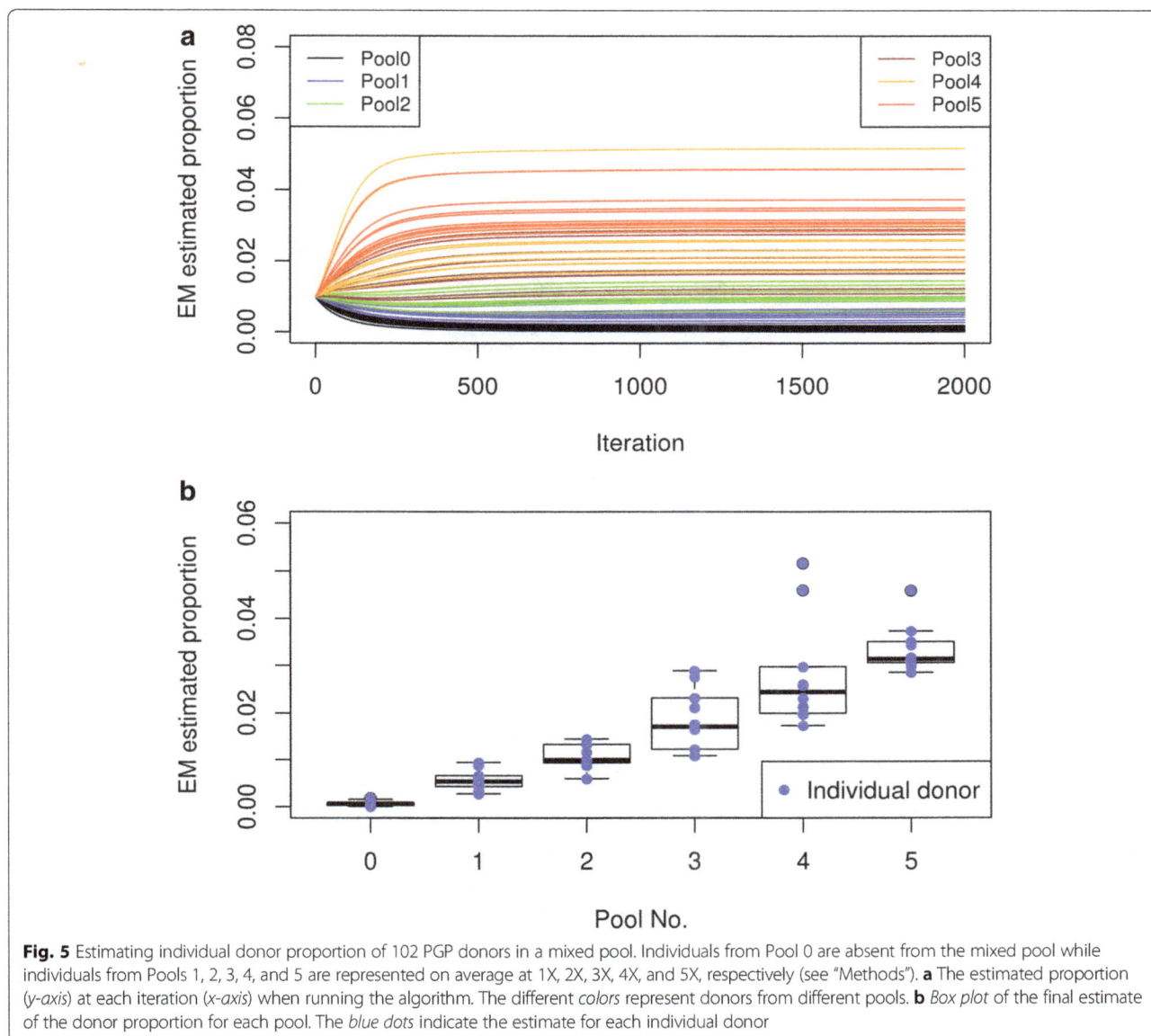

Fig. 5 Estimating individual donor proportion of 102 PGP donors in a mixed pool. Individuals from Pool 0 are absent from the mixed pool while individuals from Pools 1, 2, 3, 4, and 5 are represented on average at 1X, 2X, 3X, 4X, and 5X, respectively (see "Methods"). **a** The estimated proportion (*y-axis*) at each iteration (*x-axis*) when running the algorithm. The different *colors* represent donors from different pools. **b** *Box plot* of the final estimate of the donor proportion for each pool. The *blue dots* indicate the estimate for each individual donor

accurately reflected their actual proportions (expected proportions being 0%, 0.67%, 1.33%, 2%, 2.67%, and 3. 33%). Taken together, our results demonstrate that our method can accurately predict the proportions of real samples where the donor genotypes are known through whole-genome sequencing or otherwise.

Discussion

Various ways of pooling and sequencing DNA from multiple individuals in an effort to save costs in identifying genetic variants associated with disease status have been extensively investigated in genome-wide association studies [15]. Here, we propose a radically different use of whole-genome sequencing of pools of individuals: to enable the accurate prediction of individual donor proportion of a mixed pool of human tissue samples or cell lines. Human tissue samples and cell lines are the bedrock of biomedical research and their uses have been vital for many scientific discoveries. More recently, the development of induced pluripotent stem cells (iPSCs) derived from human tissue have allowed researchers to model a variety of cell types from any given patient [16–18]. Hence, technologies that improve our capability to perform high-throughput assays for phenotypes from cell lines will be increasingly more important, especially in the age of personalized medicine.

We described a method, which can accurately predict the individual donor proportion of a mixed pool of samples from many different donors without the need for artificial barcodes or amplification of a specific locus.

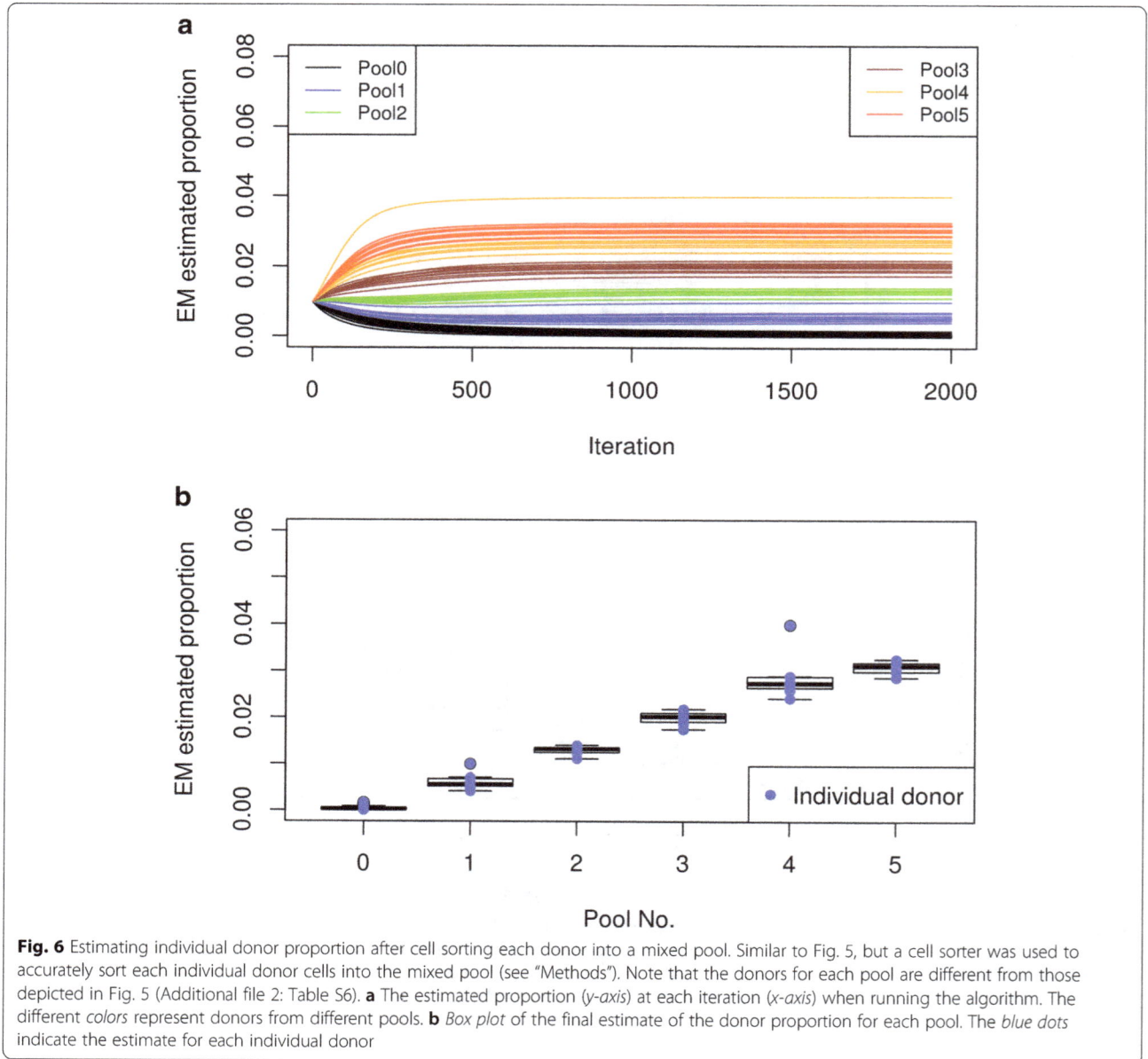

Fig. 6 Estimating individual donor proportion after cell sorting each donor into a mixed pool. Similar to Fig. 5, but a cell sorter was used to accurately sort each individual donor cells into the mixed pool (see "Methods"). Note that the donors for each pool are different from those depicted in Fig. 5 (Additional file 2: Table S6). **a** The estimated proportion (*y-axis*) at each iteration (*x-axis*) when running the algorithm. The different *colors* represent donors from different pools. **b** *Box plot* of the final estimate of the donor proportion for each pool. The *blue dots* indicate the estimate for each individual donor

Depending on the host and cell type, introducing artificial barcodes to every donor cell may not be practical or feasible to perform for large numbers of different donors. Also, PCR amplification of exogenous barcodes may potentially bias the results, as demonstrated by previous experiments when performed on mixtures of template DNA [19–22]. The use our method avoids the need to barcode every donor cell or PCR amplification of a specific locus.

As our method effectively uses many SNPs present in the host genome as input to identify donor proportion, it is not suitable for applications where such SNPs are not present. For example, previous research reported the use of 20-nt barcodes to simultaneously create and tag a library of yeast deletion mutants using mitotic recombination for high-throughput multiplex assays [23, 24]. The library of deletion mutants was created from cells from a single donor and our method would not be able to differentiate between different deletion mutants as their genome-wide SNP profile are identical. On the other hand, when multiple donor cells are used like the study that interrogated multiple cancer cell lines from different donors [7], our method would be highly effective for identifying the proportion of different donor cells without the need for DNA barcodes. Our method can also be adjusted for parallel model organism screens, i.e. pooling of cells from different organisms to be interrogated together. If the genomes of the organisms are different enough, the problem becomes trivial, as it is possible to determine the origin of each of the sequencing reads by alignment to the right host genome. However, if the genomes of the various model organisms were similar, the main genetic difference between them may not be SNPs but other polymorphisms such as insertion-deletion polymorphisms. We can incorporate these polymorphisms or other types of genetic variants into our method for such use.

Experimentally, all that is required is genomic DNA extraction and whole-genome sequencing of the extracted DNA. The prediction of individual donor proportion is then determined computationally. Our described method enables the multiplexing of phenotypic assays on multiple different donor samples in a single experiment, which significantly reduces effort and time and facilitate discoveries. Our method can be used for high-throughput measurements of various cellular phenotypes for the purpose of discovering genetic alleles associated with cellular phenotypes, similar to those performed on human traits and diseases obtained from medical record data [25–30]. While there are substantially fewer such studies of cellular phenotypes, we predict that our method would greatly accelerate such discoveries of cellular phenotypes by facilitating and enabling researchers to perform multiplexed testing of diverse donor cells *en masse*. Whether the cells are sorted via FACS or selected for via different growth conditions, the resulting proportion for each donor within the sorted or selected pool can be accurately estimated using our method, resulting in the simultaneous testing of numerous different donor cells in a single experiment (Fig. 1). Current work in our laboratory is focused on utilizing this method to perform multiple phenotype characterization on thousands of cell lines from PGP and other cohorts to uncover genetic alleles associated with these phenotypes. We have also made the software for estimating donor proportion as well as performing the simulation experiments freely available (see "Availability of data and material") so that other groups can harness our method for their research experiments as well

Conclusions

In summary, we have developed a method to accurately predict the individual proportion from a mixed pool of cells from different donors without artificial barcodes or amplification of a specific locus. The method enables the simultaneous testing of cells from a pool of different donors and is transformative for scaling up the number of donor samples used. Instead of performing lentiviral barcoding manually for each donor sample, our method relies on having whole-genome genotype information for each donor, which is now readily available for many samples. Our method lowers the costs and associated resources for performing such experiments and would help facilitate multiplexed experimentation on large cohorts of donor cells.

Abbreviations
EM: Expectation-maximization; FACS: Fluorescence-activated cell sorting; MAF: Minor allele frequency; PGP: Personal Genome Project; SNP: Single nucleotide polymorphism

Acknowledgements
We thank all the participants of the Harvard PGP for contributing cell lines and whole-genome sequencing data. We thank all staff members of the PGP for their effort in creating and maintaining the PGP. We also like to thank the Wyss Institute for Biologically Inspired Engineering for providing the necessary resources for performing cell sorting as well as general laboratory supplies for carrying out the research.

Funding
AC was funded by the Burroughs Wellcome Fund Career Award for Medical Scientists. This work was funded by grant NIH RM1HG008525 from the National Human Genome Research Institute, NIH, and the Robert Wood Johnson Foundation (grant: 74178). The views expressed here do not necessarily reflect the views of the Foundation.

Authors' contributions
YC, DBG, ETL, and GMC conceptualized the study. YC, YKC, DBG, XG, AC, and ETL performed the experiments. YC wrote the code for simulation and analysis of data. YC, YKC, and ETL wrote the initial manuscript. DBG, AC, and GMC provided critical feedback on the manuscript. GMC supervised project. All authors edited and reviewed the manuscript. All authors read and approved the final manuscript.

Competing interests
GMC holds leadership positions in many companies related to DNA sequencing technologies. A full list of these companies is available at http://arep.med.harvard.edu/gmc/tech.html. The remaining authors declare that they have no competing interests.

Author details
[1]Wyss Institute for Biologically Inspired Engineering, Harvard University, Boston, MA 02115, USA. [2]Department of Genetics, Harvard Medical School, Boston, MA 02115, USA. [3]Harvard-MIT Health Sciences and Technology, Cambridge, MA 02139, USA. [4]Department of Pathology and Cell Biology, Columbia University College of Physicians and Surgeons, New York, NY 10032, USA.

References
1. Cheung HW, Cowley GS, Weir BA, Boehm JS, Rusin S, Scott JA, et al. Systematic investigation of genetic vulnerabilities across cancer cell lines reveals lineage-specific dependencies in ovarian cancer. Proc Natl Acad Sci. 2011;108:12372–7.
2. Marcotte R, Brown KR, Suarez F, Sayad A, Karamboulas K, Krzyzanowski PM, et al. Essential gene profiles in breast, pancreatic, and ovarian cancer cells. Cancer Discov. 2012;2:172–89.
3. Cowley GS, Weir BA, Vazquez F, Tamayo P, Scott JA, Rusin S, et al. Parallel genome-scale loss of function screens in 216 cancer cell lines for the identification of context-specific genetic dependencies. Sci Data. 2014;1: 140035.
4. Li Y, Oosting M, Deelen P, Ricaño-Ponce I, Smeekens S, Jaeger M, et al. Inter-individual variability and genetic influences on cytokine responses to bacteria and fungi. Nat Med. 2016;22:952–60.

5. Quach H, Rotival M, Pothlichet J, Loh Y-HE, Dannemann M, Zidane N, et al. Genetic adaptation and neandertal admixture shaped the immune system of human populations. Cell. 2016;167:643–656.e17.

6. Nédélec Y, Sanz J, Baharian G, Szpiech ZA, Pacis A, Dumaine A, et al. Genetic ancestry and natural selection drive population differences in immune responses to pathogens. Cell. 2016;167:657–669.e21.

7. Yu C, Mannan AM, Yvone GM, Ross KN, Zhang Y-L, Marton MA, et al. High-throughput identification of genotype-specific cancer vulnerabilities in mixtures of barcoded tumor cell lines. Nat Biotechnol. 2016;34:419–23.

8. Abecasis GR, Auton A, Brooks LD, DePristo MA, Durbin RM, Handsaker RE, et al. An integrated map of genetic variation from 1,092 human genomes. Nature. 2012;491:56–65.

9. Bentley DR, Balasubramanian S, Swerdlow HP, Smith GP, Milton J, Brown CG, et al. Accurate whole human genome sequencing using reversible terminator chemistry. Nature. 2008;456:53–9.

10. Dempster AP, Laird NM, Rubin DB. Maximum likelihood from incomplete data via the EM algorithm. J R Stat Soc Ser B Methodol. 1977;39:1–38.

11. Li H. Aligning sequence reads, clone sequences and assembly contigs with BWA-MEM. 2013. http://arxiv.org/abs/1303.3997. ArXiv13033997 Q-Bio.

12. Ball MP, Thakuria JV, Zaranek AW, Clegg T, Rosenbaum AM, Wu X, et al. A public resource facilitating clinical use of genomes. Proc Natl Acad Sci. 2012; 109:11920–7.

13. Ball MP, Bobe JR, Chou MF, Clegg T, Estep PW, Lunshof JE, et al. Harvard Personal Genome Project: lessons from participatory public research. Genome Med. 2014;6:10.

14. Chan Y, Tung M, Garruss AS, Zaranek SW, Chan YK, Lunshof JE, et al. An unbiased index to quantify participant's phenotypic contribution to an open-access cohort. Sci Rep. 2017;7:46148.

15. Schlötterer C, Tobler R, Kofler R, Nolte V. Sequencing pools of individuals — mining genome-wide polymorphism data without big funding. Nat Rev Genet. 2014;15:749.

16. Burkhardt MF, Martinez FJ, Wright S, Ramos C, Volfson D, Mason M, et al. A cellular model for sporadic ALS using patient-derived induced pluripotent stem cells. Mol Cell Neurosci. 2013;56:355–64.

17. Millman JR, Xie C, Dervort AV, Gürtler M, Pagliuca FW, Melton DA. Generation of stem cell-derived β-cells from patients with type 1 diabetes. Nat Commun. 2016;7:11463.

18. Middelkamp S, van Heesch S, Braat AK, de Ligt J, van Iterson M, Simonis M, et al. Molecular dissection of germline chromothripsis in a developmental context using patient-derived iPS cells. Genome Med. 2017;9:9.

19. Polz MF, Cavanaugh CM. Bias in template-to-product ratios in multitemplate PCR. Appl Environ Microbiol. 1998;64:3724–30.

20. Hansen MC, Tolker-Nielsen T, Givskov M, Molin S. Biased 16S rDNA PCR amplification caused by interference from DNA flanking the template region. FEMS Microbiol Ecol. 1998;26:141–9.

21. Schloss PD, Gevers D, Westcott SL. Reducing the effects of PCR amplification and sequencing artifacts on 16S rRNA-based studies. PLoS One. 2011;6:e27310.

22. Kalle E, Kubista M, Rensing C. Multi-template polymerase chain reaction. Biomol Detect Quantif. 2014;2:11–29.

23. Pierce SE, Davis RW, Nislow C, Giaever G. Genome-wide analysis of barcoded *Saccharomyces cerevisiae* gene-deletion mutants in pooled cultures. Nat Protoc. 2007;2:2958.

24. Smith AM, Heisler LE, Mellor J, Kaper F, Thompson MJ, Chee M, et al. Quantitative phenotyping via deep barcode sequencing. Genome Res. 2009; 19:1836–42.

25. Wood AR, Esko T, Yang J, Vedantam S, Pers TH, Gustafsson S, et al. Defining the role of common variation in the genomic and biological architecture of adult human height. Nat Genet. 2014;46:1173–86.

26. Locke AE, Kahali B, Berndt SI, Justice AE, Pers TH, Day FR, et al. Genetic studies of body mass index yield new insights for obesity biology. Nature. 2015;518:197–206.

27. Chan Y, Salem RM, Hsu Y-HH, McMahon G, Pers TH, Vedantam S, et al. Genome-wide analysis of body proportion classifies height-associated variants by mechanism of action and implicates genes important for skeletal development. Am J Hum Genet. 2015;96:695–708.

28. Lim ET, Raychaudhuri S, Sanders SJ, Stevens C, Sabo A, MacArthur DG, et al. Rare complete knockouts in humans: population distribution and significant role in autism spectrum disorders. Neuron. 2013;77:235–42.

29. Lim ET, Liu YP, Chan Y, Tiinamaija T, Käräjämäki A, Madsen E, et al. A novel test for recessive contributions to complex diseases implicates Bardet-Biedl syndrome gene BBS10 in idiopathic type 2 diabetes and obesity. Am J Hum Genet. 2014;95:509–20.

30. Lim ET, Uddin M, De Rubeis S, Chan Y, Kamumbu AS, Zhang X, et al. Rates, distribution and implications of postzygotic mosaic mutations in autism spectrum disorder. Nat Neurosci. 2017;20:1217–24.

12

Footprints of antigen processing boost MHC class II natural ligand predictions

Carolina Barra[1†] ⓘ, Bruno Alvarez[1†], Sinu Paul[2], Alessandro Sette[2], Bjoern Peters[2], Massimo Andreatta[1], Søren Buus[3] and Morten Nielsen[1,4*]

Abstract

Background: Major histocompatibility complex class II (MHC-II) molecules present peptide fragments to T cells for immune recognition. Current predictors for peptide to MHC-II binding are trained on binding affinity data, generated in vitro and therefore lacking information about antigen processing.

Methods: We generate prediction models of peptide to MHC-II binding trained with naturally eluted ligands derived from mass spectrometry in addition to peptide binding affinity data sets.

Results: We show that integrated prediction models incorporate identifiable rules of antigen processing. In fact, we observed detectable signals of protease cleavage at defined positions of the ligands. We also hypothesize a role of the length of the terminal ligand protrusions for trimming the peptide to the MHC presented ligand.

Conclusions: The results of integrating binding affinity and eluted ligand data in a combined model demonstrate improved performance for the prediction of MHC-II ligands and T cell epitopes and foreshadow a new generation of improved peptide to MHC-II prediction tools accounting for the plurality of factors that determine natural presentation of antigens.

Keywords: MHC-II, Binding predictions, Eluted ligands, T cell epitope, Neural networks, Antigen processing, Machine learning, Mass spectrometry

Background

Major histocompatibility complex class II (MHC-II) molecules play a central role in the immune system of vertebrates. MHC-II present exogenous, digested peptide fragments on the surface of antigen-presenting cells, forming peptide-MHC-II complexes (pMHCII). On the cell surface, these pMHCII complexes are scrutinized, and if certain stimulatory conditions are met, a T helper lymphocyte may recognize the pMHCII and initiate an immune response [1].

The precise rules of MHC class II antigen presentation are influenced by many factors including internalization and digestion of extracellular proteins, the peptide binding motif specific for each MHC class II molecule, and the transport and surface half-life of the pMHCIIs. The

---
* Correspondence: mniel@bioinformatics.dtu.dk
†Carolina Barra and Bruno Alvarez contributed equally to this work.
[1]Instituto de Investigaciones Biotecnológicas, Universidad Nacional de San Martín, CP1650 San Martín, Argentina
[4]Department of Bio and Health Informatics, Technical University of Denmark, DK-2800 Kgs. Lyngby, Denmark
Full list of author information is available at the end of the article

MHC-II binding groove, unlike MHC class I, is open at both ends. This attribute facilitates peptide protrusion out of the groove, thereby allowing longer peptides (and potentially whole proteins) to be loaded onto MHC-II molecules [2, 3]. Peptide binding to MHC-II is mainly determined by interactions within the peptide binding groove, which most commonly encompass a peptide with a consecutive stretch of nine amino acids [4]. Ligand residues protruding from either side of the MHC binding groove are commonly known as peptide flanking regions (PFRs). The PFRs are variable in length and composition and affect both the peptide MHC-II binding [5] and the subsequent interaction with T cells [6–8]. The open characteristic of the MHC-II binding groove does not constrain the peptides to a certain length, thereby increasing the diversity of sequences that a given MHC-II molecule can present. Also, MHC-II molecules are highly polymorphic, and their binding motifs have appeared to be more degenerate than MHC-I motifs [9–11].

Considering all the aspects mentioned above, MHC-II motif characterization and rational identification of MHC-II ligands and epitopes is a highly challenging and costly endeavor. Because MHC-II is a crucial player in the exogenous antigen presentation pathway, considerable efforts have been dedicated in the past to develop efficient experimental techniques for MHC-II peptide binding quantification. The traditional approach to quantify peptide MHC-II binding relies on measuring binding affinity, either as the dissociation constant (Kd) of the complex [12, 13] or in terms of IC50 (concentration of the query peptide which displaces 50% of a bound reference peptide) [14]. To date, data repositories such as the Immune Epitope Database (IEDB) [15] have collected more than 150,000 measurements of peptide-MHC-II binding interactions. Such data have been used during the last decades to develop several prediction methods with the ability to predict binding affinities to the different alleles of MHC class II. While the accuracy of these predictors has increased substantially over the last decades due the development of novel machine learning frameworks and a growing amount of peptide binding data being available for training [16], state-of-the-art methods still fail to accurately predict accurately MHC class II ligands and T cell epitopes [17, 18].

Recent technological advances in the field of mass spectrometry (MS) have enabled the development of high-throughput assays, which in a single experiment can identify several thousands of peptides eluted of MHC molecules (reviewed in [19]). Large data sets of such naturally presented peptides have been beneficial to define more accurately the rules of peptide-MHC binding [20–26]. For several reasons, analysis and interpretation of MS eluted ligand data is not a trivial task. Firstly, because any given individual constitutively expresses multiple allelic variants of MHC molecules, thus, the ligands detected by MS are normally a mixture of specificities, each corresponding to a different MHC molecule. Secondly, MHC-II ligands can vary widely in length, and identification of the binding motifs requires a sequence alignment over a minimal binding core. Finally, data sets of MS ligands often contain contaminants and false spectrum-peptide identifications, which add a component of noise to the data. We have earlier proposed a method capable of dealing with all these issues, allowing the characterization of binding motifs and the assignment of probable MHC restrictions to individual peptides in such MS ligand data sets [27, 28].

Because naturally eluted ligands incorporate information about properties of antigen presentation beyond what is obtained from in vitro binding affinity measurements, large MS-derived sets of peptides can be used to generate more accurate prediction models of MHC antigen presentation [20, 21, 25]. As shown recently, generic

machine learning tools, such as NNAlign [9, 29], can be readily applied to individual MS data sets, which in turn can be employed for further downstream analyses of the immunopeptidome [30]. The amount of MHC molecules characterized by MS eluted ligand data is, however, still limited. This has led us to suggest a machine learning framework where peptide binding data of both MS and in vitro binding assays are merged in the training of the prediction method [25]. This approach has proven highly powerful for MHC class I, but has not, to the best of our knowledge, been applied to MHC class II.

Undoubtedly, antigen processing plays a critical role in generating CD4+ T cell epitopes presented by MHC class II molecules. It is assumed that endo- and exo-peptidase activities, both before and after binding to the MHC-II molecule, play a key role in the generation and trimming of MHC class II ligands [31, 32]. However, the precise rules of MHC class II antigen processing are poorly understood. Earlier works identified patterns of protein cleavage in HLA-DR ligands; Kropshofer et al. found proline at the penultimate N and C terminal position [33], and Ciudad et al. observed aspartic acid before the cleavage site and proline next to the cut sites in HLA-DR ligands [34]. In contrast, Bird et al. suggested that endolysosomal proteases have a minor and redundant role in peptide selection leading to the conclusion that the effect of processing on the generation of antigenic peptides is "relatively non-specific" [35]. Given this context, it is perhaps not surprising that limited work has been aimed at integrating processing signals into a prediction framework for MHC-II ligands.

In this work, we have analyzed large data sets of MS MHC-II eluted ligands obtained from different research laboratories covering three HLA-DR molecules with the purpose of investigating the consistency in the data, quantifying the differences in binding motifs contained with such MS eluted data compared to traditional in vitro binding data, defining a new machine learning framework capable of integrating information from MS eluted ligand and in vitro binding data into a prediction model for MHC-II peptide interaction prediction, and finally evaluating if inclusion of potential signals from antigen processing is consistent between different data sets and can be used to boost the performance of peptide-MHCII prediction models.

Methods
Data sets
HLA class-II peptidome data were obtained from two recent MS studies. Three data sets corresponding to the HLA-DRB1*01:01: DR1Ph, DR1Pm [26], and DR1Sm [24], two to DRB1*15:01: DR15-Ph and DR15-Pm, and one to the allele DRB5*01:01: DR51 Ph (for details see Table 1). Here, the data sets with subscript h correspond

Table 1 Summary of binding affinity ("Binders") and eluted ligand ("Ligands") data sets used in this work

Binders

Reference	Source	Allele	L11–19				
DR1 BA	Jensen et al. [36]	DRB1*01:01	9987				
DR15 BA	Jensen et al. [36]	DRB1*15:01	4466				
DR51 BA	Jensen et al. [36]	DRB5*01:01	4840				

Ligands

Reference	Source	Allele	Cell	Unique	GC	L11–9	Random
DR1 Ph	Ooi et al. [26]	DRB1*01:01	Human	5131	4786	3992	38115
DR1 Pm	Ooi et al. [26]	DRB1*01:01	Mouse	5744	5561	5385	55710
DR1 Sm	Clement et al. [24]	DRB1*01:01	Mouse	3216	3112	2963	30510
DR15 Ph	Ooi et al. [26]	DRB1*15:01	Human	2782	1590	1390	12870
DR51 Ph		DRB5*01:01			1087	989	9315
DR15 Pm	Ooi et al. [26]	DRB1*15:01	Mouse	4810	4486	4229	42030

Binders (upper table): data set reference name ("Reference"), data source ("Source"), MHC restriction ("Allele"), and the amount of sequences in the length range of 11 to 19 amino acids ("L11–19"). Ligands (lower table): data set reference name ("Reference"), data source ("Source"), MHC restriction ("Allele"), cell line species ("Cell"), amount of unique sequences present in the data set before filtering ("Unique") and after filtering with GibbsCluster ("GC"), quantity of sequences in the 11–19mer range ("L11–19"), number of random negatives sequences added for training ("Random"). Note that the split of the Ooi et al. human data (DR15 Pm/ DR51 Pm) was made using the GibbsCluster as described in the text

to the data obtained from human cell lines and data sets with the subscript m to the data obtained from human MHC-II molecules transfected into MHC-II deficient mice cell lines. Details on how the data were generated are provided in the original publications. Note that DR15 Ph and DR51 Ph data sets were obtained from a heterozygous EBV-transformed B lymphoblastoid cell line (BLCL), IHW09013 (also known as SCHU), which expresses two HLA-DR molecules, HLA-DRB1*15:01 and HLA-DRB5*01:01 (shortened here with the name DR15/51). The DR1 Ph data set was extracted from a BLCL culture as well (IHW09004). On the other hand, DR1 Pm, DR1 Sm, and DR15 Pm data sets were extracted from HLA transgenic mice, and therefore only cover the human alleles of interest. These cells are treated here as monoallelic.

MHC class II peptide binding affinity data was obtained from previous publications [36] for the alleles DR1 (DRB1*01:01, 9987 peptides), DR15 (DRB1*15:01, 4466 peptides), and DR51 (DRB5*01:01, 4840 peptides).

The MS-derived ligand data sets were filtered using the GibbsCluster-2.0 method with default settings as described earlier [30], to remove potential noise and biases imposed by some data containing multiple binding specificities. The details of the binding affinity (BA) and eluted ligand (EL) data sets are described in Table 1.

NNAlign modeling and architecture

Models predicting peptide-MHC interactions were trained as described earlier using NNAlign [29, 30]. Only ligands of length 11–19 amino acids were included in the training data. Random peptides of variable lengths derived from the non-redundant UniProt database were used as

negatives. The same amount of random negatives was used for each length (11 to 19) and consisted of five times the amount of peptides for the most represented length in the positive ligand data set. Positive instances were labeled with a target value of 1, and negatives with a target value of 0. Prior to training, the data sets were clustered using the common motif approach described earlier [37] with a motif length of nine amino acids to generate five partitions for cross-validation.

Two types of model were trained: one with single data type (eluted ligand or binding affinity) input, and one with a mixed input of the two data types. Single models per each data set and allele were trained as previously described with either binding affinity or eluted ligand data as input [30]. All models were built as an ensemble of 250 individual networks generated with 10 different seeds; 2, 10, 20, 40, and 60 hidden neurons; and 5 partitions for cross-validation. Models were trained for 400 iterations, without the use of early stopping. Additional settings in the architecture of the network were used as previously described for MHC class II [30]. Combined models were trained as described earlier [25] with both binding affinity and eluted ligand data as input. Training was performed in a balanced way so that on average the same number of data points of each data type (binding affinity or eluted ligand) is used for training in each training iteration.

Novel modifications were introduced to the architecture of NNAlign to better account for specific challenges associated with MHC class II ligand data. For the network to be able to learn peptide length preferences, a "binned" encoding of the peptide length was introduced, consisting of a one-hot input vector of size nine (one neuron for each of the lengths 11 to 19). In order to guide binding core identification, a burn-in period was introduced with a limited search space for the P1 binding core position. During the burn-in period, consisting of a single learning iteration, only hydrophobic residues were allowed at the P1 binding core anchor position. Starting from the second iteration, all amino acids were allowed at the P1 position (Additional file 1: Figure S1).

NetMHCII and NetMHCIIpan

NetMHCII version 2.3 [36] and NetMHCIIpan version 3.2 [36], peptide to MHC-II binding affinity prediction algorithms were employed in this work as a benchmark comparison for the new proposed model.

Sequence logos

Sequence logos for binding motifs and context information were constructed using Seg2Logo tool using weighted Kulback-Leibler logos and excluding sequence weighting [38]. Amino acids were grouped by negatively charged (red), positively charged (blue), polar (green), or hydrophobic (black).

Performance metrics

In order to assess the performance of our new model, we employed three different and well-known metrics: AUC (area under the ROC curve), AUC 0.1 (area under the ROC curve integrated up to a false positive rate of 10%), and PPV (positive predictive value). AUC is a common performance measurement for predictive models, which takes into account the relationship between true positive rates (TPR) and false positive rates (FPR) for different prediction thresholds. AUC 0.1 is similar to AUC but focuses on the high specificity range of the ROC curve. PPV is here calculated by sorting all predictions and estimating the fraction of true positives with the top N predictions, where N is the number of positives in the benchmark data set. PPV represents a good metric to benchmark on highly unbalanced data sets like MS-derived elution data, where we have approximately ten times more negatives than positives.

Results

Data filtering and motif deconvolution

We first set out to analyze the different MS data sets of eluted ligands. Data were obtained from two recent publications: Ooi et al. [26] (termed P) and Clement et al. [24] (termed S) covering the HLA-DRB1*01:01, HLA-DRB1*15:01, and HLA-DRB5*01:01 MHC class II molecules. Data were obtained from either human (termed h) or HLA-DR transfected mouse (termed m) cell lines. Using this syntax, DR1 Ph corresponds to the HLA-DRB1*01:01 data from the human cell in the study by Ooi et al. (for more details, see the "Methods" section). Here, we applied the GibbsCluster method with default

parameters for MHC class II to both filter out potential noise and to identify the binding motif(s) contained in each data set. The result of this analysis is shown in Fig. 1 and confirms the high quality of the different ligand data sets. In all data sets, less than 7% of the peptides were identified as noise (assigned to the trash cluster), and in all cases, GibbsCluster did find a solution with a number of clusters matching the number of distinct MHC specificities present in a given data set. In this context, the DR15 Ph is of particular interest, since this data set was obtained from a heterozygous cell line expressing two HLA-DR molecules, HLA-DRB1*15:01 and HLA-DRB5*01:01 (shortened here as DR15/51 Ph). Consequently, this data set contains a mixture of peptides eluted from both of these HLA-DR molecules. The GibbsCluster method was able to handle this mixed data set and correctly identified two clusters with distinct amino acid preferences at the anchor positions P1, P4, P6, and P9. Moreover, a comparison of the motifs identified from the different data sets sharing the exact same HLA-DR molecules revealed a very high degree of overlap, again supporting the high accuracy of both the MS eluted ligand data and of the GibbsCluster analysis tool.

Training prediction models on MHC class II ligand data

After filtering and deconvolution with GibbsCluster, MHC peptide binding prediction models were constructed for each of the six data sets corresponding to the majority clusters in Fig. 1. Models were trained using the NNAlign framework as described in the "Methods" section. The eluted ligand data sets (EL) were enriched with random natural peptides labeled as negatives, as described in the "Methods" section. Likewise, models were trained and evaluated on relevant and existing data sets of peptide binding affinities (BA) obtained from the IEDB [15, 36], as described in the "Methods" section. These analyses revealed a consistent and high performance for the models trained on the different eluted ligand data sets (Table 2). In accordance with what has been observed earlier for MHC class I [25], the overall cross-validated performance of models trained on binding affinity data is lower than that of models trained on eluted ligand data. Note that this observation is expected due the very different nature of the binding affinity and eluted ligand data sets: eluted ligand data are highly unbalanced, categorized, and prefiltered to remove ligands not matching the consensus binding motif.

The binding motifs captured by the different models are shown in Fig. 2. As evidenced by identical anchor positions (P1, P4, P6, and P9) and virtually identical anchor residues, highly consistent motifs were obtained from the same HLA-DR molecules irrespective of the source of the peptide (i.e., whether they were obtained from human or mouse cells, or from different laboratories). This observation to a high degree extended to the

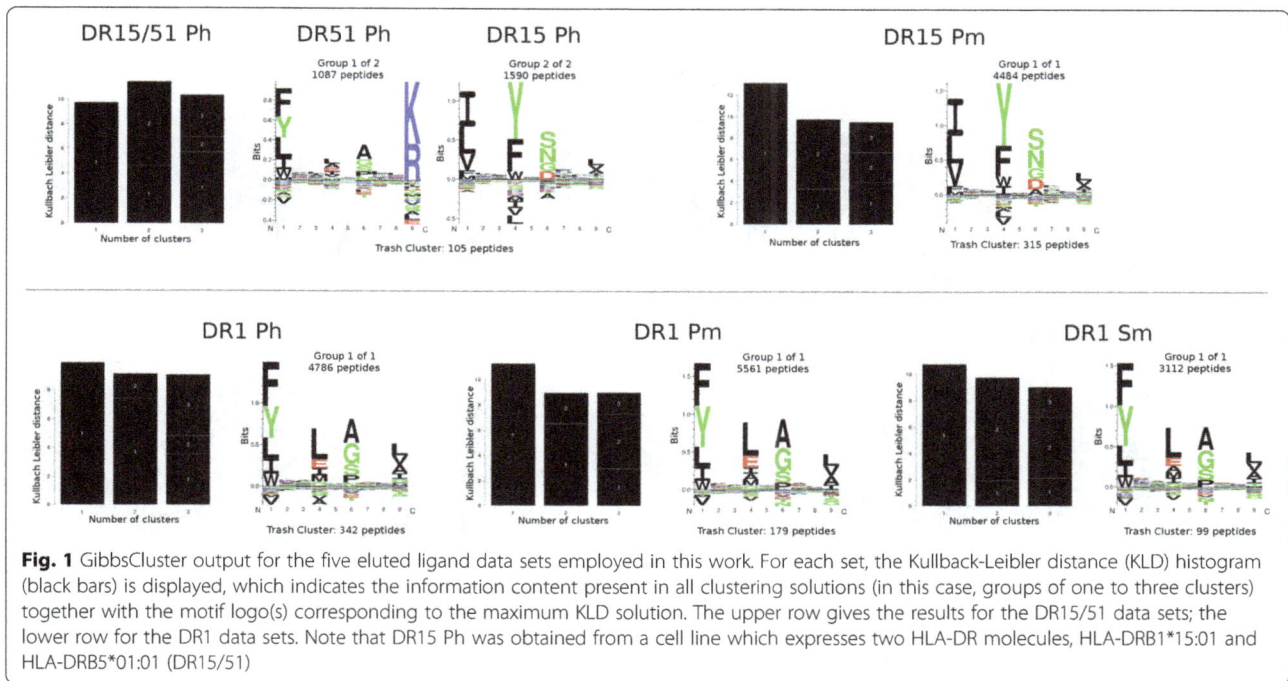

Fig. 1 GibbsCluster output for the five eluted ligand data sets employed in this work. For each set, the Kullback-Leibler distance (KLD) histogram (black bars) is displayed, which indicates the information content present in all clustering solutions (in this case, groups of one to three clusters) together with the motif logo(s) corresponding to the maximum KLD solution. The upper row gives the results for the DR15/51 data sets; the lower row for the DR1 data sets. Note that DR15 Ph was obtained from a cell line which expresses two HLA-DR molecules, HLA-DRB1*15:01 and HLA-DRB5*01:01 (DR15/51)

motifs obtained from binding affinity data, although we did observe subtle, but consistent, differences between the binding motifs derived from eluted ligand and peptide binding affinity data, exemplified for instance by the preference for E at P4 and for D at P6 in the eluted ligand motifs for DR1 and DR15, respectively. Such preferences are absent from the motifs derived from the peptide binding affinity data. To quantify differences and statistically compare the core logos shown in Fig. 2, we performed a correlation comparison of the amino acid frequency matrices of the binding motif obtained from the different models. To this end, we extracted the amino acid frequencies from the binding motifs displayed in Fig. 2, and next did a bootstrapped correlation analysis comparing the amino acid frequency values at

the four anchor positions (P1, P4, P6, and P9) of the binding core between all pairs of motifs. The results of this analysis are given in Additional file 1: Figure S2 and Table S1 and show (as expected from the logo plots of Fig. 2) that the different motifs obtained from eluted ligand data for a given HLA-DR molecule are all highly similar (and statistically indistinguishable, $P > 0.05$, Student T test), whereas motif obtained from binding affinity data are significantly different ($P < 0.001$, Student T test) from those obtained from eluted ligand motifs.

Training a combined prediction model on MHC-II binding affinity and ligand elution data

Earlier work on MHC class I has demonstrated that the information contained within eluted ligand and peptide binding affinity data is, to some degree, complementary and that a prediction model can benefit from being trained integrating both data types [25]. Here, we investigate if a similar observation could be made for MHC class II. As proposed by Jurtz et al., we extended the NNAlign neural network model to handle peptides from both binding affinity and elution assays. In short, this is achieved by including an additional output neuron to the neural network prediction model allowing one prediction for each data type. In this setup, weights are shared between the input and hidden layer for the two input types (binding affinity and eluted ligand), whereas the weights connecting the hidden and output layer are specific for each input type. During neural network training, an example is randomly selected from either data set and submitted to forward and back propagation,

Table 2 Cross-validation performance of models trained on binding affinity (BA) or eluted ligand (EL) data

BA single models			EL single models			
Training set	AUC	AUC 0.1	Training set	AUC	AUC 0.1	PPV
DR1 BA	0.84	0.374	DR1 Ph	0.96	0.819	0.773
			DR1 Pm	0.986	0.888	0.815
			DR1 Sm	0.977	0.851	0.794
DR15 BA	0.843	0.287	DR15 Ph	0.987	0.901	0.85
			DR15 Pm	0.989	0.917	0.859
DR51 BA	0.846	0.38	DR51 Ph	0.961	0.759	0.717

For BA ("BA single models"), the training performance is reported in terms of AUC and AUC 0.1. For EL ("EL single models"), values for AUC, AUC 0.1, and PPV are displayed. For references on the training sets names and compositions, refer to Table 1. For information regarding the performance metrics, see the "Performance metrics" section in the "Methods" section

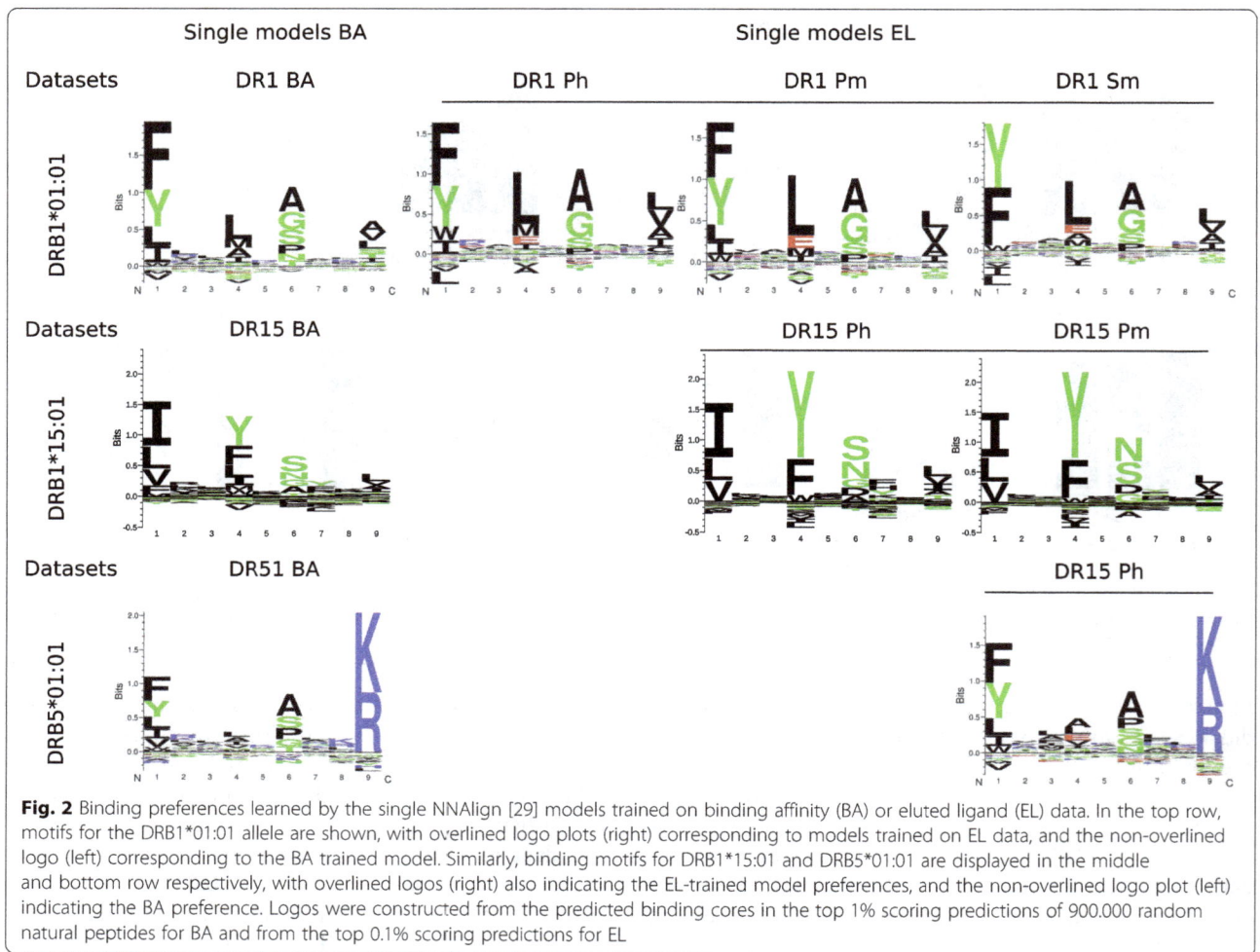

Fig. 2 Binding preferences learned by the single NNAlign [29] models trained on binding affinity (BA) or eluted ligand (EL) data. In the top row, motifs for the DRB1*01:01 allele are shown, with overlined logo plots (right) corresponding to models trained on EL data, and the non-overlined logo (left) corresponding to the BA trained model. Similarly, binding motifs for DRB1*15:01 and DRB5*01:01 are displayed in the middle and bottom row respectively, with overlined logos (right) also indicating the EL-trained model preferences, and the non-overlined logo plot (left) indicating the BA preference. Logos were constructed from the predicted binding cores in the top 1% scoring predictions of 900.000 random natural peptides for BA and from the top 0.1% scoring predictions for EL

according to the NNAlign algorithm. The weight sharing allows information to be transferred between the two data types and potentially results in a boost in predictive power (for more details on the algorithm, refer to [25]).

Models were trained and evaluated in a fivefold cross-validation manner with the same model hyper-parameters that were used for the single data type model. Comparing the performance of the single data type (Table 2), to the multiple data type models for the different data sets (Table 3), a consistent improvement in predictive performance was observed when the two data types were combined. This is the case, in particular, when looking at the PPV performance values. Here, the combined model in all cases has improved performance compared to the single data type model. This is in line to what we have previously observed for MHC class I predictions [25].

Constructing the binding motif captured by the different combined models (see Additional file 1: Figure S3) confirmed the findings from the single data type model

Table 3 Cross-validation performance for the combined NNAlign models, trained on both binding affinity (BA) and eluted ligand (EL) data

Training set		BA prediction		EL prediction		
BA	EL	AUC	AUC 0.1	AUC	AUC 0.1	PPV
DR1 BA	DR1 Ph	0.845	0.385	0.966	0.823	0.781
	DR1 Pm	0.843	0.376	0.987	0.893	0.826
	DR1 Sm	0.843	0.381	0.98	0.867	0.814
DR15 BA	DR15 Ph	0.844	0.288	0.987	0.908	0.855
	DR15 Pm	0.846	0.294	0.99	0.917	0.86
DR51 BA	DR51 Ph	0.848	0.389	0.956	0.749	0.74

Training set refers to the data set used to train the given model (BA indicated binding affinity and EL eluted ligand data). For references on the training sets names and compositions, refer to Table 1. Cross-validated performance values are reported as AUC, AUC 0.1, and PPV. For more details on these measures, refer to the "Methods" section. Note that minor variations in the BA performance values for the same molecule are due to the differences in the data partitioning in the fivefold cross-validation setup in each case (displayed in Fig. 2), with clearly defined and consistent binding motifs in all cases, and with subtle differences in the preferred amino acids at the anchor positions between motifs derived from the binding affinity and eluted ligand output value of the models.

We next turned to the issue of accurately predicting the preferred length of peptides bound to the different HLA-DR molecules. The MS eluted ligand data demonstrated a length preference for the two MHC class II molecules centered on a length around 14–16. Current prediction models such as NetMHCII and NetMHCIIpan are not able to capture this length preference and have in general a bias of assigning higher prediction values to longer peptides (data not shown). We have earlier demonstrated that including information about the peptide length in a framework integrating MS eluted ligand and peptide binding affinity data allows the model to capture the length preference of the two data types [25]. Applying a similar approach to the MHC class II data, we obtain the results shown in Fig. 3, confirming that also for class II the models are capable of approximating the preferred length preference of each molecule.

Lastly, we performed an evaluation across data sets to confirm the robustness of the results obtained and to reveal any unforeseen signal of performance overfitting. For each data set, we used the two-output model trained above to predict the other ligand data sets of the same allotype. Prior to evaluation, all data with a 9mer overlap between training and evaluation sets were removed. We observed that, in all cases, models trained on a specific data set retained high predictive performance for the prediction of ligands of the same allotype derived from a different experiment (Table 4). These results confirm the high reproducibility of the motifs across different cell lines, as well as the robustness of the prediction models derived from individual data sets.

Signals of ligand processing

Having developed improved models for prediction of MHC class II ligand binding, we next analyzed whether the models could be used to identify signals of antigen processing in the MS eluted ligand data sets. We hypothesized that information concerning antigen processing should be present in the regions around the N and C termini of the ligand. These regions comprise residues that flank the MHC binding core called peptide flanking regions (PFRs) and residues from the ligand source protein sequence located outside the ligand (see lower part of Fig. 4 for a schematic overview).

We speculate that the signals of antigen processing depend, to some degree, on the length of the PFRs on each side of the binding core. MHC-II ligands are cut and trimmed by exopeptidases, which operate according to specific motifs in prioritizing cleavage sites. However, in

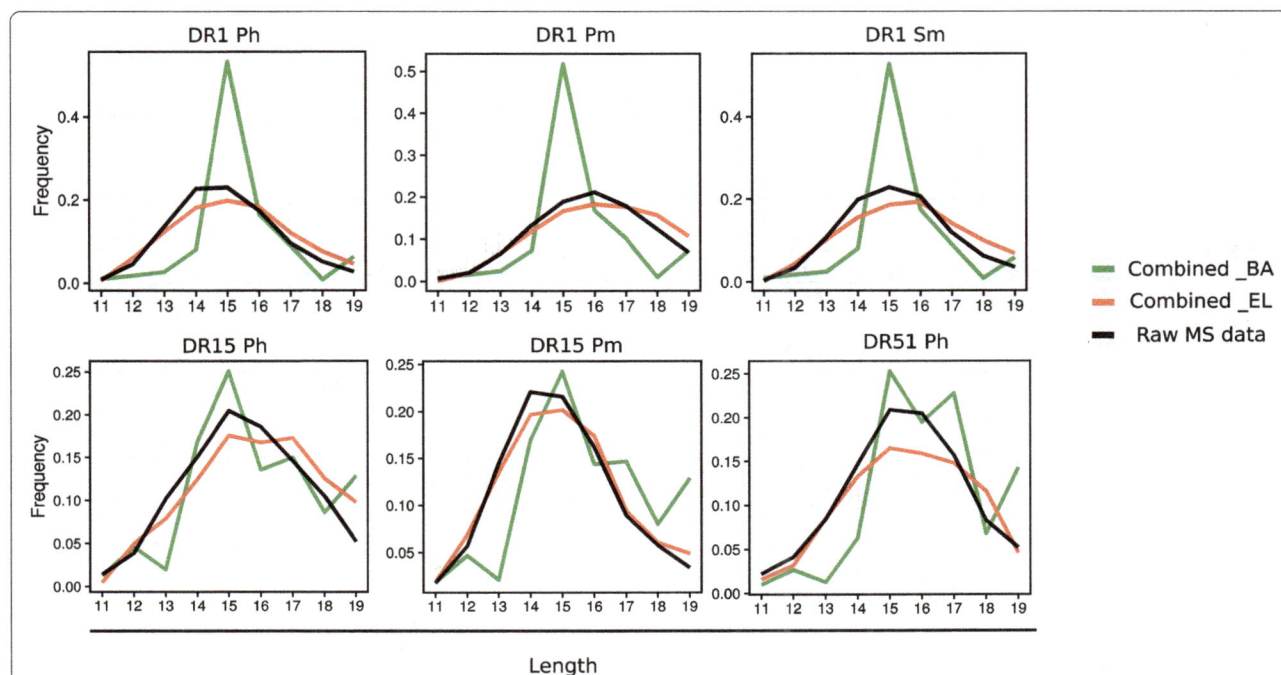

Fig. 3 Peptide length preferences learned by the six models trained on binding affinity (BA) and eluted ligand (EL) combined data. For each model, green traces represent the length histogram of the top 1% scoring predictions for the BA output neuron, on a prediction data set composed of one million random peptides; red traces refer to the length histogram of the top 0.1% scoring predictions for the EL output neuron, on the same prediction set; black traces indicate the length distribution of the raw MS data

Table 4 Independent evaluation of eluted ligand data set in terms of AUC 0.1

Training set		Eval set	BA single	BA combined	EL single	EL combined	NetMHCIIpan	NetMHCII
BA	EL							
DR1 BA	DR1 Ph	DR1 Pm	0.57	0.644	0.839	0.849	0.562	0.585
		DR1 Sm	0.573	0.648	0.81	0.813	0.576	0.578
	DR1 Pm	DR1 Ph	0.498	0.557	0.757	0.754	0.478	0.469
		DR1 Sm	0.514	0.549	0.665	0.669	0.519	0.511
	DR1 Sm	DR1 Ph	0.506	0.556	0.704	0.707	0.481	0.478
		DR1 Pm	0.568	0.636	0.824	0.835	0.54	0.57
DR15 BA	DR15 Ph	DR15 Pm	0.584	0.672	0.869	0.869	0.427	0.58
	DR15 Pm	DR15 Ph	0.615	0.71	0.888	0.889	0.459	0.583

"Training set" refers to the data sets used to train the given model (BA indicates binding affinity and EL eluted ligand data). For references on the training sets names and compositions, refer to Table 1. Cross-validated performance values are reported as AUC 0.1. "Eval set" refers to the independent eluted ligand data set from the same allotype used for evaluation. "BA single" or "EL single" refers to model trained on single data types (BA or EL respectively). "BA combined" or "EL combined" refers to the eluted ligand prediction output or binding affinity output of models trained on both data types. NetMHCIIpan or NetMHCII refers to predictions made using the NetMHCIIpan 3.2 [36], and NetMHCII 2.3 [36] publicly available prediction methods

the case of short PFRs, the MHC hinders access of the protease to the ligand, hence preventing trimming of the residues in close proximity to the MHC [39, 40]. For this reason, we expect to observe cleavage motifs only in peptides with sufficiently long PFRs, where the end-of-the-trimming signal is given by the peptide sequence rather than by MHC hindrance. To validate this hypothesis, we identified the PFRs of the ligands in the DR15 Pm EL data set, as well as three "context" residues found immediately upstream or downstream of the ligand in its source protein. To avoid over-estimation of the performance, the binding core was identified from

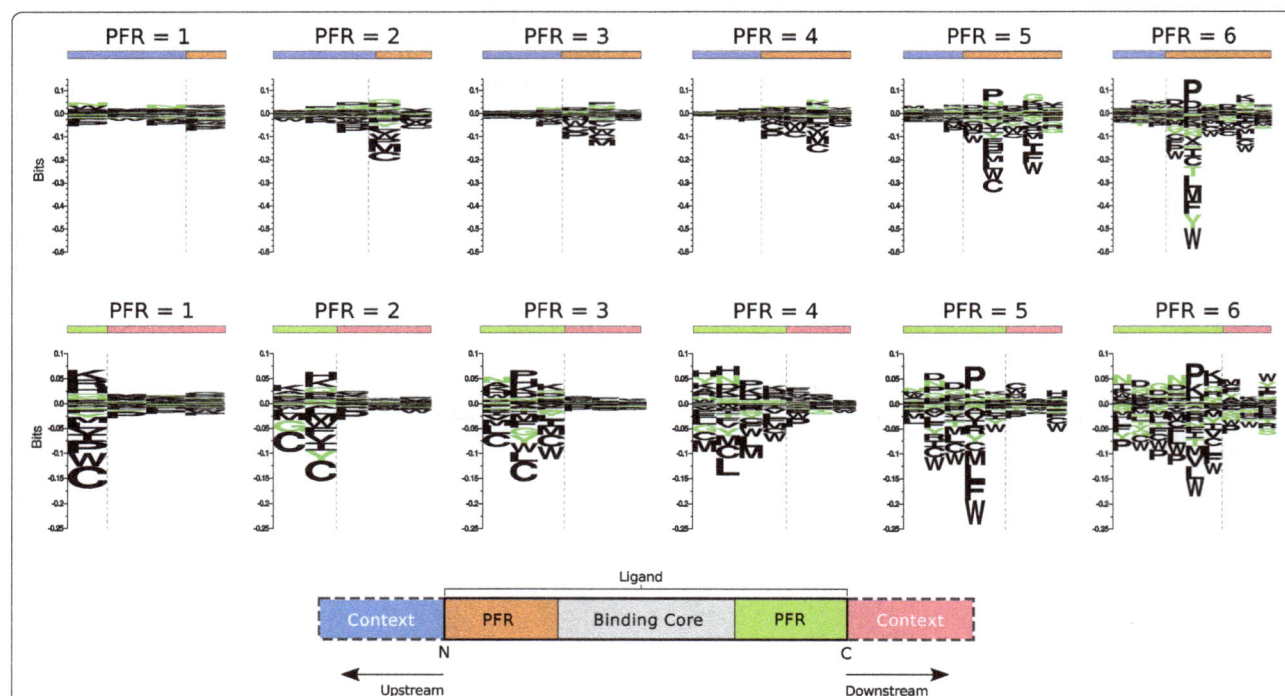

Fig. 4 Processing signals found at N and C terminus positions in the DR15 Pm data set (located at upstream and downstream regions, respectively), grouped by peptide flanking region (PFR) length. For the upstream part of the ligands (top row), the processing signal is always centered at the N terminal position, extending three positions beyond the cleavage site (upstream "context," symbolized as blue bars) and one to six positions towards the binding core, depending on the PFR length (orange bars). For the downstream region (bottom row), the disposition of elements is mirrored: the proposed processing signal is centered at C terminus and extends three positions beyond the cleavage site (downstream "context" region, pink bars) and one to six positions towards the binding core (green bars), depending on the PFR length. Amino acid background frequencies were calculated using the antigenic source protein of all the ligands present in the data set. Motifs were generated using Seq2logo, as described in the "Methods" section

the cross-validated eluted ligand predictions of the two-output model. The ligands were split into groups depending on the length of the C and N terminal PFRs, and sequence logos were generated for each ligand subset using Seq2Logo (Fig. 5).

The results displayed in Fig. 4 clearly confirm the important role of the MHC in shaping the processing signal. For both the N and C terminal data sets, we observe a clear enrichment of proline (P) at the second position from the ligand terminals only for data sets where the PFR is longer than two amino acids. This observation is confirmed from the reanalysis of a data set of peptide to HLA-DR complexes from the Protein Data Bank (PDB) previously assembled for benchmarking the accuracy for MHC-II binding core identification [41]. On this PDB data set, 29% of the entries with a N-terminal PFR longer than two amino acids contain a proline at the second position from the N terminal, and 38% of the entries with a C-terminal PFR longer than two amino acids contain a proline at the second position from the C terminal (data not shown). On the other hand, none of the bound peptides with N-terminal PFR shorter or equal than two amino acids contain a proline at the second position from N-terminal, and only 8% of peptides with C-terminal PFR shorter or equal than two amino acids exhibit a proline at the second position from the C-terminal.

To summarize these observations and construct a global motif of the processing signal, we combined the first three C and N terminal residues from all ligands with PFR length larger than two, together with the corresponding three source protein context residues at either C or N terminal side of the ligand. The processing signal at the N and C termini from DR15 Pm is shown in Fig. 5; processing motifs for all other data sets can be found in Additional file 1: Figure S4.

The processing motif confirms the strong preference for proline at the second but last position in the ligand at both N and C termini, as well as a clear signal of depletion of other hydrophobic amino acid types towards the terminals of the ligand. This cysteine depletion in the PFR is likely to be a technological artifact, as cysteines have previously been shown to be underrepresented in MS-derived peptide data sets [20, 42]. Note also that this depletion is only observed in the PFRs and not in the context residues neighboring the N and C termini. From this figure, it is also clear that processing signals present in the neighborhood (indicated as "context" in Fig. 5) of the ligand are very weak. Similar amino acid preferences were obtained in the processing motifs from the other data sets (Additional file 1: Figure S4).

Next, we investigated to what degree the processing signal was consistently identified in all data sets. To do this, the similarity between any two processing matrices was estimated in terms of the Pearson's correlation coefficient (PCC) between the two vectors of 6*20 elements (6 positions and 20 amino acid propensity scores at each position). The result of this analysis is shown in Fig. 6 in terms of a heatmap (the processing matrices from each data set are included in Additional file 1: Figure S5).

Figure 6 exhibits a clear positive correlation between the processing motif from all the data sets involved. The mean PCC score for the matrices in Fig. 6 was 0.77 for upstream and 0.73 for downstream, with the lowest PCC = 0.59 (for the DR1 Sm and DR1 Ph pair, upstream) and the maximum PCC = 0.89 (for DR15 Pm and DR1 Ph, upstream). These results suggest that the processing signals captured are, to a large degree, MHC- and even species-independent: the correlation between the two human and mouse data sets is as high as the correlation between any two data sets within the same species. To ensure that the observed correlation is not related to

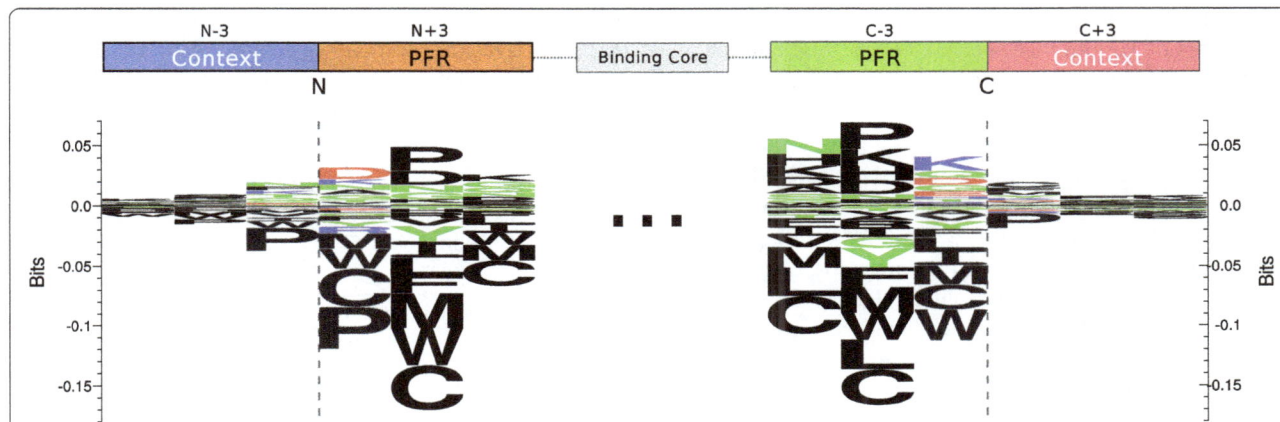

Fig. 5 Processing signals located at N and C terminal regions in the DR15 Pm data set. For each region, all ligands with PFR length lower than 3 were discarded. Then, the logos were constructed as described in the text by selecting the closest three PFR and context residues neighboring the N and C termini. For additional details on processing signal construction, refer to Fig. 4

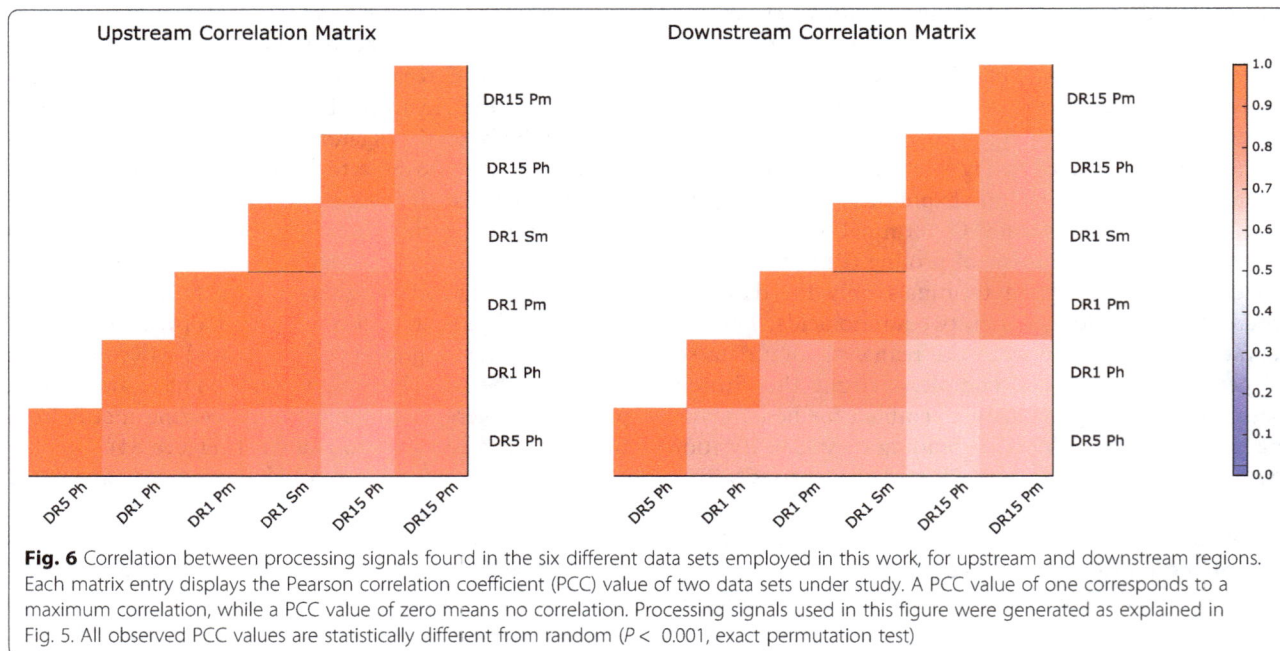

Fig. 6 Correlation between processing signals found in the six different data sets employed in this work, for upstream and downstream regions. Each matrix entry displays the Pearson correlation coefficient (PCC) value of two data sets under study. A PCC value of one corresponds to a maximum correlation, while a PCC value of zero means no correlation. Processing signals used in this figure were generated as explained in Fig. 5. All observed PCC values are statistically different from random ($P < 0.001$, exact permutation test)

MS-derived cysteine depletion, we generated the same correlation matrices removing the cysteine contribution and observed no major differences (Additional file 1: Figure S6). These results thus strongly suggest that the observed signals are related to antigen processing.

Incorporating ligand processing into a combined predictor

Having identified consistent signals associated with antigen processing, we next investigated whether these signals could be integrated into one model to boost predictive performance. The processing signals were incorporated into the machine learning framework by complementing the encoding of each ligand with the 3 N terminal context, 3 N terminal peptide, 3 C terminal context, and 3 C terminal peptide residues (see Fig. 5). For peptide binding affinity data, the context information was presented to the neural networks with three wildcard amino acids "XXX", corresponding to a vector of zeros. Two models were trained for each one of the allotypes considered in this work: one model including and one excluding the context information, both allowing integration of binding affinity and eluted ligand data. Prior to training, the complete set of data (binding affinity and eluted ligands for all three MHC-II molecules) was split into five partitions using the common motif approach as described in the "Methods" section. All model hyper-parameters were identical to the ones used earlier. The result of this benchmark is shown in Table 5 and confirms that the inclusion of context leads to a consistently improved predictive power of the models for all three data sets.

As an example of the processing signal captured by a model trained including context information, we constructed sequence motifs of the top 1% highest scoring peptides from a list of one million random natural peptides of length 10–25 and their context, for a combined model trained on the DR15 Pm data set (Additional file 1: Figure S7). As expected, the motif contained within the N and C terminal peptide flanks and context is close to identical to the motif described in Fig. 5.

T cell epitope prediction using the combined models

Having observed how prediction of naturally processed MHC ligands benefited from implementing ligand context features, we next wanted to evaluate if a similar gain could be observed when predicting T cell epitopes. We downloaded all available epitopes of length 14 to 19 (included) from the IEDB, for the molecules DRB1*01:01, DRB1*15:01, and DRB5*01:01. After filtering out entries

Table 5 Cross-validation performance for combined NNAlign models trained on single-allele data sets, with and without context information

Allele	Without context		With context		
	AUC 0.1	PPV	AUC 0.1	PPV	P value
DRB1*01:01	0.874	0.824	0.893	0.839	< 0.0001
DRB1*15:01	0.931	0.875	0.947	0.892	< 0.0001
DRB5*01:01	0.805	0.76	0.818	0.782	0.0368

"Allele" refers to the combination of all data sets for that given allele used to train the model. Cross-validated performance values are reported as AUC 0.1 and PPV. P values were estimated using bootstrapping. For more details on these measures, refer to the "Methods" section

with post translational modifications and entries lacking information about the source protein IDs, a total of 557, 411, and 114 epitopes remained for the three DR molecules, respectively. First, we evaluated this panel of epitopes in a conventional way: digesting the epitope-source protein into overlapping peptides with the length of the epitope, predicting the peptides using the different models, and calculating the AUC (area under the receiver operator curve) per source protein-epitope pair, taking peptides identical to the epitope as positives and all other peptides in the source protein as negatives. We excluded from the evaluation data sets negative peptides that shared a common motif of nine amino acids with the epitope. Four methods were included in this benchmark: EL (the eluted ligand prediction value from the model trained on the combined data without context information), EL + context (the eluted ligand prediction value from the model trained on the combined data including context signals), NetMHCII (version 2.3), and NetMHCIIpan (version 3.2). This analysis shows, in line with what we observed earlier for the eluted ligand benchmarks, a consistent improved performance of the EL model compared to both NetMHCII and NetMHCIIpan (Fig. 7a).

The benchmark however also demonstrates a substantial drop in predictive power of the EL model when incorporating the context processing signal (EL + context). This drop is however expected since the mapped T cell epitope boundaries are not a product of natural antigen processing and presentation, but

rather result from screening of overlapping peptides from a candidate antigen, or by peptides synthesized based on the results of MHC peptide binding predictions and/or in vitro binding assays. As a consequence, the N and C terminal boundaries of such epitope peptides do not necessarily contain the processing signal obtained from naturally processed ligands. However, given that the epitope was demonstrated to bind to the T cell originally induced towards a naturally processed ligand, we can assume that the sequence of the validated epitope and the original (but unknown to us) naturally processed ligand share an overlap at least corresponding to the MHC-II binding core of the validated epitope. Following this reasoning, we redefined the epitope benchmark as follows. First, we predicted a score for all 13–21mer peptides within a given source protein using the EL or EL + context models. Next, we digested the source protein into overlapping peptides of the length of the epitope and assigned a score to each of these peptides corresponding to the average prediction score of all 13–21mer peptides sharing a 9mer or more overlap with the given peptide (models where the max score was assigned were also considered, but gave consistently lower predictive performance, data not shown). Finally, we calculated as before an AUC value for the epitope-source protein pair taking peptides equal to the epitope as positives and all other peptides as negatives excluding from the

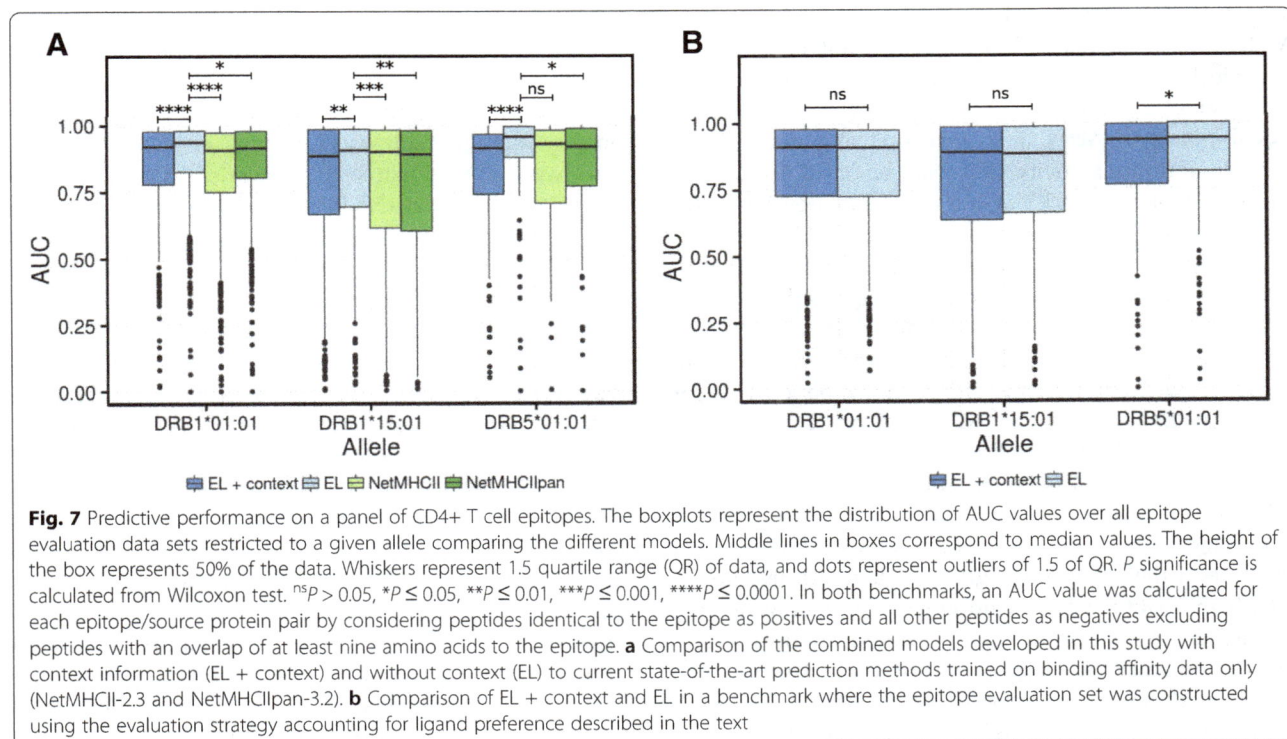

Fig. 7 Predictive performance on a panel of CD4+ T cell epitopes. The boxplots represent the distribution of AUC values over all epitope evaluation data sets restricted to a given allele comparing the different models. Middle lines in boxes correspond to median values. The height of the box represents 50% of the data. Whiskers represent 1.5 quartile range (QR) of data, and dots represent outliers of 1.5 of QR. P significance is calculated from Wilcoxon test. $^{ns}P > 0.05$, $*P \leq 0.05$, $**P \leq 0.01$, $***P \leq 0.001$, $****P \leq 0.0001$. In both benchmarks, an AUC value was calculated for each epitope/source protein pair by considering peptides identical to the epitope as positives and all other peptides as negatives excluding peptides with an overlap of at least nine amino acids to the epitope. a Comparison of the combined models developed in this study with context information (EL + context) and without context (EL) to current state-of-the-art prediction methods trained on binding affinity data only (NetMHCII-2.3 and NetMHCIIpan-3.2). b Comparison of EL + context and EL in a benchmark where the epitope evaluation set was constructed using the evaluation strategy accounting for ligand preference described in the text

evaluation set negative peptides sharing a common motif of nine amino acids with the epitope. The benchmark shows a comparable performance of the EL + context method vs EL method for the alleles analyzed in the study (Fig. 7b). Possible reasons for this lack of improved performance of the EL + context model are discussed below.

Discussion

Peptide binding to MHC II is arguably the most selective step in antigen presentation to CD4+ T cells. The ability to measure (and predict) specific CD4+ responses is crucial for the understanding of pathological events, such as infection by pathogens or cancerous transformations. Recent studies have also highlighted a potential role for CD4+ T cells for the development of cancer immunotherapies [43–45]. Characterizing peptide to MHC-II binding events has been a focal point of research over the last decades. Large efforts have been dedicated in conducting high-throughput, in vitro measurements of peptide MHC II interactions [46–48], and these data have been used to develop methods capable of accurately predicting the interaction of peptides to MHC II molecules from the sequence alone [29, 41, 49, 50]. While these approaches have proven highly successful as guides in the search for CD4 epitopes [51, 52], a general conclusion from these studies is that MHC II in vitro binding affinity (whether measured or predicted) is a relatively poor correlate of immunogenicity [53]. In other words, peptide binding affinity to MHC II is a necessary but not sufficient criterion for peptide immunogenicity. The same situation holds for MHC class I presented epitopes. Here, however, peptide binding to MHC I is a very strong correlate to peptide immunogenicity and can be used to discard the vast majority (99%) of the irrelevant peptide space while maintaining an extremely high (> 95%) sensitivity for epitope identification [25]. For MHC II, recent studies suggest that the corresponding numbers fall in the range 80% specificity and 50% sensitivity [36]. For these reasons, we suggest that other features than MHC II in vitro binding affinity may be critical for MHC II antigen presentation. Based on six MS MHC II eluted ligand data sets, we have here attempted to address and quantify this statement.

Firstly, we have demonstrated that the MS MHC II eluted ligand data sets employed in this work (generated by state-of-the-art technologies and laboratories) are of very high quality, with low noise levels and allowing very precise determination of MHC II binding motifs. Overall, the obtained binding motifs show overlap with the motifs identified from in vitro binding affinity data, with subtle differences at well-defined anchor positions.

Secondly, we demonstrated that high accuracy prediction models for peptide MHC II interaction can be constructed from the MS-derived MHC II eluted ligand data, that the accuracy of these models can be improved by training models integrating information from both binding affinity and eluted ligand data sets, and that these improved models can be used to identify both eluted ligands and T cell epitopes in independent data sets at an unprecedented level of accuracy. This observation strongly suggests that eluted ligand data contain information about the MHC peptide interaction that is not contained within in vitro binding affinity data. This notion is further supported by the subtle differences observed in the binding motifs derived from eluted ligand and in vitro binding affinity data. Similar observations have been made for MHC class I [20, 25]. We at this point have no evidence for the source of these differences, but a natural hypothesis would be that they are imposed by the presence of the molecular chaperones (such as HLA-DM) present in the eluted ligand but absent from in vitro binding assays. An alternative explanation could be that the eluted peptide ligands reflect peptide-MHC class II stability rather than affinity: something that would imply that stability is a better correlate of immunogenicity than affinity [54].

Thirdly, we analyzed signals potentially associated with antigen processing. Antigen-presenting cells employ multiple mechanisms to acquire and process antigens, making use of multiple proteases to digest the internalized proteins [55]. It is likely that the processing signals we observed are a combination of the cleavage specificities of several proteases operating in different stages of the presentation pathway. Looking for consistent patterns, we postulate that such processing signal should be influenced by the relative location of the peptide binding core compared to the N and C terminal of the given ligand. This is because the MHC II molecule may hinder the access of the protease, thus preventing trimming of the residues in close proximity to the MHC [39]. Investigating the data confirmed this hypothesis, and a relatively weak but consistent processing signal (with a preference for prolines at the second amino acid position from the N and C terminal of the ligand) was observed for ligands where the length of the region flanking the binding core was three amino acids or more. This observation was found consistently in all data sets independent of MHC II restriction and host species (human or mouse).

Lastly, we integrated this information associated with antigen processing into a machine learning framework and demonstrated a consistently improved predictive performance not only in terms of cross-validation but also when applied to independent evaluation data sets covering naturally processed MHC eluted ligands. However, we do not observe an improvement of the extended model for prediction of validated T cell epitopes. There are several possible reasons for this. In the first place, it is possible that epitope data have a bias towards current MHC class II binding prediction and/or in vitro binding assay methods, since researchers could use these tools to select which peptides to include in a T cell epitope screening or to define the MHC restriction element for a given positive epitope. Secondly, we have attempted a very simple strategy to assign a prediction score to each epitope. It might be that the conclusion is altered if alternative, more sophisticated mapping strategies were used. Thirdly, the reason might be biological: the antigen processing pathways predominantly utilized in cell lines used for ligand elution experiments which lead to the motifs we identified might not be the only ones generating T cell epitopes in vivo, where, e.g., cross-presentation might play a role. Finally, our prediction model still does not capture all properties that could determine T cell epitope immunogenicity. For example, HLA-DM and DO clearly have a role in regulating which peptides can be loaded onto MHC II [56, 57]; however, their contribution cannot be modeled based on existing data. Also, T cells themselves impose a level of antigen selection through the interaction between the TCR and the peptide-MHC complex. While approaches for peptide-MHC targets of TCR are beginning to appear [58], it is still unclear how they can be integrated in high-throughput approaches for the prediction of T cell epitopes. Future work is needed to disentangle these questions.

Conclusions

We have demonstrated how integrating MHC class II in vitro binding and MS eluted ligand data can boost the predictive performance for both binding affinity, eluted ligand, and T cell epitope predictions. To the best of our knowledge, we have also demonstrated for the first time how MHC II eluted ligand data can be used to extract signals of antigen processing and how these signals can be integrated into a model with improved predictive performance.

Our work is limited to three HLA-DR molecules, but the framework can be readily extended to additional molecules, once sufficient data become available. Also, it may become achievable to construct a pan-specific predictor as has been shown earlier for MHC class I [25], enabling predictions for any MHC molecule of known sequence.

Abbreviations

AUC 0.1: Area under the ROC curve integrated up to false positive rate of 10%; AUC: Area under the ROC curve; BA: Binding affinity data; EL: Eluted ligand data; KLD: Kullback-Leibler distance; MHC-II: Major histocompatibility complex class-II; MS: Mass spectrometry; PCC: Pearson correlation coefficient; PFRs: Peptide flanking regions; pMHCII: Peptide-MHC-II complexes; PPV: Positive predictive value; PSSM: Position-specific scoring matrix

Funding

This work was supported in part by the Federal funds from the National Institute of Allergy and Infectious Diseases, National Institutes of Health, Department of Health and Human Services, under Contract No. HHSN272201200010C, and by the Science and technology council of investigation (CONICET-Argentina).

Authors' contributions

MN designed the study. CB, BA, MA, and MN performed the experiments and statistical analysis. CB, BA, SP, AS, BP, SB, MA, and MN analyzed and interpreted the data and wrote the paper. All authors read and approved the final manuscript.

Competing interests

The authors declare that they have no competing interests.

Author details

[1]Instituto de Investigaciones Biotecnológicas, Universidad Nacional de San Martín, CP1650 San Martín, Argentina. [2]Division of Vaccine Discovery, La Jolla Institute for Allergy and Immunology, 9420 Athena Circle, La Jolla, CA 92037, USA. [3]Department of Immunology and Microbiology, Faculty of Health Sciences, University of Copenhagen, Copenhagen, Denmark. [4]Department of Bio and Health Informatics, Technical University of Denmark, DK-2800 Kgs. Lyngby, Denmark.

References

1. Rudolph MG, Stanfield RL, Wilson IA. How TCRs bind MHCs, peptides, and coreceptors. Annu Rev Immunol. 2006;24:419–66.
2. Kim A, Hartman IZ, Poore B, Boronina T, Cole RN, Song N, et al. Divergent paths for the selection of immunodominant epitopes from distinct antigenic sources. Nat Commun. 2014;5:5369.
3. Sette A, Adorini L, Colon SM, Buus S, Grey HM. Capacity of intact proteins to bind to MHC class II molecules. J Immunol. 1989;143:1265–7.
4. Andreatta M, Jurtz VI, Kaever T, Sette A, Peters B, Nielsen M. Machine learning reveals a non-canonical mode of peptide binding to MHC class II molecules. Immunology. 2017;152:255–64.
5. Lovitch SB, Pu Z, Unanue ER. Amino-terminal flanking residues determine the conformation of a peptide-class II MHC complex. J Immunol. 2006;176:2958–68.
6. Arnold PY, La Gruta NL, Miller T, Vignali KM, Adams PS, Woodland DL, et al. The majority of immunogenic epitopes generate CD4+ T cells that are dependent on MHC class II-bound peptide-flanking residues. J Immunol. 2002;169:739–49.
7. Carson RT, Vignali KM, Woodland DL, Vignali DA. T cell receptor recognition of MHC class II-bound peptide flanking residues enhances immunogenicity and results in altered TCR V region usage. Immunity. 1997;7:387–99.
8. Godkin AJ, Smith KJ, Willis A, Tejada-Simon MV, Zhang J, Elliott T, et al. Naturally processed HLA class II peptides reveal highly conserved immunogenic flanking region sequence preferences that reflect antigen processing rather than peptide-MHC interactions. J Immunol. 2001;166:6720–7.
9. Andreatta M, Schafer-Nielsen C, Lund O, Buus S, Nielsen M. NNAlign: a web-based prediction method allowing non-expert end-user discovery of sequence motifs in quantitative peptide data. PLoS One. 2011;6:e26781.

10. Hammer J, Valsasnini P, Tolba K, Bolin D, Higelin J, Takacs B, et al. Promiscuous and allele-specific anchors in HLA-DR-binding peptides. Cell. 1993;74:197–203.

11. Sturniolo T, Bono E, Ding J, Raddrizzani L, Tuereci O, Sahin U, et al. Generation of tissue-specific and promiscuous HLA ligand databases using DNA microarrays and virtual HLA class II matrices. Nat Biotechnol. 1999;17:555–61.

12. Roche PA, Cresswell P. High-affinity binding of an influenza hemagglutinin-derived peptide to purified HLA-DR. J Immunol. 1990;144:1849–56.

13. Hall FC, Rabinowitz JD, Busch R, Visconti KC, Belmares M, Patil NS, et al. Relationship between kinetic stability and immunogenicity of HLA-DR4/ peptide complexes. Eur J Immunol. 2002;32:662–70.

14. Buus S, Sette A, Colon SM, Miles C, Grey HM. The relation between major histocompatibility complex (MHC) restriction and the capacity of Ia to bind immunogenic peptides. Science. 1987;235:1353–8.

15. Vita R, Overton JA, Greenbaum JA, Ponomarenko J, Clark JD, Cantrell JR, et al. The immune epitope database (IEDB) 3.0. Nucleic Acids Res. 2015; 43(Database issue):D405–12.

16. Andreatta M, Trolle T, Yan Z, Greenbaum JA, Peters B, Nielsen M. An automated benchmarking platform for MHC class II binding prediction methods. Bioinformatics. 2018;34(9):1522–8.

17. Gowthaman U, Agrewala JN. In silico tools for predicting peptides binding to HLA-class II molecules: more confusion than conclusion. J Proteome Res. 2008;7:154–63.

18. Wang P, Sidney J, Dow C, Mothé B, Sette A, Peters B. A systematic assessment of MHC class II peptide binding predictions and evaluation of a consensus approach. PLoS Comput Biol. 2008;4:e1000048.

19. Caron E, Kowalewski DJ, Chiek Koh C, Sturm T, Schuster H, Aebersold R. Analysis of major histocompatibility complex (MHC) immunopeptidomes using mass spectrometry. Mol Cell Proteomics MCP. 2015;14:3105–17.

20. Abelin JG, Keskin DB, Sarkizova S, Hartigan CR, Zhang W, Sidney J, et al. Mass spectrometry profiling of HLA-associated peptidomes in mono-allelic cells enables more accurate epitope prediction. Immunity. 2017;46:315–26.

21. Bassani-Sternberg M, Gfeller D. Unsupervised HLA peptidome deconvolution improves ligand prediction accuracy and predicts cooperative effects in peptide-HLA interactions. J Immunol. 2016;197:2492–9.

22. Bergseng E, Dørum S, Arntzen MØ, Nielsen M, Nygård S, Buus S, et al. Different binding motifs of the celiac disease-associated HLA molecules DQ2.5, DQ2.2, and DQ7.5 revealed by relative quantitative proteomics of endogenous peptide repertoires. Immunogenetics. 2015;67:73–84.

23. Chong C, Marino F, Pak H-S, Racle J, Daniel RT, Müller M, et al. High-throughput and sensitive immunopeptidomics platform reveals profound IFNγ-mediated remodeling of the HLA ligandome. Mol Cell Proteomics MCP. 2018;17(3):533–48.

24. Clement CC, Becerra A, Yin L, Zolla V, Huang L, Merlin S, et al. The dendritic cell major histocompatibility complex II (MHC II) peptidome derives from a variety of processing pathways and includes peptides with a broad Spectrum of HLA-DM sensitivity. J Biol Chem. 2016;291:5576–95.

25. Jurtz V, Paul S, Andreatta M, Marcatili P, Peters B, Nielsen M. NetMHCpan-4.0: improved peptide-MHC class I interaction predictions integrating eluted ligand and peptide binding affinity data. J Immunol. 2017;199:3360–8.

26. Ooi JD, Petersen J, Tan YH, Huynh M, Willett ZJ, Ramarathinam SH, et al. Dominant protection from HLA-linked autoimmunity by antigen-specific regulatory T cells. Nature. 2017;545:243–7.

27. Andreatta M, Alvarez B, Nielsen M. GibbsCluster: unsupervised clustering and alignment of peptide sequences. Nucleic Acids Res. 2017;45(W1):W458–W463.

28. Andreatta M, Lund O, Nielsen M. Simultaneous alignment and clustering of peptide data using a Gibbs sampling approach. Bioinforma Oxf Engl. 2013; 29:8–14.

29. Nielsen M, Andreatta M. NNAlign: a platform to construct and evaluate artificial neural network models of receptor-ligand interactions. Nucleic Acids Res. 2017;45(W1):W344–W349.

30. Alvarez B, Barra C, Nielsen M, Andreatta M. Computational tools for the identification and interpretation of sequence motifs in immunopeptidomes. Proteomics. 2018; In Press.

31. Blum JS, Wearsch PA, Cresswell P. Pathways of antigen processing. Annu Rev Immunol. 2013;31:443–73.

32. Lippolis JD, White FM, Marto JA, Luckey CJ, Bullock TNJ, Shabanowitz J, et al. Analysis of MHC class II antigen processing by quantitation of peptides that constitute nested sets. J Immunol. 2002;169:5089–97.

33. Kropshofer H, Max H, Halder T, Kalbus M, Muller CA, Kalbacher H. Self-peptides from four HLA-DR alleles share hydrophobic anchor residues near the NH2-terminal including proline as a stop signal for trimming. J Immunol. 1993;151:4732–42.

34. Ciudad MT, Sorvillo N, van Alphen FP, Catalán D, Meijer AB, Voorberg J, et al. Analysis of the HLA-DR peptidome from human dendritic cells reveals high affinity repertoires and nonconventional pathways of peptide generation. J Leukoc Biol. 2017;101:15–27.

35. Bird PI, Trapani JA, Villadangos JA. Endolysosomal proteases and their inhibitors in immunity. Nat Rev Immunol. 2009;9:871–82.

36. Jensen KK, Andreatta M, Marcatili P, Buus S, Greenbaum JA, Yan Z, et al. Improved methods for predicting peptide binding affinity to MHC class II molecules. Immunology. 2018;154(3):394–406.

37. Hobohm U, Scharf M, Schneider R, Sander C. Selection of representative protein data sets. Protein Sci Publ Protein Soc. 1992;1:409–17.

38. Thomsen MCF, Nielsen M. Seq2Logo: a method for construction and visualization of amino acid binding motifs and sequence profiles including sequence weighting, pseudo counts and two-sided representation of amino acid enrichment and depletion. Nucleic Acids Res. 2012;40(Web Server issue):W281–7.

39. Larsen SL, Pedersen LO, Buus S, Stryhn A. T cell responses affected by aminopeptidase N (CD13)-mediated trimming of major histocompatibility complex class II-bound peptides. J Exp Med. 1996;184:183–9.

40. Mouritsen S, Meldal M, Werdelin O, Hansen AS, Buus S. MHC molecules protect T cell epitopes against proteolytic destruction. J Immunol. 1992;149:1987–93.

41. Andreatta M, Karosiene E, Rasmussen M, Stryhn A, Buus S, Nielsen M. Accurate pan-specific prediction of peptide-MHC class II binding affinity with improved binding core identification. Immunogenetics. 2015;67:641–50.

42. Bassani-Sternberg M, Chong C, Guillaume P, Solleder M, Pak H, Gannon PO, et al. Deciphering HLA-I motifs across HLA peptidomes improves neo-antigen predictions and identifies allostery regulating HLA specificity. PLoS Comput Biol. 2017;13:e1005725.

43. Kreiter S, Vormehr M, van de Roemer N, Diken M, Löwer M, Diekmann J, et al. Mutant MHC class II epitopes drive therapeutic immune responses to cancer. Nature. 2015;520:692–6.

44. Tran E, Turcotte S, Gros A, Robbins PF, Lu Y-C, Dudley ME, et al. Cancer immunotherapy based on mutation-specific CD4+ T cells in a patient with epithelial cancer. Science. 2014;344:641–5.

45. Zanetti M. Tapping CD4 T cells for cancer immunotherapy: the choice of personalized genomics. J Immunol. 2015;194:2049–56.

46. Justesen S, Harndahl M, Lamberth K, Nielsen L-LB, Buus S. Functional recombinant MHC class II molecules and high-throughput peptide-binding assays. Immunome Res. 2009;5:2.

47. Sidney J, Southwood S, Oseroff C, del Guercio MF, Sette A, Grey HM. Measurement of MHC/peptide interactions by gel filtration. Curr Protoc Immunol. 2001;Chapter 18(Unit 18):3.

48. Sidney J, Southwood S, Moore C, Oseroff C, Pinilla C, Grey HM, et al. Measurement of MHC/peptide interactions by gel filtration or monoclonal antibody capture. Curr Protoc Immunol. 2013;Chapter 18(Unit 18):3.

49. Nielsen M, Lundegaard C, Lund O. Prediction of MHC class II binding affinity using SMM-align, a novel stabilization matrix alignment method. BMC Bioinformatics. 2007;8:238.

50. Singh H, Raghava GP. ProPred: prediction of HLA-DR binding sites. Bioinforma Oxf Engl. 2001;17:1236–7.

51. Gfeller D, Bassani-Sternberg M, Schmidt J, Luescher IF. Current tools for predicting cancer-specific T cell immunity. Oncoimmunology. 2016;5: e1177691.

52. Nielsen M, Lund O, Buus S, Lundegaard C. MHC class II epitope predictive algorithms. Immunology. 2010;130:319–28.

53. Backert L, Kohlbacher O. Immunoinformatics and epitope prediction in the age of genomic medicine. Genome Med. 2015;7:119.

54. Lazarski CA, Chaves FA, Jenks SA, Wu S, Richards KA, Weaver JM, et al. The kinetic stability of MHC class II:peptide complexes is a key parameter that dictates immunodominance. Immunity. 2005;23:29–40.

55. Roche PA, Furuta K. The ins and outs of MHC class II-mediated antigen processing and presentation. Nat Rev Immunol. 2015;15(4):203–16.

56. Morris P, Shaman J, Attaya M, Amaya M, Goodman S, Bergman C, Monaco JJ, Mellins E. An essential role for HLA-DM in antigen presentation by class II major histocompatibility molecules. Nature. 1994;368(6471):551–4.

13

Prioritization and functional assessment of noncoding variants associated with complex diseases

Lin Zhou[1,2] and Fangqing Zhao[1,2,3*]

Abstract

Unraveling functional noncoding variants associated with complex diseases is still a great challenge. We present a novel algorithm, Prioritization And Functional Assessment (PAFA), that prioritizes and assesses the functionality of genetic variants by introducing population differentiation measures and recalibrating training variants. Comprehensive evaluations demonstrate that PAFA exhibits much higher sensitivity and specificity in prioritizing noncoding risk variants than existing methods. PAFA achieves improved performance in distinguishing both common and rare recurrent variants from non-recurrent variants by integrating multiple annotations and metrics. An integrated platform was developed, providing comprehensive functional annotations for noncoding variants by integrating functional genomic data, which can be accessed at http://159.226.67.237:8080/pafa.

Keywords: Complex disease, Functional annotation, Genetic variant, Variant prioritization, Noncoding variant

Background

Recent advances in sequencing technologies have enabled the identification of an increasingly large spectrum of variants within the human genome [1]. However, unraveling the genetic architecture of complex diseases is still a great challenge, particularly identifying functionally relevant variants in noncoding regions [2, 3]. Previous studies have interpreted coding variants based on our understanding of the genetic code and splicing [4]. Many existing computational approaches have been developed for prioritizing these variants, such as SIFT [5] and PolyPhen [6]. Noncoding variants, however, are noticeably understudied due to our poor understanding of noncoding regions in the human genome. Most recently, tremendous progress has been achieved in both large-scale functional genome projects (e.g., ENCODE [7] and FANTOM5 [8]) and human genome resequencing projects (e.g., 1000 Genomes Project [9]), which provide a rich resource of genomic annotations for analyzing and predicting the functional effects of both coding and noncoding variants.

Recently, several computational approaches, including both unsupervised and supervised algorithms, have been developed to prioritize noncoding variants by integrating various genomic features, including functional annotations and evolutionary conservation. To prioritize risk variants, unsupervised statistical methods (e.g., GenoCanyon [10] and Eigen [11]) construct discriminative models based on conditional probability distributions, which rely on strong model assumptions. Supervised methods (e.g., CADD [12], FATHMM series [13–15], DANN [16], GWAVA [17], and DIVAN [18]) do not rely on a priori assumptions; instead, they label the training data as deleterious or benign and fit a model that best separates the two sets. These integrative supervised methods generally outperform those based on any single individual feature [11, 12] and frequently provide more than one score depending on the regions considered (e.g., coding, noncoding) and the appropriate feature sets for that region. The scores, however, sometimes may lead to conflicting evaluation results for variants. Besides, some of these methods have intrinsic limitations in prioritizing specific categories of risk variants. For

* Correspondence: zhfq@biols.ac.cn
[1]Computational Genomics Lab, Beijing Institutes of Life Science, Chinese Academy of Sciences, Beijing 100101, China
[2]University of Chinese Academy of Sciences, Beijing 100049, China
Full list of author information is available at the end of the article

example, CADD constructed a model based on the training variants that have been under long-term selective pressure, which made it perform less well on certain disease-associated variants under weak evolutionary constraint, such as those influencing the risk of complex traits [11, 12]. LINSIGHT [19] was constructed based on the premise of inferring the selective pressure on noncoding sites and worked very well on identifying human noncoding variants associated with inherited diseases; however, this premise may not hold in all cases, such as those in which the variants increase the risk for post-reproductive diseases [19]. In addition, except for genomic annotations and conservation measures, all the currently available methods seldom consider population-level statistical measures (e.g., F statistics [20]), which may be helpful to prioritize common variants. Although supervised learning demands a representative and correctly labeled training set, a major problem for these methods is the use of mislabeled variants in the training stage, which may lead to false predictions by supervised classifiers. For example, DIVAN labeled variants from the 1000 Genomes Project as benign with few controlling or filtration steps. A considerable fraction of the variants in the 1000 Genomes is reported to be involved in various complex diseases or traits [21, 22]. CADD labeled fixed or nearly fixed derived alleles in humans as benign and simulated de novo variants as deleterious. However, such simulated de novo variants may contain a substantial proportion of benign variants, which thus may lead to false predictions.

Here, we present a novel supervised algorithm for Prioritization And Functional Assessment (PAFA) of genetic variants associated with complex diseases or traits, especially for population-specific noncoding variants. PAFA can prioritize functional variants in noncoding regions by utilizing all kinds of available annotations and metrics, including genomic annotations, evolutionary conservation metrics, and population level measures. In particular, a newly introduced feature, F_{ST}, which is frequently used as a summary of genetic differentiation among groups [20], can significantly help PAFA prioritize population-relevant functional variants in noncoding regions over background variants. In addition, to obtain more reliable training variants, PAFA utilizes training data from various curated databases, and it employs multiple filtration strategies for variant labeling. Through comprehensive evaluations of both common and rare variants, we demonstrate that PAFA exhibits a much better performance on prioritizing both common and rare complex disease-associated variants over benign variants as well as discriminating between noncoding recurrent variants and non-recurrent variants through the incorporation of multiple features and the optimization of training datasets. Moreover, a user-friendly web server (http://159.226.67.237:8080/pafa) was constructed that not only allows users to evaluate variants by PAFA but also provides comprehensive functional annotations by integrating abundant functional genomic elements.

Methods

Data and annotation sources

Genetic and genomic resources used to construct and validate the PAFA algorithm are mainly divided into three categories (Fig. 1 and Additional file 1: Figure S1). Firstly, PAFA selected variants from the 1000 Genomes Project (Phase 3) [9], ClinVar (released in 2018/3/1) [23], and GWASdb (v2) [24] as the training set of PAFA. The functional variant dataset included variants labeled "pathogenic" in ClinVar and significant SNPs associated with complex traits or diseases (cSNPs) that overlap with known genomic elements from GWASdb. Correspondingly, variants labeled "benign" in ClinVar and variants in 1000 Genomes were treated as a control dataset. The calculation of PAFA scores is based on the GRCh37/hg19 human genome assembly, as the new genome build (GRCh38) still lacks enough genomic annotations compared with GRCh37. Here, we integrated a lift-over tool [25] for users who choose GRCh38 as the reference.

Secondly, PAFA selected annotations from known databases as features to annotate training variants and to evaluate new variants. These features can be divided into three classes: evolutionary conservation metrics, genomic annotations, and population differentiation measures. For evolutionary conservation, two measures, phastCons [26] and phyloP [27], were obtained. Conservation scores based on the comparison of both 46 and 100 vertebrate genomes were used. For genomic annotations, PAFA used both genic context information, such as distance to nearest transcript start site (TSS) from GENCODE v19 annotation [28] and information from thousands of functional genomic elements across different cell types, including histone modifications, RNA polymerase binding, and transcription factor binding sites (TFBS PeakSeq). For population differentiation measures, F_{ST} and dispersion score (DS) were calculated based on allele frequencies and sample sizes of the five super populations. Based on the coding and noncoding annotations, we also built a gene-centric database to provide gene-level annotations for variants. To determine which variants may affect gene expression, we retrieved annotated exons and transcription start site information from GENCODE v19 [28] and 5'-UTR and 3'-UTR data from UTRdb [29]. The predicted enhancers that regulate the target genes were also obtained [30]. In addition, we recorded intron regions that are overlapped with any annotations, such as open chromatin and transcription factor binding sites (TFBS), from ENCODE [31]. With this integrated genomic

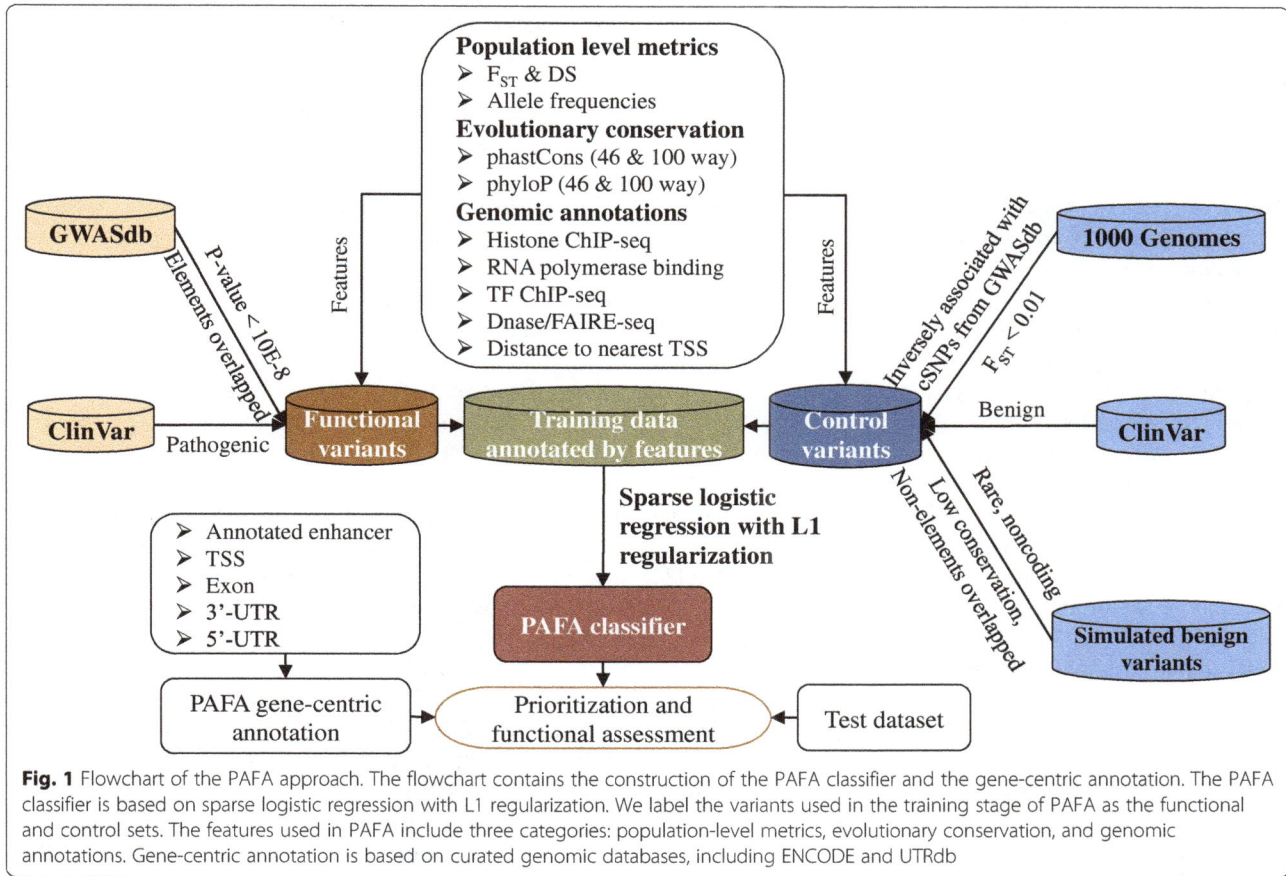

Fig. 1 Flowchart of the PAFA approach. The flowchart contains the construction of the PAFA classifier and the gene-centric annotation. The PAFA classifier is based on sparse logistic regression with L1 regularization. We label the variants used in the training stage of PAFA as the functional and control sets. The features used in PAFA include three categories: population-level metrics, evolutionary conservation, and genomic annotations. Gene-centric annotation is based on curated genomic databases, including ENCODE and UTRdb

annotation system, PAFA can link a variant to known genes or genomic elements.

Thirdly, we used test sets from seven public databases (the 1000 Genomes Project Phase 3, ClinVar, GWAS Catalog [32], COSMIC v79 [33], TCGA [34], GRASP v2.0 [35], and ICGC [36]) and variants from three recent studies including 916 breast cancer variants [37], 221 human blood metabolites variants [38], and 1764 macular telangiectasia type 2 variants [39], to compare PAFA with other available methods (Additional file 1: Figure S1). We used five different types of variant sets from four databases to perform a comprehensive evaluation, including benign and pathogenic coding variants of ClinVar, common variants with frequencies of at least 1% in the population studied in 1000 Genomes, complex diseases or trait-associated SNPs (cSNPs) of the GWAS Catalog, and recurrent noncoding variants of COSMIC. Then, we used Mendelian disease-associated variants of ClinVar and complex disease-associated variants from 560 breast cancer samples in a recent study and TCGA database to compare their performance on prioritizing coding risk variants. We used variants of GRASP, 221 variants associated with human blood metabolites, and 647 common variants associated with

macular telangiectasia type 2 to assess PAFA's performance in prioritizing noncoding variants associated with complex diseases or traits. Finally, we used variants from ICGC Cancer Genome Projects to assess PAFA's ability in discriminating both common and rare recurrent from non-recurrent variants and in prioritizing noncoding rare risk variants from adjacent common variants.

For the PAFA online platform, it was integrated with several additional utilities, including 1000 GENOMES, ANNOTATION, VSEA, and SEARCH (Additional file 1: Figure S2–5). Due to the population-scale sequencing feature of variants in the 1000 Genomes Project, the 1000 GENOMES part of the online platform utilized the population differentiation index and allele frequency of a specific variant among human populations to assist the prioritization and annotation of target variants. Correspondingly, except for known variants and genomic resources mentioned above, these utilities were also integrated with other resources. First, the ANNOTATION part of online platform integrated variants from dbSNP [40], NHLBI-Exome Sequencing Project v2 (ESP) [41], YanHuang Project [42], CNV of 100 pancreatic ductal adenocarcinomas (PDACs) [43], schizophrenia somatic deletions in brain [44], and 996 ASD rare CNVs [45] to annotate input variants. With these annotated resources, we can determine whether the input variants overlap with known variants through the online platform. Simultaneously, the ANNOTATION part also integrated with a variety of curated databases containing disease-associated genes, including Online Mendelian Inheritance in Man (OMIM) [46], the Genetic Association Database (GAD) [47], and COSMIC [33], to recognize potential disease-related variants. In addition, the VSEA part incorporated canonical pathways from the Molecular Signatures Database (MSigDB v6.1) [48], to perform enrichment analysis on variants based on these included pathways.

In total, 23 curated genetic and genomic resources were integrated into the PAFA online platform (Additional file 1: Figure S6), including known variants, various annotations, disease-associated genes, and pathways. All annotations are represented in the GRCh37 assembly of the human genome.

Construction of functional and control variant sets in PAFA

The training set of PAFA was mainly derived from curated databases, including ClinVar, GWASdb, and 1000 Genomes. Considering that these public databases may contain redundancies and erroneous or conflicted records, we employed multiple filtrations to remove low-confidence variants (Additional file 1: Figure S7). We firstly eliminated conflicted records in the training set that are labeled "benign" and "pathogenic" in ClinVar at the same time. A possible explanation is that these variants do not cause certain diseases, but they may contribute to the development of diseases in other cases [49, 50]. Therefore, they were removed from the control dataset, but they were kept in the functional dataset. In total, 30,277 "pathogenic" and 13,010 "benign" variants from ClinVar were included in PAFA. Twenty four thousand nine hundred ninety-three cSNPs from GWASdb were selected as extremely significant variants using a threshold of $p \leq 10E-8$. After removing cSNPs that share no overlap with known genomic elements, 11,570 variants from GWASdb were used in PAFA. To select non-functional variants from 1000 Genomes, we randomly selected 100,000 variants from 1000 Genomes with a low F_{ST} (< 0.01) along with the filtration of redundant records in GWASdb and constructed a regression model for cSNPs in the training set on the basis of 7131 evaluation features. L1-regularized logistic regression, which is provided by LIBLINEAR [51], was used to construct the model. Using the constructed regression model, we determined the numerical measures of these 100,000 variants with little genetic differentiation. We

ranked these variants according to their numerical output, as negative values mean variants inversely associated with cSNPs in the training set. According to their ranking, 28,837 inversely associated variants were selected as a control dataset by PAFA.

As described above, we introduced variants from ClinVar, GWASdb, and 1000 Genomes, including pathogenic/benign coding variants and common functional/benign variants. Ultimately, 41,847 functional and 41,847 control variant datasets were used by PAFA (Additional file 1: Figure S7).

Selection and analysis of features in PAFA

Based on the existing classifiers, PAFA first pre-selected 7131 features that may be sensitive to noncoding variants, which can be divided into three classes, including conservation metrics, genomic annotations, and population differentiation measures. We introduced four evolutionary conservation scores, including 46 and 100 ways of phastCons and phyloP measures. For genomic annotations, we introduced eight types of feature groups from ENCODE [7], including histone modifications (ChIP-Seq), RNA contigs (Long RNA-seq), transcription factor binding sites (TFBS PeakSeq and SPP), open chromatin (DNase-Seq and FAIRE), and transcript start site (TSS).

For population differentiation measures, we introduced allele frequencies of five super populations, including African, American, East Asian, European, and South Asian. We calculated F_{ST} and dispersion score (DS) based on allele frequencies and sample sizes of the five super populations. For a given genomic locus, consider i subpopulations (where $i = 1, ..., s$) and suppose that the observed allele frequencies are $p1, ..., ps$ and the sample sizes are $n1, ..., ns$. Let $n = \sum_{i=1}^{s} n_i$ and $\bar{n} = \sum_{i=1}^{s} n_i/s$.

Wright's unbiased F_{ST} [52] is estimated as

$$F_{ST} = \frac{MSP - MSG}{MSP + (n_c - 1) \times MSG}$$

where MSG denotes the observed mean square errors for loci within populations

$$MSG = \frac{1}{\sum_{i=1}^{s} n_i - 1} \sum_{i}^{s} n_i p_i (1 - p_i)$$

and MSP denotes the observed mean square errors for loci between populations,

$$MSP = \frac{1}{s-1} \sum_{i}^{s} n_i (p_i - \bar{p})^2$$

with $\bar{p}$ as a weighted average of p_i across populations

$$\bar{p} = n_i p_i / \sum_i n_i$$

and n_c is the average sample size across samples that also incorporates and corrects for the variance in sample size over populations.

$$n_c = \frac{1}{s-1} \sum_{i=1}^{s} n_i - \frac{\sum_i n_i^2}{\sum_i n_i}$$

The dispersion score is calculated as

$$DS = \sqrt{\frac{\sum_{i=1}^{s}(p_i - \bar{\bar{p}})^2}{n}}$$

with

$$\bar{\bar{p}} = \sum_{i=1}^{s} p_i / s$$

We constructed feature vectors for variants. These features had fixed unique sequence numbers. We performed tenfold cross-validation with the training set mentioned above to assess the pre-selected features in PAFA, including four conservation scores, seven types of feature groups for genomic annotations, and three population differentiation measures (Additional file 1: Figure S8). All annotation feature groups employed by PAFA have the ability to prioritize functional variants from a control set, with AUC values larger than 0.5. Thus, PAFA adopted all these features to annotate variants.

Model training and performance comparison

With a mass of instances and features, PAFA employed LIBLINEAR [51] to construct an ensemble discrimination model against variants. LIBLINEAR is an efficient and open source library for large-scale linear classification. PAFA treated features of a variant without an overlapping relationship as missing values and took L1 regularization to construct a sparse model. PAFA adopted the logistic regression implemented in LIBLINEAR, which was used to calculate the probability PAFA scores for variants.

To evaluate the performance of PAFA in prioritizing functional variants, seven widely used classifiers were compared with PAFA, namely, CADD, FATHMM-MKL, DANN, GWAVA, DIVAN, LINSIGHT, and Eigen. CADD has updated three versions since its publication. Here, the latest version of CADD was used to generate C scores for variants. By using different genomic annotations, FATHMM-MKL provided two different scores, namely, a "coding score" and a "noncoding score," which

were deemed to prioritize coding and noncoding variants, respectively. We used both scores for comparison. Based on different training sets from 1000 Genomes, GWAVA provided three independent scores, Region, TSS, and Unmatched, which were all used for performance comparisons. Similar to GWAVA, DIVAN also provided Region and TSS scores. Considering that DIVAN provided disease-specific scores for SNPs associated with 45 diseases or phenotypes, PAFA was compared to DIVAN on discriminating these disease- or phenotype-related variants. Moreover, Eigen provided two scores for evaluating variants by using different algorithms. To compare with Eigen, we downloaded the Eigen scores of the testing sets from its website (http://www.columbia.edu/~ii2135/download.html) and also compared with their pre-computed Eigen and Eigen-PC scores. In addition, we also obtained testing sets from the latest publications and public databases, including GRASP and TCGA. We removed all the variants that occurred in the training set of PAFA from these testing sets. We used AUC values and p values (Wilcoxon rank-sum test) to evaluate the performance of these methods.

Construction of the online platform

To facilitate the use of PAFA, we built an online platform for the navigation or batch download of target variants. This platform was developed using Java and was deployed on a Tomcat server. We developed the user interface using HTML5, JavaScript, and D3.js. In addition to conveniently accessing PAFA scores, the online platform incorporates other functions, such as evaluating target variants relying on prior databases containing disease-associated genes, providing enrichment analysis on variant set and relevant annotation information from 1000 Genomes and genomic databases, such as ENCODE and OMIM.

To evaluate variants using information from gene-disease databases (e.g., OMIM, GAD), we first mapped the variants to a range of annotated elements, such as exons, TSS, 3'-UTR, 5'-UTR, enhancers, TFBS, and open chromatin, based on the abundant annotation source integrated in our database. As variants in different types of elements cause discrepant influences on gene expression, we set empirical weights to variants based on different types of elements. In addition, the proportion of overlapping section was considered. After retrieving the involved genes, a quantitative value was assigned to the variants in the following way, according to the occurrence frequency of genes in current gene-disease databases.

Assume that the target variant overlapped with m different genes and n different elements were influenced by each gene. Then, let L_{e_j} be the ith gene's jth element's length and $L_{o_{ij}}$ be the overlapped length between variant and the ith gene's jth element. W_T represents the weight value of the type of element, which is set to 1.0 for exon and TSS, 0.5 for 3'-UTR and 5'-UTR, 0.3 for enhancer, 0.2 for TFBS (PeakSeq) and TFBS (SPP) in the gene, and 0.1 for the gene's open chromatin. s_i indicates the ith gene's frequency as it appears in gene-disease databases. The score is calculated as

$$score = \sum_{i=1}^{m} S_i$$

with

$$S_i = s_i \times min1, \sum_{j=1}^{n} \frac{L_{o_{ij}}}{L_{e_j}} \times W_T$$

To provide enrichment analysis for the target variant sets, we included background variant sets, such as variants from 1000 Genomes, genomic annotations from ENCODE, and canonical pathways in the Molecular Signatures Database (MSigDB). First, we mapped the test variants and background variants (user uploaded or selected) to a range of annotated elements. Then, we obtained genes related to the test and background variants. Next, we extracted the related pathways of these genes in MSigDB. Finally, according to the relationships among variants, genes, and pathways, we calculated the p value to estimate the enrichment degree in relevant pathways using Fisher's exact test.

Results

Population differentiation of genetic variants associated with complex diseases or traits

To explore the relationship between the population differentiation of genetic variants and common complex diseases or traits, we extracted SNPs associated with complex traits or diseases (cSNPs) from GWASdb [24]. Multiple categories of diseases/traits were chosen, including cancers, cardiovascular diseases, and mental disorders, as well as complex traits, such as hair color, adiposity, and intelligence (Fig. 2). Subsequently, we obtained population-specific allele frequencies of these

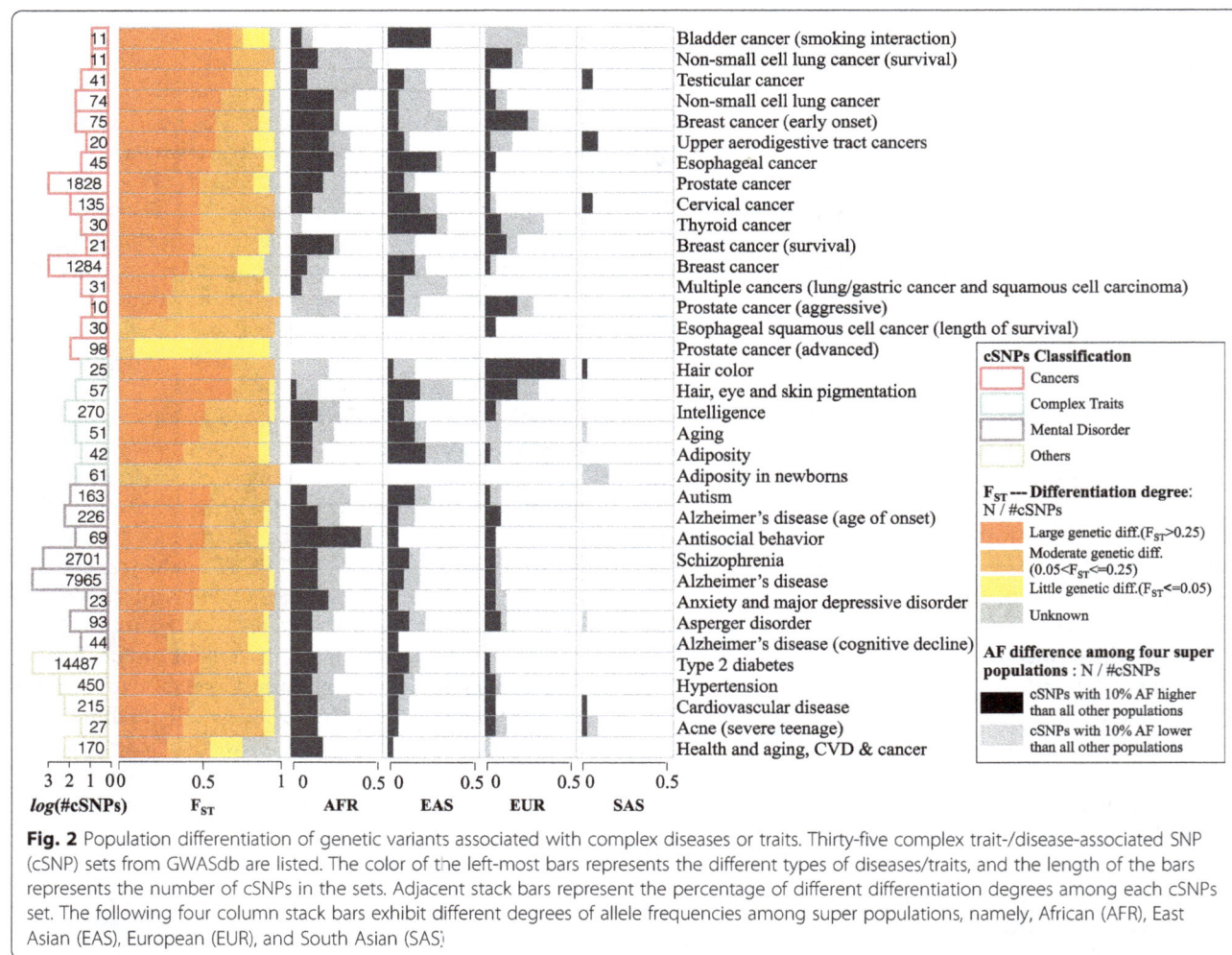

Fig. 2 Population differentiation of genetic variants associated with complex diseases or traits. Thirty-five complex trait-/disease-associated SNP (cSNP) sets from GWASdb are listed. The color of the left-most bars represents the different types of diseases/traits, and the length of the bars represents the number of cSNPs in the sets. Adjacent stack bars represent the percentage of different differentiation degrees among each cSNPs set. The following four column stack bars exhibit different degrees of allele frequencies among super populations, namely, African (AFR), East Asian (EAS), European (EUR), and South Asian (SAS)

cSNPs in four super populations (AFR, EAS, EUR, and SAS) derived from the 1000 Genomes project (Phase 3 variant calls). The corresponding allele frequency spectra in super populations for each disease/trait category were visualized in violin graphs. As shown in Additional file 1: Figure S9–12, cSNPs associated with different diseases or traits exhibited noticeably different allele frequencies, with certain diseases overrepresented in specific populations. For example, over 50% of testicular cancer-related SNPs occurred in more than half of Europeans, but in less than 25% of Africans. This is consistent with epidemiologic findings that testicular cancer incidence consistently remained the highest in Northern European populations and the lowest in African populations [53, 54]. To investigate the population genetic predispositions underlying these cSNPs, we introduced the fixation index (F_{ST}), which is a measure of population differentiation due to genetic structure. With allele frequencies and sample sizes of the five super populations available from 1000 Genomes, we calculated the unbiased estimates of F_{ST} for cSNPs. The frequency distribution of F_{ST} for each disease/trait category was shown in Additional file 1: Figure S13. According to the criteria [55] that F_{ST} lower than 0.05 means little genetic differentiation and F_{ST} larger than 0.25 means high genetic differentiation, most of the cSNPs exhibited high genetic differentiations in human populations.

Furthermore, we examined 35 cSNP sets to get a comprehensive look at the relationship between the population differentiation of cSNPs and their associated complex diseases/traits. As shown in Fig. 2, the proportion of cSNPs with large ($F_{ST} > 0.25$), moderate ($0.05 < F_{ST} \leq 0.25$), and little ($F_{ST} \leq 0.05$) genetic differentiation was displayed in different colors. The number of cSNPs with 10% allele frequencies that were higher or lower than all other populations was calculated in each category based on known allele frequencies in human populations. As illustrated in the four right-most column stack bars of Fig. 2, the dark gray bar represents the frequency of cSNPs in a super population that is higher than all other super populations, and the light gray bar represents the frequency of cSNPs in a super population that is lower than all other super populations. Clearly, the majority of cSNPs display a strong preference towards specific human populations. For example, cSNPs associated with hair color showed a high occurrence in the European population, with nearly a half of them frequently occurring in European populations, which is consistent with previous studies [56, 57]. More examples can be seen in cancer-related diseases. Of the 1828 prostate cancer-related SNPs curated from multiple literature sources, more than half showed great genetic differentiation among super populations. Out of these cSNPs, 720 were reported to likely occur in the African

population, but not in other populations. In fact, African American men have the highest prostate cancer incidence rate in the world, although the rate in the African population is unclear [58, 59]. Taken together, these examples indicate that different cSNPs exhibit various levels of population differentiation, and the incorporation of F_{ST} or other allele frequency features may help evaluate the significance of human genetic variants.

The PAFA approach

The PAFA algorithm contains two components: prioritizing functional genetic variants and annotating variants by integrating a priori functional genomic data (Fig. 1). To discriminate potential functional variants from background variants, sparse logistic regression with L1 regularization was applied to train a noncoding sensitive discriminative model. To be noncoding sensitive, PAFA utilizes training data sets located in noncoding regions and selects features with the ability to prioritize noncoding variants. First, the training variants were partly derived from ClinVar, GWASdb v2, and 1000 Genomes. PAFA classified them into two distinct variant sets (functional and control) with multiple filtration steps, including filtering duplicates and conflicting records, selecting element-overlapping SNPs associated with complex traits or diseases, and measuring the similarity between common variants from 1000 Genomes and functional variants based on various annotations. For the functional variant set, variants annotated as "pathogenic" in ClinVar were first selected; these variants are mainly located in coding regions. Considering that genome-wide association studies have reliably linked coding or noncoding genetic variants to complex diseases or traits, significant cSNPs (p value < 10E–8) in GWASdb were selected as another source of the functional variant set. Noncoding SNPs may affect target genes by disrupting their normal regulatory mechanism. To reduce the number of selected noncoding variants, we only chose the variants that overlapped with any genomic elements from ENCODE [7] and UTRdb [29]. For the control variant set, variants annotated as "benign" in ClinVar were the first data source. Common variants from 1000 Genomes were usually labeled benign by previous supervised classifiers (e.g., GWAVA [17]). However, more than 80% of curated SNPs archived in GWASdb are also present in the SNP list of 1000 Genomes, since most GWAS studies have been performed using genotyping SNP arrays based on common variants (Fig. 3a). In addition to these shared SNPs in GWASdb and 1000 Genomes, a large number of unannotated common variants in 1000 Genomes may also be clinically important, as the number of diseases and traits studied by GWAS is still not sufficiently comprehensive

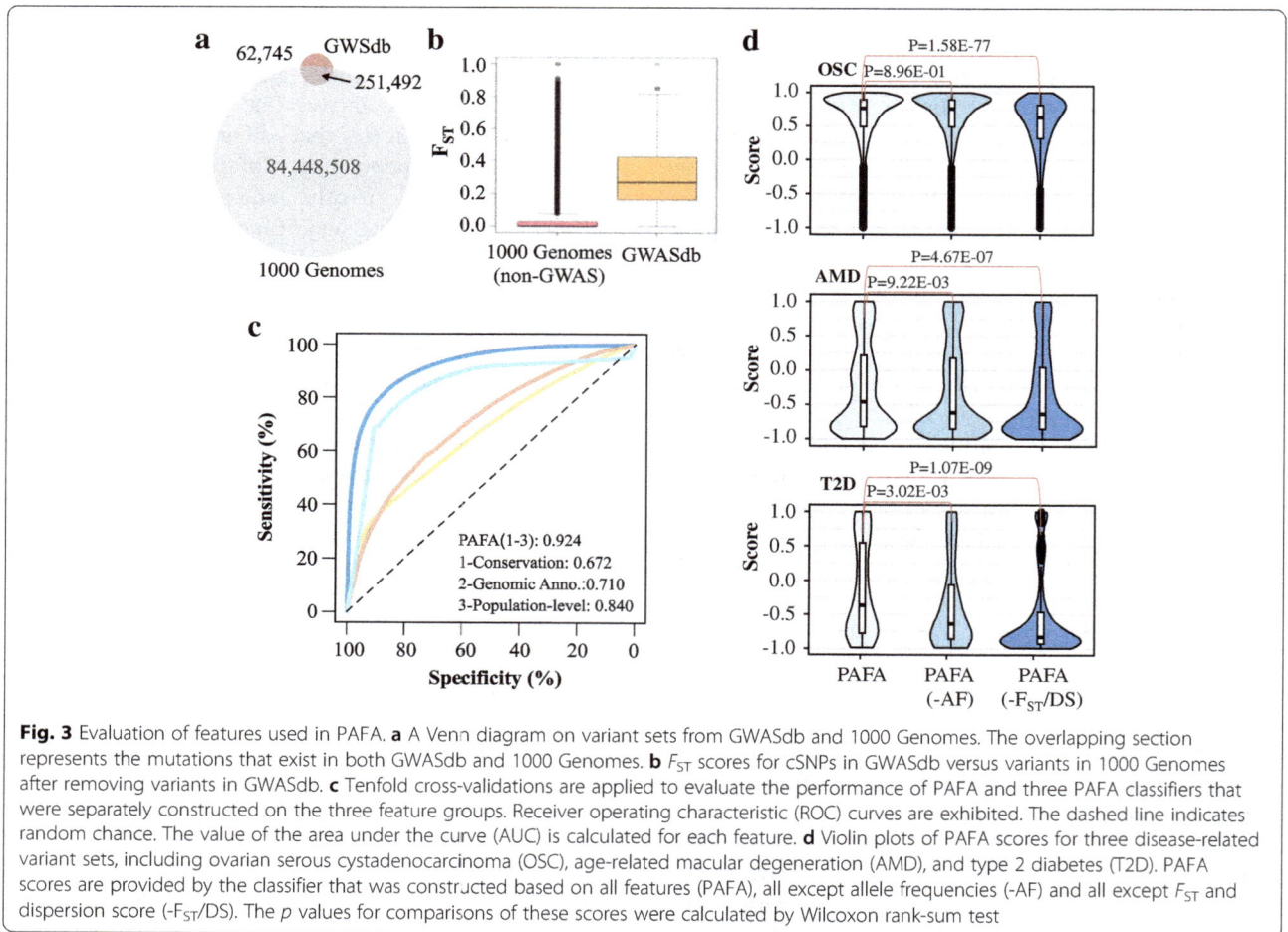

Fig. 3 Evaluation of features used in PAFA. **a** A Venn diagram on variant sets from GWASdb and 1000 Genomes. The overlapping section represents the mutations that exist in both GWASdb and 1000 Genomes. **b** F_{ST} scores for cSNPs in GWASdb versus variants in 1000 Genomes after removing variants in GWASdb. **c** Tenfold cross-validations are applied to evaluate the performance of PAFA and three PAFA classifiers that were separately constructed on the three feature groups. Receiver operating characteristic (ROC) curves are exhibited. The dashed line indicates random chance. The value of the area under the curve (AUC) is calculated for each feature. **d** Violin plots of PAFA scores for three disease-related variant sets, including ovarian serous cystadenocarcinoma (OSC), age-related macular degeneration (AMD), and type 2 diabetes (T2D). PAFA scores are provided by the classifier that was constructed based on all features (PAFA), all except allele frequencies (-AF) and all except F_{ST} and dispersion score (-F_{ST}/DS). The p values for comparisons of these scores were calculated by Wilcoxon rank-sum test

[60]. Ignoring or misclassifying these potential functional SNPs may lead to an incorrect assessment of target genetic variants. Therefore, we employed the F_{ST} index as a metric to infer the potential biological significance of variants in 1000 Genomes. We first compared the distribution of F_{ST} indexes for SNPs in 1000 Genomes with those in GWASdb, and we found that over 90% of variants in 1000 Genomes showed little genetic differentiation (Fig. 3b). In contrast, more than half of the cSNPs in GWASdb displayed enhanced genetic differentiation. A considerable fraction of variants (over 6 million out of 84 million) show high population differentiation indices (> 0.25) in 1000 Genomes, the number of which is much larger than the total number of variants presented in GWASdb. To generate the control variant set, we first constructed a regressive model based on various features of the cSNPs used in the training stage. Then, we selected variants with very low F_{ST} values (< 0.01) from 1000 Genomes. The constructed regressive model was used to rank the selected low-F_{ST} variants. According to the rank of variants, we selected the variants that were inversely

associated with cSNPs utilized by PAFA as another source for the control variant set. Finally, PAFA incorporated simulated rare benign variants as part of the control variant set.

The features used in PAFA can be classified into three categories: population-level metrics, evolutionary conservation, and genomic annotations. These features show distinct patterns in the functional and control variant sets and exhibit certain abilities in annotating noncoding variants. Among these features, population-level metrics consist of fixation index (F_{ST}), allele frequencies, and dispersion score (DS) that is calculated based on allele frequencies. F_{ST}, which is frequently used as a summary of genetic differentiation among groups, was first introduced as a feature to distinguish between functional and background variants. DS was also incorporated, as standard deviation is by far the most widely used measure of dispersion. As shown in Fig. 3c, the population-level features alone exhibited better performance than all other feature groups, with an AUC of 0.840 (tenfold cross-validation). To reveal which feature has a stronger impact in the PAFA model, we selected three variants sets related to complex diseases, including 6147 variants related to ovarian serous cystadenocarcinoma (OSC) from the TCGA database [34], 1339 variants associated with age-related macular degeneration in East Asians [61], and 150 variants related to type 2 diabetes from European populations [62]. These diseases are all reported to be population-relevant [63–66]. As shown in Fig. 3d, the constructed model based on the combination of F_{ST}, DS, and allele frequencies exhibited much better performance in evaluating these variants associated with complex diseases than the model based on allele frequencies or F_{ST} alone. In addition, the PAFA classifiers without features of F_{ST} and DS exhibited a poorer performance than the classifiers without allele frequencies, according to the p values calculated by a Wilcoxon rank-sum test (Fig. 3d).

In addition to prioritizing functional variants, PAFA also provides gene-centric annotations for both coding and noncoding variants. PAFA integrates genetic elements, including annotated enhancer, TSS, exon, 3′-UTR, and 5′-UTR, from curated databases, including ENCODE. To test the reliability of the annotated genomic elements, functional enrichment analysis was performed on 10,143 de novo mutations identified from 200 autism spectrum disorder (ASD) parent-child trios [67]. Among these mutations, 5635 variants do not have any overlap with annotated coding regions. We obtained the affected genes of coding and noncoding variants through the gene-centric database of PAFA, and we performed enrichment analysis on these genes separately using DAVID [68]. All enriched pathways listed in Additional file 1: Figure S14 were reported to be closely related to ASD in previous studies. Several pathways were apparently enriched in the affected gene sets of both coding and noncoding variants, indicating that these noncoding variants may cooperate with coding variants in the development of ASD. For example, the affected gene sets of both coding and noncoding variants were enriched in the cAMP pathway, with Benjamini-adjusted p values of 3.31E–05 and 5.81E–05, respectively. The affected gene sets of coding and noncoding variants are not consistent, with several enriched pathways that are specific to noncoding variants (Additional file 1: Figure S14).

Performance comparison on prioritizing functional variants

To evaluate the performance of PAFA on prioritizing functional variants from background variants, we compared PAFA with seven widely used prioritization methods, CADD [12], FATHMM-MKL [13], DANN [16], GWAVA [17], DIVAN [18], Eigen [11], and LINSIGHT [19]. A detailed comparison of these tools is shown in Additional file 1: Table S1. Considering that FATHMM-MKL provides two different scores by using

different features, namely, a "coding score" and a "noncoding score," PAFA was compared with both of them. Eigen provides Eigen and Eigen-PC scores by using different algorithm strategies, and GWAVA provides Region, TSS, and Unmatched scores by using different training datasets; thus, all these scores were included in the comparison. Similarly, the Region and TSS scores provided by DIVAN were also included. For comparison, we downloaded pre-computed GWAVA (v1.0), DANN (Oct 10, 2014), DIVAN (Dec 6, 2016), Eigen (Jan 4, 2016), and LINSIGHT (Aug 15, 2016) scores from their source websites, and we obtained CADD (v1.3) and FATHMM-MKL (Jan 11, 2015) scores through their online retrieval systems.

We first performed a comprehensive evaluation of seven tools (PAFA, Eigen, CADD, GWAVA, DANN, FATHMM-MKL, and LINSIGHT) by assessing five different types of variant sets, including benign and pathogenic coding variants, common variants with frequencies of at least 1% in the populations studied in 1000 Genomes, cSNPs, and recurrent noncoding variants (Fig. 4). LINSIGHT was not involved in assessing pathogenic and benign coding variants because it mainly inferred the selective pressure on noncoding sites and only provided scores for noncoding sites. We randomly selected 12,035 variants in chromosome 22 from the 1000 Genomes project (Phase 3 variant calls), and we downloaded the variant data sets used in the Eigen paper, which presented the four other types of variant data sets. In total, we obtained 16,545 pathogenic/likely pathogenic variants and 3482 benign or likely benign nonsynonymous variants from the ClinVar database, 121,507 recurrent somatic noncoding variants in the COSMIC database [1], and 14,915 cSNPs that were found to be genome-wide significant and were reported in the GWAS Catalog at the National Human Genome Research Institute (NHGRI). After removing the variants used in the training dataset, the common variants were reduced to a total of 11,035 variants, and the benign/likely benign variants and pathogenic/likely pathogenic variants were reduced to 1671 and 2429, respectively. Similarly, the number of recurrent variants and cSNPs from the GWAS Catalog were reduced to 120,437 and 11,570, respectively. After generating these five datasets, PAFA and the six other tools were used to compute scores to evaluate these variants.

As shown in Additional file 1: Table S2, all tested tools (except for GWAVA, which aims to predict the functional impact of noncoding genetic variants) perform well in distinguishing pathogenic coding variants from benign ones, with AUC values ranging from 0.702 to 0.885. However, when we evaluated their abilities in prioritizing recurrent noncoding variants and cSNPs from common variants in the 1000

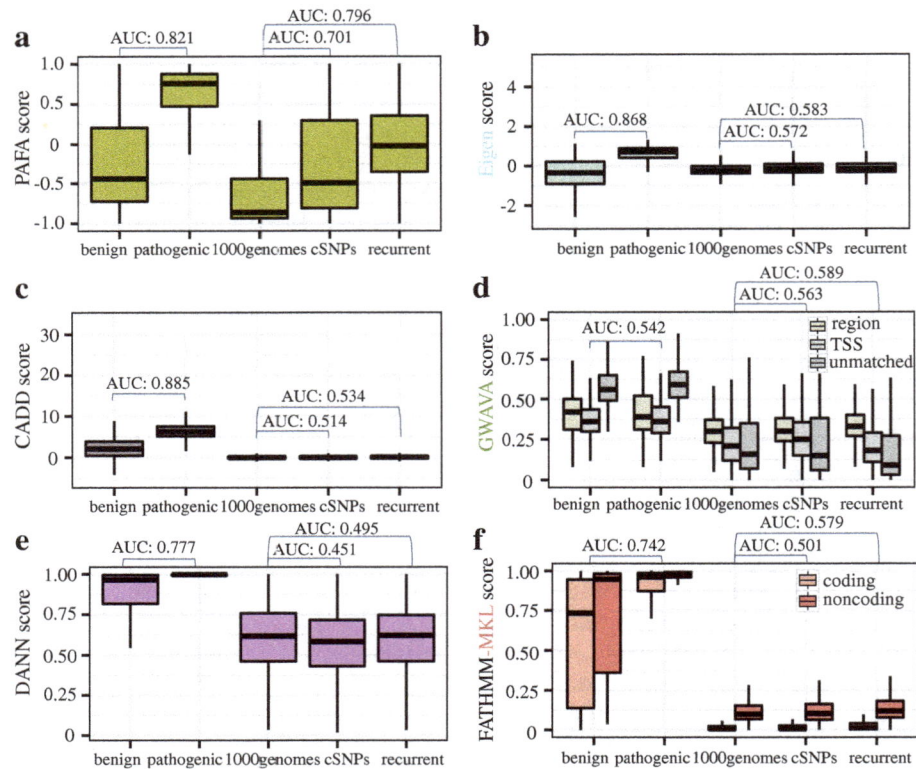

Fig. 4 Performance comparison on prioritizing functional variants. Distribution of scores for evaluating five different variant sets, from left to right: variants labeled "benign/likely benign" in ClinVar, variants labeled "pathogenic/likely pathogenic" in ClinVar, randomly selected variants from 1000 Genomes, significant trait-/disease-associated SNPs (cSNPs) from GWAS Catalog and recurrent cancer-related mutations in noncoding regions from COSMIC. **a** Boxplot for PAFA scores. **b** Boxplot for Eigen scores. **c** Boxplot for *C* scores of CADD v1.3. **d** Boxplot for Region, TSS, and Unmatched scores of GWAVA. **e** Boxplot for DANN scores. **f** Boxplot for coding and noncoding scores of FATHMM-MKL. Area under the curve (AUC) values were calculated for each tool to evaluate their performance on (1) prioritizing pathogenic variants from benign ones, most of which are located in coding regions; (2) prioritizing cSNPs from common variants in 1000 Genomes; and (3) prioritizing noncoding recurrent variants from common variants in 1000 Genomes. As GWAVA and FATHMM-MKL provide more than one score, we display the AUC value with the best performance

Genomes, some tools exhibited decreased performance with AUC values < 0.5 (Fig. 4e and Additional file 1: Table S2). Besides PAFA, which performed well with an AUC value of 0.701 (Fig. 4a), Region score of GWAVA, Eigen, coding, and noncoding scores of FATHMM-MKL and CADD exhibited moderate performance in distinguishing recurrent noncoding variants from common variants with AUC values ranging from 0.534 to 0.589 (Fig. 4 b–d, f). In general, among these supervised and unsupervised algorithms, PAFA achieved comparable performance to CADD and Eigen on pathogenic coding variants, with an AUC value of 0.821. Remarkably, PAFA exhibited the best performance in discriminating multiple types of variants associated with complex diseases or traits, with an AUC value of 0.796 for prioritizing recurrent noncoding variants and an AUC value of 0.701 for prioritizing cSNPs (Fig. 4a and Additional file 1: Table S2).

Prioritizing coding risk variants

We first compared the performance of PAFA, Eigen, CADD, GWAVA, FATHMM-MKL, and DANN on prioritizing coding variants from five well-studied genes (MLL2, CFTR, BRCA1, BRCA2, and TERT) associated with Kabuki syndrome, cystic fibrosis, breast cancer, or aggressive thyroid tumor, respectively. After removing variants used in the training stage of PAFA, we obtained 37 disease-associated variants in BRCA1, 15 in BRCA2, 41 in CFTR, 92 in MLL2, and 42 in TERT. At the same time, variants of these genes that were labeled benign in ClinVar were obtained for comparison. The *p* values were determined by comparing the scores of disease-associated variants with those of benign variants using a Wilcoxon rank-sum test. As shown in Additional file 1: Table S3, for variants in BRCA1, CFTR, and MLL2, most tools could identify risk variants from benign ones with *p* values smaller than 0.05. However, for variants in BRCA2 and TERT, PAFA outperformed all other methods by prioritizing more variants with much more significant p values.

We further evaluated PAFA's performance in prioritizing risk coding variants from adjacent variants utilizing two cancer-related coding variant sets. The first dataset includes 916 driver variants that were identified from 560 breast cancer samples in a recent study [37]. These driver variants are all located in coding regions. Correspondingly, variants adjacent to these disease-related variants (50 bp upstream and downstream) were extracted from 1000 Genomes and were used as the control dataset. As shown in Additional file 1: Figure S15A, previous methods, such as CADD, DANN, and FATHMM-MKL, exhibited good performance on prioritizing rare pathogenic variants from adjacent common variants, with AUC values larger than 0.8. PAFA exhibited the best performance with an AUC value of 0.947. Without population-level metrics, the PAFA classifier exhibited a decreased AUC value dropping to 0.714 (Additional file 1: Figure S16A–16B), which indicates that population-level metrics can greatly improve the performance of PAFA in discriminating coding risk variants from common variants. To further explore the role of various features used in the PAFA classifier, we constructed three models using different features. As shown in Additional file 1: Figure S16C–16E, all three features, including evolutionary conservation, genomic annotations, and population-level metrics, exhibited the ability to prioritize these breast cancer-related variants. Among them, population-level metrics showed an AUC value of 0.969, where common variants with low population differentiation indexes were assigned relatively low scores, and rare variants exhibited an even distribution of scores. In the following, we constructed five different models using various combinations of the training datasets (Additional file 1: Figure S16F–16J). After removing pathogenic rare variants from the training datasets, the PAFA classifier cannot distinguish breast cancer-related rare variants from adjacent common variants, with an AUC value of 0.052 (Additional file 1: Figure S16F).

The second dataset contains 6133 ovarian serous cystadenocarcinoma (OSC)-related variants that were obtained from the TCGA database [69]. More than 97% of these variants overlapped with exons. Correspondingly, we generated rare noncoding variants as the control dataset by simulating variants of the number of OSC-associated variants ten times; these variants are adjacent to the risk rare variants (50 bp upstream and downstream). PAFA, CADD, FATHMM-MKL, and LINSIGHT exhibited an ability to discriminate OSC-associated variants from simulated rare noncoding variants, with AUC values ranging from 0.565 to 0.682

(Additional file 1: Figure S15B), and PAFA exhibited the best performance. We constructed different PAFA classifiers to test feature groups as described above (Additional file 1: Figure S17A–E). The PAFA classifier that was constructed based on genomic annotations exhibited fairly good performance, with an AUC value of 0.747 (Additional file 1: Figure S17C), and the classifier constructed based on evolutionary conservation features had a moderate performance, with an AUC value of 0.543 (Additional file 1: Figure S17D). As expected, when the PAFA classifier utilized population-level metrics alone, it had no ability in discriminating risk rare variants from simulated ones, with an AUC value of 0.48 (Additional file 1: Figure S17E), since we only had population differentiation information of variants with frequencies of at least 1% in the populations studied in the 1000 Genomes. However, PAFA performed better than the PAFA classifier without population-level features (Additional file 1: Figure S17A–B). In addition, we found that the pathogenic rare variants and simulated rare benign noncoding variants in the training datasets also contributed to the performance of PAFA (Additional file 1: Figure S17F–17J).

Applying PAFA to noncoding genetic variants associated with complex diseases

To assess PAFA's performance in prioritizing noncoding variants associated with complex diseases and traits, we first compared PAFA with seven tools, namely, DIVAN, LINSIGHT, Eigen, GWAVA, CADD, DANN, and FATHMM-MKL. The tools were used to prioritize diseases or traits related to variants in the GRASP database [35], which includes approximately 8.87 million SNPs identified from 2082 GWAS. Considering that DIVAN constructed a specific classifier for each disease and only provided scores for variants related to 45 diseases, we selected 36 matched variant sets in GRASP as a test dataset; over 85% of these variants were noncoding common variants. The corresponding benign variants were randomly selected by sampling all the risk variants from the 1000 Genomes ten times; all GRASP variants were excluded from sampling. As shown in Fig. 5a, CADD, DANN, FATHMM-MKL, and the Region scores provided by GWAVA exhibited poor ability in prioritizing common variants associated with complex diseases/traits. Unsupervised methods, namely, LINSIGHT and Eigen, exhibited moderate performance in some diseases/traits, such as heart failure and ulcerative colitis, with AUC values larger than 0.55. PAFA achieved the best performance out of all methods, with AUC values in the range of 0.738–0.858 (median 0.799), followed by the performance of TSS and Region scores provided by DIVAN and Unmatched and TSS scores provided by GWAVA. DIVAN achieved comparable performance with PAFA in

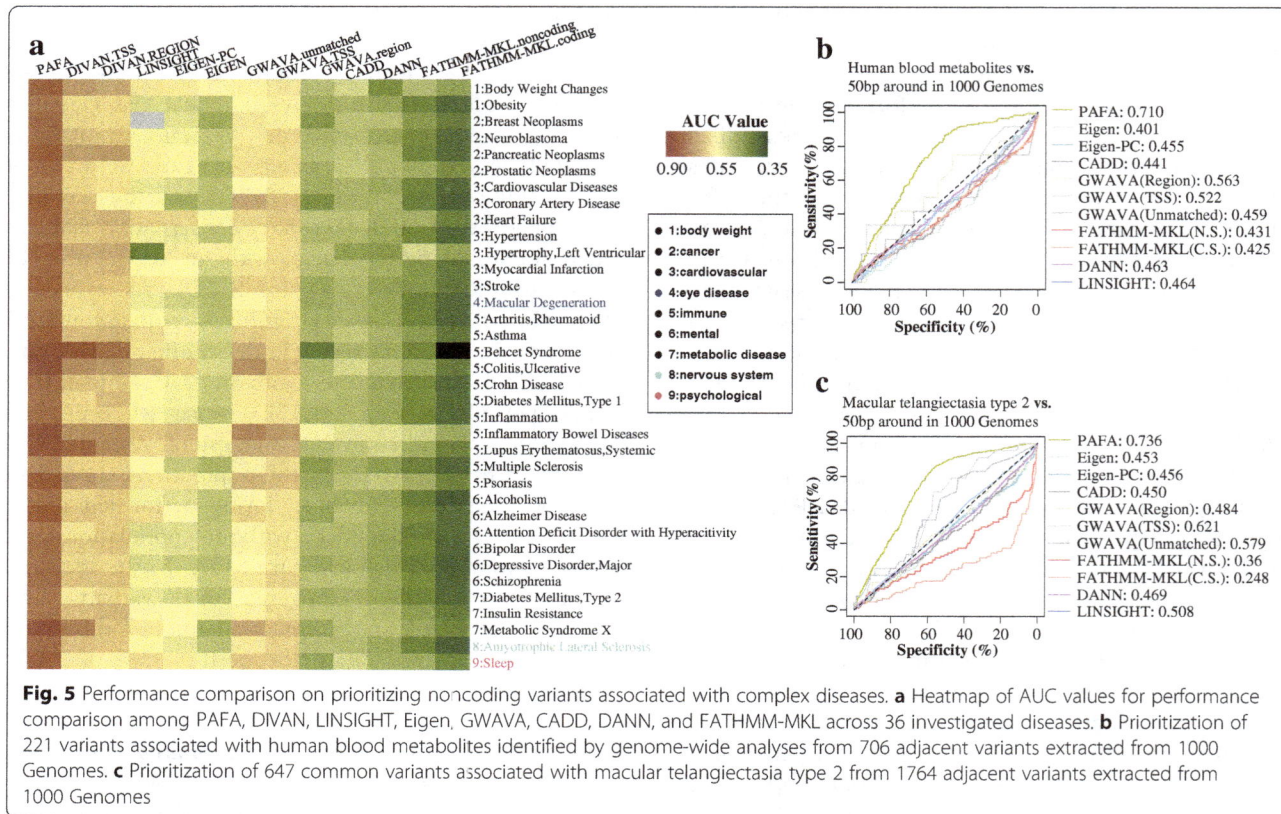

Fig. 5 Performance comparison on prioritizing noncoding variants associated with complex diseases. **a** Heatmap of AUC values for performance comparison among PAFA, DIVAN, LINSIGHT, Eigen, GWAVA, CADD, DANN, and FATHMM-MKL across 36 investigated diseases. **b** Prioritization of 221 variants associated with human blood metabolites identified by genome-wide analyses from 706 adjacent variants extracted from 1000 Genomes. **c** Prioritization of 647 common variants associated with macular telangiectasia type 2 from 1764 adjacent variants extracted from 1000 Genomes

several immune diseases, such as Behcet syndrome and systemic lupus erythematosus. Moreover, we found that PAFA outperformed all other methods in prioritizing variants associated with immune-related diseases, cancers, and cardiovascular diseases, with a median AUC value of 0.810.

Next, we selected two of the most recently published functional variant sets identified by genome-wide association studies to further evaluate the performance of PAFA. The first dataset includes 221 variants associated with human blood metabolites [38], among which 150 are common noncoding variants. The second dataset contains 647 common variants associated with macular telangiectasia type 2 [39], among which are 554 common noncoding variants. For each dataset, variants adjacent to the disease-related variants were extracted from 1000 Genomes and were used as the corresponding control dataset. Ultimately, we obtained 706 variants for human blood metabolites and 1764 for macular telangiectasia type 2 as control datasets. As shown in Fig. 5b, c, PAFA exhibited the best performance out of all the tools in prioritizing these complex disease/traits related to variants identified by whole-genome sequencing, with an AUC of 0.710 for human blood metabolites and 0.736 for macular telangiectasia type 2. The Region scores provided by GWAVA exhibited moderate performance

in prioritizing blood metabolites, with an AUC of 0.563. The TSS and Unmatched scores provided by GWAVA exhibited an ability to prioritize macular telangiectasia type 2, with AUC values of 0.621 and 0.579, respectively. Except for PAFA and GWAVA, the other tools exhibited a poor ability to prioritize the two functional variant datasets identified from GWAS. Genomic annotations and conservation metrics were not efficient to discriminate common noncoding functional variants from common noncoding neutral variants (Additional file 1: Figure S18A–18B, S19A–19B). For blood metabolites and macular telangiectasia type 2, the PAFA classifier constructed based on population-level metrics had improved performance, with AUC values of 0.884 and 0.826, respectively (Additional file 1: Figure S18C, S19C). In addition, the training data from GWASdb and 1000 Genomes also contributed to the performance of PAFA (Additional file 1: Figure S18F–18G, S19F–19G). Without the training data from GWASdb or 1000 Genomes, the PAFA classifier exhibited a dramatic decrease in its ability to prioritize common variants associated with diseases from adjacent common variants, with AUC values of 0.405 and 0.556, respectively, for human blood metabolite-related variants and AUC values of 0.350 and 0.559, respectively, for macular telangiectasia type 2-related variants.

Applying PAFA to cancer-related noncoding variants

To assess PAFA's ability in discriminating common recurrent from non-recurrent variants, we selected ten cancer-related variant sets from ICGC Cancer Genome Projects [36] (Additional file 1: Table S4). We selected variants located in noncoding regions as well as those recorded in 1000 Genomes, obtaining 127~74,685 noncoding common variants for each cancer dataset. Here, we deemed a noncoding variant that was observed in at least two donors of a specific cancer as a recurrent noncoding variant. As shown in Fig. 6a, for common variants from THCA-SA, most of the methods exhibited an ability to prioritize recurrent variants from non-recurrent ones, with AUC values ranging from 0.5 to 0.56. However, except for PAFA, these methods exhibited poor performance for variants from other projects. For variants from BTCA-JP, BOCA-FR, LAML-KR, PAEN-AU, PAEN-IT, and EOPC-DE, most of the previous methods (LINSIGHT, Eigen, FATHMM-MKL, CADD,

and DANN) could not discriminate recurrent from non-recurrent noncoding variants, with AUC values ranging from 0.369 to 0.496. PAFA, however, exhibited better performance in prioritizing recurrent noncoding variants, with AUC values larger than 0.5 for seven out of ten samples.

To explore the role of population-level metrics on common noncoding variants introduced in the PAFA classifier, we tested its ability in prioritizing recurrent variants from non-recurrent ones by removing population-level features. Under default settings, the PAFA classifier exhibited better performance in discriminating common recurrent variants according to ten cancer-related variant sets from ICGC (Fig. 6b). After removing population-level features, however, recurrent variants tended to have more decreased scores than non-recurrent variants (Fig. 6c).

To assess PAFA's ability in discriminating rare recurrent variants, we first compared PAFA's performance in

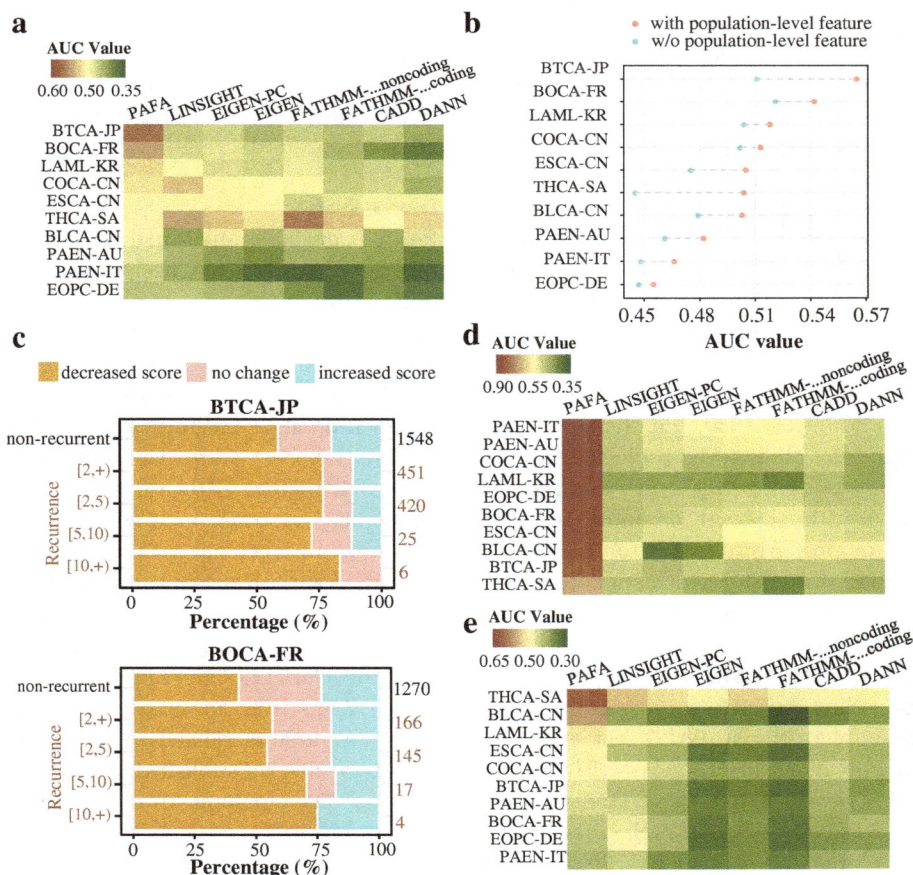

Fig. 6 Performance evaluation on cancer-related noncoding risk variants. **a** Common recurrent noncoding variants versus common non-recurrent noncoding variants. **b** Prioritizing recurrent variants from non-recurrent variants using PAFA with or without population-level features across ten cancer-related variant sets from ICGC. **c** Alteration of PAFA scores after removing population-level features in BTCA-JP and BOCA-FR. **d** Rare noncoding variants versus adjacent common noncoding variants extracted from 1000 Genomes. **e** Rare recurrent noncoding variants versus rare non-recurrent noncoding variants

prioritizing noncoding rare risk variants from adjacent common variants with other algorithms. For variants from ICGC, we selected variants located in noncoding regions as well as those not recorded in 1000 Genomes, and we obtained 963, 242,564, 5408, 129,975, 31,632, 76,763, 95,741, 25,388, 1181, and 111,088 noncoding rare variants for BLCA-CN, COCA-CN, ESCA-CN, PAEN-AU, BOCA-FR, EOPC-DE, PAEN-IT, BTCA-JP, THCA-SA, and LAML-KR, respectively (Additional file 1: Table S4). For each of the ten variant sets from ICGC, benign variants adjacent to the cancer-related variants (50 bp upstream and downstream) were extracted from 1000 Genomes and were used as control datasets. As shown in Fig. 6d, the previous methods exhibited unstable and relatively poor performance in discriminating noncoding rare risk variants from adjacent common variants. For example, CADD, DANN, Eigen, and FATHMM-MKL exhibited an ability to prioritize rare risk variants from PAEN-IT, PAEN-AU, BOCA-FR, and ESCA-CN, with AUC values ranging from 0.502 to 0.561, but they could not discriminate cancer-related variants from LAML-KR and THCA-SA, with AUC values ranging from 0.414 to 0.488. PAFA outperformed all other methods in all ten variant sets, with AUC values ranging from 0.682 to 0.877. As shown in Additional file 1: Figure S20, the good performance of PAFA relied on the introduction of population differentiation features. Because these benign common variants are close to the cancer-related variants, prioritization methods that were solely based on genomic annotations did not perform well. According to LINSIGHT scores, noncoding rare risk variants from ESCA-CN, BLCA-CN, and BTCA-JP exhibited higher degrees of evolutionary constraint than adjacent common variants, with AUC values ranging from 0.509 to 0.539, but the noncoding rare risk variants from the other seven projects exhibited indistinguishable or lower degrees of evolutionary constraint compared with adjacent common variants, with AUC values ranging from 0.452 to 0.5. Moreover, we assessed the six tools' performance in prioritizing rare recurrent noncoding variants, which are population-irrelevant. As shown in Fig. 6e, all current methods exhibited poor performance in prioritizing rare recurrent noncoding variants from non-recurrent ones. Among these algorithms, PAFA achieved the best performance in THCA-SA, BLCA-CN, LAML-KR, ESCA-CN, COCA-CN, BTCA-JP, and PAEN-AU. LINSIGHT, CADD, DANN, Eigen, and FAHMM-MKL exhibited an ability to discriminate rare recurrent noncoding variants in THCA-SA, with AUC values larger than 0.5. LINSIGHT also exhibited a slight discrimination ability for variants from BLCA-CN, COCA-CN, and EOPC-DE, with AUC values of 0.503, 0.503, and 0.51, respectively.

An integrated online platform for PAFA

We developed an online platform to facilitate the use of PAFA. Precomputed PAFA scores for all 231 million variants of dbSNP and 2.68 billion single nucleotide variants throughout the human genome are integrated into this online platform, where users can access these precomputed PAFA scores through batch download or can submit a list of genomic locations or variants of interest to obtain target PAFA scores and gene-centric annotations. As shown in Additional file 1: Figure S6, this platform provides a simple and intuitive interface to help users determine the functional significance of variants. Its major functions include performing enrichment analysis for variants; annotating variants with known risk variants, genomic annotations, disease-associated genes, and pathways recorded in curated databases (e.g., ClinVar, COSMIC, and ENCODE); and providing scores for target variants based on their associated genes' occurrence frequency in disease-related databases. Moreover, for variants that are found in 1000 Genomes, population-level information is also shown, including the F_{ST} index, allele frequency spectrum, and associated genomic elements. All curated knowledge data have been stored in MySQL, the platform was developed in JAVA, and the interactive interface was created with HTML5 and JavaScript.

Discussion

PAFA is an integrative method for prioritizing clinically relevant variants from background variants by concentrating on factors associated with population-specific diseases/traits and common variants with weak effect. Through extensive evaluations, we demonstrated that PAFA consistently outperforms the latest published supervised and unsupervised methods. First, PAFA exhibits the best performance in discriminating significant cSNPs in the GWAS Catalog and recurrent somatic noncoding variants in the COSMIC database from common variants in 1000 Genomes. Second, PAFA exhibits high sensitivity and specificity in prioritizing pathogenic variants related to Mendelian diseases as well as prioritizing coding risk variants from both adjacent common variants and simulated noncoding variants. Third, PAFA has an increased capability to prioritize common variants related to 36 complex diseases/traits and two newly published variant sets identified by genome-wide analyses from background variants with population-level metrics. It also outperforms previous methods in discriminating recurrent common noncoding variants from non-recurrent noncoding variants. In addition, PAFA also provides gene-centric functional annotations for variants based on the integrated annotated functional elements. To facilitate its usage, we developed a user-friendly online platform that not only allows users to evaluate variant sets by PAFA but also provides multiple functions, including enrichment analysis on target variant sets and comprehensive annotations for variants/genes.

Previous supervised classifiers are good at prioritizing coding functional variants but have limited ability to prioritize and annotate noncoding variants. As an unsupervised method, Eigen avoids the problem caused by erroneous labeling, but it still cannot distinguish complex disease-/trait-associated variants from the background variants. PAFA exhibited much better performance in prioritizing noncoding variants than the currently available approaches, no matter supervised or unsupervised methods, under comprehensive evaluations. Its good performance can be attributed to three types of improvements. First, PAFA employs a population differentiation index to prioritize population-specific associations of common risk variants for complex diseases. This feature relies on the variants in Phase 3 of 1000 Genomes and considers both population difference and diversity within populations by calculating F_{ST} and dispersion score (DS). It improves the performance of PAFA in prioritizing common functional noncoding variants from background variants. Second, the optimization of training datasets from GWASdb and 1000 Genomes helps PAFA prioritize common functional variants and reduce its false-positive rate. Due to the limited amount of verified functional noncoding variants, we introduced cSNPs from GWAS, which is composed of tens of thousands of loci associated with various human diseases and traits. Since noncoding variants are suspected of disrupting the normal regulatory control mechanisms of target genes [18], we selected significant cSNPs that overlap genomic elements from GWASdb as functional variants in the training stage. Considering that 1000 Genomes may contain a large number of functionally or clinically important variants, we selected likely benign variants from 1000 Genomes utilizing multiple filtration strategies. Based on the cSNPs used in the training stage, we constructed a regressive model and selected variants from 1000 Genomes with the least similarity and low population differentiation indices as control variants. Third, we integrated multiple genomic annotations and selected verified pathogenic variants from ClinVar as a part of PAFA's training set, and the results showed that PAFA exhibited improved performance in prioritizing recurrent from non-recurrent variants and performed well in discriminating noncoding risk variants.

In this work, we describe PAFA, an effective method for the prioritization and functional assessment of genetic variants associated with complex traits or diseases, particularly population-relevant noncoding variants. PAFA employs a sophisticated model for feature integration by combining multiple features, including genomic annotations, evolutionary conservation metrics, and population differentiation metrics. The population differentiation index is adopted to improve predictive performance due to the high genetic differentiation of cSNPs among human populations. Genomic annotations help PAFA discriminate risk variants by the information of genomic elements the variants overlapped. Functional regions are more likely to have higher evolutionary conservation degree than neutral regions. These features work together by employing a sparse logistic regression algorithm with L1 regularization, and this algorithm is fit for sparse matrices by ignoring missing values. In addition, to avoid strong model assumptions, PAFA employs an integrative supervised approach. Considering that the number of verified noncoding variants is limited, PAFA selects the training set from curated databases with multiple filtration strategies. This combination of more efficient features and reliable training sets makes PAFA more powerful and robust than existing state-of-the-art methods, both supervised and unsupervised, in detecting functional noncoding variants. However, as a correctly labeled training set is the key to improving the sensitivity and accuracy of prioritization methods, more verified annotated noncoding variants are still expected. Pre-computed PAFA pathogenicity scores for 2.68 billion human SNVs based on the GRCh37/hg19 assembly are now available for batch download through our constructed online platform. Users can navigate variants based on either GRCh37/hg19 or GRCh38 using the lift-over tool integrated in PAFA. We will update the PAFA tool and its web portal when new versions of annotated noncoding variants and genomic annotations (e.g., ClinVar and ENCODE) are available. New released resources, like gnomAD frequency data [70], are expected to be integrated in a future update. We believe that PAFA will be an indispensable tool for prioritizing and annotating functional noncoding variants that are associated with complex traits or diseases.

Conclusion

This study presents a novel supervised algorithm for prioritization and functional assessment of genetic variants associated with complex diseases or traits, especially for noncoding variants. It introduces measures to evaluate genetic differentiation of variants among different population groups. PAFA also recalibrates abundant training variants from curated databases with multiple new filtration strategies. Through comprehensive performance evaluations, as well as compared with previous methods, we demonstrated that PAFA exhibits a much better performance on prioritizing both coding and noncoding risk variants as well as discriminating recurrent from non-recurrent variants. We further constructed a user-friendly web server, which not only allows users to evaluate variants using PAFA but also provides comprehensive functional annotations by integrating abundant functional genomic elements.

Availability and requirements

The availability and requirements are listed as follows:

Project name: PAFA

Project home page: http://159.226.67.237:8080/pafa; http://bioinfo.biols.ac.cn

Operating system(s): platform independent.

Programming language: Java, MySQL, JavaScript, HTML5.

Other requirements: Chrome, Firefox, Safari.

Additional files

Additional file 1: Table S1. A tabular comparison between PAFA and seven other ensemble classifiers aimed at detecting functional/deleterious variants from background variants. Table S2. Comparisons among PAFA, Eigen, CADD, GWAVA, DANN, FATHMM-MKL, and LINSIGHT in evaluating variants from four curated databases, including ClinVar, 1000 Genomes, GWAS Catalog, and COSMIC. Table S3. Comparisons among PAFA, Eigen, CADD, GWAVA, FATHMM-MKL, and DANN in discriminating pathogenic variants from benign variants associated with Mendelian diseases. Table S4. Statistics often cancer-related variant sets from ICGC projects. Figure S1. Genetic and genomic resources used in PAFA and their screenshots. Figure S2. Genetic and genomic resources used in the 1000 GENOMES part of the PAFA online platform and their screenshots. Figure S3. Genetic and genomic resources used in the ANNOTATION part of the PAFA online platform and their screenshots. Figure S4. Genetic and genomic resources used in the VSEA part of the PAFA online platform and their screenshots. Figure S5. Genetic and genomic resources used in the SEARCH part of the PAFA online platform and their screenshots. Figure S6. An integrated PAFA online platform for variant prioritization and functional annotation. Figure S7. Flowchart of selecting and filtering training variants used in PAFA. Figure S8. Tenfold cross-validations are applied to evaluate the performance of features used in PAFA. Figure S9. Distribution of allele frequencies for 24 cancer-associated variant sets from GWASdb among super populations. Figure S10. Distribution of allele frequencies for nine complex trait-associated variant sets from GWASdb among super populations. Figure S11. Distribution of allele frequencies for eight mental disorder-associated variant sets. Figure S12. Distribution of allele frequencies for 17 complex disease-associated variant sets. Figure S13. Distribution of F_{ST} values for variant sets associated with complex diseases and traits. Figure S14. Enriched pathways of genes associated with coding and noncoding variants. Figure S15. Sensitivity and specificity of tools in distinguishing coding risk variants from adjacent variants. Figure S16. Distributions of PAFA scores for breast cancer-related variants and adjacent variants from the 1000 Genomes. Figure S17. Distributions of PAFA scores for OSC-related variants from TCGA and simulated noncoding rare variants. Figure S18. Distributions of PAFA scores for human blood metabolite-related variants and adjacent variants from 1000 Genomes. Figure S19. Distributions of PAFA scores for macular telangiectasia type 2-related variants and adjacent variants from 1000 Genomes. Figure S20. Distributions of PAFA scores for bladder cancer-related variants and adjacent variants from 1000 Genomes.

Funding

This work was supported by grants from the National Natural Science Foundation of China [31722031, 31671364, 91531306] and National Key R&D Program [2016YFC1200804].

Authors' contributions

FZ conceived the study. FZ and LZ designed the methods. LZ carried out the analysis. LZ and FZ wrote the manuscript. Both authors read and approved the final manuscript.

Competing interests

The authors declare that they have no competing interests.

Author details

[1]Computational Genomics Lab, Beijing Institutes of Life Science, Chinese Academy of Sciences, Beijing 100101, China. [2]University of Chinese Academy of Sciences, Beijing 100049, China. [3]Center for Excellence in Animal Evolution and Genetics, Chinese Academy of Sciences, Kunming 650223, China.

References

1. Mardis ER. A decade's perspective on DNA sequencing technology. Nature. 2011;470:198.
2. Todorovic V. Genetics. Predicting the impact of genomic variation. Nat Methods. 2016;13:203.
3. Saint Pierre A, Genin E. How important are rare variants in common disease? Brief Funct Genomics. 2014;13:353–61.
4. Cooper GM, Shendure J. Needles in stacks of needles: finding disease-causal variants in a wealth of genomic data. Nat Rev Genet. 2011;12:628–40.
5. Kumar P, Henikoff S, Ng PC. Predicting the effects of coding non-synonymous variants on protein function using the SIFT algorithm. Nat Protoc. 2009;4:1073–81.
6. Adzhubei IA, Schmidt S, Peshkin L, Ramensky VE, Gerasimova A, Bork P, Kondrashov AS, Sunyaev SR. A method and server for predicting damaging missense mutations. Nat Methods. 2010;7:248–9.
7. Consortium EP. An integrated encyclopedia of DNA elements in the human genome. Nature. 2012;489:57–74.
8. Andersson R, Gebhard C, Miguel-Escalada I, Hoof I, Bornholdt J, Boyd M, Chen Y, Zhao X, Schmidl C, Suzuki T, et al. An atlas of active enhancers across human cell types and tissues. Nature. 2014;507:455–+.
9. Altshuler DM, Durbin RM, Abecasis GR, Bentley DR, Chakravarti A, Clark AG, Donnelly P, Eichler EE, Flicek P, Gabriel SB, et al. A global reference for human genetic variation. Nature. 2015;526:68–+.
10. Lu QS, Hu YM, Sun JH, Cheng YW, Cheung KH, Zhao HY. A statistical framework to predict functional non-coding regions in the human genome through integrated analysis of annotation data. Sci Rep. 2015;5:10576.
11. Ionita-Laza I, McCallum K, Xu B, Buxbaum JD. A spectral approach integrating functional genomic annotations for coding and noncoding variants. Nat Genet. 2016;48:214–20.
12. Kircher M, Witten DM, Jain P, O'Roak BJ, Cooper GM, Shendure J. A general framework for estimating the relative pathogenicity of human genetic variants. Nat Genet. 2014;46:310–5.
13. Shihab HA, Rogers MF, Gough J, Mort M, Cooper DN, Day INM, Gaunt TR, Campbell C. An integrative approach to predicting the functional effects of non-coding and coding sequence variation. Bioinformatics. 2015;31:1536–43.
14. Shihab HA, Gough J, Cooper DN, Stenson PD, Barker GL, Edwards KJ, Day IN, Gaunt TR. Predicting the functional, molecular, and phenotypic consequences of amino acid substitutions using hidden Markov models. Hum Mutat. 2013;34:57–65.
15. Rogers MF, Shihab HA, Mort M, Cooper DN, Gaunt TR, Campbell C. FATHMM-XF: accurate prediction of pathogenic point mutations via extended features. Bioinformatics. 2018;34:511–3.
16. Quang D, Chen Y, Xie X. DANN: a deep learning approach for annotating the pathogenicity of genetic variants. Bioinformatics. 2015;31:761–3.
17. Ritchie GR, Dunham I, Zeggini E, Flicek P. Functional annotation of noncoding sequence variants. Nat Methods. 2014;11:294–6.
18. Chen L, Jin P, Qin ZHS. DIVAN: accurate identification of non-coding disease-specific risk variants using multi-omics profiles. Genome Biol. 2016;17:252.
19. Huang YF, Gulko B, Siepel A. Fast, scalable prediction of deleterious noncoding variants from functional and population genomic data. Nat Genet. 2017;49:618–24.

20. Jakobsson MEMD, Rosenberg NA. The relationship between FST and the frequency of the most frequent allele. Genetics. 2013;193:515–28.

21. Gonzaga-Jauregui C, Lupski JR, Gibbs RA. Human genome sequencing in health and disease. Annu Rev Med. 2012;63:35–61.

22. Zhang F, Lupski JR. Non-coding genetic variants in human disease. Hum Mol Genet. 2015;24:R102–10.

23. Landrum MJ, Lee JM, Benson M, Brown G, Chao C, Chitipiralla S, Gu B, Hart J, Hoffman D, Hoover J, et al. ClinVar: public archive of interpretations of clinically relevant variants. Nucleic Acids Res. 2016;44:D862–8.

24. Li MJ, Liu ZP, Wang PW, Wong MP, Nelson MR, Kocher JPA, Yeager M, Sham PC, Chanock SJ, Xia ZY, Wang JW. GWASdb v2: an update database for human genetic variants identified by genome-wide association studies. Nucleic Acids Res. 2016;44:D869–76.

25. Casper J, Zweig AS, Villarreal C, Tyner C, Speir ML, Rosenbloom KR, Raney BJ, Lee CM, Lee BT, Karolchik D, et al. The UCSC Genome Browser database: 2018 update. Nucleic Acids Res. 2018;46:D762–9.

26. Siepel A, Bejerano G, Pedersen JS, Hinrichs AS, Hou MM, Rosenbloom K, Clawson H, Spieth J, Hillier LW, Richards S, et al. Evolutionarily conserved elements in vertebrate, insect, worm, and yeast genomes. Genome Res. 2005;15:1034–50.

27. Pollard KS, Hubisz MJ, Rosenbloom KR, Siepel A. Detection of nonneutral substitution rates on mammalian phylogenies. Genome Res. 2010;20:110–21.

28. Harrow J, Frankish A, Gonzalez JM, Tapanari E, Diekhans M, Kokocinski F, Aken BL, Barrell D, Zadissa A, Searle S, et al. GENCODE: the reference human genome annotation for the ENCODE Project. Genome Res. 2012;22:1760–74.

29. Grillo G, Turi A, Licciulli F, Mignone F, Liuni S, Banfi S, Gennarino VA, Horner DS, Pavesi G, Picardi E, Pesole G. UTRdb and UTRsite (RELEASE 2010): a collection of sequences and regulatory motifs of the untranslated regions of eukaryotic mRNAs. Nucleic Acids Res. 2010;38:D75–80.

30. Yip KY, Cheng C, Bhardwaj N, Brown JB, Leng J, Kundaje A, Rozowsky J, Birney E, Bickel P, Snyder M, Gerstein M. Classification of human genomic regions based on experimentally determined binding sites of more than 100 transcription-related factors. Genome Biol. 2012;13:R48.

31. Ma W, Yang Y, Qi LT, Zhao F, Zhang BW, Meng L, Zhang Y, Jiang J, Li JP, Zhu SN, et al. Association between serum uric acid and brachial ankle pulse wave velocity in Beijing community residents. Zhonghua Xin Xue Guan Bing Za Zhi. 2012;40:204–8.

32. MacArthur J, Bowler E, Cerezo M, Gil L, Hall P, Hastings E, Junkins H, McMahon A, Milano A, Morales J, et al. The new NHGRI-EBI Catalog of published genome-wide association studies (GWAS Catalog). Nucleic Acids Res. 2017;45:D896–901.

33. Forbes SA, Beare D, Gunasekaran P, Leung K, Bindal N, Boutselakis H, Ding MJ, Bamford S, Cole C, Ward S, et al. COSMIC: exploring the world's knowledge of somatic mutations in human cancer. Nucleic Acids Res. 2015;43:D805–11.

34. Bell D, Berchuck A, Birrer M, Chien J, Cramer DW, Dao F, Dhir R, DiSaia P, Gabra H, Glenn P, et al. Integrated genomic analyses of ovarian carcinoma. Nature. 2011;474:609–15.

35. Eicher JD, Landowski C, Stackhouse B, Sloan A, Chen WJ, Jensen N, Lien JP, Leslie R, Johnson AD. GRASP v2.0: an update on the Genome-Wide Repository of Associations between SNPs and phenotypes. Nucleic Acids Res. 2015;43:D799–804.

36. International Cancer Genome Consortium, Hudson TJ, Anderson W, Artez A, Barker AD, Bell C, Bernabe RR, Bhan MK, Calvo F, Eerola I, et al. International network of cancer genome projects. Nature. 2010;464:993–8.

37. Nik-Zainal S, Davies H, Staaf J, Ramakrishna M, Dominik ZXQ, Martincorena I, Alexandrov LB, Martin S, Wedge DC, et al. Landscape of somatic mutations in 560 breast cancer whole-genome sequences. Nature. 2016;534:47.

38. Long T, Hicks M, Yu HC, Biggs WH, Kirkness EF, Menni C, Zierer J, Small KS, Mangino M, Messier H, et al. Whole-genome sequencing identifies common-to-rare variants associated with human blood metabolites. Nat Genet. 2017;49:568–78.

39. Scerri TS, Quaglieri A, Cai C, Zernant J, Matsunami N, Baird L, Scheppke L, Bonelli R, Yannuzzi LA, Friedlander M, et al. Genome-wide analyses identify common variants associated with macular telangiectasia type 2. Nat Genet. 2017;49:559–67.

40. Sherry ST, Ward MH, Kholodov M, Baker J, Phan L, Smigielski EM, Sirotkin K. dbSNP: the NCBI database of genetic variation. Nucleic Acids Res. 2001;29:308–11.

41. Emond MJ, Louie T, Emerson J, Zhao W, Mathias RA, Knowles MR, Wright FA, Rieder MJ, Tabor HK, Nickerson DA, et al. Exome sequencing of extreme phenotypes identifies DCTN4 as a modifier of chronic Pseudomonas aeruginosa infection in cystic fibrosis. Nat Genet. 2012;44:886–+.

42. Li GQ, Ma LJ, Song C, Yang ZT, Wang XL, Huang H, Li YR, Li RQ, Zhang XQ, Yang HM, et al. The YH database: the first Asian diploid genome database. Nucleic Acids Res. 2009;37:D1025–8.

43. Waddell N, Pajic M, Patch AM, Chang DK, Kassahn KS, Bailey P, Johns AL, Miller D, Nones K, Quek K, et al. Whole genomes redefine the mutational landscape of pancreatic cancer. Nature. 2015;518:495–501.

44. Kim J, Shin JY, Kim JI, Seo JS, Webster MJ, Lee D, Kim S. Somatic deletions implicated in functional diversity of brain cells of individuals with schizophrenia and unaffected controls. Sci Rep. 2014;4:3807.

45. Pinto D, Pagnamenta AT, Klei L, Anney R, Merico D, Regan R, Conroy J, Magalhaes TR, Correia C, Abrahams BS, et al. Functional impact of global rare copy number variation in autism spectrum disorders. Nature. 2010;466:368–72.

46. Hamosh A, Scott AF, Amberger JS, Bocchini CA, McKusick VA. Online Mendelian Inheritance in Man (OMIM), a knowledgebase of human genes and genetic disorders. Nucleic Acids Res. 2005;33:D514–7.

47. Becker KG, Barnes KC, Bright TJ, Wang SA. The Genetic Association Database. Nat Genet. 2004;36:431–2.

48. Liberzon A. A description of the Molecular Signatures Database (MSigDB) web site. Methods Mol Biol. 2014;1150:153–60.

49. Marek-Yagel D, Bar-Joseph I, Pras E, Berkun Y. Is E148Q a benign polymorphism or a disease-causing mutation? J Rheumatol. 2009;36:2372–3.

50. Cao ZM, Petroulakis E, Salo T, TriggsRaine B. Benign HEXA mutations, C739T(R247W) and C745T(R249W), cause beta-hexosaminidase A pseudodeficiency by reducing the alpha-subunit protein levels. J Biol Chem. 1997;272:14975–82.

51. Fan RE, Chang KW, Hsieh CJ, Wang XR, Lin CJ. Liblinear: a library for large linear classification. J Mach Learn Res. 2008;9:1871–4.

52. Weir BS, Cockerham CC. Estimating F-statistics for the analysis of population-structure. Evolution. 1984;38:1358–70.

53. Znaor A, Lortet-Tieulent J, Jemal A, Bray F. International variations and trends in testicular cancer incidence and mortality. Eur Urol. 2014;65:1095–106.

54. Chia VM, Quraishi SM, Devesa SS, Purdue MP, Cook MB, McGlynn KA. International trends in the incidence of testicular cancer, 1973–2002. Cancer Epidemiol Biomark Prev. 2010;19:1151–9.

55. Hartl DL, Clark AG. Principles of population genetics. 3rd ed. Sunderland: Sinauer Associates, Inc; 1997.

56. Eriksson N, Macpherson JM, Tung JY, Hon LS, Naughton B, Saxonov S, Avey L, Wojcicki A, Pe'er I, Mountain J. Web-based, participant-driven studies yield novel genetic associations for common traits. PLoS Genet. 2010;6:e1000993.

57. Zhang MF, Song FJ, Liang LM, Nan HM, Zhang JW, Liu HL, Wang LE, Wei QY, Lee JE, Amos CI, et al. Genome-wide association studies identify several new loci associated with pigmentation traits and skin cancer risk in European Americans. Hum Mol Genet. 2013;22:2948–59.

58. Chu LW, Ritchey J, Devesa SS, Quraishi SM, Zhang H, Hsing AW. Prostate cancer incidence rates in Africa. Prostate Cancer. 2011;2011:947870.

59. Xu X, Wu J, Xiao J, Tan Y, Bao Q, Zhao F, Li X. PlasmoGF: an integrated system for comparative genomics and phylogenetic analysis of Plasmodium gene families. Bioinformatics. 2008;24:1217–20.

60. Zheng-Bradley X, Flicek P. Applications of the 1000 Genomes Project resources. Briefings in functional genomics. 2016;16:163–70.

61. Cheng CY, Yamashiro K, Chen LJ, Ahn J, Huang LL, Huang LZ, Cheung CMG, Miyake M, Cackett PD, Yeo IY, et al. New loci and coding variants confer risk for age-related macular degeneration in East Asians. Nat Commun. 2015;6:6063.

62. Qi Q, Hu FB. Genetics of type 2 diabetes in European populations. J Diabetes. 2012;4:203–12.

63. Albain KS, Unger JM, Crowley JJ, Coltman CA, Hershman DL. Racial disparities in cancer survival among randomized clinical trials patients of the southwest oncology group. J Natl Cancer Inst. 2009;101:984–92.

64. Bradley CJ, Given CW, Roberts C. Race, socioeconomic status, and breast cancer treatment and survival. J Natl Cancer Inst. 2002;94:490–6.

65. Wong WL, Su XY, Li X, Cheung CMG, Klein R, Cheng CY, Wong TY. Global prevalence of age-related macular degeneration and disease burden projection for 2020 and 2040: a systematic review and meta-analysis. Lancet Global Health. 2014;2:E106–16.

66. Ma RCW, Chan JCN. Type 2 diabetes in East Asians: similarities and differences with populations in Europe and the United States. Ann N Y Acad Sci. 2013;1281:64–91.

67. Krishnan A, Zhang R, Yao V, Theesfeld CL, Wong AK, Tadych A, Volfovsky N, Packer A, Lash A, Troyanskaya OG. Genome-wide prediction and functional characterization of the genetic basis of autism spectrum disorder. Nat Neurosci. 2016;19:1454–62.

14

Integrative analysis of DNA methylation and gene expression reveals hepatocellular carcinoma-specific diagnostic biomarkers

Jinming Cheng[1,2] ⓘ, Dongkai Wei[3], Yuan Ji[4], Lingli Chen[4], Liguang Yang[2], Guang Li[3], Leilei Wu[1,2], Ting Hou[2], Lu Xie[5], Guohui Ding[2*], Hong Li[2*] and Yixue Li[1,2,5*]

Abstract

Background: Hepatocellular carcinoma (HCC) is the one of the most common cancers and lethal diseases in the world. DNA methylation alteration is frequently observed in HCC and may play important roles in carcinogenesis and diagnosis.

Methods: Using the TCGA HCC dataset, we classified HCC patients into different methylation subtypes, identified differentially methylated and expressed genes, and analyzed *cis-* and *trans-*regulation of DNA methylation and gene expression. To find potential diagnostic biomarkers for HCC, we screened HCC-specific CpGs by comparing the methylation profiles of 375 samples from HCC patients, 50 normal liver samples, 184 normal blood samples, and 3780 samples from patients with other cancers. A logistic regression model was constructed to distinguish HCC patients from normal controls. Model performance was evaluated using three independent datasets (including 327 HCC samples and 122 normal samples) and ten newly collected biopsies.

Results: We identified a group of patients with a CpG island methylator phenotype (CIMP) and found that the overall survival of CIMP patients was poorer than that of non-CIMP patients. Our analyses showed that the *cis-*regulation of DNA methylation and gene expression was dominated by the negative correlation, while the *trans-*regulation was more complex. More importantly, we identified six HCC-specific hypermethylated sites as potential diagnostic biomarkers. The combination of six sites achieved ~ 92% sensitivity in predicting HCC, ~ 98% specificity in excluding normal livers, and ~ 98% specificity in excluding other cancers. Compared with previously published methylation markers, our markers are the only ones that can distinguish HCC from other cancers.

Conclusions: Overall, our study systematically describes the DNA methylation characteristics of HCC and provides promising biomarkers for the diagnosis of HCC.

Keywords: Hepatocellular carcinoma, Methylation, CpG island methylator phenotype, Gene regulation, Specific diagnostic biomarker

Background

Hepatocellular carcinoma (HCC) is the sixth most common cancer and the third leading cause of cancer deaths in the world [1]. Most cases of HCC occur in developing countries, such as China, and the leading cause of HCC is chronic infection with hepatitis B virus (HBV); in contrast, the main cause in developed countries, such as the USA, is infection with hepatitis C virus (HCV) [2]. Other risk factors for developing HCC include exposure to aflatoxin, excessive alcohol consumption, tobacco smoking, and diabetes [1]. After being affected by one or more of these risk factors, both genetic and epigenetic alterations will emerge, which may result in the activation of oncogenes and the inactivation of tumor suppressor genes, leading to the occurrence of hepatocellular carcinoma. The 5-year survival rate is > 70% if patients

* Correspondence: gwding@sibs.ac.cn; lihong01@sibs.ac.cn; yxli@sibs.ac.cn
[2]Key Lab of Computational Biology, CAS-MPG Partner Institute for Computational Biology, Shanghai Institutes for Biological Sciences, Chinese Academy of Sciences, Shanghai, China
[1]Department of Bioinformatics and Biostatistics, School of Life Sciences and Biotechnology, Shanghai Jiao Tong University, Shanghai, China
Full list of author information is available at the end of the article

are diagnosed at an early stage [3], while the 5-year survival rate decreases to approximately 10% for advanced HCC patients [4]. Therefore, early detection of HCC is important for increasing the chances for effective treatment and improving the survival rate.

Alpha-fetoprotein (AFP) combined with ultrasonography is a widely used method for the screening and diagnosis of HCC. Marrero et al. [5] reported the diagnostic performance of serum AFP when using a cut-off of 20 ng/mL. Its sensitivity is 59% and specificity 90% for all HCC patients. Additionally, the sensitivity is 53% and the specificity 90% for early-stage HCC [5]. Due to the lack of diagnostic accuracy, the American Association for the Study of Liver Diseases and the European Association for the Study of the Liver do not recommend AFP for HCC diagnosis [6, 7]. The development of omics technologies has allowed researchers to choose a single molecule or a panel of multiple molecules as potential diagnostic biomarkers. Des-γ-carboxy prothrombin (DCP) is a promising serum biomarker. It achieved 74% sensitivity and 70% specificity in all HCC patients, as well as 61% sensitivity and 70% specificity for early-stage HCC at the level of 150 mAU/mL [5]. Another serum biomarker, Dickkopf-1 (DKK1), has similar sensitivity (~ 70%) and specificity (~ 90%) in all HCC patients and for early-stage HCC at a cut-off of 2.153 ng/mL [8]. Although many candidate biomarkers have been reported, few of them are currently used in clinical practice. More effective biomarkers are urgently needed to increase the accuracy of HCC diagnosis.

DNA methylation alteration has been observed in various cancers and is considered to be a cause of carcinogenesis. Global hypomethylation is frequently seen in highly and moderately repeated DNA sequences and plays a key role in chromosomal instability [9, 10]. Hypermethylation in gene promoter regions, such as in tumor suppressor genes, is usually related to gene silencing [9, 11]. Some DNA methylation is involved in the early stage of carcinogenesis, such as RASSF1A in ovarian cancer [12]. Additionally, DNA methylation is relatively stable over time [13] and can be non-invasively detected in blood. Therefore, DNA methylation has a great potential to become an early diagnostic biomarker of cancers. An increasing number of methylation-based biomarkers have been developed to aid in the early diagnosis of cancers [14]. The FDA-approved "Epi proColon test" is based on the SEPT9 promoter methylation status in the plasma. This diagnostic test had a sensitivity of 36.6 to 95.6% and a specificity of 81.5 to 99.0% for colorectal cancer [15]. Zheng et al. [16] reported that using the DNA methylation of ten CpGs could achieve good performance to discriminate tumors from normal tissues in HCC patients, with a sensitivity of more than 86% and a specificity of almost 100%. Xu et al. [17] found

that the circulating tumor DNA (ctDNA) methylation of another ten CpGs could also discriminate HCC patients from healthy individuals with a sensitivity of more than 83% and a specificity of more than 90%. Both CpG sets could be good biomarkers for the diagnosis of HCC, but neither of these research groups considered whether other cancer types could have similar methylation alterations; hence, these biomarkers may not be HCC-specific, and specific biomarkers are absent and needed.

In this study, we first classified HCC patients into different methylation subtypes and analyzed the *cis*- and *trans*-regulation of DNA methylation and gene expression. Then, we identified six HCC-specific methylation biomarkers by comparing HCC with normal livers and other cancer types. The combinations of two and six markers achieved 84.8–92.0 and 90.9–92.4% sensitivity and 97.0–100% and 97.0–100% specificity, respectively, in three independent datasets.

Methods
Data preparation
DNA methylation, gene expression, and clinical HCC data were collected from The Cancer Genome Atlas (TCGA) project (https://portal.gdc.cancer.gov/). The methylation level of CpGs was represented as β values (375 HCC and 50 normal; β = Intensity of the methylated allele (M)/[Intensity of the unmethylated allele (U) + Intensity of the methylated allele (M) + 100], ranging from 0 to 1) [18]. Gene expression was defined using the raw read count or log2 transformed normalized count (369 HCC and 41 normal). Moreover, the methylation levels for another ten tumor types were collected from TCGA: BLCA (409 tumor, 21 normal), BRCA (774 tumor, 82 normal), COAD (292 tumor, 38 normal), GBM (126 tumor, 2 normal), HNSC (523 tumor, 45 normal), KIRC (316 tumor, 160 normal), LUAD (455 tumor, 32 normal), LUSC (365 tumor, 41 normal), READ (95 tumor, 7 normal) and UCEC (425 tumor, 46 normal), which have both tumor and normal tissues.

Additionally, four methylation array datasets were collected from the Gene Expression Omnibus (GEO) database: GSE69270 [19] (blood of 184 young Finns), GSE54503 [20] (66 paired HCC and adjacent normal), GSE89852 [21] (37 paired HCC and adjacent normal), and GSE56588 [22] (224 HCC, nine cirrhotic, and ten normal). The array platform was the HumanMethylation450 BeadChip (GPL13534). The CpG annotations were downloaded from GEO.

CpG island methylator phenotype
To find CIMP in HCC, we selected CpGs in the promoter region that have a high standard deviation (SD > 0.2) of the methylation level in 375 tumor tissues and a low methylation level (mean β value < 0.05) in 50

normal tissues, similar to the results of previous studies [23, 24]. K-means-based consensus clustering was performed using the R package ConsensusClusterPlus [25]. Overall survival of the CIMP group and other groups was estimated using the Kaplan-Meier method. Fisher's exact test was performed to associate the clinical characteristics with each cluster.

Differential analysis of DNA methylation and gene expression

Fifty of the 375 patients from TCGA have both HCC and normal methylation profiles, and the paired HCC and normal methylation data were used for differential methylation analysis. CpGs with more than 10% missing values were removed. The remaining missing values were imputed with the Bioconductor package impute. Then, a paired *t*-test was used to identify differentially methylated CpGs between the tumor and adjacent normal tissue. *P* values were adjusted using the false discovery rate (FDR) method. CpGs in chromosomes X and Y were ignored. The CpGs with an FDR less than 0.05 and an absolute value of the β difference greater than 0.2 were considered to be differentially methylated. When a CpG mapped to more than one gene, the first gene was taken as the reference.

Of the 50 patients from TCGA, 41 have both HCC and normal expression profiles, and the paired HCC and normal expression data were used for differential expression analysis. The Bioconductor package edgeR [26] was used to identify differentially expressed (DE) genes from raw read counts. Genes with an FDR less than 0.05 and an absolute value of $\log_2$ (fold change) greater than 1 were considered to be differentially expressed.

Correlation between DNA methylation and gene expression

The 369 tumor samples with matched methylation and expression data were used for correlation analysis. First, we investigated the correlation between DNA methylation and gene expression (*cis*-regulation). As one gene contains multiple CpGs, Pearson correlation coefficients were calculated between the expression value and the methylation level of each CpG site. Correlation was significant if the correlation coefficient was greater than 0.3 and FDR was less than 0.05. Second, we investigated the correlation of one gene's methylation and another gene's expression (*trans*-regulation) using a similar method. Only differentially expressed genes were used to analyze *trans*-regulation, and the DNA methylation was focused on CpGs that were located simultaneously in differentially methylated and differentially expressed genes.

Identification of candidate diagnostic biomarkers

TCGA datasets were used to screen potential methylation sites as diagnostic biomarkers of HCC. First, 50 paired HCC and normal samples were compared to select hypermethylated CpGs of low-expression genes in HCC. Second, 375 HCC and 50 normal tissues were compared. CpGs without significantly different methylation were filtered out. Third, 375 HCC tissues were compared with blood samples from individuals without HCC (GSE69270); we removed CpGs that had higher average methylation levels in blood than in HCC tissues. Fourth, HCC-specific hypermethylated sites were selected by removing CpGs whose mean methylation levels were higher than 0.1 in tumor or normal samples of another ten tumor types. The remaining CpGs were candidate diagnostic biomarkers of HCC. Finally, information gain-based feature selection was used to decrease the number of candidate diagnostic biomarkers.

Evaluation of candidate diagnostic biomarkers

The TCGA HCC dataset was taken as the training set, while three other independent datasets (GSE54503, GSE89852, and GSE56588) were used as test sets. A logistic regression model was built based on the methylation levels of the candidate diagnostic biomarkers. This model was used to predict the tumor and normal samples. Sensitivity and specificity were calculated to evaluate the accuracy of the prediction model. Modeling and prediction were performed in the data mining tool WEKA [27].

Bisulfite sequencing PCR experiments

Surgical biopsies were collected from ten Chinese patients diagnosed with HCC. This study was approved by the ethical committee of the Zhongshan hospital. All patients signed written informed consent to donate their tissue samples for research. Fresh tumor and normal tissues were subjected to bisulfite sequencing PCR (BSP) and quantitative PCR (qPCR) experiments.

Genomic DNA was extracted from tissue samples using a QiaAmp DNA Mini Kit (Qiagen, Valencia, CA, USA) according to the manufacturer's manual. The DNA sample quality and integrity were determined by the A260/280 ratio and agarose gel electrophoresis using Nanodrop2000 (Thermo Scientific, USA) and Horizontal Electrophoresis Systems (Bio-Rad, USA). The BSP primers were designed using online websites with customization, and all PCR products were approximately 400 bp. The CpGs we were interested in were designed at almost the middle of the PCR product. Additionally, 250 ng of genomic DNA was converted using an EZ DNA Methylation-Gold Kit™ (Zymo Research, USA) according to the manufacturer's manual. Bisulfite PCR amplification was performed with KAPA Uracil+ PCR

Ready Mix (KAPA Biosystems, USA) and BSP PCR primers, and the PCR conditions were optimized. The PCR product was directly sequenced on an ABI 3730× system (Thermo Scientific, USA) using the same primers as the BSP amplification. The results from direct sequencing were analyzed with Sequencing Scanner 2 (Thermo Scientific, USA) using $C/(C + T)$ peak ratios to define a CpG site methylation rate for each CpG dinucleotide within the covered region.

Gene expression experiments

Total RNA was isolated with an RNeasy Plus Mini kit (Qiagen, Valencia, CA, USA) with DNase I digestion, and cDNA was synthesized by using a PrimeScript RT Reagent Kit (TaKaRa, Japan) according to the manufacturer's manual. PCR primers were designed using Primer3 online tools. Quantitative PCR was performed using SYBR GREEN (Bio-Rad, USA) on an Eco qPCR system (Illumina, USA). Target mRNA expression was compared between the samples by normalization to beta-actin (ACTB) mRNA expression.

Results

Methylation landscape of HCC

DNA methylation profiles of 375 HCC tumor samples and 50 adjacent normal tissue samples were obtained from TCGA. We selected the 591 most variable CpGs and performed unsupervised consensus clustering. HCC samples were classified into seven clusters (Fig. 1a). The methylation level of cluster 2 was the lowest. Cluster 7 (4.3%) showed widespread hypermethylation of promoter-associated CpGs and was considered to have the CpG island methylator phenotype. To determine whether the methylation subtypes are related to prognosis, the overall survival of each cluster was estimated using the Kaplan-Meier method. The p value obtained from the log-rank test is approximately 0.12, indicating there were differences in prognosis among the different subtypes (Fig. 1b). Furthermore, we compared the survival probability of CIMP patients (cluster 7) with those of other patients (clusters 1–6). The CIMP subgroup showed poorer prognosis ($P = 0.0185$; Fig. 1d).

We next examined whether the subtypes were significantly associated with clinical characteristics. The significant characteristics of cluster 1 were that there were more male ($P = 0.0054$) and virus-infected (HBV and HCV, $P = 0.0012$) patients. The genetic background of cluster 3 included mainly Asians ($P = 0.0034$). Cluster 2 had more patients without virus infection ($P = 0.0055$) and showed low methylation. Cluster 4 had more male patients ($P = 1.21e-06$) and cluster 6 had more female patients ($P = 0.014$). No significant characteristics were found for cluster 5. The CIMP group had more stage III ($P = 0.0141$) and HCV-infected ($P = 0.0330$) patients than

the other clusters. To understand whether the poor prognosis of CIMP was due to more stage III patients, we compared the survival probability of stage III patients in the CIMP group and stage III patients in the non-CIMP group. We found that stage III patients in the CIMP group had a much poorer prognosis than stage III patients in the non-CIMP group (Fig. 1e). Hence, the poor prognosis of CIMP is possibly associated with global hypermethylation.

Differential analysis of methylation and expression

Methylation data of 50 paired samples from TCGA were used for differential methylation analysis ($|\beta$ value difference$| > 0.2$ and FDR < 0.05). There were 7372 hypermethylated and 39,995 hypomethylated CpGs in HCC, which correspond to 2222 hypermethylated and 5478 hypomethylated genes. Then we analyzed the distribution of differentially methylated (DM) CpGs and genes in different genomic regions (Fig. 2a, d). Hypomethylation occurred globally in the whole genome, involving 84% of CpGs and 71% of genes. However, 61% of the CpGs (73% of genes) were hypermethylated in CpG-rich regions (CpG islands), and 91% of the CpGs (93% of genes) were hypermethylated in the CpG islands of the promoter regions. When we considered the distance of the probes to CpG islands, the percentage of hypermethylation was highest in the CpG island. This percentage decreased when the probes were far away from the CpG islands (Fig. 2b). The gene body was dominated by hypomethylation, while hypermethylation occurred preferentially in the regions around the transcription start sites (Fig. 2c). Such hypomethylation of the whole genome and hypermethylation of the promoter CpG islands are general characteristics of solid tumors. Expression data of 41 paired samples from TCGA were used for differential expression analysis ($|\log_2$ (fold change)$| > 1$ and FDR < 0.05). We found 662 highly expressed ("DE-high") and 1553 lowly expressed ("DE-low") genes in HCC.

Roles of methylation in regulating gene expression

First, we analyzed the intersection between differentially expressed genes and differentially methylated genes (Fig. 3a). Methylation alterations of the genes were assigned based on the status of the promoter methylation. Genes were called "DM-high" if at least one promoter CpG had a higher methylation level in HCC than in normal tissues. Similarly, "DM-low" genes had at least one hypomethylated promoter CpG. The promoter methylation defined 881 DM-high genes and 2550 DM-low genes. In total, 293 genes were differentially methylated and differentially expressed: 97 genes were hypermethylated with low expression in HCC, 32 genes were hypomethylated with high expression, 20 genes were hypermethylated with high expression, and 144

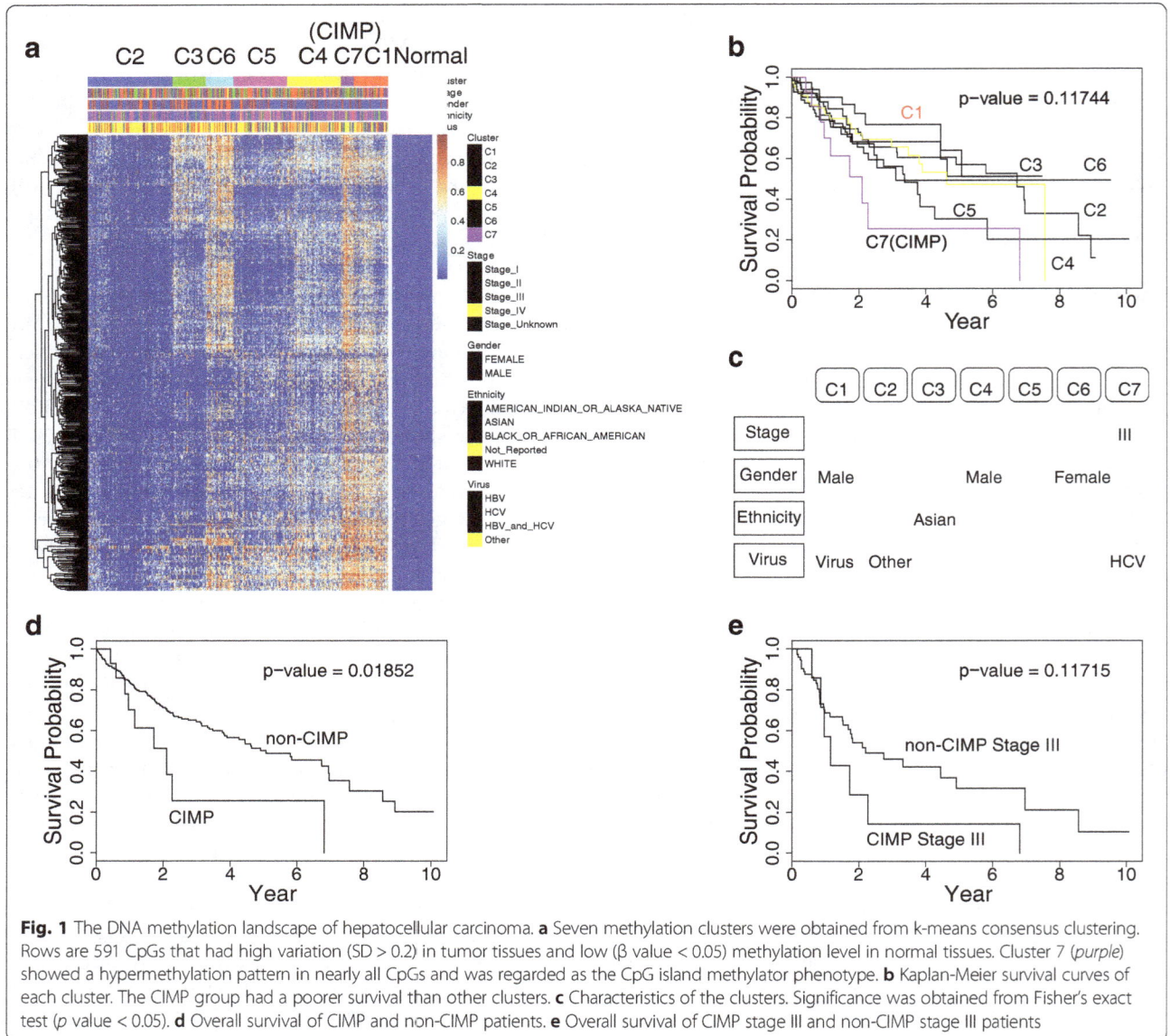

Fig. 1 The DNA methylation landscape of hepatocellular carcinoma. **a** Seven methylation clusters were obtained from k-means consensus clustering. Rows are 591 CpGs that had high variation (SD > 0.2) in tumor tissues and low (β value < 0.05) methylation level in normal tissues. Cluster 7 (*purple*) showed a hypermethylation pattern in nearly all CpGs and was regarded as the CpG island methylator phenotype. **b** Kaplan-Meier survival curves of each cluster. The CIMP group had a poorer survival than other clusters. **c** Characteristics of the clusters. Significance was obtained from Fisher's exact test (*p* value < 0.05). **d** Overall survival of CIMP and non-CIMP patients. **e** Overall survival of CIMP stage III and non-CIMP stage III patients

genes were hypomethylated with low expression (Fig. 3a). Since promoter hypermethylation plays important roles in the inactivation of cancer-related genes [28], we are particularly interested in the 97 highly methylated and lowly expressed genes, and in the subsequent analysis we used these genes to screen candidate diagnostic biomarkers.

To study the effect of DNA methylation on the expression of the same gene (*cis*-regulation), Pearson correlation coefficients were calculated between promoter methylation and gene expression. Among 16,206 genes with methylation and expression profiles, promoter methylation of 2798 (877) genes was significantly negatively (positively) correlated with gene expression (Fig. 3b). *Cis*-regulation was dominated by the negative correlation between promoter methylation and gene

expression (Fig. 3b), which was consistent with previous reports [29, 30].

Furthermore, we investigated whether DNA methylation was related to the expression of other genes (*trans*-regulation). We focused on 512 CpGs in 287 differentially methylated and differentially expressed genes, analyzing their correlation with 2215 differentially expressed genes (Fig. 3c). The methylation of DM-high genes was predominantly negative correlated with gene expression while the methylation of DM-low genes was more likely to be positively correlated with gene expression.

Identification HCC-specific methylation markers
To find sensitive and specific methylation biomarkers for HCC, we designed a workflow to strictly screen

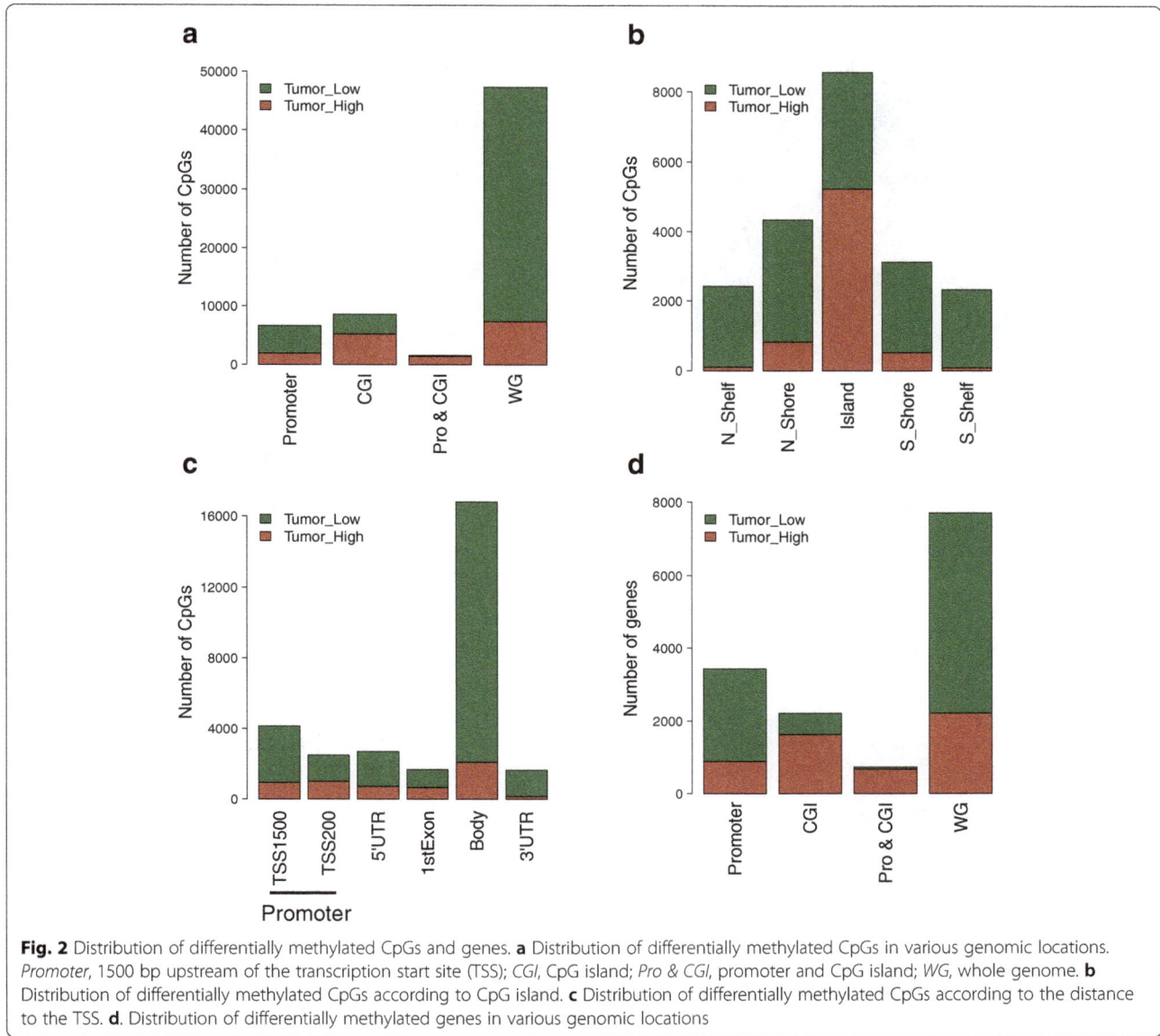

Fig. 2 Distribution of differentially methylated CpGs and genes. **a** Distribution of differentially methylated CpGs in various genomic locations. *Promoter*, 1500 bp upstream of the transcription start site (TSS); *CGI*, CpG island; *Pro & CGI*, promoter and CpG island; *WG*, whole genome. **b** Distribution of differentially methylated CpGs according to CpG island. **c** Distribution of differentially methylated CpGs according to the distance to the TSS. **d**. Distribution of differentially methylated genes in various genomic locations

biomarkers by comparing HCC with normal livers and other cancers (Fig. 4a). We started from 185 hypermethylated CpGs that were located in 97 lowly expressed genes. First, 130 CpGs remained after requiring hypermethylation in 375 HCC tissues. Second, the methylation data from blood of healthy people was used for filtering, and 109 CpGs were selected which were lowly methylated in healthy people and highly methylated in HCC. Figure 4b illustrates the methylation levels of these 109 CpGs in TCGA and three independent datasets (Additional file 1). Tumor samples could be well discriminated from normal tissue and blood samples, indicating the robustness of our results. Third, 109 CpGs were further filtered, requiring hypermethylation only in HCC but not in ten other cancers in TCGA, and six HCC-specific CpGs were obtained (Fig. 4c).

The six HCC-specific CpGs are mapped to four genes: NEBL (cg23565942), FAM55C (cg21908638, cg11223367, and cg03509671), GALNT3 (cg05569109), and DSE (cg11481534). Since the methylation status of CpGs is usually similar in neighboring regions [18], we investigated other CpG sites in the promoter of these four genes (Additional file 2: Figure S1). Most of the CpGs were also hypermethylated in HCC compared to normal tissues, consistent with the six specific CpGs. Next, we compared the methylation status of patients in different stages. The results showed that six HCC-specific CpGs are significantly hypermethylated even in stage I patients (Additional file 2: Figure S2). Therefore, these six CpGs are good candidates for the early detection of HCC.

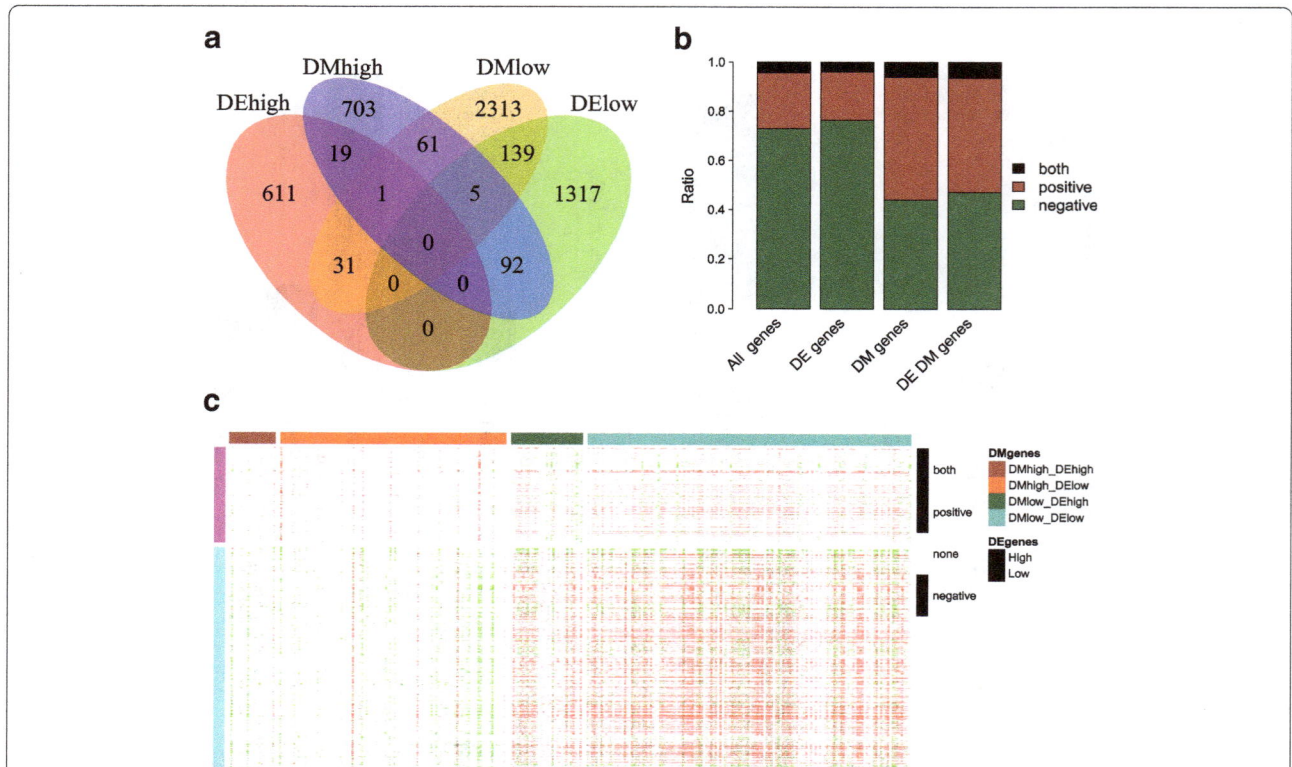

Fig. 3 Relationship between DNA methylation and gene expression. **a** Comparison of differentially methylated genes and differentially expressed genes. Genes were considered differentially methylated if at least one promoter CpG site was significantly differentially methylated. **b** Correlation between gene expression and its promoter methylation. Correlations were calculated using all 16,206 genes, 2215 differentially expressed (DE) genes, 3364 differentially methylated (DM) genes, or 287 both DE and DM genes. The vertical axis shows the percentage of negatively correlated genes (*green*), positively correlated genes (*red*), and genes with both negative and positive correlation (*black*). **c** Correlation between promoter methylation and other gene expression. This analysis focused on the promoter methylation of 287 DM and DE genes (columns) and the gene expression of 2215 DE genes (rows). Positive and negative correlations are shown in *red* and *green*, respectively

Evaluation of diagnostic accuracy in independent datasets

Methylation data of the 50 paired HCC and normal tissues from TCGA were used as a training set. Three independent methylation datasets of HCC (GSE54503, GSE89852, and GSE56588) were used as test sets, including 327 HCC samples and 122 normal samples. Information gain-based feature selection was performed on the six CpGs to rank them. A logistic regression model was used to predict HCCs from one CpG to the combination of six CpGs. The ROC area associated with using one CpG to the combination of six CpGs to predict HCC in three independent datasets is shown in Fig. 5a. The performance using a combination of six HCC-specific CpGs was very good, with ROC areas of 0.972, 0.945, and 0.957 in GSE54503, GSE89852, and GSE56588, respectively. When using a combination of two specific CpGs (cg23565942 and cg21908638), the ROC area was higher than 0.92 in all three test sets. Hence, using a combination of two specific CpGs as markers could be more cost-effective.

Then, we compared our results with previously published methylation markers. Logistic regression models were built based on different feature sets: six or two CpGs from our study, nine CpGs from Zheng et al. [16], and seven CpGs from Xu et al. [17] (Additional file 3). The sensitivity and specificity of distinguishing HCC from normal livers were high and similar among the different feature sets (Table 1), while the number of CpGs we used was the least. Next, we compared the ability of different methylation markers to distinguish HCC from other cancers. Tumor and normal tissues from other cancers were seldom (0–12%, median 0.15%) predicted as HCC when using two or six HCC-specific CpGs in our study. However, 32.5 to 100% (median 92.85%) of tumor and 0 to 100% (median 48.95%) of normal tissues were predicted as HCC when using the CpGs of Zheng et al. and Xu et al. as feature sets (Fig. 5b). Therefore, our study found more cost-effective and specific biomarkers for HCC diagnosis.

To verify whether the six HCC-specific CpGs could be stably detected by cheaper technologies, BSP was used

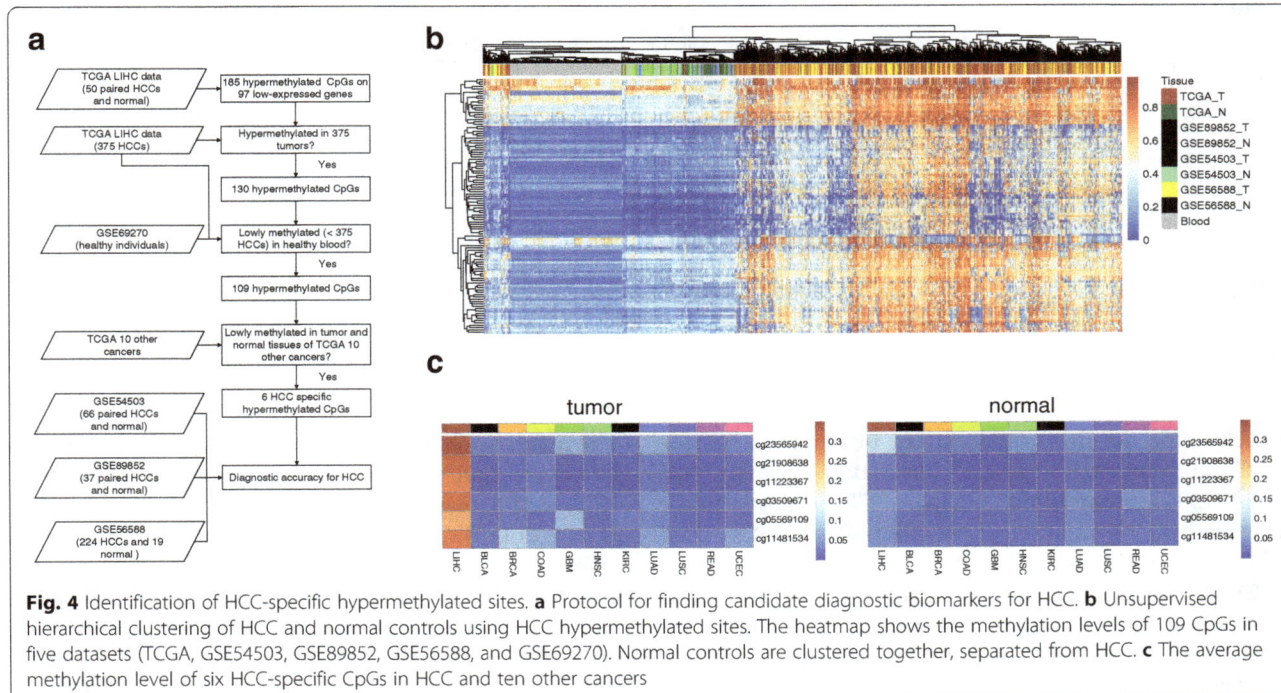

Fig. 4 Identification of HCC-specific hypermethylated sites. **a** Protocol for finding candidate diagnostic biomarkers for HCC. **b** Unsupervised hierarchical clustering of HCC and normal controls using HCC hypermethylated sites. The heatmap shows the methylation levels of 109 CpGs in five datasets (TCGA, GSE54503, GSE89852, GSE56588, and GSE69270). Normal controls are clustered together, separated from HCC. **c** The average methylation level of six HCC-specific CpGs in HCC and ten other cancers

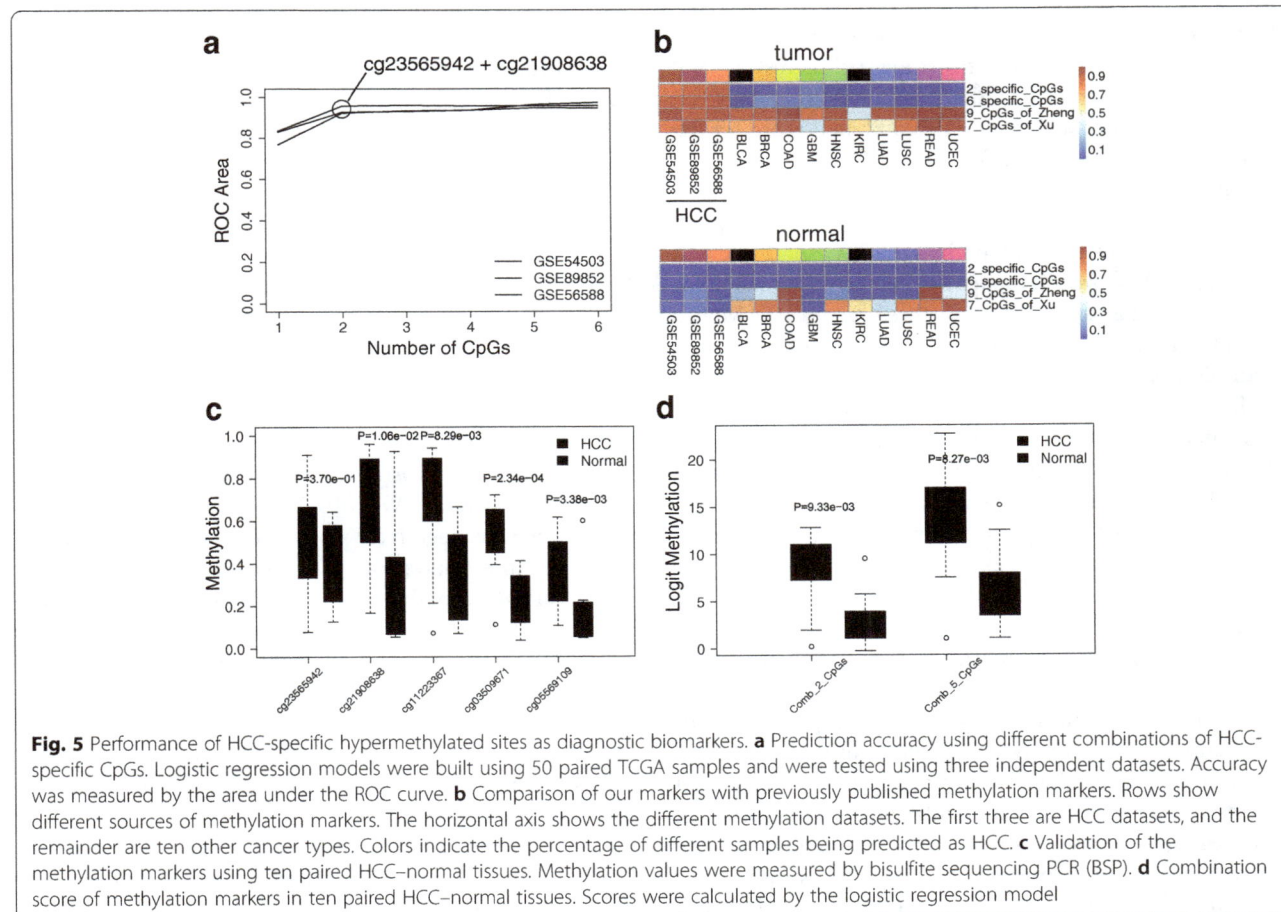

Fig. 5 Performance of HCC-specific hypermethylated sites as diagnostic biomarkers. **a** Prediction accuracy using different combinations of HCC-specific CpGs. Logistic regression models were built using 50 paired TCGA samples and were tested using three independent datasets. Accuracy was measured by the area under the ROC curve. **b** Comparison of our markers with previously published methylation markers. Rows show different sources of methylation markers. The horizontal axis shows the different methylation datasets. The first three are HCC datasets, and the remainder are ten other cancer types. Colors indicate the percentage of different samples being predicted as HCC. **c** Validation of the methylation markers using ten paired HCC–normal tissues. Methylation values were measured by bisulfite sequencing PCR (BSP). **d** Combination score of methylation markers in ten paired HCC–normal tissues. Scores were calculated by the logistic regression model

Table 1 Comparison of the performance of different methylation markers for classifying HCC and normal tissues

Markers	Two HCC-specific CpGs	Six HCC-specific CpGs	Nine CpGs of Zheng et al.[a]	Seven CpGs of Xu et al.[b]
Sensitivity				
GSE54503	0.848	0.909	0.970	0.833
GSE89852	0.892	0.919	0.919	0.946
GSE56588	0.920	0.924	0.942	0.741
Specificity				
GSE54503	0.970	0.970	0.970	0.955
GSE89852	0.973	0.973	0.892	0.919
GSE56588	1.000	1.000	1.000	1.000

[a]Zheng et al. [16] reported ten CpGs as HCC diagnostic markers. Nine of them had methylation values in TCGA HCC dataset
[b]Xu et al. [17] reported ten CpGs as HCC diagnostic markers. Seven of them had methylation values in TCGA HCC dataset

to determine the methylation status of ten fresh frozen HCC and normal tissues. The BSP primers of cg11481534 cannot amplify enough PCR products; thus, the methylation status of another five CpGs was analyzed (Additional file 4). Four specific CpGs (cg21908638, cg11223367, cg03509671, and cg05569109) were significantly hypermethylated ($P < 0.05$), as determined using the paired t-test. Another CpG (cg23565942) also showed some difference between the tumor and normal samples, although the p value ($P = 0.37$) was not significant (Fig. 5c). Then we combined the methylation of two specific CpGs and five specific CpGs according to the formula obtained from logistic regression and compared the difference in the combined score between the tumor and normal tissues. The combined score for the two and five CpGs was significantly higher in tumor tissues than in normal tissues, with p values of 0.009 and 0.008, respectively (Fig. 5d). Additionally, we validated the expression of the four genes mapped by six HCC-specific CpGs in the paired fresh frozen tissues by qPCR (Additional file 2: Figure S3). The expression of three genes (FAM55C, GALNT3, and DSE) was significantly ($p < 0.05$) lower in tumor tissues than in normal tissues. The expression of NEBL was also lower in the tumor, but the difference was not significant ($p = 0.17$). The phenomenon of hypermethylation and low expression of these genes in the fresh frozen tissues is concordant with that in TCGA HCC datasets. Thus, the specific CpGs identified in our study are promising diagnostic biomarkers specific for HCC.

Discussion

In this study, we systematically analyzed the DNA methylation and gene expression data of hepatocellular carcinoma. We identified a subgroup of patients with CIMP and observed the poor prognosis of these patients. We found that methylation was negatively correlated with gene expression in *cis*-regulation. The patterns of *trans*-regulation are more complex; generally, the methylation of hypermethylated genes was negatively correlated with gene expression, while the methylation of hypomethylated genes was positively correlated with gene expression. Furthermore, we identified six CpGs as HCC-specific diagnostic biomarkers by comparing HCC, normal controls, and non-HCC cancers. These sites achieved ~91% sensitivity and ~97% specificity when predicting HCC. Our diagnostic biomarkers are more sensitive and more specific than most of the previously reported protein markers or methylation markers. These results provide new insights into the roles of DNA methylation in gene regulation and diagnosis.

CIMP is a phenomenon of simultaneous methylation of a group of genes in a subset of tumors [23] and has been studied in multiple cancer types, such as colorectal cancer (22.4%) [31], papillary renal-cell carcinoma (5.6%) [24], and glioblastoma (8.8%) [23]. It has been associated with prognosis, but the impact of CIMP on prognosis is not consistent among different cancers. We found that 4.3% of HCC patients had CIMP. Compared to other cancer types, the fraction of CIMP is smaller in HCC. However, the CIMP group needs special attention due to their poor prognosis. Somatic mutations of IDH1 and IDH2 have been reported to be associated with glioma CIMP [23]. Due to the low mutation frequencies of these genes in HCC, we did not observe a significant association between them and the CIMP group.

DNA methylation is an important epigenetic regulator of gene expression. We observed that *cis*-regulation is predominantly negatively correlated, which is concordant with the views of gene expression silenced by promoter DNA methylation [28, 32]. Promoter methylation of a hypermethylated gene was mainly negatively correlated with the expression of other genes, but promoter methylation of a hypomethylated gene was prone to being positively correlated with the expression of other genes. The reason for the inconsistent relationship of hypermethylated and hypomethylated genes in *trans*-regulation is unclear.

The most important finding of this study is the identification of several methylated CpGs as candidate diagnostic biomarkers of HCC. An ideal diagnostic biomarker should have high sensitivity, enabling the detection of HCC at an early stage; should be specific to HCC and not detected in other tumor types or premalignant liver diseases; should be measurable by non-invasive and cost-effective technology; and should be validated across different populations. Here, we discovered six HCC-specific hypermethylated sites whose sensitivity and specificity are better than the widely used serum biomarker AFP and another candidate serum biomarker, DKK1. Moreover, their methylation levels can be measured by relatively cheap PCR-based technology. However, we have not validated their diagnostic ability using non-invasive biospecimens. To resolve this problem, we will first develop a sensitive technology to detect methylation in cell-free ctDNA. Then, we will compare the consistency of methylation between tissues and blood and validate the prediction ability of the candidate biomarkers by measuring DNA methylation in the blood. Another problem is whether the methylation-based biomarkers could distinguish HCC from other liver diseases. In the future, we plan to investigate methylation profiles during the progression of liver cancers, including non-alcoholic fatty liver, hepatocirrhosis, and early HCC. Additionally, we are also interested in the downstream biological functions of methylation biomarkers, which may help us to understand the roles of methylation in carcinogenesis.

Conclusions

DNA methylation plays important roles in gene regulation and carcinogenesis in HCC. We discovered several methylation-based biomarkers by analyzing the genome-wide methylation data of 375 HCC samples, 50 normal liver samples, 3780 samples of cancers of other sites, and 474 normal samples of other organs. The candidate biomarkers were validated in three independent datasets with more than 300 HCC samples and 100 normal liver samples. Then, BSP-based experimental validation was performed in ten HCC patients. The candidate biomarkers achieved high diagnostic ability and have the potential to be translated into clinical application. Future translational research will accelerate the clinical validation of candidate biomarkers and promote the early detection of HCC. A similar analysis method could be used for other tumor types to find more associations between methylation and cancer diagnosis.

Abbreviations
AFP: Alpha-fetoprotein; BSP: Bisulfite sequencing PCR; CIMP: CpG island methylator phenotype; ctDNA: Circulating tumor DNA; DCP: Des-γ-carboxy prothrombin; DE: Differentially expressed; DKK1: Dickkopf-1; FDR: False discovery rate; GEO: Gene Expression Omnibus; HBV: Hepatitis B virus; HCC: Hepatocellular carcinoma; HCV: Hepatitis C virus; DM: Differentially methylated; TCGA: The Cancer Genome Atlas; TSS: Transcription start site

Acknowledgements
We would like to thank all the patients who contributed samples for this research.

Funding
This work was supported by grants from National Key Research and Development Plan (2016YFC0902400) and National Natural Science Foundation of China (NSFC, 31771472, 31501077).

Authors' contributions
JC collected and analyzed methylation data, screened candidate diagnostic markers, and built prediction models. LY, LW, and TH helped in data analysis. JC and HL wrote the manuscript. DW, GL, and GD designed and performed experimental validation. YJ and LC provided patients' samples for validation. LX, HL, GD, and YL designed the study and revised the manuscript. All authors read and approved the final manuscript.

Competing interests
The authors declare that they have no competing interests.

Author details
[1]Department of Bioinformatics and Biostatistics, School of Life Sciences and Biotechnology, Shanghai Jiao Tong University, Shanghai, China. [2]Key Lab of Computational Biology, CAS-MPG Partner Institute for Computational Biology, Shanghai Institutes for Biological Sciences, Chinese Academy of Sciences, Shanghai, China. [3]Basepair biotechnology Co. LTD, Suzhou, China. [4]Department of Pathology, Zhongshan Hospital, Fudan University, Shanghai, China. [5]Shanghai Center for Bioinformation Technology, Shanghai Academy of Science and Technology, Shanghai, China.

References
1. Forner A, Llovet JM, Bruix J. Hepatocellular carcinoma. Lancet. 2012; 379(9822):1245–55.
2. Jemal A, Bray F, Center MM, Ferlay J, Ward E, Forman D. Global cancer statistics. CA Cancer J Clin. 2011;61(2):69–90.
3. Wang JH, Wang CC, Hung CH, Chen CL, Lu SN. Survival comparison between surgical resection and radiofrequency ablation for patients in BCLC very early/early stage hepatocellular carcinoma. J Hepatol. 2012;56(2):412–8.
4. Altekruse SF, McGlynn KA, Reichman ME. Hepatocellular carcinoma incidence, mortality, and survival trends in the United States from 1975 to 2005. J Clin Oncol. 2009;27(9):1485–91.
5. Marrero JA, Feng Z, Wang Y, Nguyen MH, Befeler AS, Roberts LR, Reddy KR, Harnois D, Llovet JM, Normolle D, et al. Alpha-fetoprotein, des-gamma carboxyprothrombin, and lectin-bound alpha-fetoprotein in early hepatocellular carcinoma. Gastroenterology. 2009;137(1):110–8.
6. Bruix J, Sherman M. American Association for the Study of Liver D: Management of hepatocellular carcinoma: an update. Hepatology. 2011; 53(3):1020–2.
7. European Association for the Study of the Liver, European Organisation for Research and Treatment of Cancer. EASL-EORTC clinical practice guidelines: management of hepatocellular carcinoma. J Hepatol. 2012;56(4):908–43.
8. Shen QJ, Fan J, Yang XR, Tan YX, Zhao WF, Xu Y, Wang N, Niu YD, Wu Z, Zhou J, et al. Serum DKK1 as a protein biomarker for the diagnosis of hepatocellular carcinoma: a large-scale, multicentre study. Lancet Oncol. 2012;13(8):817–26.
9. Ehrlich M. DNA methylation in cancer: too much, but also too little. Oncogene. 2002;21(35):5400–13.
10. Eden A, Gaudet F, Waghmare A, Jaenisch R. Chromosomal instability and tumors promoted by DNA hypomethylation. Science. 2003;300(5618):455.
11. Yang B, Guo M, Herman JG, Clark DP. Aberrant promoter methylation profiles of tumor suppressor genes in hepatocellular carcinoma. Am J Pathol. 2003;163(3):1101–7.

12. Si JG, Su YY, Han YH, Chen RH. Role of RASSF1A promoter methylation in the pathogenesis of ovarian cancer: a meta-analysis. Genet Test Mol Biomarkers. 2014;18(6):394–402.

13. Laird PW. The power and the promise of DNA methylation markers. Nat Rev Cancer. 2003;3(4):253–66.

14. Leygo C, Williams M, Jin HC, Chan MWY, Chu WK, Grusch M, Cheng YY. DNA methylation as a noninvasive epigenetic biomarker for the detection of cancer. Dis Markers. 2017;2017:3726595.

15. Song LL, Li YM. Current noninvasive tests for colorectal cancer screening: An overview of colorectal cancer screening tests. World J Gastrointest Oncol. 2016;8(11):793–800.

16. Zheng Y, Huang Q, Ding Z, Liu T, Xue C, Sang X, Gu J. Genome-wide DNA methylation analysis identifies candidate epigenetic markers and drivers of hepatocellular carcinoma. Brief Bioinform. 2016;19(1):101–8.

17. Xu RH, Wei W, Krawczyk M, Wang W, Luo H, Flagg K, Yi S, Shi W, Quan Q, Li K, et al. Circulating tumour DNA methylation markers for diagnosis and prognosis of hepatocellular carcinoma. Nat Mater. 2017;16(11):1155–61.

18. Bibikova M, Barnes B, Tsan C, Ho V, Klotzle B, Le JM, Delano D, Zhang L, Schroth GP, Gunderson KL, et al. High density DNA methylation array with single CpG site resolution. Genomics. 2011;98(4):288–95.

19. Kananen L, Marttila S, Nevalainen T, Jylhava J, Mononen N, Kahonen M, Raitakari OT, Lehtimaki T, Hurme M. Aging-associated DNA methylation changes in middle-aged individuals: the Young Finns study. BMC Genomics. 2016;17:103.

20. Shen J, Wang S, Zhang YJ, Wu HC, Kibriya MG, Jasmine F, Ahsan H, Wu DPH, Siegel AB, Remotti H, et al. Exploring genome-wide DNA methylation profiles altered in hepatocellular carcinoma using Infinium HumanMethylation 450 BeadChips. Epigenetics-Us. 2013;8(1):34–43.

21. Kuramoto J, Arai E, Tian Y, Funahashi N, Hiramoto M, Nammo T, Nozaki Y, Takahashi Y, Ito N, Shibuya A, et al. Genome-wide DNA methylation analysis during non-alcoholic steatohepatitis-related multistage hepatocarcinogenesis: comparison with hepatitis virus-related carcinogenesis. Carcinogenesis. 2017;38(3):261–70.

22. Villanueva A, Portela A, Sayols S, Battiston C, Hoshida Y, Mendez-Gonzalez J, Imbeaud S, Letouze E, Hernandez-Gea V, Cornella H, et al. DNA methylation-based prognosis and epidrivers in hepatocellular carcinoma. Hepatology. 2015;61(6):1945–56.

23. Noushmehr H, Weisenberger DJ, Diefes K, Phillips HS, Pujara K, Berman BP, Pan F, Pelloski CE, Sulman EP, Bhat KP, et al. Identification of a CpG island methylator phenotype that defines a distinct subgroup of glioma. Cancer Cell. 2010;17(5):510–22.

24. Cancer Genome Atlas Research Network, Linehan WM, Spellman PT, Ricketts CJ, Creighton CJ, Fei SS, Davis C, Wheeler DA, Murray BA, Schmidt L, et al. Comprehensive molecular characterization of papillary renal-cell carcinoma. N Engl J Med. 2016;374(2):135–45.

25. Wilkerson MD, Hayes DN. ConsensusClusterPlus: a class discovery tool with confidence assessments and item tracking. Bioinformatics. 2010;26(12):1572–3.

26. Robinson MD, McCarthy DJ, Smyth GK. edgeR: a Bioconductor package for differential expression analysis of digital gene expression data. Bioinformatics. 2010;26(1):139–40.

27. Hall M, Frank E, Holmes G, Pfahringer B, Reutemann P, Witten IH. The WEKA data mining software: an update. ACM SIGKDD Explorations Newslett. 2009;11(1):10–8.

28. Herman JG, Baylin SB. Gene silencing in cancer in association with promoter hypermethylation. N Engl J Med. 2003;349(21):2042–54.

29. Wagner JR, Busche S, Ge B, Kwan T, Pastinen T, Blanchette M. The relationship between DNA methylation, genetic and expression inter-individual variation in untransformed human fibroblasts. Genome Biol. 2014;15(2):R37.

30. Yang IV, Pedersen BS, Rabinovich E, Hennessy CE, Davidson EJ, Murphy E, Guardela BJ, Tedrow JR, Zhang Y, Singh MK, et al. Relationship of DNA methylation and gene expression in idiopathic pulmonary fibrosis. Am J Respir Crit Care Med. 2014;190(11):1263–72.

31. Hinoue T, Weisenberger DJ, Lange CP, Shen H, Byun HM, Van Den Berg D, Malik S, Pan F, Noushmehr H, van Dijk CM, et al. Genome-scale analysis of aberrant DNA methylation in colorectal cancer. Genome Res. 2012;22(2):271–82.

32. Jones PA. Functions of DNA methylation: islands, start sites, gene bodies and beyond. Nat Rev Genet. 2012;13(7):484–92.

15

Cross-genetic determination of maternal and neonatal immune mediators during pregnancy

Michela Traglia[1], Lisa A. Croen[2], Karen L. Jones[3,4], Luke S. Heuer[3,4], Robert Yolken[5], Martin Kharrazi[6], Gerald N. DeLorenze[2], Paul Ashwood[4,7], Judy Van de Water[3,4] and Lauren A. Weiss[1*] iD

Abstract

Background: The immune system plays a fundamental role in development during pregnancy and early life. Alterations in circulating maternal and neonatal immune mediators have been associated with pregnancy complications as well as susceptibility to autoimmune and neurodevelopmental conditions in later life. Evidence suggests that the immune system in adults not only responds to environmental stimulation but is also under strong genetic control.

Methods: This is the first genetic study of > 700 mother-infant pairs to analyse the circulating levels of 22 maternal mid-gestational serum-derived and 42 neonatal bloodspot-derived immune mediators (cytokines/chemokines) in the context of maternal and fetal genotype. We first estimated the maternal and fetal genome-wide SNP-based heritability (h^2_g) for each immune molecule and then performed genome-wide association studies (GWAS) to identify specific loci contributing to individual immune mediators. Finally, we assessed the relationship between genetic immune determinants and ASD outcome.

Results: We show maternal and neonatal cytokines/chemokines displaying genetic regulation using independent methodologies. We demonstrate that novel fetal loci for immune function independently affect the physiological levels of maternal immune mediators and vice versa. The cross-associated loci are in distinct genomic regions compared with individual-specific immune mediator loci. Finally, we observed an interaction between increased IL-8 levels at birth, autism spectrum disorder (ASD) status, and a specific maternal genotype.

Conclusions: Our results suggest that maternal and fetal genetic variation influences the immune system during pregnancy and at birth via distinct mechanisms and that a better understanding of immune factor determinants in early development may shed light on risk factors for developmental disorders.

Keywords: Cytokines, Chemokines, Immune system, Maternal and fetal genetics, GWAS, SNP-based heritability, Early brain development, Autism

Background

Women experience dramatic changes in immune system status during pregnancy. Tolerance for fetal-placental antigens allowing for healthy development of the fetus must be balanced with the ability of the mother to fight infections. Further, immune dysregulation during pregnancy can lead to outcomes such as preeclampsia, fetal growth retardation, and miscarriage [1, 2]. However, little is known about inter-individual differences in immune status during pregnancy. Similarly, immune protection in early infancy is thought to be accomplished by a combination of maternal transfer and fetal production of soluble immune molecules, but the extent of maternal contribution has not been worked out for many immune molecules.

Among the soluble molecules that mediate the immune response, cytokines and chemokines are particularly important for regulating inflammation, immune cell proliferation and differentiation, and for influencing the progression of some chronic inflammatory conditions [3, 4]. Cytokines are small peptides involved in most phases

* Correspondence: Lauren.Weiss@ucsf.edu
[1]Department of Psychiatry and Institute for Human Genetics, University of California, San Francisco, San Francisco, CA, USA
Full list of author information is available at the end of the article

of immune response, and chemokines are specific cytokines that are also important in controlling white blood cell trafficking and attracting cells to an infection site.

Immune responses to environmental stimuli (e.g., infections) are tightly regulated by genetics. Several studies have shown genetic variation associated with RNA or protein levels of immune mediators [5–7] and substantial heritability of immune cell counts [6]. Moreover, a recent study [8] identified 27 specific loci associated with circulating levels of 41 cytokines/chemokines, mainly in genes that encode the proteins and/or their receptors, and that were also associated with inflammatory and autoimmune diseases. However, despite this strong evidence for genetic control of immune system status, no study has analysed the genetic regulation of maternal immune mediator levels during pregnancy, neonatal levels at birth, or the intersection of genetic determinants of either with chronic disorders.

To fill the gaps in our current understanding of genetic regulation of the immune system during pregnancy and at birth, we first hypothesize that maternal mid-gestational mediator levels will be regulated by maternal genetics, some of which could be unique to pregnancy. Second, we define two possible scenarios for neonatal immune system status. At birth, the neonatal immune system might be at least partially determined by the mother; so, we hypothesize that maternal genetics could regulate not only maternal mediator levels but also contribute to neonatal mediator levels. In the second scenario, we hypothesize that the neonatal genome would exert independent influence on neonatal mediator levels.

Increasing evidence shows that during pregnancy, fetal genetics also contributes to different aspects of maternal physiology, such as blood pressure, gestational diabetes, metabolism, and preeclampsia [9–11]. We previously showed that some maternal circulating toxicant levels in pregnancy are in part regulated by fetal genetics [12]. However, there has been no study looking at the potential fetal genetic influences on maternal immune status during pregnancy. Thus, we also hypothesize that genetic variation in the fetus and placenta might influence the mother's immune system function during pregnancy.

Understanding patterns of genetic regulation of circulating maternal and neonatal immune mediators might elucidate important mechanisms for immune system status and disease susceptibilities. Beyond their classical roles in immune function, recent evidence suggests that some cytokines show pleiotropic effects in the central nervous system (CNS), acting as neuromodulators, growth and survival factors [13], neurodevelopmental organizers [14], and ultimately influencing behavior and cognition. Animal models [15] of maternal immune activation (MIA) during pregnancy demonstrate behavioral abnormalities in offspring, proposed to be mediated via cytokines [16–18]. In addition,

peripheral abnormalities of circulating cytokine levels have been observed in individuals affected by neuropsychiatric disorders, such as major depression, bipolar disorder, schizophrenia, and autism spectrum disorder (ASD) [19–23].

Among neurodevelopmental disorders, ASD is thought to originate in early development. ASD is a highly heritable complex disease, with both genetic and non-genetic risk factors, proposed to include maternal infection [24] and fever [25, 26] and maternal and neonatal immune system dysregulation [27–30]. Elevated peripheral cytokine profiles in pregnancy [31] and at birth have been associated with ASD diagnosis in childhood [32, 33]. A study in our Early Markers for Autism (EMA) maternal dataset found elevated maternal cytokine levels during mid-gestation associated with an increased risk of ASD with intellectual disability [34]. We have also observed elevated levels of cytokines/chemokines in neonatal bloodspots from ASD-affected children compared to controls. However, neither our studies nor others implicating immune mediators in ASD have included measurement of genetics to distinguish inborn from environmentally stimulated variation in immune molecules.

To test our hypotheses, we applied several methodologies to a large set of maternal and neonatal soluble immune mediators (SIMs), specifically cytokines and chemokines, in combination with genetic markers in the EMA cohort, a population-based nested case-control study of ASD. This dataset utilizes samples from a maternal prenatal screening program and neonatal bloodspots from the sampled pregnancies to measure genetic and immune molecules (with no direct measurement or record of infection or illness). (Note that we define the genetic contribution from the fetus during pregnancy and from the neonate at birth as 'fetal genetics' for consistency of terminology and to represent the likely timing of genetic regulation, although the genetic data were collected shortly after birth). We first estimated heritability to determine the extent to which an individual's cytokine/chemokine levels might be genetically regulated. We next performed genome-wide association identifying specific contributing loci. We also used several approaches to investigate whether neonatal cytokines/chemokines might be influenced by maternal genetic variation and/or maternal cytokines/chemokines could be influenced by fetal genetic variation. Finally, in order to understand the intersection of genetic determinants of maternal and/or fetal immune function with developmental disorders, we studied the potential for interaction between an immune mediator and genetic variation on ASD outcome.

Methods
Study population and blood sampling
The Early Markers for Autism (EMA) study is a population-based nested case-control study [35, 36] that

includes a population of pregnant women (15–20 weeks) and their babies from Orange, San Diego and Imperial Counties, California, who were enrolled in the State's Prenatal Expanded Alphafetoprotein Screening Program and delivered a live-born infant in 2000–2003. We used prenatal (maternal blood) and newborn (neonatal blood spot) specimens from each mother-baby matching pair. The offspring outcome of ASD was ascertained from the client files of two regional centers (RCs) and verified by study clinician expert review of records according to a protocol developed by the Metropolitan Atlanta Developmental Disabilities Surveillance Program, as described previously [12, 36]. The controls were randomly sampled from the birth certificate files after past or current RC clients had been excluded, matched to ASD cases by sex, birth month, and birth year [36]. Maternal blood samples were collected in serum separator tubes at 15–20 weeks gestation and stored as part of Project Baby's Breath. Serum was stored in cryovials and cell pellets stored in SSTs at − 20 °C. Newborn blood spots were collected on filter paper 1–2 days after birth and stored at − 20 °C and maintained by the Genetic Disease Screening Program, California Department of Public Health.

Cytokine and chemokine measurement

Maternal mid-gestational serum concentrations of 22 cytokines and chemokines were determined using a commercially available multiplex bead-based kit (MILLIPLEX MAP Human Cytokine/Chemokine Kit; Millipore, Billerica, MA, USA) in accordance with the kit-specific protocols provided by Millipore and as already described [34] (see more details in Additional file 1: Supplemental methods). We measured 16 cytokines and six chemokines reported in Additional file 2: Table S1. The neonatal levels of peripheral blood immune markers were extracted from filter spots as described in Additional file 1: Supplemental methods and determined using a commercially available, slightly modified, Luminex multiplex assay. We combined a Bio-Plex Pro Human Chemokine kit (Bio-Rad, Hercules, CA) containing a mix of 40 different immune markers with two individual single-plex beads from the same company, interleukin (IL)-12p70 and IL-13 (see more details in Additional file 1: Supplemental methods). We measured 12 cytokines and 30 chemokines reported in Additional file 2: Table S1. All study procedures were approved by the institutional review boards of the California Health and Human Services Agency and Kaiser Permanente Northern California; it was determined at UCSF Committee on Human Research that the institution was not engaged in human subject research.

DNA extraction and genotyping

The QIAGEN QIAamp 96 DNA Blood Kit was used to extract DNA from a subset of maternal and neonatal blood samples and the Invitrogen Quant-iT DNA Assay Kit to measure the DNA concentration by the biomedical laboratory at Utah State University, as previously described [36]. Maternal and neonatal samples were genotyped using the Affymetrix Axiom (Affymetrix 2011) EUR array (675,000 SNPs across the genome) by the Genomics Core Facility (GCF) at UCSF, using standard protocols. Genotype calling was carried out using Affymetrix Power-Tools ('Affymetrix Power Tools, Affymetrix Website'), as previously described [36]. Individual-based and marker-based quality controls, such as detection of Mendelian errors and HWE assessment, were performed with PLINK software [37] as reported in Tsang et al. [36]. Additionally, we extracted only common SNPs (MAF ≥ 1%). Two high quality datasets were used in our analysis: the first dataset included 790 maternal samples of varied ancestry (390 ASD cases, 400 controls) and 629,686 genotyped markers, and the second dataset included 764 neonatal samples (385 ASD cases, 379 controls) and 622,716 genotyped markers. Most of these were related pairs of maternal-neonatal samples (366 case pairs, 369 control pairs). The maternal dataset was a subset of those with immune mediator levels reported in Jones et al. [34].

Ancestry analysis

We reported in Traglia et al. [12] the genome-wide multidimensional scaling (MDS) analysis on high-quality markers genotyped in mothers and in infants included in our dataset. The resulting maternal and fetal genetic matrices included ten principal coordinates that summarized the genetic distance between each maternal and neonatal sample and that captured 90% and 89% of the maternal and fetal genetic variance. The distribution of maternal race/ethnicity based on the birth certificate was: 42% Hispanic, 35% non-Hispanic Caucasian, 15% Asian, 3% South Asian, and 3% African American. The ten maternal and fetal principal coordinates showed highly significant pairwise correlation with ρ ranging between 0.82 and 0.95 (Spearman's test in R 3.2.0 environment [38] $P < 0.05$; Additional file 2: Table S2).

Confounding factors for maternal and neonatal immune mediator levels and linear correlations

We analysed the log-transformed levels of the 22 maternal and 42 neonatal cytokines and chemokines with > 60% of values greater than their limit of detection (LOD) defined as the fluorescence intensity signal 2 standard deviations above the background signal, as reported in the assay manual (see Additional file 1: Supplemental methods and Additional file 2: Table S1). The values below LOD were replaced with $LOD/\sqrt{2}$ before the normalization, as reported in Jones et al. [34]. We applied a threshold of 3 or 4 SD from the mean to exclude outliers. The number of extreme values is reported in Additional file 2: Table S3.

We analysed the effects of available socio-demographic and technical covariates on maternal and neonatal immune mediator levels with linear regression models in the genotyped mothers and infants using R 3.2.0 [38]. In all the maternal analyses, we included potential confounding factors that were nominally associated with at least three maternal immune mediators ($P < 0.05$), such as maternal country of birth (USA, Mexico, others), age at mid-pregnancy (15–45 years old), maternal gestational days and weight, year of birth, maternal educational attainment (elementary, high school, college, post-graduate), and maternal genetic ancestry (the first ten coordinates) (Additional file 3: Figure S1). No variables nominally significant in one immune mediator ($0.01 < P < 0.05$) would survive multiple testing correction. We also used confounding factors associated with at least three neonatal immune mediators in all the neonatal analyses: offspring sex, bloodspot time after birth, birth type (spontaneous, C-section) and weight, birth month and year, maternal gestational days, maternal and paternal age and educational attainment, number of prenatal visits, number of previous live births, assay plate number, neonatal TSH levels, and neonatal genetic ancestry (1–10 coordinates) (Additional file 3: Figure S1). In both datasets, we used offspring ASD status as an additional covariate for quantitative cytokine analyses. The statistics for the residual

levels of each cytokine/chemokine after adjustment for confounding factors are reported in Additional file 2: Table S3. Finally, we performed a Shapiro-Wilk normality test in the R 3.2.0 [38] and reported in Additional file 2: Table S3. We assessed the linear correlation across 22 maternal cytokines/chemokines and 42 neonatal cytokines/chemokines, including 15 overlapping molecules measured in both datasets, using the Spearman's test implemented in R 3.2.0 'corrplot' package (Fig. 1, Additional file 2: Tables S4, S5, and S6).

SNP-based heritability and genetic correlation
The final set of maternal and fetal autosomal high quality markers were used to generate genetic relationship matrices and calculate SNP-based additive heritability (h^2_g) for each maternal and neonatal cytokine/chemokine level with a Restricted Maximum Likelihood (REML) model implemented in GCTA software [39], taking into account each specific set of covariates. The heritability estimation indicates the proportion of the total phenotypic variance of each cytokine/chemokine level (σ_p) accounted for by the genetic variance (σ_g/σ_p) after the exclusion of the effect of the sociodemographic, ancestry, and case/control status covariates. For each maternal and neonatal cytokine/chemokine, we used both maternal and fetal genotypes to assess the

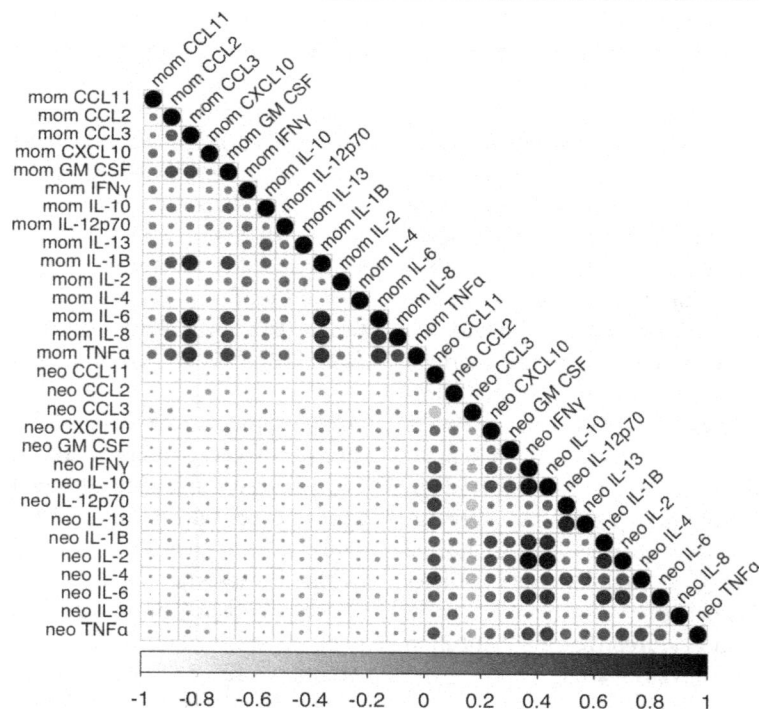

Fig. 1 Linear non-parametric correlation coefficients for 15 overlapping maternal and neonatal cytokines and chemokines. Correlation coefficients were calculated with Spearman's test. From weakest to strongest, positive correlation coefficients are represented in a dark grey gradient; negative correlation coefficients are displayed in a light grey gradient

heritability for the same cytokine/chemokine. We estimated that our dataset has low power to detect moderate heritability via the REML approach with GCTA-GREML Power Calculator [40]. To validate that our approach is suitable to adjust for population stratification, we used permutations swapping the phenotype labels for each individual 100 times, and we estimated 100 SNP-based permuted heritability models for the significantly heritable immune mediators. Most of the significant maternal and fetal h^2_g are in the top 5% of the permuted h^2_g distributions, and the medians are close to zero, suggesting little bias from population structure. To determine whether the significantly heritable maternal and neonatal cytokines/chemokines shared genetic determinants, we estimated the genetic correlations (r_g) between all possible pairs within the two datasets using the estimated heritability (h^2_g) for each heritable immune mediator in a bivariate REML [41] model in GCTA software [39] and compared to the linear correlations across each pair with cor.test() in the R 3.2.0 'stats' package [38]. We applied Fisher's z transformation test in the R 3.2.0 environment [38] to assess significant differences between estimated correlation coefficients (Additional file 2: Table S7). For each cytokine/chemokine that shows both significant maternal and fetal heritability, we assessed whether both individuals independently contribute to the phenotypic variance. We used PLINK software [37] and ad hoc bash scripts to compare each maternal allele to the matching fetal allele for the same locus ($a1a2$), and we replaced each maternal genotype with the one maternal allele not transmitted to offspring and each fetal genotype with one allele not inherited from the maternal lineage (i.e. for SNP1 maternal $a1a2$ = AA and fetal $a1a2$ = AG, A is the maternal non-transmitted allele and G is the fetal non-maternal allele). We set to 0 (missing genotype) all the SNPs for which we were unable to determine which allele was maternal (heterozygous genotype in both mother and offspring). This approach may affect the estimate of the genetic contribution by introducing missing genotypes among the more common SNPs; thus, we interpret having significant heritability as meaningful but do not interpret the estimates as precise. We used PLINK software [37] to merge the individual pairs and create two new sets of independent maternal and fetal genotypes (--make-bed). In the genetic analysis, we wanted to take into account the haploid status, so we also replaced the sex of all individuals with 1 (male) and the chromosome with X (--update-sex; --update-chr), and we coded the entire maternal and fetal independent haploid genomes as male pseudo-X chromosomes. Two genetic matrices that include only the maternal-specific alleles and the fetal-specific alleles and that look like X-chromosomes were generated from PLINK bed files with GCTA software [39] using a no dosage compensation (ND) model (--dc 0; --make-grm-xchr)

and used in cytokine-specific REML models. The ND model assumes that each allele has a similar effect on the trait. The genetic relationship matrix (A_X) for the X chromosome is redefined as $A_X^{ND} = 1/2A_X$ for male-male pairs [39]. We applied the Fisher scoring approach as implemented in GCTA (--reml alg 1) for models that did not converge. It should be noted that the estimates might be overestimated by using only one haploid genetic matrix in the model in addition to the low power of moderate heritability detection. Thus, in the text, these estimates are not considered as 'heritability' in a classic sense, but, when significant, as an indication of maternal and/or fetal genetic contribution to the trait.

Genome-wide association study

We performed immune mediator-specific genome-wide association studies (GWAS) for maternal and fetal SNPs using a linear model implemented in PLINK software [37] (--linear) using each specific set of covariates including ten PCs. To validate that our approach is suitable to adjust for stratification 'within' and 'across' populations, we also performed a meta-analysis of four separate association tests in homogeneous sub-populations with ten population-specific PCs and we found consistent results for top SNPs (Additional file 2: Table S8). We also extracted the meta-analysis top hits ($P < 5 \times 10^{-8}$) and we observed a similar trend (Additional file 2: Table S8). Then, we used the LocusZoom tool [42] to generate regional genomic plots and assess linkage disequilibrium (LD) among associated SNPs. We use the genome-wide significance threshold ($P < 5 \times 10^{-8}$) and suggestive threshold ($P < 1 \times 10^{-7}$) to account for approximate independent common polymorphism testing per GWAS [43, 44]. We have tested many correlated cytokines/chemokines in related mothers and offspring; because the tests are not completely independent, we were unable to calculate the exact correction for study-wide significance and present uncorrected P values.

Maternal and fetal contribution to the associated loci

For each cytokine/chemokine that showed a genome-wide significant maternal and/or fetal locus that is also suggestively associated in the paired individual's genetics, we assessed whether the associations were controlled by maternal and/or fetal genetics. We performed separate linear regression models including the entire maternal- and/or fetal-specific set of covariates and the genotypes of maternal- and fetal-associated SNPs (for three maternal immune mediators ~ maternal SNP + fetal SNP + maternal covariates; for ten neonatal immune mediators ~ fetal SNP + maternal SNP + fetal covariates), and we assessed the residual association for maternal and fetal genotypes.

Offspring ASD outcome association with immune mediators

We tested for differences between the residuals for maternal cytokines/chemokines in mothers of ASD cases and mothers of controls and for neonatal cytokines/chemokines in ASD-affected neonates and control neonates with a two-sample Mann-Whitney Wilcoxon test in R 3.2.0 [38].

Genetic interaction between chemokine levels and ASD association

We assessed whether genetic determinants associated with chemokines that showed statistically significant associations with ASD might drive the association between chemokines and ASD or show interaction effects. Thus, we selected each maternal and fetal cytokine-specific top (GW or suggestive) SNPs for maternal and neonatal chemokines that are associated with ASD. We included each genotype in logistic regression models for ASD outcome and we assessed whether the top SNPs interact with ASD in cytokine-specific models. We compared the levels of chemokines in the individuals with different genotypes for ASD-interacting SNPs using a two-sample Mann-Whitney Wilcoxon test in the R 3.2.0 environment [38].

Results

Maternal immune mediators

To assess our ability to identify genetic contributions of circulating maternal immune mediators, we first analysed distributions of the log-transformed concentrations of 16 cytokines and six chemokines surveyed in mid-gestational maternal blood. We applied adjustment for potential maternal and neonatal confounding factors, including offspring ASD outcome (Additional file 3: Figure S1) to obtain residuals, as we first wanted to assess cytokine/chemokine levels independent of outcome. After excluding a few extreme residual values for 11 of 22 mediators (outliers < 4% of the total individuals, mean = 1%; see the 'Methods' section), we observed approximately normally distributed residuals for most cytokine/chemokine levels (Additional file 2: Table S2). The observation of unimodal distributions suggested continuous inter-individual variation in immune mediator levels, rather than distinct classes of individuals with low/high levels, such as immune-activated vs. non-activated, within the study population. Thus, all 22 maternal cytokines and chemokines could be used as quantitative traits for genetic analysis. Some maternal immune mediators appeared interrelated, as 22 of 231 pairs (9.5%) demonstrated high correlations ($\rho > 0.5$) (Additional file 2: Table S4).

High maternal heritability contributes to two maternal immune mediator levels

We estimated SNP-based maternal heritability for 22 maternal mid-gestational mediator residual levels via mixed linear model. CXCL10 (or IP-10) and IL-7 were significantly regulated by genome-wide maternal SNP effects (Table 1). The additive maternal polygenic contribution is estimated to account for 79% and 84% of the total CXCL10 and IL-7 phenotypic variance ($P = 4.4 \times 10^{-3}$ and $P = 2.1 \times 10^{-3}$, respectively). We are not able to determine whether the remaining immune mediators might be heritable because our dataset has low power to detect moderate heritability.

Maternal loci associated with maternal mediators

We performed genome-wide association studies (GWAS) for maternal cytokine/chemokine levels via linear regression. The maternal cytokines sIL-2Ra and IL-1α and the chemokine CCL11, were significantly ($P < 5 \times 10^{-8}$) associated with specific maternal loci (Table 2 and Additional file 3: Figure S2A–C). CCL11 (or eotaxin-1) is associated with a low-frequency polymorphism, rs115463265, which maps on chromosome 3p24.2 in a lincRNA between *THRB* and *RARB* genes encoding receptors for thyroid hormone. Soluble IL-2Ra is associated with rs12778662, an intronic variant located in a RNA binding protein gene (*RBM17*) and near the gene encoding the IL-2 receptor (*IL2RA*) on chromosome 10p15.1. Finally, IL-1α is associated with rs1562064 near the *SMAD1* gene which encodes a member of the bone morphogenetic protein (BMP) pathway on chromosome 4q31.21.

Neonatal immune mediators

We analysed the log-transformed concentrations of 12 cytokines and 30 chemokines measured in neonatal bloodspots at birth in the genotyped EMA sample. As reported in Additional file 2: Table S2, 15 out of 42

Table 1 SNP-based maternal and fetal heritability for maternal and neonatal chemokines and cytokines

SIM	Dataset	Maternal genetics			Fetal genetics		
		h^2_g	SE	P value	h^2_g	SE	P value
Chemokines							
CXCL10	Mothers	0.79	0.28	4.4×10^{-3}	0.99	0.38	5.8×10^{-4}
CCL1	Infants	0.72	0.35	2.9×10^{-2}	0.98	0.35	1.6×10^{-2}
CCL3	Infants	0.60	0.33	4.6×10^{-2}	0.72	0.43	5.0×10^{-2}
CCL17	Infants	0.59	0.37	0.09	0.99	0.42	1.0×10^{-2}
CCL19	Infants	0.69	0.36	4.0×10^{-2}	0.99	0.42	7.8×10^{-3}
CCL22	Infants	0.92	0.32	3.8×10^{-3}	0.97	0.43	2.0×10^{-2}
CCL25	Infants	0.50	0.33	0.07	0.70	0.42	5.0×10^{-2}
CXCL5	Infants	0.88	0.34	1.4×10^{-2}	0.92	0.43	2.0×10^{-2}
Cytokines							
IL-4	Infants	0.76	0.37	3.2×10^{-2}	0.05	0.49	NS
IL-7	Mothers	0.84	0.28	2.1×10^{-3}	0.90	0.37	1.0×10^{-2}

NS not significant

Table 2 Maternal and fetal genome-wide significant association of maternal and neonatal cytokines/chemokines

SNP	gen	chr	A1	MAF	Beta	SE	P value	Locus	SIM	Set	P value match-gen
rs12327057	Fetal	18p11	C	0.18	− 0.42	0.07	1.4×10^{-8}	ADCYAP1	sIL2R-α	M	9.4×10^{-4}
rs75885714	Fetal	3p24.3	C	0.08	− 0.53	0.05	8.6×10^{-21}	PLCL2	CCL17	I	3.8×10^{-6}
rs75885714	Fetal	3p24.3	C	0.08	− 0.48	0.05	3.3×10^{-20}	PLCL2	CCL19	I	3.8×10^{-6}
rs75885714	Fetal	3p24.3	C	0.08	− 0.36	0.04	2.8×10^{-19}	PLCL2	CXCL9	I	5.4×10^{-6}
rs75885714	Fetal	3p24.3	C	0.08	− 0.23	0.03	8.2×10^{-13}	PLCL2	CCL7	I	1.1×10^{-3}
rs75885714	Fetal	3p24.3	C	0.08	− 0.24	0.03	5.2×10^{-12}	PLCL2	IFN-γ	I	6.0×10^{-3}
rs75885714	Fetal	3p24.3	C	0.08	− 0.27	0.04	2.1×10^{-12}	PLCL2	IL-2	I	1.5×10^{-3}
rs75885714	Fetal	3p24.3	C	0.08	− 0.26	0.04	1.7×10^{-11}	PLCL2	IL-6	I	9.7×10^{-4}
rs75885714	Fetal	3p24.3	C	0.08	− 0.20	0.03	1.8×10^{-11}	PLCL2	IL-10	I	3.8×10^{-4}
rs75885714	Fetal	3p24.3	C	0.08	− 0.22	0.03	3.5×10^{-10}	PLCL2	IL-1β	I	1.4×10^{-3}
rs75885714	Fetal	3p24.3	C	0.08	− 0.17	0.03	9.3×10^{-10}	PLCL2	CXCL13	I	1.3×10^{-4}
rs75885714	Fetal	3p24.3	C	0.08	− 0.16	0.03	2.0×10^{-8}	PLCL2	CX3CL1	I	9.8×10^{-4}
rs1003645	Fetal	17q12	C	0.28	− 0.63	0.02	2.5×10^{-100}	CCL23	CCL23	I	3.4×10^{-24}
rs854625	Fetal	17q12	A	0.12	0.47	0.04	4.6×10^{-25}	CCL15	CCL15	I	1.1×10^{-6}
rs3921	Fetal	4q21.1	C	0.29	0.24	0.03	2.0×10^{-14}	CXCL9/10/11	CXCL11	I	1.2×10^{-3}
rs16850073	Fetal	4q13.3	T	0.32	0.10	0.02	6.4×10^{-9}	CXCL6	CXCL6	I	6.8×10^{-6}
rs73359750	Fetal	7q11.23	T	0.08	0.86	0.16	4.9×10^{-8}	CCL24	CCL24	I	NS
rs41272321	Fetal	3q22.1	G	0.13	− 0.20	0.03	2.8×10^{-10}	ACKR4	CCL21	I	3.3×10^{-4}
rs2228467	Fetal	3p22.1	C	0.04	0.29	0.05	2.8×10^{-8}	ACKR2	CXCL9	I	0.01
rs2228467	Fetal	3p22.1	C	0.04	0.42	0.07	4.4×10^{-9}	ACKR2	CCL19	I	0.03
rs2228467	Fetal	3p22.1	C	0.04	0.48	0.07	1.8×10^{-10}	ACKR2	CCL17	I	0.02
rs74331971	Fetal	8p23.3	A	0.03	− 0.40	0.07	1.9×10^{-9}	FBXO25/TDRP	IL-4	I	0.03
rs4303899	Fetal	3q13.32	G	0.12	− 0.09	0.02	1.7×10^{-8}	lincRNA	CXCL12	I	NS
rs115463265	Maternal	3p24.2	T	0.02	− 1.50	0.24	1.6×10^{-9}	THRB/RARB	CCL11	M	NS
rs12778662	Maternal	10p15.1	T	0.07	0.65	0.11	3.7×10^{-9}	IL2R	sIL2R-α	M	0.04
rs1562064	Maternal	4q31.21	G	0.32	− 0.74	0.13	2.1×10^{-8}	near SMAD1	IL1-α	M	1.5×10^{-3}
rs34642455	Maternal	7q22.1	C	0.13	− 2.17	0.38	3.1×10^{-8}	CYP3A4	CXCL5	I	3.6×10^{-3}
rs72751339	Maternal	15q26.2	T	0.02	− 1.52	0.25	1.3×10^{-8}	MCTP2	CCL24	I	1.7×10^{-3}
rs17159338	Maternal	5q21.3	C	0.03	− 0.36	0.06	1.2×10^{-9}	near EFNA5	IL-16	I	NS

gen genetics, chr chromosomal region, A1 tested allele, MAF minor allele frequency, Set dataset, M mothers, I infants and NS not significant

cytokines/chemokines measured in the neonates overlapped with those measured in maternal serum. After applying adjustment for a set of maternal and neonatal confounding factors (described in the 'Methods' section) and exclusion of extreme values (outliers < 7% of the total individuals, mean = 1%, Additional file 2: Table S3 and Additional file 3: Figure S1), neonates showed significantly less variance than mothers for the immune mediators measured in both individuals (F test, $P < 0.05$) and particularly tight but approximately normal distributions and high correlations among most of the immune mediators (Additional file 2: Tables S3 and S5). We did not observe any significant correlation (or coefficients $\rho > 0.15$) between the 15 cytokines/chemokines measured in the maternal dataset and the same 15 mediators measured in the neonatal dataset (Fig. 1). Nor did we

find other correlated maternal-neonatal immune mediator pairs, considering all combinations in case we could infer a relationship with a non-measured cytokine/chemokine (Additional file 2: Table S6).

High fetal heritability regulates the levels of seven neonatal chemokines

In order to assess whether the infant immune mediator levels measured at birth might be genetically regulated independently of the maternal immune system, we measured SNP-based fetal heritability for 42 neonatal cytokine/chemokine levels after adjustment for potential confounding factors (including ASD status) via mixed linear modelling. We were able to identify seven neonatal chemokines that showed significant fetal genetic contribution (heritability = 70–99%; Table 1). To assess whether the subset of heritable neonatal chemokines shared genetic determinants, we calculated the co-heritability (genetic correlation) between all the possible pairs of the seven neonatal chemokines, and we compared genetic correlations to linear correlations. We expected that genetic correlation might be higher than linear correlation if there were differences in environmental determinants but similar genetic determinants of both immune mediators. In contrast, significantly lower genetic correlations than linear correlations might indicate a similar response to the shared environment but distinct genetic determinants involved. We found seven out of 21 chemokine pairs that showed significant genetic correlations ($\rho > 0.50$) and four were significantly higher compared to the linear correlations (Additional file 2: Table S7). Thus, our results allowed us to define a set of neonatal immune mediators with strong genetic control that includes CCL1, CCL3, CCL17, CCL19, CCL22, and CCL25. Our results support the hypothesis that some neonatal chemokines are under strong fetal genetic control early in life.

PLCL2 is a novel fetal locus for several neonatal immune mediators

Next, we performed genome-wide association studies for the 42 neonatal cytokine/chemokine levels via linear regression analyses. We observed a SNP (rs75885714, MAF = 7%) located on chromosome 3p24.3 that was highly associated with 11 neonatal cytokines and chemokines (Table 2 and Additional file 2: Table S5). The strongest association was with the chemokine CCL17 (or TARC, $\beta = -0.53$, SE = 0.05, $P = 8.6 \times 10^{-21}$). This SNP was also associated with a number of inflammatory cytokines and chemokines: IFNγ, IL-2, CCL7, CXCL9, and CCL19. We next asked whether the rs75885714 locus is independently associated with each immune mediator or whether it drives the regulation of the entire set of correlated mediators. Regression models including CCL17 with each other cytokine/chemokine separately suggest that CXCL9 might independently account for the association between rs75885714 and the other correlated cytokines/chemokines. To confirm this, we performed a linear regression model for CXCL9 after including the entire set of ten correlated cytokines/chemokines and we still observed a residual association between rs75885714 and CXCL9. Thus, the association of the locus with the cytokines/chemokines is driven by CXCL9 (rs75885714, $\beta = -0.36$, SE = 0.04, $P = 2.8 \times 10^{-19}$), for which the SNP was responsible for 13% of the total CXCL9 phenotypic variance. The polymorphism rs75885714 maps to the *PLCL2* gene, which encodes phospholipase C (Fig. 2a). A second SNP in the same locus (rs12496141 CXCL9, $\beta = -0.21$, SE = 0.03, $P = 1.5 \times 10^{-9}$; MAF = 10%; variance explained = 19%) shows high linkage disequilibrium (LD) with rs75885714 in our dataset

($r^2 = 0.68$, comparable to LD estimated in Hispanic ancestry populations included in 1000 Genomes Project [45] with ENSEMBL [46]; Fig. 2b). After a conditional analysis using the individual genotypes of rs75885714 as covariate, the second SNP, rs12496141, showed no association.

A large set of other neonatal immune mediators was associated with specific fetal loci. Most of the genome-wide significant loci were near the gene encoding the associated neonatal cytokine/chemokine or its receptor (Table 2 and Additional file 3: Figure S2D–H). Additionally, we found an association with *ACKR4* (atypical chemokine receptor 4) and *ACKR2* (atypical chemokine receptor 2) loci encoding receptors that serve several chemokines (Table 2 and Additional file 3: Figure S2I–J).

We identified two additional novel loci genome-wide significantly associated with immune molecule levels (Table 2 and Additional file 3: Figure S2K–L) not near molecule- or receptor-encoding genes: IL-4 levels were associated with the low-frequency SNP rs74331971 that maps between *FBXO25* and *TDRP* on chromosome 8p23.3 ($\beta = -0.40$, SE = 0.07, $P = 1.9 \times 10^{-9}$), and the levels of CXCL12 (or SDF-1) were associated with rs4303899, located in LINC02024, a long non-coding RNA on chromosome 3q13.32 between *LSAMP* and *IGSF11* ($\beta = -0.09$, SE = 0.02, $P = 1.7 \times 10^{-8}$).

Neonatal immune mediators show evidence for maternal heritability

We performed similar genetic analyses using the 42 neonatal cytokine/chemokine levels, but instead of fetal genotype data, we substituted maternal genotype data. We defined the cytokines and chemokines measured in the neonatal dataset with maternal genetic contribution and vice versa as 'cross-heritable'. Six neonatal cytokines and chemokines showed significant contribution of maternal heritability, ranging between 60% for CCL3 (or MIP-1α) and 92% for CCL22 (or MDC). Five of these six were also neonatally heritable; additionally, the neonatal level of the cytokine IL-4 was not influenced by fetal genetics but only by maternal heritability (Table 1). The high standard error did not allow us to distinguish whether both maternal and fetal genomes contribute independently or only one individual's genome exerts influence (but the other shares 50% of alleles by inheritance).

To differentiate between the contributions of the maternal and neonatal genome, we identified the offspring alleles not inherited from the maternal lineage at conception (fetal-specific alleles) and the maternal alleles not transmitted to the offspring (maternal-specific alleles) (see the 'Methods' section) and we calculated genetic contribution using maternal-specific alleles and fetal-specific alleles. (Note that we are using haploid genomes, so significant values are interpreted as evidence for independent genetic contribution rather than as a

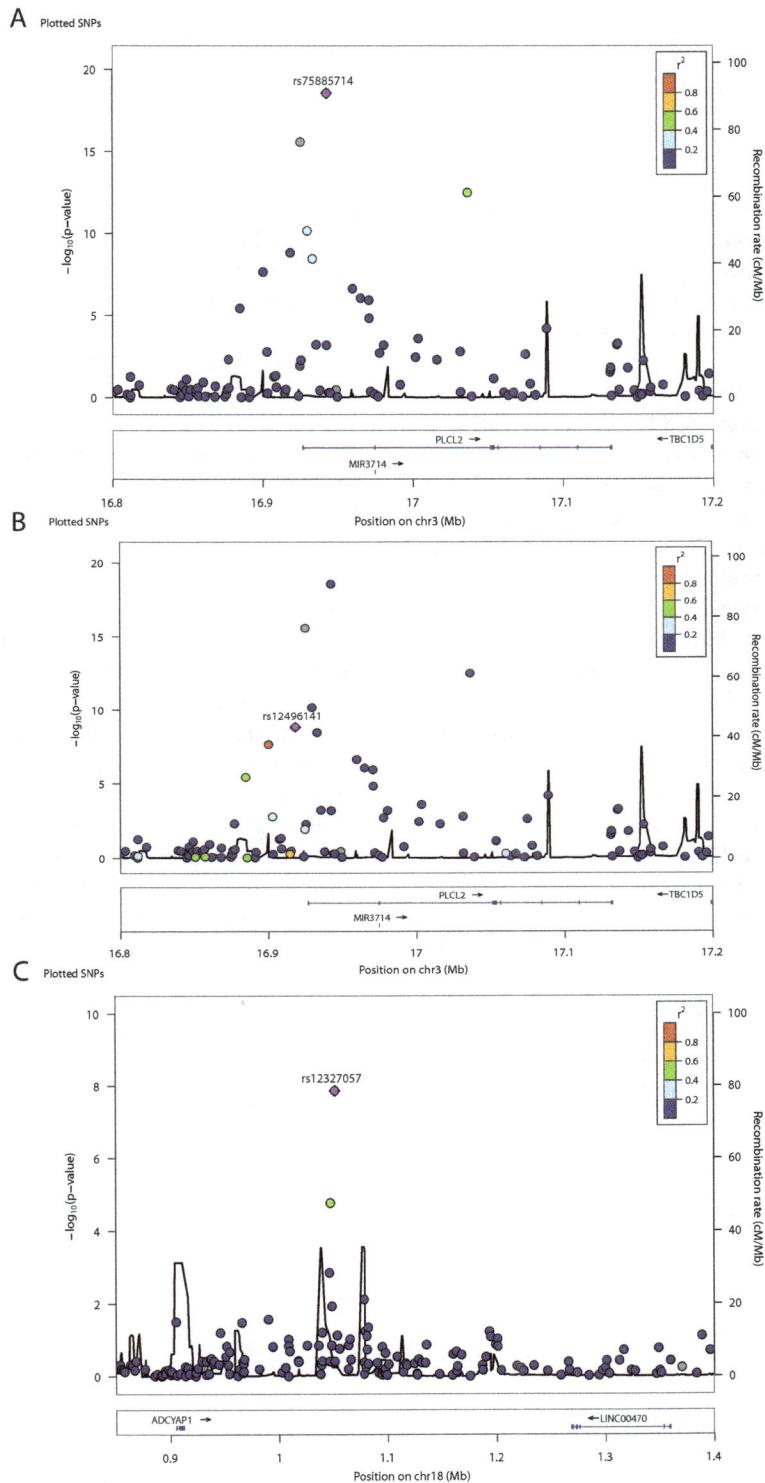

Fig. 2 (See legend on next page.)

Fig. 2 Linkage disequilibrium regional genomic plot of fetal genome-wide associated SNPs with maternal serum levels of sIL2R-α and 11 neonatal immune mediators. **a** Fetal rs75885714 on chromosome 3p24.3 associated with CCL17 ($\beta = -0.53$, SE = 0.05, $P = 8.6 \times 10^{-21}$); **b** The independent fetal SNP rs12496141 which maps in the *PLCL2* gene and (**c**) Fetal rs12327057 on chromosome 18p11 associated with sIL2R-α maternal levels ($\beta = -0.42$, SE = 0.07, $P = 1.4 \times 10^{-8}$) maps to a lincRNA *ADCYAPi* gene. The x-axis represents the genomic position; the y-axis shows the negative logarithm of the observed association P value for each tested SNP. Plotted with LocusZoom tool [42]

traditional 'heritability' estimate). We observed that three out of six cross-heritable neonatal cytokine/chemokine levels were significantly estimated as controlled by both maternal and fetal genetics, as well as CXCL5 only by maternal genetics (CCL1 and IL-4 estimate were not significant; Table 3).

Maternal genome-wide associated loci for the levels of three neonatal immune mediators

In order to determine whether maternal variation in the cytokine/chemokine- or receptor-encoding genes associated with maternal cytokine/chemokines also contributed to neonatal cytokine/chemokine levels, or whether different maternal loci are involved via a separate mechanism, we mapped specific maternal loci associated with neonatal cytokine/chemokines levels. We interestingly identified, via GWAS, three independent low-frequency significant maternal loci (MAF range 1–3%; $P < 3.1 \times 10^{-8}$) affecting three neonatal immune mediators. Neonatal levels of CCL24 were associated with the SNP rs72751339 in *MCTP2* on chromosome 15q26.2. The levels of IL-16 were associated with rs17159338 in the lincRNA *LINC01950* near the *EFNA5* gene (Ephrin-A5) on chromosome 5q21.3. Finally, CXCL5 (or ENA-78) was associated with rs34642455 in the cytochrome P450 3A4

gene (*CYP3A4*) on chromosome 7q22.1 (Table 2 and Additional file 3: Figure S2M–O). CCL24 showed distinct fetal- and maternal-associated loci whereas IL-16 and CXCL5 did not show significant fetal loci. These maternal SNPs were not associated with any maternal immune mediator ($P < 0.05$), except rs17159338 with IL-4 at $P = 0.02$.

High fetal SNP-based contribution to maternal CXCL10 and IL-7

We also estimated whether the fetal genome affects maternal mid-gestational circulating cytokine/chemokine levels. About 99% of the maternal phenotypic variance of CXCL10 (SE = 37%, $P = 5.8 \times 10^{-4}$) and 90% of IL-7 (SE = 38%, $P = 0.02$) were explained by fetal heritability, compared to 79% and 84% maternal heritability estimates, respectively (Table 1). Once again, the high standard errors did not allow us to distinguish the exact maternal and fetal contributions or their independence. Thus, we estimated the proportion of the maternal circulating cytokine/chemokine levels regulated by fetal-specific alleles and by maternal-specific alleles. Maternal IL-7 and CXCL10 levels were significantly regulated by both maternal-specific alleles and fetal-specific alleles (Table 3).

Table 3 Maternal-specific allele-based proportion of genetic variance and fetal-specific allele-based proportion of genetic variance for maternal and neonatal chemokines and cytokines under a no dosage compensation model

SIM	Dataset	Maternal-only non transmitted allele			Fetal-only non inherited allele		
		$V_{(g)}/Vp$	SE	P value	$V_{(g)}/Vp$	SE	P value
Chemokines							
CXCL10	Mothers	0.81	0.19	7.1×10^{-3}	0.81	0.20	0.01
CCL1	Infants	0.63	0.31	*0.09*	0.75	0.26	0.04
CCL3	Infants	0.47	0.40	NS	0.41	0.44	NS
CCL17	Infants	0.75	0.25	0.05	0.81	0.22	0.02
CCL19	Infants	0.80	0.23	0.03	0.83	0.21	0.01
CCL22	Infants	0.95	0.16	2.8×10^{-3}	0.83	0.22	0.02
CCL25	Infants	0.48	0.37	NS	0.39	0.44	NS
CXCL5	Infants	0.87	0.20	0.025	0.45	0.41	NS
Cytokines							
IL-4	Infants	0.49	0.40	NS	0.00	0.73	NS
IL-7	Mothers	0.79	0.21	0.0163	0.99#	0.17	< 0.01

$V_{(g)}/Vp$ proportion of genetic variance over phenotypic variance
#Fisher's test applied for non converging models
NS not significant

One fetal locus contributes to maternal soluble IL-2 receptor levels

We performed genome-wide association analysis using the fetal genome for each maternal mediator level. Supporting our heritability evidence of an active role of fetal genetics on the maternal immune system, the fetal locus rs12327057 (MAF = 18%) on chromosome 18p11 in RP11-78F17.1, a long noncoding RNA, near *ADCYAP1* (Fig. 2c and Table 2), was associated with soluble maternal interleukin-2 receptor levels ($\beta = -0.42$, SE = 0.07, $P = 1.4 \times 10^{-8}$). The adenylate cyclase activating polypeptide 1 gene encodes secreted processed peptides involved in transcriptional activation of target genes. We did not measure sIL2R-α in neonates so we are not able to determine whether variation near the fetal *ADCYAP1* gene might affect the neonatal soluble immune receptor levels. However, maternal sIL2R-α levels were associated with variation at the *IL2RA* maternal locus, but not at the fetal *IL2RA* locus, supporting the interpretation that both maternal and fetal genetics might contribute to immune mediator variability, and specifically that fetal genetics influences maternal cytokines not via direct transfer of fetal-derived cytokines during pregnancy but via different pathways. This SNP was not associated with any neonatal immune mediator ($P < 0.05$), except with CCL24 at a nominal level ($P = 5.0 \times 10^{-3}$).

Independent contribution of maternal- and fetal-associated loci to immune mediator variance

Most of the 17 genome-wide significant loci that were associated with cytokine/chemokine levels showed strong association when analysing either the contribution from fetal or maternal genetics but had reduced associations when considering paired mother/offspring genetics. We tested whether at these specific loci, fetal genetics contributes independently from maternal genetics to maternal immune mediators and whether fetal genetics contributes independently from maternal genetics to neonatal immune mediators. In nine out of 11 fetal genome-wide significant associated loci with maternal and neonatal immune mediators reported in Table 2, nominal maternal genetic association was observed; and in four out of six associated maternal loci with both maternal and fetal immune mediators, nominally significant fetal effects were seen (Table 2). When conditioning each associated immune mediator with both maternal and fetal genotypes, we observed no residual association in the mother/offspring with less significant initial evidence for association (Table 2 and Additional file 2: Table S9). Additionally, most of the maternal top SNPs ($P < =5 \times 10^{-4}$) do not overlap with the fetal top SNPs ($P < =5 \times 10^{-4}$) for the same immune mediators (Additional file 3: Figure S3).

Interleukin-8 and CCL2 levels are associated with ASD outcome

Consistent with previous findings using a quartile analysis approach in the full EMA sample [34, 47, Heuer LS, Jones KL, Yoshida CK, Hansen R, Yolken R, Zerbo O, Ashwood P, de WJ CLAV. An examination of neonatal cytokines and chemokines as predictors of autism risk: the early markers for autism study [In preparation]. We observed two borderline negative associations between maternal mid-gestational levels of the chemokines IL-8 and CCL2 (MCP1) with ASD (Wilcoxon test, $P = 9.3 \times 10^{-3}$ and $P = 0.02$, respectively) and a positive association between neonatal IL-8 and ASD ($P = 8.6 \times 10^{-3}$) (Table 4 and Fig. 3), after adjustment for the effects of covariates (Additional file 3: Figure S1). No additional significant association was detected.

Interleukin-8 levels interact with maternal genotype to show association with ASD

We hypothesized that the specific genetic factors that contribute to CCL2 and IL-8 might drive the association observed with ASD outcome (Table 4). Since no genome-wide significant associated loci emerged for CCL2 and IL-8 (Table 2), we selected the most suggestively associated maternal and fetal SNPs: three maternal SNPs (maternal CCL2: rs1869714, $\beta = 0.20$, SE = 0.04, $P = 4.3 \times 10^{-6}$; maternal IL-8: rs60587996, $\beta = -0.77$, SE = 0.16, $P = 3.1 \times 10^{-6}$, neonatal IL-8: rs55823040, $\beta = 0.24$, SE = 0.05, $P = 3.6 \times 10^{-7}$) and three fetal SNPs (maternal CCL2: rs17504601, $\beta = 0.28$, SE = 0.06, $P = 5.0 \times 10^{-7}$; maternal IL-8: rs1252145, $\beta = -0.66$, SE = 0.13, $P = 5.3 \times 10^{-7}$, neonatal IL-8: rs80166972, $\beta = 0.47$, SE = 0.09, $P = 4.3 \times 10^{-7}$). These SNPs were not themselves associated in logistic models with ASD outcome ($P > 0.1$), but we observed a significant interaction ($\beta = -0.22$ SE = 0.11, $P = 0.04$) between ASD outcome and maternal SNP rs55823040 (MAF = 0.09), which was associated ($P = 3.6 \times 10^{-7}$) with neonatal IL-8 levels. Our analysis showed that neonatal IL-8 levels were significantly increased only in ASD offspring of mothers with the CT genotype for rs55823040 (Fig. 4) (few TT homozygotes were observed). This SNP had only interaction effects and not main effects with ASD outcome.

Discussion

We report here the first genome-wide multi-approach study to provide insight into potential patterns of

Table 4 ASD outcome association with CCL2 and IL-8 in mothers and infants after adjustment for sociodemographic covariates and for maternal and fetal genetic ancestry

SIM	Dataset	N	Beta	SE	OR	[95% CI]	P value
CCL2	Mothers	707	− 0.135	0.058	0.874	[0.78–0.98]	0.019
IL-8	Mothers	707	− 0.243	0.112	0.784	[0.63–0.98]	0.030
IL-8	Infants	649	0.082	0.041	1.090	[1.00–1.18]	0.046

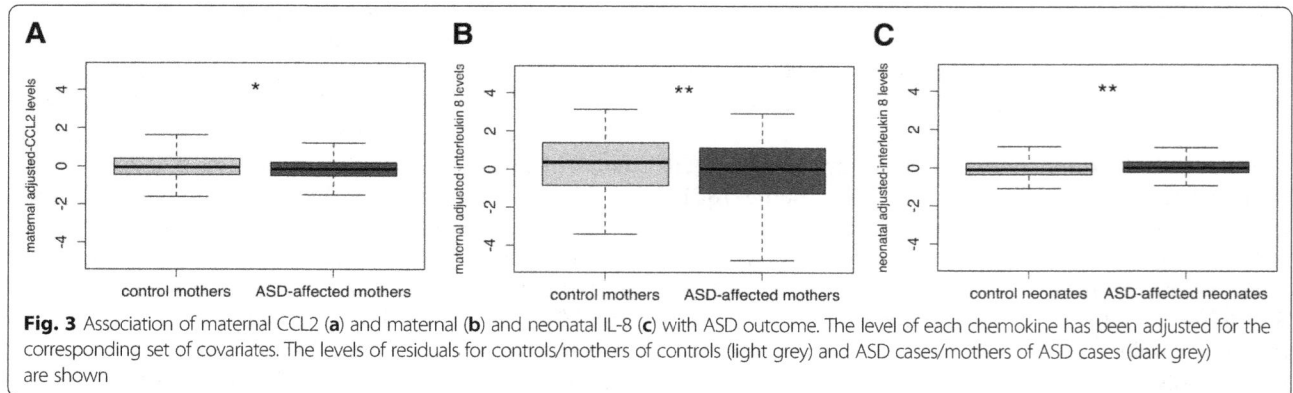

Fig. 3 Association of maternal CCL2 (**a**) and maternal (**b**) and neonatal IL-8 (**c**) with ASD outcome. The level of each chemokine has been adjusted for the corresponding set of covariates. The levels of residuals for controls/mothers of controls (light grey) and ASD cases/mothers of ASD cases (dark grey) are shown

maternal-fetal genetic control of immune mediator status in the prenatal and neonatal periods (Fig. 5). We discuss specific significant findings, some of which may be unique to these life stages. In addition, we detail our observations supporting the interpretation that cross-genetic associations represent independent maternal and fetal influence on one another and that this influence occurs via a distinct mechanism rather than direct exchange of soluble factors.

We showed that the circulating levels of CXCL10 (IP-10) and IL-7 during mid-gestation were strongly regulated by the maternal genome. These results were consistent with two studies analysing the SNP-based heritability and twin-based heritability of immune molecules [48, 49]. Many of the immune mediators without significant estimated genetic contribution showed significant GWAS associations, suggesting genetic influence beyond what we could detect as heritability. We

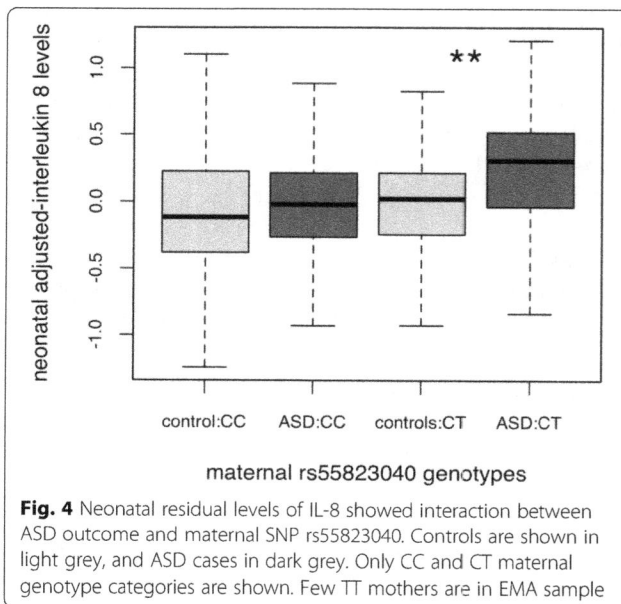

Fig. 4 Neonatal residual levels of IL-8 showed interaction between ASD outcome and maternal SNP rs55823040. Controls are shown in light grey, and ASD cases in dark grey. Only CC and CT maternal genotype categories are shown. Few TT mothers are in EMA sample

identified three maternal loci that were potentially involved in mid-gestational immune system status. A SNP (rs12778662) was associated with soluble levels of IL-2 receptor alpha and maps near the gene encoding *IL2RA* (Fig. 5). This association has previously been observed in healthy adults [8]. In addition, the chemokine CCL11, a strong activator of eosinophils, was associated with a novel SNP located between *THRB* (encoding the thyroid hormone receptor β) and *RARB* (encoding retinoic acid receptor β), which is effective at controlling inflammatory and inducing tolerogenic immune responses. Finally, maternal levels of the inflammatory cytokine IL1-α were associated with a novel SNP near *SMAD1*, which encodes one of the SMAD proteins involved in the TGF-β signalling pathway. These latter two associations were not observed ($P > 0.05$) in large populations of healthy adults studied [8].

We also assessed neonatal cytokine/chemokine levels and their potential genetic control in early life. The reduced variance observed in the distributions of neonatal cytokines suggests that stressful events during birth did not unduly impact neonatal immune mediator levels, allowing for the detection of genetic influence. Moreover, there were low correlations between neonatal and maternal cytokine/chemokine levels. Although the samples are taken months apart, should they reflect baseline genetically-determined levels, we might expect correlation if neonatal immune mediators were directly transferred from the maternal bloodstream. Thus, our observations suggest that maternal cytokines and chemokines are not directly populating the neonatal blood at birth. However, since the neonatal levels reflect both serum and lysed cells, and the maternal levels were measured only in serum, the levels measured may not be directly comparable. Note that the difference in variation observed in maternal and neonatal immune mediator distributions may be biological variation (e.g. influence of long-term environmental exposure in mothers) or it may be technical noise (e.g. serum vs. bloodspot or

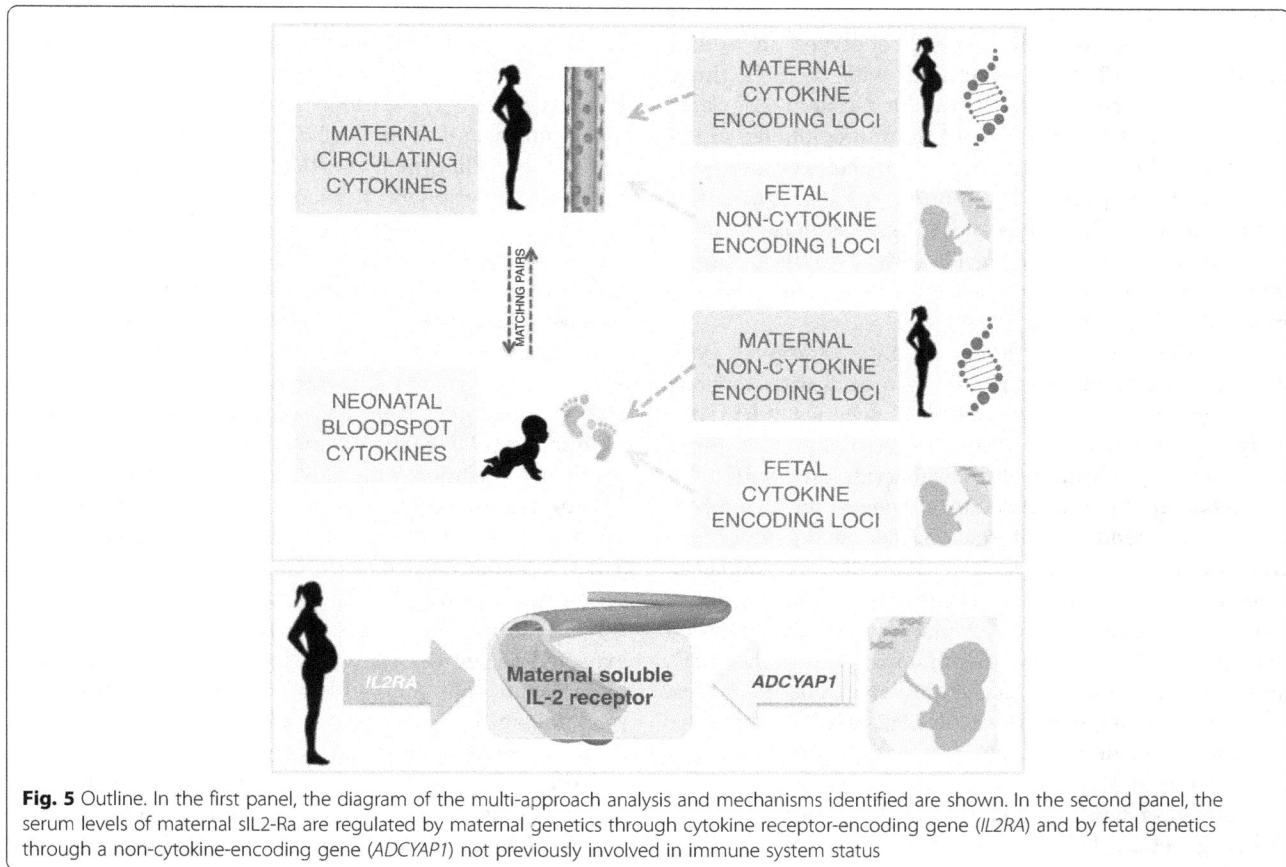

Fig. 5 Outline. In the first panel, the diagram of the multi-approach analysis and mechanisms identified are shown. In the second panel, the serum levels of maternal sIL2-Ra are regulated by maternal genetics through cytokine receptor-encoding gene (*IL2RA*) and by fetal genetics through a non-cytokine-encoding gene (*ADCYAP1*) not previously involved in immune system status

different assay properties); however, either of these explanations are non-genetic and thus will have the same impact on our genetic analyses.

Genome-wide association analysis identified ten fetal loci associated with 19 circulating neonatal immune mediators at birth (Table 2). We defined a set of six neonatal chemokines, CCL1, CCL3, CCL17, CCL19, CCL22, and CCL25, controlled by shared common fetal genetic factors. Interestingly, a single large-impact SNP (variance explained about 13%) rs75885714 was associated with CXCL9, which drives the association with ten other highly correlated ($\rho > 0.90$) neonatal cytokines/chemokines including the heritable CCL17 and CCL19. The marker rs75885714 maps in *PLCL2*, which encodes a phospholipase involved in the regulation of calcium-protein kinase C signalling pathway. In studies of *Plcl2*-deficient mice, it has been shown that *Plcl2* acts as a negative regulator of B cell receptor signalling and humoral immune responses [50], and in humans is involved in metabolism [51] and implicated in autoimmune diseases such as psoriasis [52], rheumatoid arthritis [53], and systemic sclerosis [54]. However, this is the first study to show *PLCL2* associated with

quantitative levels of immune molecules, which could reflect a developmental observation.

Seven other fetal loci associated with neonatal cytokine and chemokine levels were located in the gene encoding the receptor of that cytokine/chemokine. Among these seven loci, our study found evidence for association with a cluster of atypical chemokine receptors (ACKRs) and confirms evidence shown in a recently published study [8]. The study analysing an adult human population from Finland showed association between *ACKR1* and *ACKR2* and other immune molecules but did not replicate our neonatal finding in *ACKR4*. Our neonatal EMA sample replicates at a nominally significant level the association of *ACKR1* (CXCL11; $P = 9.0 \times 10^{-3}$) in adults, but we did not replicate all previously-implicated SNPs [8], likely due to differences between the two studies, such as the age of the recruited participants and/or the genetic make-up of the Finnish population.

Finally, two other fetal SNPs were identified in loci not attributable so far to any known immune function. In particular, one SNP that was associated with neonatal IL-4 levels, maps near to *TDRP*, a gene that encodes a testis development related protein that is expressed in the thyroid gland and placenta, and has not previously been associated with immune phenotypes in adults. Finally, CXCL12 was associated with a SNP in a lincRNA between *LSAMP* (limbic system-associated membrane protein) and *IGSF11* (immunoglobulin superfamily member 11), both involved in cell-cell adhesion and may be important in immune synapse formation. Although this SNP has not been associated at a genome-wide significant level with cytokines/chemokines previously, it did show modest signal with several molecules ($P_{min} = 8 \times 10^{-4}$) [8].

Since the circulating levels of mid-gestational cytokines and chemokines were not correlated with neonatal levels, we asked whether maternal genetics might directly regulate neonatal cytokines/chemokines at birth. We found significant maternal genetic contribution for six neonatal immune mediators, suggesting a combination of independent maternal and neonatal genetic control for most of those. IL-4 showed only maternal evidence for heritability. In pregnancy, IL-4 is produced [55] by immune cells of the placenta, by the maternal decidua, amniochorionic membranes, cytotrophoblasts, and both maternal and fetal endothelial cells. IL-4 is an archetypal cytokine involved in TH2-mediated adaptive immunity and during pregnancy is thought to help reduce the risk of miscarriage. Our result suggests that neonatal IL-4 levels might be actively regulated by maternal genetics. However, what those genetic mechanisms are, we were unable to determine. We found only one maternal SNP (rs7546782) that was significantly associated with neonatal IL-4 at borderline levels ($P = 7.7 \times 10^{-8}$) and maps to a region in chromosome 1 that is rich in regulatory elements (see the full set of summary statistics-level results available at DOI: https://doi.org/10.5281/zenodo.1321338).

Three maternal GW-associated loci regulate neonatal mediator levels. The neonatal chemokine CCL24 is associated with a maternal SNP in *MCTP2*, which encodes a transmembrane protein that binds to Ca^{2+}. MCTP2 is involved in intercellular signal transduction and synapse function and potentially metabolic processes as it is associated with body mass index [56, 57]. Variation near maternal *EFNA5*, a member of the ephrin family, is associated with the neonatal cytokine IL-16. Ephrin ligands and receptors are observed in lymphocytes, monocytes, and dendritic cells, and their expression levels change during inflammation. Finally, the neonatal chemokine CXCL5 is associated with a maternal locus in the cytochrome P450 3A4 gene (*CYP3A4*), one of the most important effectors of oxidative metabolism in humans. None of these loci have previously been associated with adult immune phenotypes [8].

Previous evidence showed that fetal genetics could also regulate several maternal phenotypes during pregnancy

[10, 11]. In our sample, maternal IL-7 and CXCL10 were under the control of independent contributions from maternal-specific and fetal-specific non-overlapping alleles. We further identified one fetal locus associated with maternal sIL2R-α, *ADCYAP1*, or *PACAP*, which encodes a signalling neuropeptide widely expressed in the central and peripheral nervous systems. PACAP is also expressed in different parts of the placenta and the umbilical cord where it affects cell survival, angiogenesis, and proliferation of trophoblast cells [58]. This locus was not associated with any fetal cytokine/chemokine, nor has it previously been associated with adult immune phenotypes [8].

Across our results, the cross-genetic associated loci map to genes that were not already associated with the analysed cytokines/chemokines and they showed independent association with only maternal or fetal genetics, but the same locus never showed evidence for both maternal and fetal effects. As summarized in Fig. 5, our genetic data suggest that the cross-genetic influence between mother and fetus is not simply a redistribution of soluble immune mediators, in which case we would have expected to see the same loci contributing to the same mediator in both genetic datasets, and that these would predominantly encode genes directly relevant to each cytokine/chemokine or its receptor. Our alternative hypothesis (Fig. 5) is that most of the maternal-fetal impact occurs via distinct regulatory or indirect placental mechanisms such as signalling at the placental interface and through a different set of genes than currently implicated in inflammation. Moreover, these mechanisms could potentially be responsible for the pregnancy-specific regulation of the cytokines/chemokines produced by maternal and/or fetal placental tissues within the tissues of pregnancy [59] and possibly in the peripheral blood.

Finally, we observed that maternal levels of the chemokines IL-8 and CCL2 were significantly lower in mothers of ASD-affected children compared to mothers of control children. We also identified a positive association with neonatal IL-8 levels that is consistent with our findings in a larger EMA sample. Other studies implicating IL-8 include measuring IL-8 in the plasma of young (2–5 years of age) ASD children [19] and one showing increased expression of the IL-8 gene in brains of ASD children [60]. Interestingly, we demonstrated that the neonatal levels of IL-8 were significantly associated with ASD outcome only in children of mothers heterozygous for SNP rs55823040, which was suggestively associated with overall neonatal IL-8 levels. This SNP maps near the pseudogene *CACYBPP2*, between the nucleoporin *NUP35* and the zinc finger protein ZNF804A, a candidate for ASD, schizophrenia [61], and other neuropsychiatric disorders [62]. This SNP did not show main effects with ASD outcome but only the observed interaction with IL-8 levels. It will be important to replicate this finding in additional studies.

This study has several limitations, including sample size and lack of information about infection or illness at the time of sampling. The population sampled also includes heterogeneous genetic ancestries. While this introduces methodological challenges and does not allow for heritability estimates precise for a homogenous population, we have used a number of approaches to ensure that our study design did not introduce false positives into our results. Overall, we believe studying a representative US population (Southern California) is a significant strength of this study, as our results are more likely to be applicable across genetic populations.

Conclusions

Taking advantage of a unique set of mother-infant matching pairs, this study shows patterns of genetic variation regulating cytokine/chemokine status during pregnancy and at birth. We identified a total of 17 specific maternal and fetal loci contributing to one or more cytokine and chemokine status at the two different time points. Several of these are novel and may be shown to be specific to pregnancy and newborn periods upon further study. Our cross-genetic analysis identified distinct maternal loci in novel regions independently associated with cytokine/chemokine levels in our neonatal dataset and that fetal loci in novel regions were independently associated with maternal cytokine/chemokine levels. We speculate that this pattern of cross-genetic influences at non-cytokine, non-chemokine, and non-receptor encoding loci and exclusively at loci not previously implicated for adult immune molecule levels implies a major influence of variation in placental biology on cytokine and chemokine levels. Interestingly, the observation of an association between increased IL-8 and ASD status only in the presence of a specific maternal SNP genotype suggests that future studies should consider the cross-genetic interaction involved in early risk for neurodevelopmental disorders.

Additional files

Additional file 1 Supplemental methods. Neonatal filter extraction and validity of the multiplex assay for maternal and neonatal immune mediators.
Additional file 2 Table S1. Statistics for 22 maternal immune mediator levels and 42 neonatal immune mediator levels after adjustment for individual-specific confounding factors. **Table S2.** Spearman's correlation coefficient (φ) across ten maternal principal coordinates and ten fetal principal coordinates. **Table S3.** Statistics for 22 maternal immune mediator levels and 42 neonatal immune mediator levels after adjustment for individual-specific confounding factors. **Table S4.** Spearman's correlation coefficient (φ) across cytokines and chemokines within mothers. **Table S5.** Spearman's correlation coefficient (φ) across cytokines and chemokines within infants. Table S6. Spearman's correlation coefficient (φ) across 15 overlapping immune molecules measured in maternal and neonatal datasets. **Table S7.** Significant genetic correlation across heritable covariate-adjusted neonatal immune cytokine/chemokine levels and corresponding linear correlation. **Table S8.** Comparison of maternal and fetal genome-

wide significant associations (Table 2) and meta-analysis across populations. **Table S9.** Combined effects of maternal-fetal SNPs in linear regression models.

Additional file 3 Figure S1. Significance levels of each confounding factor across the entire set of maternal and neonatal immune mediators. **Figure S2.** Linkage disequilibrium regional genomic plots. **Figure S3.** Maternal and fetal SNPs ($P <= 5 \times 10^{-4}$) from maternal sIL2R-a and neonatal CCL24 summary statistics.

Abbreviations
ASD: Autism spectrum disorder; chr: Chromosome; CI: Confidence interval; EMA: Early Markers for Autism; gen: Genetics; GWAS: Genome-wide association study; h^2_g: SNP-based heritability; I: Infants; LD: Linkage disequilibrium; LOD: Limit of detection; M: Mothers; MAF: Minor allele frequency; MDS: Multidimensional scaling; MIA: Maternal immune activation; OR: Odds ratio; SE: Standard error; SIM: Soluble immune mediator

Acknowledgments
We acknowledge Dr. Anthony Torres, for the preparation of maternal and infant DNA, and Cathleen Yoshida, for the data preparation and management. The findings and conclusions in this report are those of the authors and do not necessarily represent the views of the California Department of Public Health (CDPH).

Funding
This work was supported by NIEHS R01 ES016669 (Croen) and an IMHRO/Staglin Family Professorship (Weiss).

Authors' contributions
LAW, JVW, and LAC conceived the project. MK and GND were involved in sample collection and study design. KLJ, LSH, and JVW provided immune analyte data, and LAW provided genotype data. MT and LAW designed the genetic analyses, and MT conducted the analysis. PA and RY contributed helpful interpretation of data. The manuscript was written by MT and LAW, with critical input from LAC, PA, and JVW. All authors read and approved the final manuscript for publication.

Ethics approval and consent to participate
All study procedures were approved by the institutional review boards of the California Health and Human Services Agency and Kaiser Permanente Northern California. Study activities were also approved by the CA State Committee for the Protection of Human Subjects. It was determined at the CDC that the agency was not engaged in human subject research. It was also determined at UCSF Committee on Human Research that the institution was not engaged in human subject research. Samples used in this study were coded, no one at the CDC or UCSF has access to identifiable information, and there are IRB-approved policies prohibiting the release of the key. The study conforms to the Declaration of Helsinki.
Consent forms for the California's prenatal expanded alpha-fetoprotein (XAFP) screening program were obtained at the time of the maternal sampling and included privacy notifications, which stipulated that specimens and data from prenatal testing could be used for legitimate research purposes given appropriate institutional review board (IRB) approval. Newborn bloodspot specimens were obtained from the archives of the Genetic Disease Screening Program (GDSP), which distributes a 'Notice of Information Practices' describing how personal and medical information from newborn screening may be used without additional consent for legitimate research purposes, given appropriate institutional review board (IRB) and GDSP approval.

Competing interests

The authors declare that they have no competing interests.

Author details

[1]Department of Psychiatry and Institute for Human Genetics, University of California, San Francisco, San Francisco, CA, USA. [2]Divison of Research, Kaiser Permanente Northern California, Oakland, CA, USA. [3]Department of Internal Medicine, Division of Rheumatology, Allergy, and Clinical Immunology, University of California Davis, Davis, CA, USA. [4]MIND Institute, University of California Davis, Davis, CA, USA. [5]Stanley Division of Developmental Neurovirology, Department of Pediatrics, Johns Hopkins University School of Medicine, Baltimore, MD, USA. [6]Division of Environmental and Occupational Disease Control, California Department of Public Health, Richmond, CA, USA. [7]Department of Medical Microbiology and Immunology, University of California Davis, Davis, CA, USA.

References

1. Lyall K, Schmidt RJ, Hertz-Picciotto I. Environmental factors in the preconception and prenatal periods in relation to risk for ASD. In: Volkmar FR, Paul R, Rogers SJ, Pelphrey KA, editors. Handbook of autism and pervasive developmental disorders, fourth edition: assessment, interventions, policy, the future. Fourth ed. Hoboken: Wiley; 2014. p. 424–56.
2. Hsu P, Nanan RK. Innate and adaptive immune interactions at the fetal-maternal interface in healthy human pregnancy and pre-eclampsia. Front Immunol. 2014;5:125.
3. Neurath MF. Cytokines in inflammatory bowel disease. Nat Publ Gr. 2014;14: 329–42.
4. Kallaur AP, Oliveira SR, Simao ANC, Alfieri DF, Flauzino T, Lopes J, et al. Cytokine profile in patients with progressive multiple sclerosis and its association with disease progression and disability. Mol Neurobiol. 2017; 54(4):2950–60.
5. Li Y, Oosting M, Smeekens SP, Wijmenga C, Kumar V, Netea MG, et al. A functional genomics approach to understand variation in cytokine production in humans. Cell. 2016;167(4):1099–1110.e14.
6. Orru V, Steri M, Sole G, Sidore C, Virdis F, Dei M, et al. Genetic variants regulating immune cell levels in health and disease. Cell. 2013;155:242–56.
7. Roederer M, Quaye L, Mangino M, Beddall MH, Mahnke Y, Chattopadhyay P, et al. The genetic architecture of the human immune system: a bioresource for autoimmunity and disease pathogenesis. Cell. 2015;161:387–403.
8. Ahola-Olli A, Würtz P, Havulinna AS, Aalto K, Pitkänen N, Lehtimäki T, et al. Genome-wide association study identifies 17 new loci influencing concentrations of circulating cytokines and growth factors. Am J Hum Genet. 2017;100(1):40–50.
9. Liu N, Archer E, Srinivasasainagendra V, Allison DB. A statistical framework for testing the causal effects of fetal drive. Front Genet. 2014;5:464.
10. Petry CJ, Ong KK, Dunger DB. Does the fetal genotype affect maternal physiology during pregnancy? Trends Mol Med. 2007;13:414–21.
11. Petry CJ, Beardsall K, Dunger DB. The potential impact of the fetal genotype on maternal blood pressure during pregnancy. J Hypertens. 2014;32:1553–61. discussion 1561
12. Traglia M, Croen LA, Lyall K, Windham GC, Kharrazi M, DeLorenze GN, et al. Independent maternal and fetal genetic effects on mid-gestational circulating levels of environmental pollutants. G3 (Bethesda). 2017;7(4):1287–99.
13. Deverman BE, Patterson PH. Cytokines and CNS development. Neuron. 2009;64:61–78.
14. Mokhtari R, Lachman HM. The major histocompatibility complex (MHC) in schizophrenia: a review. J Clin Cell Immunol. 2016;7:417–24.e5.
15. Ponzio NM, Servatius R, Beck K, Marzouk A, Kreider T. Cytokine levels during pregnancy influence immunological profiles and neurobehavioral patterns of the offspring. In: Annals of the New York Academy of Sciences; 2007. p. 118–28.
16. Choi GB, Yim YS, Wong H, Kim S, Kim H, Kim SV, et al. The maternal interleukin-17a pathway in mice promotes autism-like phenotypes in offspring. Science (80-). 2016;351:933–9.
17. Smith SEP, Li J, Garbett K, Mirnics K, Patterson PH. Maternal immune activation alters fetal brain development through interleukin-6. J Neurosci. 2007;27:10695–702.
18. Girard S, Tremblay L, Lepage M, Sebire G. IL-1 receptor antagonist protects against placental and neurodevelopmental defects induced by maternal inflammation. J Immunol. 2010;184:3997–4005.
19. Ashwood P, Krakowiak P, Hertz-Picciotto I, Hansen R, Pessah I, Van de Water J. Elevated plasma cytokines in autism spectrum disorders provide evidence of immune dysfunction and are associated with impaired behavioral outcome. Brain Behav Immun. 2011;25:40–5.
20. Goldsmith DR, Rapaport MH, Miller BJ. A meta-analysis of blood cytokine network alterations in psychiatric patients: comparisons between schizophrenia, bipolar disorder and depression. Mol Psychiatry. 2016;21:1696–709.
21. Dowlati Y, Herrmann N, Swardfager W, Liu H, Sham L, Reim EK, et al. A meta-analysis of cytokines in major depression. Biol Psychiatry. 2010;67:446–57.
22. Miller BJ, Buckley P, Seabolt W, Mellor A, Kirkpatrick B. Meta-analysis of cytokine alterations in schizophrenia: clinical status and antipsychotic effects. Biol Psychiatry. 2011;70:663–71.
23. Modabbernia A, Taslimi S, Brietzke E, Ashrafi M. Cytokine alterations in bipolar disorder: a meta-analysis of 30 studies. Biol Psychiatry. 2013;74:15–25.
24. Zerbo O, Qian Y, Yoshida C, Grether JK, Van de Water J, Croen LA. Maternal infection during pregnancy and autism spectrum disorders. J Autism Dev Disord. 2015;45:4015–25.
25. Zerbo O, Qian Y, Yoshida C, Fireman BH, Klein NP, Croen LA. Association between influenza infection and vaccination during pregnancy and risk of autism spectrum disorder. JAMA Pediatr. 2017;171:e163609.
26. Hornig M, Bresnahan MA, Che X, Schultz AF, Ukaigwe JE, Eddy ML, et al. Prenatal fever and autism risk. Mol Psychiatry. 2018;23(3):759-66.
27. Bilbo SD, Schwarz JM. The immune system and developmental programming of brain and behavior. Front Neuroendocrinol. 2012;33:267–86.
28. Goines P, Haapanen L, Boyce R, Duncanson P, Braunschweig D, Delwiche L, et al. Autoantibodies to cerebellum in children with autism associate with behavior. Brain Behav Immun. 2011;25:514–23.
29. Mead J, Ashwood P. Evidence supporting an altered immune response in ASD. Immunol Lett. 2015;163:49–55.
30. Wong H, Hoeffer C. Maternal IL-17A in autism. Exp Neurol. 2018;299(Pt A): 228-240
31. Goines PE, Croen LA, Braunschweig D, Yoshida CK, Grether J, Hansen R, et al. Increased midgestational IFN-γ, IL-4 and IL-5 in women bearing a child with autism: a case-control study. Mol Autism. 2011;2:13.
32. Masi A, Glozier N, Dale R, Guastella AJ. The immune system, cytokines, and biomarkers in autism spectrum disorder. Neurosci Bull. 2017;33:194–204.
33. Krakowiak P, Goines PE, Tancredi DJ, Ashwood P, Hansen RL, Hertz-Picciotto I, et al. Neonatal cytokine profiles associated with autism spectrum disorder. Biol Psychiatry. 2017;81(5):442-51.
34. Jones KL, Croen LA, Yoshida CK, Heuer L, Hansen R, Zerbo O, et al. Autism with intellectual disability is associated with increased levels of maternal cytokines and chemokines during gestation. Mol Psychiatry. 2017;22:273–9.
35. Croen LA, Goines P, Braunschweig D, Yolken R, Yoshida CK, Grether JK, et al. Brain-derived neurotrophic factor and autism: maternal and infant peripheral blood levels in the early markers for autism (EMA) study. Autism Res. 2008;1:130–7.
36. Tsang KM, Croen LA, Torres AR, Kharrazi M, Delorenze GN, Windham GC, et al. A genome-wide survey of transgenerational genetic effects in autism. PLoS One. 2013;8(10):e76978.
37. Purcell S, Neale B, Todd-Brown K, Thomas L, Ferreira MAR, Bender D, et al. PLINK: a tool set for whole-genome association and population-based linkage analyses. Am J Hum Genet. 2007;81:559–75.
38. Core Team R. R: a language and environment for statistical computing. Vienna: R Foundation for Statistical Computing; 2014.
39. Yang J, Lee SH, Goddard ME, Visscher PM. GCTA: a tool for genome-wide complex trait analysis. Am J Hum Genet. 2011;88:76–82.
40. Visscher PM, Hemani G, Vinkhuyzen AAE, Chen GB, Lee SH, Wray NR, et al. Statistical power to detect genetic (co)variance of complex traits using SNP data in unrelated samples. PLoS Genet. 2014;10(4):e1004269.
41. Lee SH, Wray NR, Goddard ME, Visscher PM. Estimating missing heritability for disease from genome-wide association studies. Am J Hum Genet. 2011;88:294–305.

42. Pruim RJ, Welch RP, Sanna S, Teslovich TM, Chines PS, Gliedt TP, et al. LocusZoom: regional visualization of genome-wide association scan results. Bioinformatics. 2011;27:2336–7.

43. Risch N, Merikangas K. The future of genetic studies of complex human diseases. Science. 1996;273:1516–7.

44. Pe'er I, Yelensky R, Altshuler D, Daly MJ. Estimation of the multiple testing burden for genomewide association studies of nearly all common variants. Genet Epidemiol. 2008;32:381–5.

45. Sudmant PH, Rausch T, Gardner EJ, Handsaker RE, Abyzov A, Huddleston J, et al. An integrated map of structural variation in 2,504 human genomes. Nature. 2015;526:75–81.

46. Zerbino DR, Achuthan P, Akanni W, Amode MR, Barrell D, Bhai J, et al. Ensembl 2018. Nucleic Acids Res. 2018;46:754–61.

47. Zerbo O, Traglia M, Yoshida C, Heuer LS, Ashwood P, Delorenze GN, et al. Maternal mid-pregnancy C-reactive protein and risk of autism spectrum disorders: the early markers for autism study. Transl Psychiatry. 2016;6(4): e783.

48. Enroth S, Enroth SB, Gyllensten U. Strong effects of genetic and lifestyle factors on biomarker variation and use of personalized cutoffs. Nat Commun. 2014;5:4684.

49. Brodin P, Jojic V, Gao T, Bhattacharya S, Angel CJL, Furman D, et al. Article variation in the human immune system is largely driven by non-heritable influences. Cell. 2015;160:37–47.

50. Takenaka K, Fukami K, Otsuki M, Nakamura Y, Kataoka Y, Wada M, et al. Role of phospholipase C-L2, a novel phospholipase C-like protein that lacks lipase activity, in B-cell receptor signaling role ofphospholipase C-L2, a novel phospholipase C-like protein that lacks lipase activity, in B-cell receptor signaling. Mol Cell Biol. 2003;23:7329–38.

51. Hirokawa M, Morita H, Tajima T, Takahashi A, Ashikawa K, Miya F, et al. A genome-wide association study identifies PLCL2 and AP3D1-DOT1L-SF3A2 as new susceptibility loci for myocardial infarction in Japanese. Eur J Hum Genet. 2015;23:374–80.

52. Tsoi LC, Spain SL, Ellinghaus E, Stuart PE, Capon F, Knight J, et al. Enhanced meta-analysis and replication studies identify five new psoriasis susceptibility loci. Nat Commun. 2015;6:7001.

53. Bowes J, Ho P, Flynn E, Ali F, Marzo-Ortega H, Coates LC, et al. Comprehensive assessment of rheumatoid arthritis susceptibility loci in a large psoriatic arthritis cohort. Ann Rheum Dis. 2012;71:1350–4.

54. Arismendi M, Giraud M, Ruzehaji N, Dieudé P, Koumakis E, Ruiz B, et al. Identification of NF-κB and PLCL2 as new susceptibility genes and highlights on a potential role of IRF8 through interferon signature modulation in systemic sclerosis. Arthritis Res Ther. 2015;17:71.

55. Chatterjee P, Chiasson VL, Bounds KR, Mitchell BM. Regulation of the anti-inflammatory cytokines interleukin-4 and interleukin-10 during pregnancy. Front Immunol. 2014;5:253.

56. Locke A, Kahali B, Berndt S, Justice A, Pers T. Genetic studies of body mass index yield new insights for obesity biology. Nature. 2015;518:197–206.

57. Hromatka BS, Tung JY, Kiefer AK, Do CB, Hinds DA, Eriksson N. Genetic variants associated with motion sickness point to roles for inner ear development, neurological processes and glucose homeostasis. Hum Mol Genet. 2015;24:2700–8.

58. Oride A, Kanasaki H, Mijiddorj T, Sukhbaatar U, Yamada T, Kyo S. Expression and regulation of pituitary adenylate cyclase-activating polypeptide in rat placental cells. Reprod Sci. 2016;23:1080–6.

59. Bowen JM, Chamley L, Mitchell MD, Keelan JA. Cytokines of the placenta and extra-placental membranes: biosynthesis, secretion and roles in establishment of pregnancy in women; 2002. p. 239–56.

60. Li X, Chauhan A, Sheikh AM, Patil S, Chauhan V, Li XM, et al. Elevated immune response in the brain of autistic patients. J Neuroimmunol. 2009;207:111–6.

61. Tao R, Cousijn H, Jaffe AE, Burnet PWJ, Edwards F, Eastwood SL, et al. Expression of ZNF804A in human brain and alterations in schizophrenia, bipolar disorder, and major depressive disorder. JAMA Psychiatry. 2014;71:1112.

62. Cross-Disorder Group of the Psychiatric Genomics Consortium. Identification of risk loci with shared effects on five major psychiatric disorders: a genome-wide analysis. Lancet. 2013;381:1371–9.

63. Traglia M, Croen LA, Jones LK, Heuer LS, Yolken R, Kharrazi M, et al: Dataset from: cross-genetic determination of maternal and neonatal immune mediators during pregnancy [dataset] Zenodo. 2018. https://doi.org/10.5281/zenodo.1321338.

Permissions

List of Contributors

Renato Polimanti
Department of Psychiatry, Yale School of Medicine and VA CT Healthcare Center, 950 Campbell Avenue, West Haven, CT 06516, USA

Joel Gelernter
Department of Psychiatry, Yale School of Medicine and VA CT Healthcare Center, 950 Campbell Avenue, West Haven, CT 06516, USA
Departments of Genetics and Neuroscience, Yale School of Medicine, New Haven, CT, USA

Manfred H. Kayser
Department of Genetic Identification, Erasmus University Medical Center, Rotterdam, Rotterdam, the Netherlands

Mikhail V. Pogorelyy, Alla D. Fedorova, Dmitri V. Bagaev and Anna E. Koneva
Department of Genomics of Adaptive Immunity, IBCH RAS, Moscow, Russia

Alexey V. Eliseev and Ivan V. Zvyagin
Department of Genomics of Adaptive Immunity, IBCH RAS, Moscow, Russia
Department of Molecular Technologies, Pirogov Russian National Research Medical University, Moscow, Russia

Mikhail Shugay
Department of Genomics of Adaptive Immunity, IBCH RAS, Moscow, Russia
Department of Molecular Technologies, Pirogov Russian National Research Medical University, Moscow, Russia
Center for Data-Intensive Biomedicine and Biotechnology, Skoltech, Moscow, Russia

Artem I. Mikelov
Department of Genomics of Adaptive Immunity, IBCH RAS, Moscow, Russia
Center for Data-Intensive Biomedicine and Biotechnology, Skoltech, Moscow, Russia

Dmitry M. Chudakov
Department of Genomics of Adaptive Immunity, IBCH RAS, Moscow, Russia
Department of Molecular Technologies, Pirogov Russian National Research Medical University, Moscow, Russia
Center for Data-Intensive Biomedicine and Biotechnology, Skoltech, Moscow, Russia

Central European Institute of Technology, CEITEC, Brno, Czech Republic

James E. McLaren and Kristin Ladell
Division of Infection and Immunity, Cardiff University School of Medicine, Cardiff, UK

David A. Price
Division of Infection and Immunity, Cardiff University School of Medicine, Cardiff, UK
Systems Immunity Research Institute, Cardiff University School of Medicine, Cardiff, UK

Angela Mo, Urko M. Marigorta, Dalia Arafat and Greg Gibson
Center for Integrative Genomics and School of Biological Sciences, Georgia Institute of Technology, Engineered Biosystems Building, EBB 2115, 950 Atlantic Drive, Atlanta, GA 30332, USA

Lai Hin Kimi Chan, Lori Ponder, Se Ryeong Jang, Jarod Prince, Subra Kugathasan and Sampath Prahalad
Department of Pediatrics, Emory University School of Medicine and Children's Healthcare of Atlanta, 1760 Haygood Dr NE, Atlanta, GA 30322, USA

Vinay K. Kartha and Stefano Monti
Bioinformatics Program, Boston University, Boston, MA, USA
Division of Computational Biomedicine, Boston University School of Medicine, Boston, MA, USA

Khalid A. Alamoud, Khikmet Sadykov, Bach-Cuc Nguyen, Manish V. Bais and Maria A. Kukuruzinska
Department of Molecular and Cell Biology, Goldman School of Dental Medicine, Boston University School of Medicine, 72 East Concord Street, E4, Boston, MA 02118, USA

Fabrice Laroche and Hui Feng
Department of Pharmacology and Experimental Therapeutics, Boston University School of Medicine, Boston, MA, USA

Jina Lee, Sara I. Pai
Department of Surgery, Massachusetts General Hospital, Harvard Medical School, Boston, MA, USA

Xaralabos Varelas
Department of Biochemistry, Boston University School of Medicine, Boston, MA, USA

Ann Marie Egloff
Department of Surgery, Brigham and Women's Hospital, Boston, MA, USA

Anna C. Belkina
Flow Cytometry Core Facility, Boston University School of Medicine, Boston, MA, USA

Jennifer E. Snyder-Cappione
Flow Cytometry Core Facility, Boston University School of Medicine, Boston, MA, USA
Department of Microbiology, Boston University School of Medicine, Boston, MA, USA

Amy P. Webster
Arthritis Research UK Centre for Genetics and Genomics, Centre for Musculoskeletal Research, The University of Manchester, Manchester, Uk
Department of Cancer Biology, UCL Cancer Institute, University College London, London, UK

Anne Barton and Jane Worthington
Arthritis Research UK Centre for Genetics and Genomics, Centre for Musculoskeletal Research, The University of Manchester, Manchester, Uk
NIHR Manchester Biomedical Research Centre Manchester Academy of Health Sciences, Manchester University Foundation Trust, Manchester, UK

Simone Ecker and Stephan Beck
Department of Cancer Biology, UCL Cancer Institute, University College London, London, UK

Andrew Feber
Department of Cancer Biology, UCL Cancer Institute, University College London, London, UK
Division of Surgery and Interventional Science, University College London, London, UK

Darren Plant
NIHR Manchester Biomedical Research Centre Manchester Academy of Health Sciences, Manchester University Foundation Trust, Manchester, UK

Flore Zufferey, Jordana T. Bell and Frances M. K. Williams
Department of Twin Research and Genetic Epidemiology, King's College London, London, UK

Dirk S. Paul
MRC/BHF Cardiovascular Epidemiology Unit, Department of Public Health and Primary Care, University of Cambridge, Cambridge, UK

Praneeth Reddy Devulapally and Hans-Jörg Warnatz
Otto Warburg Laboratory Gene Regulation and Systems Biology of Cancer, Max Planck Institute for Molecular Genetics, Berlin, Germany

Marie-Laure Yaspo
Otto Warburg Laboratory Gene Regulation and Systems Biology of Cancer, Max Planck Institute for Molecular Genetics, Berlin, Germany
Alacris Theranostics GmbH, Berlin, Germany

Thorsten Mielke
Microscopy and Cryo-Electron Microscopy Service Group, Max Planck Institute for Molecular Genetics, Berlin, Germany

Jörg Bürger
Microscopy and Cryo-Electron Microscopy Service Group, Max Planck Institute for Molecular Genetics, Berlin, Germany
Institut für Medizinische Physik und Biophysik, Charité-Universitätsmedizin, Berlin, Germany

Zoltán Konthur
Department of Biomolecular Systems, Max Planck Institute of Colloids and Interfaces, Potsdam, Germany

Hans Lehrach
Alacris Theranostics GmbH, Berlin, Germany
Dahlem Centre for Genome Research and Medical Systems Biology, Berlin, Germany

Jörn Glökler
Department of Molecular Biotechnology and Functional Genomics, Institute of Applied Biosciences, Technical University of Applied Sciences Wildau, Wildau, Brandenburg, Germany

Cherry S. Leung, Kevin Y. Yang, Xisheng Li and Vicken W. Chan
Department of Chemical Pathology, Prince of Wales Hospital, The Chinese University of Hong Kong, Hong Kong, China

Jason C. H. Tsang, Yuk Ming Dennis Lo and Kathy O. Lui
Department of Chemical Pathology, Prince of Wales Hospital, The Chinese University of Hong Kong, Hong Kong, China
Li Ka Shing Institute of Health Sciences, Prince of Wales Hospital, The Chinese University of Hong Kong, Hong Kong, China

Manching Ku
Department of Paediatrics and Adolescent Medicine, Division of Paediatric Hematology and Oncology, Faculty of Medicine, Medical Center, University of Freiburg, Freiburg im Breisgau, Germany

Herman Waldmann
Sir William Dunn School of Pathology, University of Oxford, Oxford, UK

Shohei Hori
Laboratory of Immunology and Microbiology, Graduate School of Pharmaceutical Sciences, The University of Tokyo, Tokyo, Japan

Romain Guérillot, Lucy Li, Sarah Baines, Brian Howden, Ian Monk, Sacha J. Pidot, Wei Ga and Stefano Giulieri
Department of Microbiology and Immunology, The University of Melbourne at the Doherty Institute for Infection and Immunity, Melbourne, Victoria, Australia

Timothy P. Stinear
Department of Microbiology and Immunology, The University of Melbourne at the Doherty Institute for Infection and Immunity, Melbourne, Victoria, Australia
Doherty Applied Microbial Genomics, The University of Melbourne at the Peter Doherty Institute for Infection and Immunity, Melbourne, Victoria, Australia

Mark B. Schultz and Anders Gonçalves da Silva
Department of Microbiology and Immunology, The University of Melbourne at the Doherty Institute for Infection and Immunity, Melbourne, Victoria, Australia
Doherty Applied Microbial Genomics, The University of Melbourne at the Peter Doherty Institute for Infection and Immunity, Melbourne, Victoria, Australia
Microbiological Diagnostic Unit Public Health Laboratory, The University of Melbourne at the Peter Doherty Institute for Infection and Immunity, Melbourne, Victoria, Australia

Benjamin P. Howden
Department of Microbiology and Immunology, The University of Melbourne at the Doherty Institute for Infection and Immunity, Melbourne, Victoria, Australia
Doherty Applied Microbial Genomics, The University of Melbourne at the Peter Doherty Institute for Infection and Immunity, Melbourne, Victoria, Australia
Microbiological Diagnostic Unit Public Health Laboratory, The University of Melbourne at the Peter Doherty Institute for Infection and Immunity, Melbourne, Victoria, Australia
Infectious Diseases Department, Austin Health, Heidelberg, Victoria, Australia

Anthony D'Agata and Takehiro Tomita
Microbiological Diagnostic Unit Public Health Laboratory, The University of Melbourne at the Peter Doherty Institute for Infection and Immunity, Melbourne, Victoria, Australia

Torsten Seemann
Melbourne Bioinformatics, The University of Melbourne, Melbourne, Victoria, Australia
Doherty Applied Microbial Genomics, The University of Melbourne at the Peter Doherty Institute for Infection and Immunity, Melbourne, Victoria, Australia

Anton Y. Peleg
Department of Infectious Diseases, The Alfred Hospital and Central Clinical School, Monash University, Melbourne, Victoria, Australia
Infection and Immunity Theme, Monash Biomedicine Discovery Institute, Department of Microbiology, Monash University, Clayton, Victoria, Australia

Qian Zhang, Matthew R Robinson and Allan F McRae
Institute for Molecular Bioscience, The University of Queensland, Brisbane, QLD 4072, Australia

Naomi R Wray and Peter M Visscher
Institute for Molecular Bioscience, The University of Queensland, Brisbane, QLD 4072, Australia
The Queensland Brain Institute, The University of Queensland, St Lucia, QLD 4072, Australia

Riccardo E Marioni
Centre for Cognitive Ageing and Cognitive Epidemiology, University of Edinburgh, Edinburgh EH8 9JZ, UK
Medical Genetics Section, Centre for Genomic and Experimental Medicine, Institute of Genetics and Molecular Medicine, University of Edinburgh, Edinburgh EH4 2XU, UK

Ian J Deary
Centre for Cognitive Ageing and Cognitive Epidemiology, University of Edinburgh, Edinburgh EH8 9JZ, UK
Department of Psychology, University of Edinburgh, Edinburgh EH8 9JZ, UK

Jon Higham
Medical Research Council Human Genetics Unit, Medical Research Council Institute of Genetics and Molecular Medicine, University of Edinburgh, Edinburgh EH4 2XU, UK

Duncan Sproul
Medical Research Council Human Genetics Unit, Medical Research Council Institute of Genetics and Molecular Medicine, University of Edinburgh, Edinburgh EH4 2XU, UK
Edinburgh Cancer Research Centre, Medical Research Council Institute of Genetics and Molecular Medicine, University of Edinburgh, Edinburgh EH4 2XU, UK

John Welch
Division of Oncology, Department of Medicine, Washington University, St. Louis, MO 63108, USA

Sohini Sengupta, Sam Q. Sun, Kuan-lin Huang, Clara Oh, Matthew H. Bailey and Matthew A. Wyczalkowski
Division of Oncology, Department of Medicine, Washington University, St. Louis, MO 63108, USA

McDonnell Genome Institute, Washington University, St. Louis, MO 63108, USA

Michael C. Wendl
Division of Oncology, Department of Medicine, Washington University, St. Louis, MO 63108, USA
McDonnell Genome Institute, Washington University, St. Louis, MO 63108, USA
Department of Mathematics, Washington University, St. Louis, MO 63108, USA
Department of Genetics, Washington University, St. Louis, MO 63108, USA

Cynthia Ma
Division of Oncology, Department of Medicine, Washington University, St. Louis, MO 63108, USA
Department of Genetics, Washington University, St. Louis, MO 63108, USA

Li Ding
Division of Oncology, Department of Medicine, Washington University, St. Louis, MO 63108, USA
McDonnell Genome Institute, Washington University, St. Louis, MO 63108, USA
Department of Genetics, Washington University, St. Louis, MO 63108, USA
Siteman Cancer Center, Washington University, St. Louis, MO 63108, USA

Reid R. Townsend and John F. Dipersio
Division of Oncology, Department of Medicine, Washington University, St. Louis, MO 63108, USA
Siteman Cancer Center, Washington University, St. Louis, MO 63108, USA

Joshua F. McMichael,
McDonnell Genome Institute, Washington University, St. Louis, MO 63108, USA

Rajees Varghese, Jie Ning and Piyush Tripathi
Division of Nephrology, Department of Medicine, Washington University, St. Louis, MO 63108, USA

Feng Chen
Division of Nephrology, Department of Medicine, Washington University, St. Louis, MO 63108, USA
Department of Genetics, Washington University, St. Louis, MO 63108, USA

Kimberly J. Johnson
Brown School, Washington University, St. Louis, MO 63105, USA

Cyriac Kandoth
Marie-Josée and Henry R. Kravis Center for Molecular Oncology, Memorial Sloan Kettering Cancer Center, New York, NY, USA

Samuel H. Payne
Biological Sciences Division, Pacific Northwest National Laboratory, Richland, WA 99352, USA

David Fenyö
Department of Biochemistry and Molecular Pharmacology, New York University Langone School of Medicine, New York, NY 10016, USA
Institute for Systems Genetics, New York University Langone School of Medicine, New York, NY 10016, USA

Yingleong Chan, Ying Kai Chan, Xiaoge Guo, Elaine T. Lim and George M. Church
Wyss Institute for Biologically Inspired Engineering, Harvard University, Boston, MA 02115, USA
Department of Genetics, Harvard Medical School, Boston, MA 02115, USA

Daniel B. Goodman
Wyss Institute for Biologically Inspired Engineering, Harvard University, Boston, MA 02115, USA
Department of Genetics, Harvard Medical School, Boston, MA 02115, USA
Harvard-MIT Health Sciences and Technology, Cambridge, MA 02139, USA

Alejandro Chavez
Department of Pathology and Cell Biology, Columbia University College of Physicians and Surgeons, New York, NY 10032, USA

Carolina Barra, Bruno Alvarez and Massimo Andreatta
Instituto de Investigaciones Biotecnológicas, Universidad Nacional de San Martín, CP1650 San Martín, Argentina

Morten Nielsen
Instituto de Investigaciones Biotecnológicas, Universidad Nacional de San Martín, CP1650 San Martín, Argentina
Department of Bio and Health Informatics, Technical University of Denmark, DK-2800 Kgs. Lyngby, Denmark

Sinu Paul, Alessandro Sette and Bjoern Peters
Division of Vaccine Discovery, La Jolla Institute for Allergy and Immunology, 9420 Athena Circle, La Jolla, CA 92037, USA

Søren Buus
Department of Immunology and Microbiology, Faculty of Health Sciences, University of Copenhagen, Copenhagen, Denmark

Lin Zhou
Computational Genomics Lab, Beijing Institutes of Life Science, Chinese Academy of Sciences, Beijing 100101, China

University of Chinese Academy of Sciences, Beijing 100049, China

Fangqing Zhao
Computational Genomics Lab, Beijing Institutes of Life Science, Chinese Academy of Sciences, Beijing 100101, China
University of Chinese Academy of Sciences, Beijing 100049, China
Center for Excellence in Animal Evolution and Genetics, Chinese Academy of Sciences, Kunming 650223, China

Jinming Cheng and Leilei Wu
Department of Bioinformatics and Biostatistics, School of Life Sciences and Biotechnology, Shanghai Jiao Tong University, Shanghai, China
Key Lab of Computational Biology, CAS-MPG Partner Institute for Computational Biology, Shanghai Institutes for Biological Sciences, Chinese Academy of Sciences, Shanghai, China

Dongkai Wei and Guang Li
Basepair biotechnology Co. LTD, Suzhou, China

Yixue Li
Department of Bioinformatics and Biostatistics, School of Life Sciences and Biotechnology, Shanghai Jiao Tong University, Shanghai, China
Key Lab of Computational Biology, CAS-MPG Partner Institute for Computational Biology, Shanghai Institutes for Biological Sciences, Chinese Academy of Sciences, Shanghai, China
Shanghai Center for Bioinformation Technology, Shanghai Academy of Science and Technology, Shanghai, China

Liguang Yang, Ting Hou, Guohui Ding and Hong Li
Key Lab of Computational Biology, CAS-MPG Partner Institute for Computational Biology, Shanghai Institutes for Biological Sciences, Chinese Academy of Sciences, Shanghai, China

Yuan Jiand Lingli Chen
Department of Pathology, Zhongshan Hospital, Fudan University, Shanghai, China

Lu Xie
Shanghai Center for Bioinformation Technology, Shanghai Academy of Science and Technology, Shanghai, China

Michela Traglia and Lauren A. Weiss
Department of Psychiatry and Institute for Human Genetics, University of California, San Francisco, San Francisco, CA, USA

Lisa A. Croen and Gerald N. DeLorenze
Divison of Research, Kaiser Permanente Northern California, Oakland, CA, USA

Karen L. Jones, Luke S. Heuer and Judy Van de Water
Department of Internal Medicine, Division of Rheumatology, Allergy, and Clinical Immunology, University of California Davis, Davis, CA, USA
MIND Institute, University of California Davis, Davis, CA, USA

Paul Ashwood
MIND Institute, University of California Davis, Davis, CA, USA
Department of Medical Microbiology and Immunology, University of California Davis, Davis, CA, USA

Robert Yolken
Stanley Division of Developmental Neurovirology, Department of Pediatrics, Johns Hopkins University School of Medicine, Baltimore, MD, USA

Martin Kharrazi
Division of Environmental and Occupational Disease Control, California Department of Public Health, Richmond, CA, USA

Index